Medical Herbalism: Principles and Practices

Medical Herbalism: Principles and Practices

Edited by Melissa Gould

MURPHY & MOORE
www.murphy-moorepublishing.com

Published by Murphy & Moore Publishing,
1 Rockefeller Plaza,
New York City, NY 10020, USA
www.murphy-moorepublishing.com

Medical Herbalism: Principles and Practices
Edited by Melissa Gould

International Standard Book Number: 978-1-63987-359-3 (Hardback)

Cataloging-in-Publication Data

Medical herbalism : principles and practices / edited by Melissa Gould.
p. cm.
Includes bibliographical references and index.
ISBN 978-1-63987-359-3
1. Herbs--Therapeutic use. 2. Medicinal plants. 3. Botany, Medical.
4. Materia medica, Vegetable. I. Gould, Melissa.

RM666.H33 M43 2022
615.321--dc23

TABLE OF CONTENTS

PREFACE

Every book is a source of knowledge and this one is no exception. The idea that led to the conceptualization of this book was the fact that the world is advancing rapidly; which makes it crucial to document the progress in every field. I am aware that a lot of data is already available, yet, there is a lot more to learn. Hence, I accepted the responsibility of editing this book and contributing my knowledge to the community.

The use of plants for medicinal purposes refers to as medical herbalism. It includes the use of fungal products, bee products, animal products, shells, etc. It is generally used for the treatment of chronic diseases such as diabetes, cancer, end-stage kidney disease, asthma, etc. A liquid or herbal tea is the most common form of medication formulated from herbs. They can be further classified into infusions, maceration and decoction. The alcoholic extraction of herbs is known as tinctures. Herbs can also be applied directly to the skin in the form of essential oils, balms and lotions. The inhalation of herbs for therapeutic purposes is known as aromatherapy. Pharmacognosy also falls under the domain of medical herbalism. It is concerned with the study of plants as a potential source of drugs. This book traces the progress of this field and highlights some of its key concepts and applications. The various advancements in medical herbalism are glanced at and their applications as well as ramifications are looked at in detail. Those in search of information to further their knowledge will be greatly assisted by this book.

While editing this book, I had multiple visions for it. Then I finally narrowed down to make every chapter a sole standing text explaining a particular topic, so that they can be used independently. However, the umbrella subject sinews them into a common theme. This makes the book a unique platform of knowledge.

I would like to give the major credit of this book to the experts from every corner of the world, who took the time to share their expertise with us. Also, I owe the completion of this book to the never-ending support of my family, who supported me throughout the project.

Editor

1

Anti-angiogenesis effect of *Crocous sativus* L. extract on matrix metalloproteinase gene activities in human breast carcinoma cells

Marzieh Mousavi[1], Javad Baharara[2*], Majid Asadi-Samani[3]

[1]Young Researchers and Elite Club, Mashhad Branch, Islamic Azad University, Mashhad, Iran
[2]Research Center for Animal Development Applied Biology, Mashhad Branch, Islamic Azad University, Mashhad, Iran
[3]Medical Plants Research Center, Shahrekord University of Medical Sciences, Shahrekord, Iran

ARTICLE INFO

Keywords:
Crocous Sativus L
Angiogenesis
Matrix metalloproteinase
MCF-7 Cell Line
Cancer

ABSTRACT

Introduction: There is an interest in *Crocous sativus* L. (Saffron) mainly because of its biological properties. Biomedical research has focused on saffron as a powerful antioxidant, anti-inflammatory and anti-tumor, but its mechanism has not yet been thoroughly clarified. In this study, the effects of saffron aqua extract on matrix metalloproteinases (MMP) gene expression were investigated.

Methods: In this experimental study, the saffron was extracted using water as solvent. MCF-7 cells in RPMI1640 medium were supplemented with 10% FBS and incubated at 37 °C with 5% CO2. After 24 h, the cells were treated by saffron extract at concentrations of 100, 200, 400 and 800 µg/ml. 48 h after treatment, total RNA was extracted and cDNA was synthesized using specific primer. Synthesized products were analyzed by Real Time PCR to determine expression level of MMP.

Results: Data analysis showed inhibitory effect of saffron at concentrations of 100 to 800 µg/ml on MMP gene expression in comparison with control group. Reduction for 100, 200, 400 and 800 µg/ml were 5%, 18%, 15%, 11%, respectively. According to data analysis treating MCF-7 cells with saffron at concentration of 200 µg/ml caused the highest decrease, with 18% reduction in gene expression ($P<0.001$).

Conclusion: Results indicate decrease in the expression of MMP compared with controls revealing induction of inhibitory effects of saffron on angiogenesis which might be also considered as a promising chemotherapeutic agent in breast cancer treatment.

Implication for health policy/practice/research/medical education:
In this study saffron decreased the expression of MMP revealing an inhibitory effect on angiogenesis. This might be considered as a promising chemotherapeutic agent in breast cancer treatment.

Introduction

First blood vessels in a process, known as vasculogenesis, is formed from endothelial progenitor cells with novel specific patterns and gradually begin to spread, develop and form new branches (1). Formation of new blood vessels in adults is controlled precisely than previous vessels and angiogenesis just occurs in a physiological conditions such as pregnancy and specific pathological conditions such as wound healing, diabetic retinopathy, rheumatoid arthritis or cancer. Since angiogenesis is happened in pathological condition such as tumor growth and metastasis and plays an important role, it can also be targeted for antitumor therapy. In general, the process of angiogenesis is considered to have 10 stages

***Corresponding author**: Javad Baharara, Rahnamaie Ave, Street No. 24. Research Center for Animal Development Applied Biology,M ashhad Branch, Islamic Azad University, Mashhad, Iran.
E-mail: baharara@mshdiau.ac.ir

which one or more sequential steps could be targeted by angiogenesis inhibitors or simulators (2). This process is extensively depend on interactions between different cells and molecules and also is controlled by a variety of peptides and moderating factors (3). Several factors, such as vascular endothelial growth factor (VEGF), fibroblast growth factor (FGF), placental transforming growth factor (PTGF), signal transducer and activator of transcription 3 (STAT 3) are involved in this pathway (4). VEGF binding to vascular endothelial growth factor receptor 2 (VEGFR-2) triggers the specific activation of tyrosine amino acid residues within intra cytoplasmatic tail of the receptor inducing multiple signaling networks that result in endothelial cell survival, proliferation, migration, focal adhesion turnover, actin remodeling and vascular permeability. Signaling through mitogen-activated protein kinase and phosphatidylinositol 3' kinase is a common receptor tyrosine kinase activation pattern. Additional signaling pathways are also triggered upon VEGFR-2 activation, i.e., phospholipase C gamma, protein kinase focal adhesion kinase and T Cell-Specific Adaptor-Src kinase which are linked to migration and vascular permeability (5,6). Under hypoxic conditions, reduction of oxygen pressure is crucial and tissues start synthetizing and releasing angiogenic factors such as endothelial cell growth factors after binding to their special receptors, activating them which may lead to secretion of metalloproteinase from endothelial cells to digest and decompose basement membrane in the region. By reaching this aim endothelial cells would be able to migrate and proliferate. In addition, the molecule of adhesion such as integrins $\alpha_7\beta_5$ and $\alpha_3\beta_7$ are helpful in the process of pulling forward and bud blood vessels develop. In the next steps in the process of angiogenesis, matrix metalloproteinases (MMP) degrade extracellular matrix and start the production or reconstruction. By the interaction of the Tie-2 with angiopoietin tube formation begins at a later stage, EphB (ephrin B) also regulates formation of tubes, finally smooth muscle cells and pericytes as well as inducing the stabilization of newly formed blood vessel structure (7,8).

MMPs degrade and modify the extracellular matrix (ECM) as well as cell-ECM and cell-cell contacts, facilitating detachment of epithelial cells from the surrounding tissues (9). MMPs play key functions in embryonic development and mammary gland branching morphogenesis, but they are also up-regulated in breast cancer, where they stimulate tumorigenesis, cancer cell invasion and metastasis (10).

Rising cancer resistance to chemical therapies increased effort to find out new drugs in cancer therapy with fewer side effects and resistance (11). Cancer is growing in the world, and causes death of more than 6 million people each year, and breast cancer has the highest rates of mortality at ages of 40 (12,13). This cancer is hormone-dependent, which many of risk factors are known (14). Some of these risk factors are: geographic diversity, age, family history, pregnancy history, pregnancy, benign breast disease, exogenous estrogens, oral contraceptive drugs, obesity, high-fat diet, alcohol consumption, smoking and radiation chest out (15,16).

Interfering with normal function of at least 4 to 6 genes by genetic and epigenetic mechanisms can lead to breast cancer, which disturb the balance between proliferation, apoptosis and differentiation, and also regulation of steroid receptors, binding cells and angiogenesis (17,18).

Saffron, the stigma of *Crocus sativus* L. (Iridaceae), is currently used as spice, source of food additives, colorants and as a component of traditional medicines (19). This biomedical herb contains many constituents such as crocetin, picrocrocin and volatile compounds including safranal, crocins and crocetin (20,21). Saffron has been evaluated for its pharmacological activities such as anti-cancer, and antitumor and its constituents showed antioxidant activity in different organs such as muscle, kidney and hippocampus. Recent studies demonstrated the antitumor properties of saffron both *in vitro* and *in vivo* (22).

As regards to identification an effective strategy by using new agents from natural sources to treatment cancers, and since matrix metalloproteinase (MMP) is potent endothelial mitogen that up regulated in number of tumor types, including breast cancer, the aim of this study was to investigated the effect of saffron aqueous extract on level of MMP in human breast cancer cell line (MCF-7).

Materials and Methods

Saffron sample preparation

Original Iranian saffron (*Crocus sativus* L.) which is widely grown and gathered at autumn in south of Khorasan province was purchased from Novin Zaferan Co (Mashhad, Iran) and was identified by a plant taxonomist from the Herbarium Division of the College of Ferdowsi University. The stigma's aqueous extract was prepared as follow: 3 g dried stigmas was extracted with 250 ml sterile distilled water by soxhlet apparatus. The mixtures were transferred to Rotary to remove water. In order to dry, the extract lyophilization was done by using freeze dryer.

Cell culture and treatment

MCF7 cells were obtained from Pasteur Institute, Iran. Cells were cultured in RPMI medium (Biosera, Iran) with 10% fetal bovine serum (Gibco, USA), 100 units/ml penicillin, and 100 μg/ml streptomycin (Sigma, France) and also 1 ml L-glutamine (Sigma, France). Then, it was incubated at 37 °C with 5% CO_2. 24 h after cell culture and insurance about cell adhesion to flask, cells were treated with aqueous extract of saffron at concentrations of 100, 200, 400 and 800 micrograms per ml. Then to evaluate the viability, Trypan blue (Sigma, France) test was used and pictures captured with a digital camera with invert microscope (Dinocapture) for 5 days to investigate cell morphological changes.

RNA extraction

RNA was extracted by total RNA purification kit (Bioscience, Germany). After 48 h of treatment, the total RNA was purified and stored at -20 °C until cDNA synthesis. To measure the amount of RNA, Nanodrop was used by wavelengths 260, 280 and 320 nm and data were measured and analyzed. These data indicate the concentration of the extracted RNA which was used for cDNA synthesis as follow:

RNA concentration = (OD 260 - OD 320) × 40 × 100

cDNA synthesis

cDNA was synthesized by Bioneer Kit (Korea), the temperature of synthesis was according to Table 1.

Synthesis of primers

The sequence of genes was received from NCBI site and the bio-informatic validation of RT-PCR primers were done in PRIMER BLAST and delivered Bioneer Company (Korea). Primers were designed according to Table 2.

Evaluation of gene expression using real time PCR

Process of real time PCR to study gene expression was done according to the protocol by Bioneer kit (South Korea) by Applied Biosystem. According to the protocol, Master Mix firstly was prepared and added to strip cap microtube and then the cDNA was added to it. Application temperature according Tm of designed primers and the characteristics of the different phases in polymerase chain reaction were determined.

Gene expression levels of MMP in samples exposed low frequency electromagnetic field in comparison with control samples were analyzed by SPSS (V.16). P-value of less than 0.05 and CI (Confidence Interval) 95% were accepted as significant. In this project, we used relative quantitative based on expression of target gene to the reference gene via comparing the target gene efficiency with control sample. The primer and the temperature of binding primer are essential factors in the optimization of Real Time PCR reaction. So condition of reaction was optimized in which no nonspecific products produced. This optimized condition observed by mono peak in melting curve and also electrophoresis in agar gel by looking single sharp band. The mean ± SD were determined for each study group. Data were analyzed by ANOVA & Tukey multiple comparison procedure to calculate the significance. P<0.05 value between study groups was taken as statistically significant.

Table 1. The temperature required for the synthesis of cDNA

Steps	Temperature	Time (min)
Primer annealing	Tm of specific primer	1
cDNA synthesis	42-70 °C	10 – 60
Heat inactivation	95 °C	5

Table 2. Sequences of genes

Gene	Forward 5'→3'	Reverse 5'→3'	Chromosomal location
Beta actin	CCC GCC GCC AGC TCA CCA TGG	AAG GTC TCA AAC ATG ATC TGG GTC	7p22
MMP	CTG CAT CCT CAG CAG GTTG	GTC TCG GAT AGT CTT TAT CC	1q 26422762-26426467bp

Results

Gene expression studies showed a significant reduction in the gene expression levels of MMP gene treated with concentrations of 100 (P<0.05), 200 (P<0.001), 400 (P<0.05) and 800 (P<0.05) micrograms per ml of cells in comparison with the control group (Figure 1). Also data analysis showed inhibitory effect of saffron extract at concentrations of 100, 200, 400 and 800 μg/ml on MMP gene expression with 5%, 18%, 15% and 11% respectively in MCF-7 cell line in comparison with control group. As data indicate significant inhibitory effect on gene expression of MMP was 18% in 200 μg/ml of saffron extract.

Since the PCR reaction efficiency between the target gene and the housekeeping gene (beta-actin) was the same, the comparative threshold cycle (CT) was used in this project. It was examined whether the CT variance scale down by using dilution standard samples with quantity of 100, 10, 0.1, and 0.01 or not? Data analysis revealed that by dilution of samples CT changed and scale down. Acceptable data with high efficiency are represented in Figure 2.

Discussion

In this research, we investigated the effect of saffron extract on MMP level in human breast cancer cells. Since extracellular proteolysis mediates tissue homeostasis and in cancer, altered proteolysis leads to unregulated tumor growth, tissue remodeling, inflammation, tissue invasion, and metastasis, so the MMPs represent the most prominent family of proteinases associated with tumorigenesis. Also while MMPs regulate signaling pathways that control cell growth, inflammation, or angiogenesis, the study of MMP function may be new approaches to cancer therapy (23).

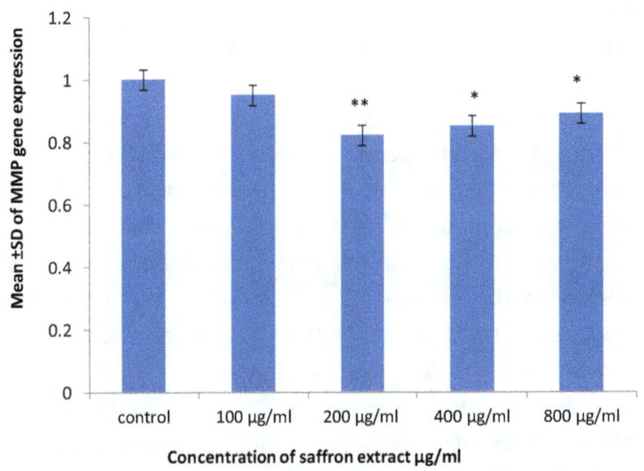

Figure 1. MMP gene expression in samples treated with saffron aqueous extract in different concentration compared with control group; * P<0.05, **P<0.001.

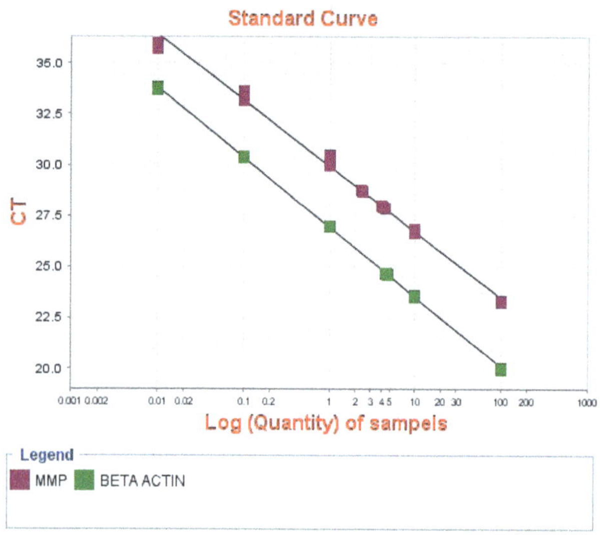

Figure 2. CT scale down by using dilution standard samples with quantity of 100, 10, 0.1, and 0.01.

Previously it was revealed that inhibition of MMP with two murine models could lead to decrease angiogenesis and MMPs may be a target in cancer treatment and inhibition of metastasis (24). Another research in 2009 indicated EGFR activation led to enhanced MMP expression and/or function, and suggested that modulating the expression or activity of the EGFR and/or matrix metalloproteinases offers opportunity for targeted intervention in patients with metastatic disease (25).

It has been demonstrated that saffron's main component such as crocin, crocetin and safranal could inhibit neurons erosion and depression (21). Result of a research in 2009 revealed that angiogenesis inhibition with natural products seemed to be useful and promising method in order to encounter less resistance (22). There are several mechanisms for the antitumor effect of saffron and its components, including inhibition of nucleic acid, scavenging free radical, effect on the expression of topoisomerase 2, and induction of programmed cell death. Furthermore, it could reduce cancer, decline the rate of tumor cell and significantly increase the lifelong of animal (26). It is indicated that saffron in different tumors, including leukemia, ovarian and breast carcinoma had anticancer and selective cytotoxic effect on different malignant cells (27). Moreover, saffron had cancer-preventive and anti genotoxic potential, so it would be used in combination with chemotherapy. Saffron has been shown reduce potential against lipid peroxidation and at the same time increase the enzymatic antioxidants like superoxide dismutase and catalase and non-enzymatic antioxidants such as liver glutathione regeneration (28). In addition, safranal increased tissue oxygen which have sweeping effect on free radicals and could inhibit oxidative stress of genotoxic compounds. Safranal also had protective effect on lipid peroxidation; since angiogenesis shows direct relation with tissue oxygen and hypoxia is one of the most important simulator of angiogenesis, increasing tissue oxygen accompanied. Saffron treatment may explain some part of anti-angiogenic effect of this herb (29). Results of another research represented that saffron had antitumor effects on TCC cell line (related to bladder cancer) in a time- and dose-dependent manner in a way that in high concentration the percentage of vital cells declined dramatically (30). Results of these researches were consistent with the findings of the present project. Influential potential of saffron on the induction or inhibition of gene expression in few cases has been studied so far. However, Mousavi *et al.* studied the effect of saffron extract on the level of protein which was related to apoptosis such as bax protein and enzyme as influential as caspase in breast cancer cells and represent that using saffron extract could reduce cell viability dose-dependently (31). The result on the induction of apoptosis of saffron extract depicts that on hepatocarcinoma and cervix cells extract showed significant cytotoxic effects (32). These results were coincided with our findings and cancer cell growth inhibited by the extract on concentration-dependent manner. In this research, saffron extract could reduce the level of MMP and gene expression decline which shows conformity with other data that reveals cytotoxic and anticancer effect of saffron.

Conclusion

The results of this study indicate reduction in MMP gene expression in breast cancer cells treated with the saffron aqueous extract. This may show the anti-angiogenic potential of this medical herb as a promising chemotherapeutic agent, and its potential in prevention of angiogenesis and metastasis.

Acknowledgments

The authors gratefully thank the colleagues in Research Center for Animal Development Applied Biology of Islamic Azad University of Mashhad (Mashhad, Iran) and also Department of Biophysics for their help and kind support.

Authors' contributions

JB designed and supervised the experiments, analyzed the data and wrote the paper; MM performed experiments, analyzed data and wrote the paper; MAS designed, analyzed data and wrote and edited the paper.

Conflict of interests

The authors declare no conflict of interest.

Ethical considerations

Ethical issues (including plagiarism, misconduct, data fabrication, falsification, double publication or submission, redundancy) have been completely observed by the authors.

Funding/Support
This work was financially supported by the Research Center for Animal Development Applied Biology, Mashhad Branch, Islamic Azad University, Mashhad, Iran

References

1. Hendrix MJ, Seftor EA, Seftor REB. Vasculogenic Mimicry: Angiogenesis in Disguise? In: Forough R, editor. New Frontiers in Angiogenesis. Netherlands: Springer; 2006.
2. Fayette J, Soria JC, Armand JP. Use of angiogenesis inhibitors in tumour treatment. Eur J Cancer 2005; 41(8):1109–16.
3. Breier G. Vasculogenesis. In: Unsicker K, Krieglstein K, editors. Cell Signaling and Growth Factors in Development: From Molecules to Organogenesis. 1 ed. Weinheim, Germany: Wiley-VCH Verlag GmbH; 2008.
4. Guo S, Colbert LS, Fuller M, Zhang Y, Gonzalez-Perez RR. Vascular endothelial growth factor receptor -2 in breast cancer. Biochim Biophys Acta 2010; 1806(1): 108-21.
5. Olsson AK, Dimberg A, Kreuger J, Claesson-Welsh L. VEGF receptor signalling— in control of vascular function. Nat Rev Mol Cell Biol 2006; 7(5): 359–71.
6. Solowiej J, Bergqvist S, McTigue MA, Marrone T, Quenzer T, Cobbs M, *et al.* Characterizing the effects of the juxtamembrane domain on vascular endothelial growth factor receptor-2 enzymatic activity, autophosphorylation, and inhibition by axitinib. Biochemistry 2009; 48(29):7019-31.
7. Singh AJ, Meyer RD, Band H, Rahimi N. The carboxyl terminus of VEGFR-2 is required for PKC-mediated down-regulation. Mol Biol Cell 2005; 16(4):2106-18.
8. Brooks SA, Lomax-Browne HJ, Carter TM, Kinch CE, Hall DM. Molecular interactions in cancer cell metastasis. Acta Histochem 2010; 112(1):3-25.
9. Nisato RE, Hosseini G, Sirrenberg C, Butler GS, Crabbe T, Docherty AJ, *et al.* Dissecting the role of matrix metalloproteinases (MMP) and integrin αvβ3 in angiogenesis in vitro: absence of hemopexin C domain bioactivity, but membrane-type 1-MMP and αvβ3 are critical. Cancer Res 2005; 65(20):9377-87.
10. Radisky ES, Radisky DC. Matrix Metalloproteinase-Induced Epithelial-Mesenchymal Transition in Breast Cancer. J Mammary Gland Biol Neoplasia 2010; 15(2):201–12.
11. Bhat TA, Singh RP. Tumor angiogenesis – A potential in cancer chemoprevention. Food Chem Toxicol 2008; 46(4):1334-45.
12. Kummalue T. Molecular mechanism of herbs in human lung cancer cells. J Med Assoc Thai 2005; 88(11):1725-34.
13. Mousavi SM, Montazeri A, Mohagheghi MA, Jarrahi AM, Harirchi I, Najafi M, *et al.* Breast cancer in Iran: an epidemiological review. Breast J 2007; 13(4):383-91.
14. Harirchi I, Karbakhsh M, Kashefi A, Momtahen AJ. Breast cancer in Iran: results of a multi-center study. Asian Pac J Cancer Prev 2004; 5(1):24-7.
15. Cristofanilli M, Broglio KR, Guarneri V, Jackson S, Fritsche HA, Islam R, *et al.* Circulating tumor cells in metastatic breast cancer biology staging beyond tumor burden. Clin Breast Cancer 2007; 7(6):471-9.
16. Rudel RA, Fenton SE, Ackerman JM, Euling SY, Makris SL. Environmental exposures and mammary gland development: state of the science, public health implications, and research recommendations. Environ Health Perspect 2011; 119(8):1053.
17. Fernández JA, Pandalai S. Biology, biotechnology and biomedicine of saffron. Recent Res Devel Plant Sci 2004; 2:127-59.
18. Kaefer CM, Milner JA. The role of herbs and spices in cancer prevention. J Nutr Biochem 2008; 19(6): 347-61.
19. Melnyk JP, Wang S, Marcone MF. Chemical and biological properties of the world's most expensive spice: saffron. Food Res Int 2010; 43(8):1981-9.
20. Ochiai T, Shimeno H, Mishima K, Iwasaki K, Fujiwara M, Tanaka H, *et al.* Protective effects of carotenoids from saffron on neuronal injury invitro and invivo. Biochim Biophys Acta 2007; 1770(4): 578-84.
21. Premkumar K, Thirunavukkarasu C, Abraham SK, Santhiya ST, Ramesh A. Protective effect of saffron (Crocus sativus L.) aqueous extract against genetic damage induced by anti-tumor agents in mice. Hum Exp Toxicol 2006; 25(2):79-84.
22. Abd Majid FA, Sarmidi MR, SH C. Impact of saffron as an anti-cancer and anti-tumor herb. Afr J Pharma Pharmacol 2010;4(11):834-40.
23. Kessenbrock K, Plaks V, Werb Z. Matrix metalloproteinases: regulators of the tumor microenvironment. Cell 2010; 141(1):52-67.
24. Naglich JG, Jure-Kunkel M, Gupta E, Fargnoli J, Henderson AJ, Lewin AC, *et al.* Inhibition of angiogenesis and metastasis in two murine models by the matrix metalloproteinase inhibitor, BMS-275291. Cancer Res 2001; 61(23):8480-5.
25. Hudson LG, Moss NM, Stack MS. EGF-receptor regulation of matrix metalloproteinases in epithelial ovarian carcinoma. Future Oncol 2009; 5(3):323–38.
26. Schmidt M, Betti G, Hensel A. Saffron in phytotherapy: pharmacology and clinical uses. Wien Med Wochenschr 2007; 157(13-14):315-9.
27. Melnyk JP, Wang S, Marcone MF. Chemical and biological properties of the world's most expensive spice: saffron. Food Res Int 2010; 43(8):1981-9.
28. Ochiai T, Soeda S, Ohno S, Tanaka H, Shoyama Y, Shimeno H. Crocin prevents the death of PC-12 cells through sphingomyelinase-ceramide signaling by increasing glutathione synthesis. Neurochem Int 2004; 44(5):321-30.
29. Holloway GM, Gainer JL. The carotenoid crocetin enhances pulmonary oxygenation. J Appl Physiol 1988; 65(2):683-6.
30. Feizzadeh B, Afshari JT, Rakhshandeh H, Rahimi A, Brook A, Doosti H. Cytotoxic effect of saffron stigma aqueous extract on human transitional cell carcinoma and mouse fibroblast. Urol J 2008; 5 (3):161-7.
31. Mousavi SH, Tavakkol-Afshari J, Brook A, Jafari-Anarkooli I. Role of caspases and Bax protein in saffron-induced apoptosis in MCF-7 cells. Food Chem Toxicol 2009; 47(8):1909-13.
32. Tavakkol-Afshari J, Brook A, Mousavi SH. Study of cytotoxic and apoptogenic properties of saffron extract in human cancer cell lines. Food Chem Toxicol 2008; 46(11):3443-7.

2

Formulation and physicochemical evaluation of toothpaste formulated with *Thymus vulgaris* essential oil

Mohammad Kiani[1,2], **Farzin Firoozian**[3], **Shirin Moradkhani**[1,2*]

[1]Medicinal Plants and Natural Products Research Center, Hamadan University of Medical Sciences, Hamadan, Iran
[2]Department of Pharmacognosy and Pharmaceutical Biotechnology, School of Pharmacy, Hamadan University of Medical Sciences, Hamadan, Iran
[3]Department of Pharmaceutics, School of Pharmacy, Hamadan University of Medical Sciences, Hamadan, Iran

ARTICLE INFO

Keywords:
Thymus vulgaris
Essential oil
Herbal toothpaste
Drug formulation
Physicochemical properties

ABSTRACT

Introduction: *Streptococcus mutans* is the most common cause of tooth decay. Parabens, and other commonly used as anti-*Streptococcus* agents in toothpaste industry have numerous side effects such as discoloration of teeth. *Thymus vulgaris* essential oil has profound antimicrobial activity against a wide range of species. The aim of present study was the aim of the present study was to formulate and evaluate the physicochemical properties of a kind of toothpaste formulated with Thymus vulgaris essential oil. Thyme oil components were also analyzed using gas chromatography–mass spectrometry (GC-MS).
Methods: Toothpaste was formulated in forms of gel and opaque and Thyme essence was added to it. The formulation was evaluated in terms of stability in different temperatures, pH, consistency, uniformity, taste, smell, and compatibility with special packaging for toothpaste at three temperatures. Profilometry was used to determine abrasivity. The rate of contaminations with lead and arsenic was determined by atomic absorption. The amount of fluoride was measured by potentiometry.
Results: Forty-one different components, representing 99.64% of the total oil were identified in essential oil. Addition of thyme essence to formulation had no deleterious effect in stability, consistency, taste and smell. The pH of opaque and gel formulations was 7.02 and 7.45, respectively. The abrasiveness of opaque and gel formulations was in standard ranges. The fluoride content was 1000 ppm. Lead and arsenic were not detected at all.
Conclusion: Formulation of toothpaste with *T. vulgaris* essential oil was acceptable and might be considered as a desirable herbal toothpaste.

Implication for health policy/practice/research/medical education:
Addition of *T. vulgaris* essential oil to toothpaste and evaluation of the physicochemical properties of this new formulation was the aim of present study. Addition of herbal components such as *T. vulgaris* essential oil to toothpastes may make them interesting for introducing new candidates in oral hygiene products.

Introduction

The oral cavity infections are the most common types of infections. Dental caries, an infectious disease, results in damage and infection of enamel and dentine (1). If left untreated, the infection continues and will lead to tooth loss. The mouth normal flora consists of opportunistic bacteria which are normally non-pathogenic. The imbalance of this situation creates infection and tooth decay. *Streptococcus mutans* is considered as the main species involved in the development of dental caries (2). *S. mutans,* acid producing bacteria, causes fermentation of carbohydrates which results in tooth decay (3). Toothpaste, toothbrush, mouthwash, and toothpaste that contain antimicrobial agents are commonly used as products which improve oral hygiene. Their uses dates back to ancient times and continues up to now (4). Toothpaste, as an irreplaceable agent in effective home care system, is a gel or paste dentifrice used with a toothbrush as an accessory to clean and maintain health of teeth in order to enhance oral hygiene (5).

Thymus vulgaris (*Lamiaceae),* or thyme as common name, contains a useful essential oil. It has antiseptic, expectorant, antispasmodic and carminative activities (6). Thyme oil consists of high amounts of phenolic monoterpenes. These compounds have strong antimicrobial activity against *S. mutans* and a wide range of

***Corresponding author:** Shirin Moradkhani,
Email: shirin.moradkhani@yahoo.com

viruses, bacteria and fungi (6,7). Considering the ongoing use of plants, their lower side effects in comparison to synthetic substances and the wide range of antimicrobial activities of thyme oil, the aim of the present study was to formulate and evaluate the physicochemical properties of a kind of toothpaste formulated with *T. vulgaris* essential oil. Thyme oil components were also analyzed using gas chromatography–mass spectrometry (GC-MS).

Materials and methods

All substances were dental grade and purchased from Goltash Company (Iran). The essence was prepared from Giahessence Company (Iran).

Thymus vulgaris essential oil components identification

One microliter of oil was injected to GC-MS. The volatile compounds were analyzed by GC/MS (TRACE MS-Thermo Finnegan Polaris Q). The capillary column type was DB-5 (30 m * 0.25 mm * 0.25 µm). The oven temperature was programmed (60°C for 1 minute, then 5°C/min to 250°C, and then left at 250°C for 5 minutes). The injection port temperature was 250°C and that of the detector was 280°C (split ratio: 1/100). The carrier gas was helium (99.995% purity) with a flow rate of 1.1 mL/min. The MS conditions were as follow: ionization voltage, 70 eV; ion source temperature, 200°C; electron ionization mass spectra were acquired over the mass range 40 to 460 m/z.

Formulation of clear gel and opaque toothpaste

In this study, 4 gel and 4 opaque toothpastes were formulated. Three formulations of each type had thyme oil and one in each type contained methyl and propyl parabene. The amounts of oil used in the formulations were based on microbial studies and measurement of minimum inhibitory concentration (MIC) and minimum bactericidal concentration (MBC). The formulated toothpastes were packaged in laminate tubes.

Determination of physicochemical properties

pH

The pH of formulations was measured by the methods described in ISO3996 (grade 3) (13).

Homogeneity

Determination of homogeneity was studied by applying normal force to containers at 27±2°C (14).

Tube inertness

Tube inertness was examined by cutting the tubes and investigating internal surface for any signs of deterioration in different storage conditions including normal and heating temperature at 45±2°C for 180 days (14).

Sharp and edge abrasive particles

This test was performed considering the extradition of the content of 10 tubes and investigating the presence of sharp and hard edged abrasive particles (14).

Stability

The stability study was performed by soring formulations in three different temperatures and humidity conditions, viz. 4°C, 25°C± 2°C/60% ± 5% RH, 40°C ± 2°C/75% ± 5% RH for a period of 6 months considering ICH guidelines (15).

Fluoride ion

Potentiometry with fluoride ion sensitive electrodes was used for determination of fluoride ions.

Calculation: a graph was plotted on a log scale, taking the concentration of fluoride (y-axis) versus potential in mV (x-axis). From the calibration curve, the fluoride ion concentration (in ppm) of test solution was measured. Fluoride ion concentration (ppm) was calculated from the graph (16).

Heavy metals quantification

Sample preparation was carried out according to USP 231. Determination of heavy metals was done by atomic absorption spectrophotometer (17,18).

Dentine and enamel abrasion

Sample preparation was performed by use of brush machine and according to ISO 11609:2010 (16). The nominal Ra values were tabulated and analyzed using descriptive statistical software (SPSS version 18.0, IBM Corporation). The data of surface roughness were compared between the 2 experimental groups in each experimental period (standard formulation was control test and compared with F1 & F2 formulation roughness) using paired *t* test. $P<0.05$ was considered significant. Variation in roughness was calculated and compared with the 2 experimental groups by the same tests mentioned above.

Results

Thyme oil components identification

Analyzing thyme oil by means of GC-MS resulted in identification of 41 different components, representing 99.64% of the total oil (Figure 1 and Table 1). Identification was done by calculating the Kovats index for each

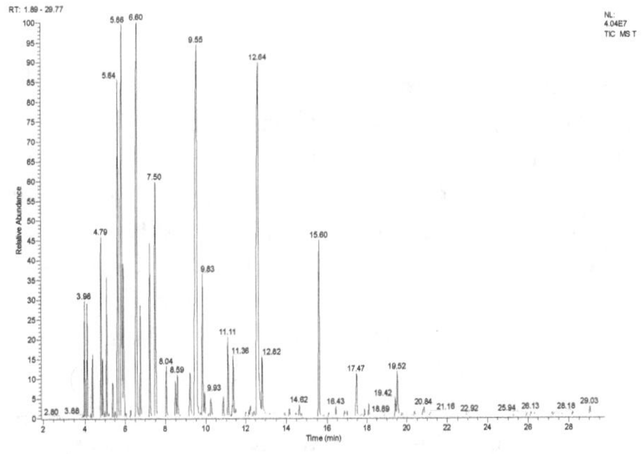

Figure 1. *Thymus vulgaris* oil components in GC-MS chromatogram.

Table 1. *Thymus vulgaris* chemical composition result

Peak Number	Compound	Retention time (RT)	Retention index (RI)	Percent
1	α-Thujene	3.98	926	1.2
2	α-Pinene	4.11	934	1.25
3	Camphene	4.37	949	0.7
4	Sabinene	4.79	974	2.34
5	β-Pinene	4.87	978	0.69
6	β-Myrcene	5.08	991	1.77
7	α-Phellandrene	5.38	1006	0.46
8	α-Terpinene	5.64	1018	6.19
9	p-Cymene	5.86	1028	12.09
10	Limonene	5.92	1031	2.48
11	1,8-Cineole	5.95	1032	0.49
12	γ-Terpinene	6.59	1061	11.61
13	cis-Sabinene hydrate	6.76	1069	1.56
14	α-Terpinolene	7.22	1090	2.63
15	Linalool	7.50	1102	5.23
16	cis-p-Menth-2-en-1-ol	8.04	1124	0.76
17	1-Terpineol	8.49	1141	0.62
18	Camphor	8.59	1145	0.63
19	Borneol	9.21	1170	1
20	4-Terpineol	9.55	1184	16.55
21	α-Terpineol	9.83	1195	2.6
22	cis-Piperitol	9.93	1199	0.37
23	trans-Piperitol	10.23	1211	0.39
24	Thymol, methyl ether	10.86	1235	0.29
25	Carvacrol, methyl ether	11.11	1245	1.3
26	trans-Sabinene hydrate acetate	11.31	1253	0.13
27	linalyl acetate	11.36	1255	1.02
28	Anethole<E->	12.24	1289	0.21
29	Thymol	12.64	1305	15.95
30	Carvacrol	12.82	1312	1.05
31	Neryl acetate	14.14	1364	0.1
32	Geranyl acetate	14.62	1383	0.17
33	E-Caryophyllene	15.60	1423	3.32
34	α-Humulene	16.43	1457	0.14
35	Bicyclogermacrene	17.47	1499	0.9
36	γ-Cadinene	17.88	1517	0.1
37	δ-Cadinene	18.09	1526	0.18
38	Spathulenol	19.42	1582	0.32
39	Caryophyllene oxide	19.52	1587	0.94
40	Iso-Spathulenol	20.80	1643	0.09
41	α-epi-Cadinol	20.84	1645	0.2

compound comparing the results with the library of mass apparatus and with those reported in the literature.

Physicochemical properties result

The results of physicochemical tests indicate the stability of both formula of Opaque and Jelly at room temperature (the temperature of 4°C of refrigerated and temperature of 40°C with germinator and 75% humidity). Also the formulations were satisfactory in terms of the status of consistency, uniformity, taste and smell. Also, there was no fermentation in two formulations (Figures 2 and 3). Also both formula had not any sharp and hard edged abrasive particles. The toothpaste container did not produce any corrosion or deterioration and Thymus vulgaris essential oil had perfect compatibility with container. Also, formulation F7 with parabens and without essence was stable and had proper consistency that was expected.

pH

At first the pH of Opaque and Jelly formulations before stability test was respectively 6.82 and 6.78. After stability test for a period of 6 months, the pH was 7.02 and 7.54 which were in the standard range.

Heavy metal content

The heavy metals of lead and arsenic test results indicated the absence of the two metals in the formulation and since the standard level of lead is less than 20 μg/g and arsenic is less than 2 μg/g, hence, both are in the standard range (Table 2).

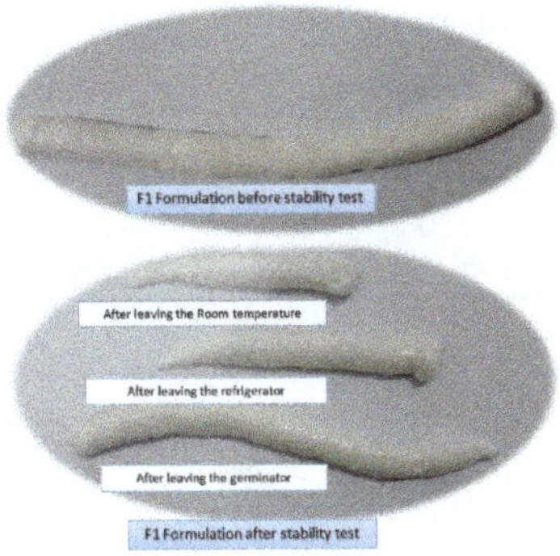

Figure 2. Physicochemical properties result of F1 formulation

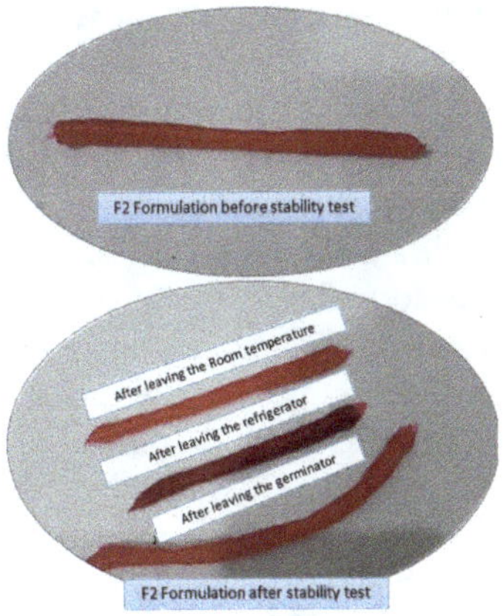

Figure 3. Physicochemical properties result of F2 formulation

Fluoride ion content

The graph was plotted for content of fluoride ion against potential difference on semi-logarithmic paper (Figure 4). The potential difference, in millivolts, was plotted on the X axis and the fluoride ion, in milligrams, on the Y axis. The amount of fluoride formulation was 1000 ppm according to fluoride ion that formulation was standard and acceptable (Table 3).

Toothpaste roughness on enamel and dentine

The amounts of abrasive of the formulations were determined. In opaque formula the amounts of dentin and enamel were 0.15, and 0.5 times of reference toothpaste, respectively, these amounts in Jelly formulas were 0.8 and 1.07 times of reference toothpaste, respectively. The abrasiveness of both formulae was acceptable and standard (Table 4). Also independent sample *t* tests were carried out to compare between F1 and F2 dentine and enamel roughness.

Independent sample *t* test was carried out to compare between F1 and F2 roughness in an effort to establish approximate differences in mean values between

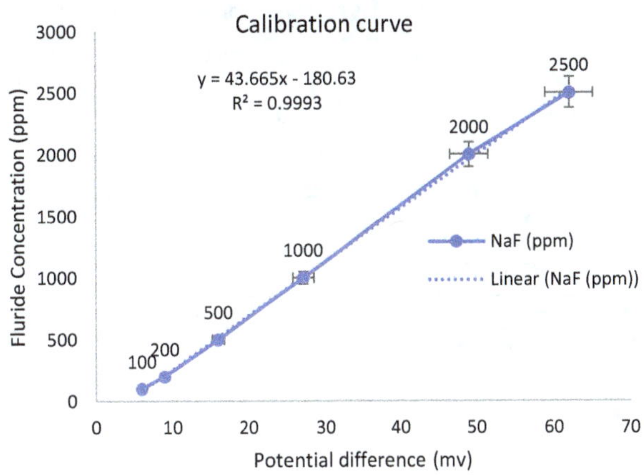

Figure 4. Fluoride ion calibration curve

Table 3. Content of NaF (ppm)

Sample	Measured potential difference (mv)	NaF (ppm)
Standard 1	6	100
Standard 2	9	200
Standard 3	16	500
Standard 4	27.1	1000
Standard 5	49	2000
Standard 6	62	2500
F1 & F2 Fluoride (ppm)	27.1	1000

dentifrices that were statistically significant (Table 5) ($P < 0.05$).

Discussion

The results of GC-MS analysis showed that *T. vulgaris* essential oil contained 15.95 % thymol and 1% carvacrol. In this way, Thyme oil effectiveness on *S. mutans* bacteria that causes oral infections is clear. The results of the initial investigation and after thermal & cooling physicochemical tests showed no changes in physical stability of formula. Also the pH of formula after tests did not change and remained in the range of 7 to 7.5 which indicates the stability of the *T. vulgaris* essential oil. Formulations containing *T. vulgaris* essential oil as preservative compared to formulations containing parabens had appropriate stability. A previous study on a cream made with *T. vulgaris* essential oil indicated appropriate and consistent formulation stability (19). *T. vulgaris* essential oil has been proven to possess antioxidant properties. This property is due to various components such as α pinen, β pinen, γ terpinen, 1,8 cineol, para-cimen, linalool, sabinen, eugenol and phellandrene. The antioxidant capacity of this components has previously proven (20,21).

Table 2. Determination of heavy metal content

Formulation/Heavy metal	Lead	Arsenic	Standard range	LOD	LOQ	Result
F1	Not detect	Not detect	Pb: <20 μg/g & As_2O_3: <2 μg/g	0.3 ppm	1 ppm	In rang
F2	Not detect	Not detect				In rang

Table 4. Formulated toothpastes roughness on enamel and dentine in comparison to standard toothpaste

Group	Dentine roughness (µm) Mean ± SD	Roughness compared to standard (times)	Enamel roughness (µm) Mean ± SD	Roughness compared to standard (times)
Standard	0.324±0.011	-	0.315±0.007	-
F1 (Dicalcium phosphate)	0.463±0.011	0.15	0.360±0.008	0.5
F2 (Hydrated silica)	0.561±0.007	0.8	0.666±0.019	1.07

Table 5. Independent samples of statistical *t* test results

Formulation	Roughness Mean	Standard error	*P* value
F1 (Dicalcium phosphate)	0.36	0.009	P< 0.001*
F2 (Hydrated silica)	0.56	0.009	

*Significant at a significance level of 5%.

Periodontal disease is associated with an increase in reactive oxidative species (ROS) in the body and this increase in free radicals in the body causes chronic and worsens the symptoms. The essence of *T. vulgaris* can be used in oral products as a good antioxidant to improve inflammatory and infectious diseases of oral tissue (22). Preliminary results of this study showed that F1 formula had appropriate and suitable stability. In F3 formulation carbapol gelling agent was exchanged with CMC. In the gel formulation stability and consistency became lost so that it could not be packaged in its own tube. Carbapol has been shown to be not suitable for the opaque toothpaste formulation and affects the stability of toothpaste (23). Our findings in this study was consistent with that results. Also the study of Wilkinson and Moore in 1996 showed that CMC was a suitable gelling agent for the preparation of opaque toothpaste (24).

In F5 formulation abrasive silica was used instead of dicalcium phosphate. Due to changes form a paste formulation and heterogeneous particles in the formulation this change is not considered desirable. Kitchin about the history of the use of dicalcium phosphate abrasive showed that the abrasive since 1940 is used as an abrasive in opaque toothpaste (25).

The results of this study are consistent with the above findings. According to the dentine & enamel roughness result, the abrasivity of formulations F1 (dicalcium phosphate) and F2 (hydrated silica) both dentin and enamel roughness was in the range of standard, and both were good. After ensure the standardization of both samples F1 and F2 wear rate were compared with each other through statistical test (Tables 4 and 5). Thus it can be concluded that the average abrasivity of formulations with hydrated silica is more than the average abrasivity of formulations with dicalcium phosphate and repeating about the test result of the change cannot be achieved. Also, a study on 26 commercial toothpastes indicated that the roughness of toothpaste with hydrated silica abrasive (like Brill smile) was significantly different from that of toothpaste containing calcium phosphate (26).

Conclusion

An ideal plant dentifrice should provide optimum physicochemical, cleaning and polishing properties with maximum compatibility with dental tissue and minimum abrasion to the dental hard tissues. The formulated toothpaste with *T. vulgaris* essential oil was successfully evaluated using different standard parameters including testing pH, consistency, uniformity, change in colors, change in smell, standard roughness, temperature and tolerance. The formulated toothpaste may be safer compared to fully synthetic toothpastes and can be used as desirable toothpaste in terms of stability and physicochemical properties in the pharmaceutical market.

Acknowledgments

This article is a part of the thesis of Mohammad Kiani for the fulfillment of Pharm. D. degree in School of Pharmacy, Hamadan University of Medical Sciences, Hamadan, Iran. The authors are grateful to deputy of vice chancellor of research and technology for financial supports.

Authors' contributions

SM and FF were the supervisors of the thesis project, respectively. MK performed the experiments. All read and confirmed the manuscript.

Conflict of interests

The authors declare that there is no conflict of interest.

Funding/ Support

This study was financially supported by deputy of vice chancellor of research and technology, Hamadan University of Medical Sciences, Hamadan, Iran.

References

1. Bowen WH, Koo H. Biology of *Streptococcus mutans* derived glucosyltransferases: Role in extracellular matrix formation of cariogenic biofilms. Caries Res. 2011;45:69 86.
2. Wright JT, Hart TC. The genome projects: implications for dental practice and education. J Dent Educ. 2002;66:659-71.
3. Freedman ML, Tanzer JM. Dissociation of plaque formation from glucan-induced Agglutination in Mutants of *Streptococcus mutans*. Infect Immun. 1974;10(1):189-196.
4. Davies R, Scully C, Preston AJ. Dentifrices - an update. Med Oral Patol Oral Cir Bucal. 2010;15(6): 976-82.
5. Namba T, Tsunezuka M, Hattori M. Dental caries prevention by traditional Chinese medicines. Part II. Potent

antibacterial action of Magnoliae cortex extracts against *Streptococcus mutans.* Planta Med. 1982;44(2):100-6.

6. Zargari A. Herbal Medicine. Iran: Publishing and Printing Institute of Tehran University; 1996:353. [Persian].
7. Abdulsattar BA, Hassan AM, Hassan AS. In vitro antimicrobial activity of *Thymus vulgaris, Origanum vulgare* and *Rosmarinus officinalis* Against Dental Caries Pathogens. Haitham J Pure Appl Sci. 2011;25(2):1-7.
8. Richardson LM. International collaborative research of fluride. J Dent Res. 2000;79:893-904.
9. Kielbassa AM, Gillmann L, Zantner C, Meyner-Lueckel H. Profilometric and microradiographic studies on the effects of toothpastes and acidic gel roughness on sound and demineralized bovine dental enamel. Caries Res. 2005;39:380-6.
10. Amartey EO, Asumadu-Sakyi AB, Adjei CA, Quashie FK, Duodu GO, Bentil NO. Determination of heavy metals concentration in hair pomades on the Ghanaian market using atomic absorption spectrometry technique. Br J Pharmacol Toxicol. 2011;2(4):192-98.
11. Butler H, Poucher's Perfumes Cosmetics and Soaps. 9th ed. Netherlands: Kluwer Academic Publishers; 2000:981-6.
12. ISO E. 3696: Water for analytical laboratory use. Specification and test methods; 1997.
13. Benzian H, Holmgren C, Buijs M, van Loveren C, van der Weijden F, van Palenstein-Helderman W. Total and free available fluoride in toothpastes in Brunei, Cambodia, Laos, the Netherlands and Suriname. Int Dent J. 2012;62(4):213-21.
14. Bureau of Indian standard. 2001. https://law.resource.org/pub/in/bis/S11/is.6356.2001.pdf. Accessed September 2010.
15. Pope DG. Accelerated stability testing for prediction of drug product stability. 2. Drug & Cosmetic Industry; 1980; 127(6):48.
16. International Standard organization. https://www.iso.org/obp/ui/#iso:std:38010:en. Accessed September 2010.
17. US Pharmacopeia. Heavy metal analysis in toothpastes, 1990:1523-4.
18. British Pharmacopeia. Heavy metal analysis in toothpastes. 1990:87-8.
19. Manou I, Bouillard L, Devleescherouwer MJ, Barel AO. Evaluation of the preservative properties of *Thymus vulgaris* essential oil in topically applied formulations under a challenge test. J Appl Microbiol. 1998;84:368-78.
20. Przygodzka M, Zielińska D, Ciesarová Z, Kukurová K, Zieliński H. Comparison of methods for evaluation of the antioxidant capacity and phenolic compounds in common spices. LWT-Food Science and Technology. 2014; 58(2):321-6.
21. Nikolić M, Glamočlija J, Ferreira IC, et al. Chemical composition, antimicrobial, antioxidant and antitumor activity of *Thymus serpyllum* L., *Thymus algeriensis* Boiss. and Reut and *Thymus vulgaris* L. essential oils. Ind Crops Prod. 2014;52:183-90.
22. Tamaki N, Tomofuji T, Ekuni D, Yamanaka R, Yamamoto T, Morita M. Short-term effects of non-surgical periodontal treatment on plasma level of reactive oxygen metabolites in patients with chronic periodontitis. J Periodontol.2009;80(6):901-6.
23. Saeidi M, Azadbakht M. Formulation of herbal toothpaste from chamomile and myrah, apreliminary clinical evaluation on bleeding gum. Journal of Mazandaran University of Medical Science. 2003;13(40):61-9.
24. Wilkinson JB, Moore RJ: Harry's Cosmeticology. 7th ed. London: Longman Scientific & Technical; 1996:613.
25. Kitchin PC, Robinson HBG. How abrasive need a dentifrice be? J Dent Res. 1948;27:501-6.
26. Schemehorn BR, Moore MH, Putt MS. Abrasion, polishing, and stain removal characteristics of various commercial dentifrices in vitro. J Clin Dent. 2011;22(1):11.

3

Synergistic effect of pulsed electromagnetic fields and saffron extract on osteogenic differentiation of bone marrow mesenchymal stem cells

Javad Baharara[1*], Tayebeh Ramezani[2], Marzieh Mousavi[1], Majid Asadi-Samani[3]

[1]Research Center for Animal Development Applied Biology, Mashhad Branch, Islamic Azad University, Mashhad, Iran
[2]Faculty of Biological Sciences, Kharazmi University, Tehran, Iran
[3]Medical Plants Research Center, Shahrekord University of Medical Sciences, Shahrekord, Iran

ARTICLE INFO

Keywords:
Osteogenesis
Saffron
Pulsed electromagnetic fields
Differentiation

ABSTRACT

Introduction: Pulsed electromagnetic fields (PEMFs) are usually used to treat non-union fractures. Saffron is a medicinal plant with various pharmacologic effects. In the present study, the synergistic effect of PEMF and saffron aqueous extract on osteogenic differentiation of bone marrow mesenchymal stem cells (BMSCs) was evaluated
Methods: BMSCs were isolated from rat femur. After purification, the cells were divided into four groups including control group (did not receive any treatment), saffron alone (800 μg/mL), PEMF alone (50 Hz, 3 times a weak, 2 hours for every time, for 2 weeks), and saffron plus PEMF. Cytotoxicity was measured using MTT assay. After calculating the IC50 value for saffron extract (1.5 mg/mL), a lower concentration (800 μg/mL) was combined with PEMF. The differentiation of each cell group was evaluated using alkaline phosphatase (ALP) enzyme activity, alizarin red staining and reverse transcribed polymerase chain reaction (RT-PCR) method.
Results: Saffron aqueous extract decreased dose-dependently the cell viability but the PEMF had not any significant effects on cell viability. The PEMF, saffron extract and their combination increased the ALP activity on day 10 but the increase was significant in synergist group. Alizarin red staining showed that mineralization groups were higher at day 14. RT-PCR results demonstrated that on the day 14 the group treated with both PEMF and saffron expressed osteogenic genes.
Conclusion: Saffron extract combined with PEMFs could promote osteogenesis at the initial stage (the commitment of undifferentiated mesenchymal stem cells into osteoblast), hence, its usage might be beneficial in these patients

Implication for health policy/practice/research/medical education:
Saffron in combination with PEFMs is able to promote osteogenesis at the initial stage in a synergic manner and this combination might be used as a new approach in differentiation of stem cells into bone cells.

Introduction

Bone defects resulting from resorption trauma, both pathological and physiological, are still a main challenge in orthopedic surgery. The limits of bone regeneration continue to result in failure to fully recover function and quality of life in many people (1). However, in recent decade, the use of stem cells has helped to develop promising cell-based therapies for osseous defects. The use of human embryonic stem cells could be unethical, and hence the use of pluripotent adult stem cells, such as bone marrow mesenchymal stem cells (BMSCs), in engineering medicine has been considered (2). Recently, autologous cell therapy for bone engineering has been recommended as an interesting choice. The concept of such therapies is based on the especial effect of stem cells to differentiate into osteoblast. BMSCs are most accessible source of stem cells for many tissue engineering and regenerative medicine applications (3). BMSCs can be isolated and easily expanded from a small bone marrow aspirate. In addition, allogeneic transplant of BMSCs is

***Corresponding author:** Javad Baharara, Professor, Research Center for Animal Development Applied Biology, Mashhad Branch, Islamic Azad University, Mashhad, Iran.
Email: baharara@yahoo.com

possible with no high risk of immune rejection because of their ability to modulate immune responses (4). Growth factors including platelet-derived growth factor, bone morphogenetic proteins (BMPs) and transforming growth factor-β (TGF-β) showed promising effects in differentiation of stem cells into bone cells (5). However, the high cost and rapid degradation of such growth factors have led to limited use of them (6). Therefore, alternative osteogenic agents with lower costs compared to growth factors should be expanded (6).

Low frequency pulsed electromagnetic fields (PEMFs) can be used to treat diseases characterized by pain, inflammation and regeneration (7). PEMFs have a significant potential as a non-invasive physical therapy. PEMFs are effective adjunct to manage non-union long-bone fractures (8). PEMFs are able to stimulate bone tissue to remodel itself. PEMFs have been extensively used in the treatment of skeletal diseases such as osteoporosis and non-union fracture. PEMFs have some physiological effects on cells and tissues, including the up-regulation transcription of collagen type II, preservation of the extracellular matrix (ECM) integrity and increasing prostaglandin E_2, vascular endothelial growth factor and tumor growth factor-b_3 (TGF-b_3) production (9,10).

In recent years, use of natural products especially medicinal plants has increased. *Crocus sativus* L., commonly known as saffron, is a member of the Iridaceae family. This plant is extensively cultivated in some countries including Iran, India and Greece (11). The main component of saffron is crocetin. Other components of saffron include picrocrocin and safranal which are responsible for its color, flavor and aroma. Anthocyanins, flavonoids, vitamins, amino acids, proteins, starch, minerals and other chemical compounds have been also found in saffron (12). Previous studies have shown that retinoids may have useful effects in prevention of osteoporosis through both enhancing bone formation and suppressing osteoclast activity (13).

Due to the effects of magnetic fields and saffron extract compounds on osteogenic differentiation, in this study the effect of 50 Hz electromagnetic field with 200 g intensity and saffron aquatic extract on osteogenic differentiation of BMSCs from Wistar rats was investigated.

Material and Methods

Design PEMF exposure system

Generator of electromagnetic field was designed and manufactured in the laboratory of developmental biology, Islamic Azad University of Mashhad, Iran. This special circuit included coil, three rheostats, capacitors and ampermeter. To build a coil, around a tube, made of PVC, a suitable amount of copper wire was wrapped. Intensity was calculated according to the equation $B=\mu nI$ (B = the magnetic field intensity by Tesla, $\mu=4\pi\times10$, n = t he number of cycles per unit length, I = amperage). Intensity was controlled by the gauss meter. Culture flasks and plates were placed into solenoid; left and right sides of solenoid were closed and a humidified atmosphere of 5% CO_2 and 95% air at 37°C were established. In this configuration, the magnetic fields were parallel to the flasks and plates.

Preparation of plant extract

Crocus sativa stigmas were collected from Ghaen (Khorasan province, northeast Iran). Stigmas were dried and pulverized. Pulverized stigma of saffron was dissolved in distilled water and soaked for 24 hours at 4°C. The extract was filtered and concentrated by a rotary evaporator and dried by freeze dryer. The extract then was dissolved in deionized water to a final concentration of 100 mg/mL and diluted in culture medium to the working solution prior to use.

Isolation and Expansion of BMSCs

Bone marrow cells were harvested by flushing of femurs bone marrow of 6- to 8-week-old rats with Dulbecco's modified Eagle's medium (DMEM). Then the cells were centrifuged, suspended in DMEM and cultured in DMEM containing 10% FBS and 1% penicillin-streptomycin. Cells were incubated at 37°C in 5% humidified CO_2 for 24 hours until the medium was replaced to remove non-adherent cells. When cells reached 90% confluency, they were trypsinized with 0.25% trypsin for 5 minutes at 37°C. After centrifugation, the cells were re-suspended and used for other analyses.

Flow cytometry

To confirm that the used cells are stem cells, flow cytometry method agonist stem cell specific markers were done. After cells separation from bottom of the flask, they were centrifuged. The primary antibodies including CD44, CD31 and CD45 were conjugated with isothiocyanate and added to the cells. They were washed with PBS and fixed with formalin. Then, analysis was done by flow cytometer.

In vitro cytotoxicity

Cytotoxicity of saffron extract was evaluated by MTT assay. In this method the cleavage and the conversion of the soluble yellowish MTT into the insoluble purple formazan by active mitochondrial dehydrogenase of living cells is used to develop an assay system for cell proliferation measurement. Briefly, harvested cells were seeded into a 24-well plate (4×10^5 cell/mL) at various amounts of saffron extract (0.5, 1, 1.5 and 2 mg/mL) and exposed to PEMF at 200 g intensity for 2 hours. At the completion of incubations, 100 µL of MTT solution (5 mg/mL in PBS) was added to each well and left for 4 hours in darkness. Subsequently, the produced insoluble formazan was dissolved with 1 mL of dimethyl sulfoxide and left at room temperature for 20 minutes. Finally, the solution optical density was read by multi well scanning spectrophotometer (Epoch, US) at 570 nm wavelength. The cell viability was calculated using the following equation: Cell viability (%) = $(A_{treated}/A_{control}) \times 100$ where $A_{treated}$ and $A_{control}$ are the absorbance of the treated and untreated cells, respectively.

Treatment of BMSCs with PEMF and saffron

BMSCs were seeded in 24-well plates (5×10^4). When over 80% confluence was reached, osteogenesis was induced by 50 Hz PEMF three times a week (2 hours for every time) for 2 weeks. In some groups 800 μg/mL saffron alongside with PEMF was added. The medium was replaced once every three days and treated with saffron again. On day 10, cells were collected for measuring alkaline phosphatase (ALP) activity and on day 14, reverse transcribed polymerase chain reaction (RT-PCR) analysis and alizarin red staining were done. Control group was put in off generator in a condition same as experimental groups.

Alizarin red staining

Cells were fixed with 4% paraformaldehyde at room temperature for 10 minutes. After washing with distilled water once, 1 mL alizarin red solution (2%, pH 4.2) was added to each well in a 24-well plate. The staining solution was removed after 10 minutes. Each well was washed with distilled water 4 to 5 times. Finally it was observed by an inverted microscope (Biomed, Korea).

Measurement of alkaline phosphatase activity

BMSCs were cultured in 6-well plate dishes for 24 hours as described previously and then were treated with 50 Hz 200 g intensity three days a week for 10 days. To determine ALP activity level, total cell protein was extracted by 200 μl NP40 buffer (Sigma, UK). The lysate was then centrifuged at 14000×g at 4°C for 15 minutes. The protein concentrations were determined by the border of Ford assay reagent. ALP activity was measured by ALP assay kit (Parsazmun, Iran) using p-nitrophenyl phosphate as substrate and ALP provided in the kit as standard.

Semi-quantification RT-PCR analysis

Osteocalcin mRNA expression was analyzed by RT-PCR. For this propose RNA was extracted from approximately $10^{10}\times6$ BMSCs treated with PEMF, saffron and a combination of both using RNEasy per the manufacturer's instructions. The mRNA was reverse transcribed to CDNA using advantage RT-for-PCR per the manufacturer's instructions. After initial denaturation at 94°C for 5 minutes, cDNA was amplified using a termocycler (Perkin Elmer Applied Biosystems, Boston, MA) at 94°C for 40 seconds, 56°C for 50 seconds and 72°C for 60 seconds for 35 cycles. Primers used for amplification are forward primers shown in Table 1. The PCR products were analyzed by the electrophoresis of samples in 1.5% agarose gels stained with ethidium bromide. Results were analyzed by Image J software for measurement of band density.

Statistical analysis

Data were expressed as mean ± standard deviation (SD). Statistical analyses were done by analysis of variance (ANOVA) test. $P<0.05$ was considered as significant level.

Results

Flow cytometric results confirmed presence of BMSCs. Cells were positive for CD44 but negative for CD45 and CD31 (Figure 1).

Cytotoxicity study results

Saffron extract led to time and dose-dependent inhibition of viability at 24 hours and 48 hours. Inhibitory

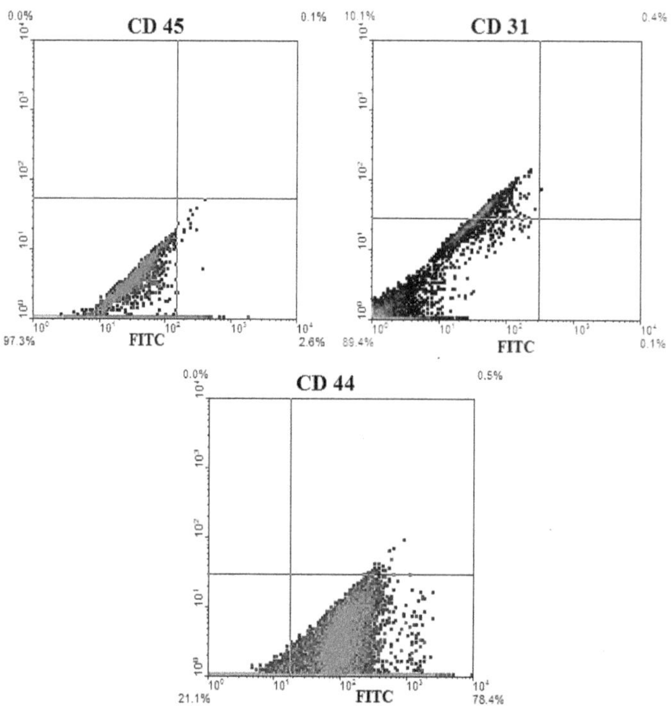

Figure 1. Flow cytometric analysis of isolated BMSCs.
BMSCs were expression specific surface marker CD44 but they were not hematopoietic marker (CD45); endothelial marker (CD31).

Table 1. Sequencing of used primers

Gene	Forward	Reverse
Beta Actin	5'CCCGCCGCCAGCTCACCATGG3'	5'AAGGTCTCAAACATGATCTGGGTC3'
OCN	5'GTGCAGAGTCCAGCAAAGGT3'	5'CGATAGGCCTCCTGAAAGC3'
OPN	5'ACAGCCAGGACTCCATTGAC3'	5'ACACTATCACCTCGGCCATC3'

concentration (IC50) that decreased half of the cells viability was about 1.5 mg/mL (Figure 2). The lower IC50 value (800 µg/mL) was used to induce osteoblast differentiation. The BMSCs viability values were around 80% when treated with 800 µg/mL of saffron extract. The viability of cells that exposed to PEMF did not show significant change compared to the control groups.

Alizarin red staining results

Matrix mineralization showed that PEMF and saffron extract had positive effects on osteogenic differentiation of BMSCs. However the greatest difference was observed in the PEMF+saffron extract groups compared to the control, PEMF and saffron extract groups (Figure 3).

ALP activity measurement results

In the present study ALP activity was detected using Naphthol AS-MX Phosphate stain. The results showed that ALP activity increased at day 10 compared to the control. However in PEMF+saffron extract group, increase was significant compared to saffron extract and PEMF groups (Figure 4).

Semi-quantification RT-PCR results

Significant up regulation of osteocalcin expression was seen in the groups treated with saffron extract and PEMF+saffron. However in the groups treated with PEMF alone, osteopontin gene (OPN) expression did not show any significant changes. However osteocalcin gene (OCN) expression in all the experimental groups increased but this increase was not statistically significant compared to the control group (Figure 5).

Discussion

Bone cells and mineralized matrix comprise two main components of bone. Osteoblasts are main bone cells. They produce organic bone's matter and lead mineralization of matrix (14,15). The biological activity and proliferation rate of the osteoblasts have been directly correlated with the bone formation rate. However, for bone repair and osteoporosis treatment osteoblast proliferation is main factor. BMSCs are the source of bone-forming osteoblasts (2). Hence it is necessary to identify factors that enhance the differentiated stem cell into osteoblast. Stimulatory effects of the PMEF on hard tissues such as bone and soft tissue such as muscles, tendons and nerves, have been demonstrated. Saffron is a medical plant with different pharmacological effects. In the present

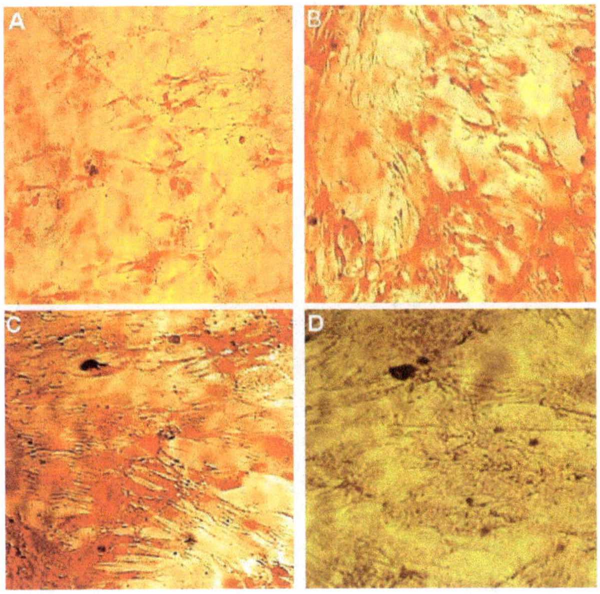

Figure 3. Alizarin red staining of BMSCs. Exposure to PEMF (A), saffron extract (800 µg/mL) (B) and saffron extract with PEMF after 14 days (C) comparing with untreated group (D). Synergic use of saffron extract and PEMF induced osteogenic differentiation more efficiency than each one.

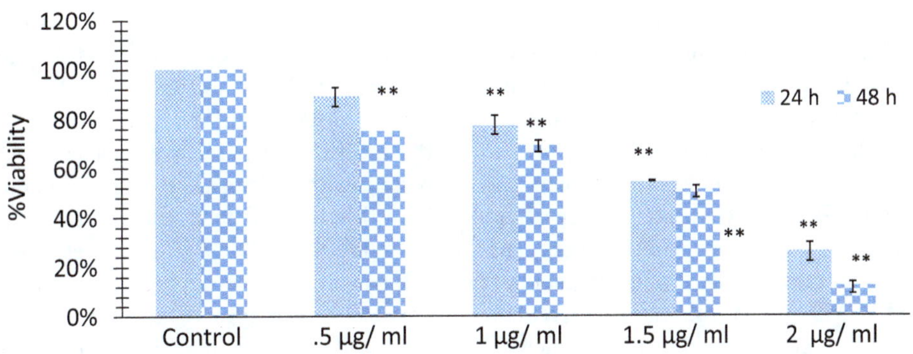

Figure 2. Cytotoxicity of saffron extract.
Saffron extract decreased cell viability dose dependently. Data are indicated as Mean ± SEM; * $P < 0.05$, ** $P < 0.01$.

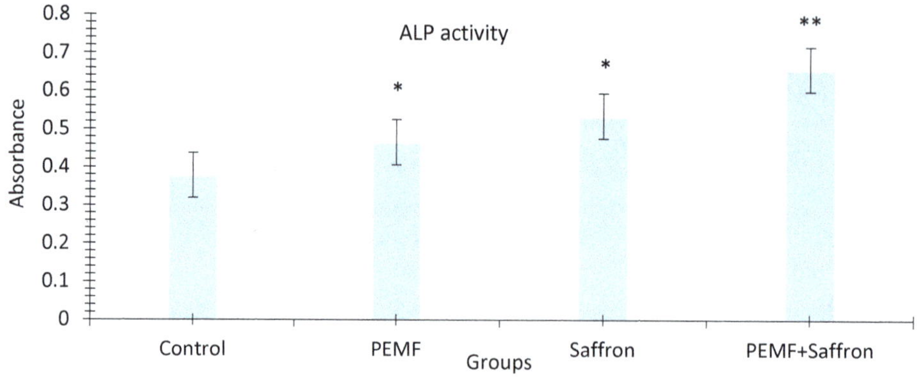

Figure 4. Diagram of the measurement alkaline phosphatase activity in different groups at 10th days, compared to control groups.

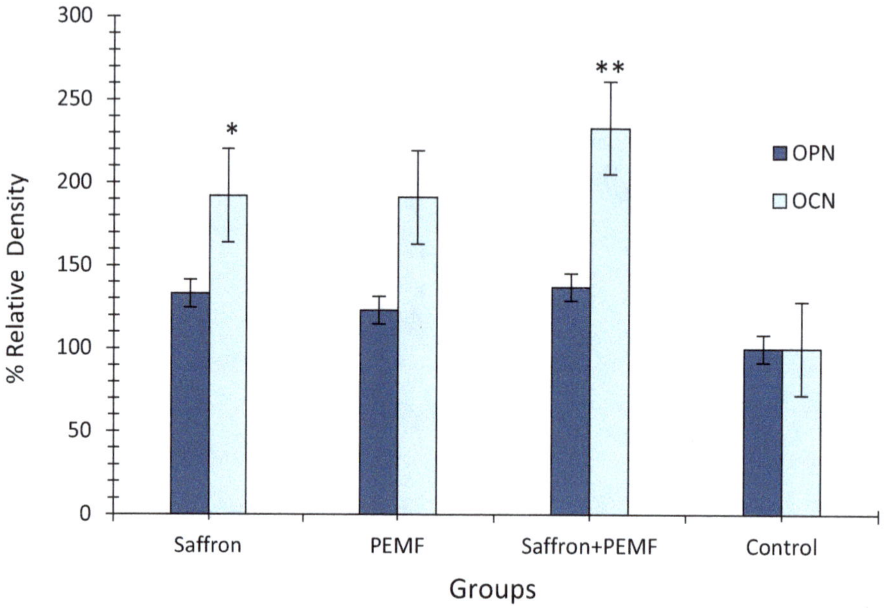

Figure 5. Comparison of osteogenic genes (OPN and OCN) expression on BMSCs treated with saffron extract, PEMF and PEMF plus saffron. The expression of OPN and OCN in the group treated with PEMF and saffron together increased significantly. Data are indicated as Mean ± SEM; * $P < 0.05$, ** $P < 0.01$.

study, differentiation effects of non-invasion PEMF and aqueous extract of saffron on BMSCs was investigated. Differentiation of stem cells was assessed by alizarin red staining, ALP activity and semi quantification RT-PCR. Alizarin red is widely used to detect MSCs differentiation into osteoblast. At the end of the day 14, alizarin red staining was evaluated to detect stem cells differentiation. In another research it was reported that sinusoidal EMF of 15 Hz, 1 mT in promoted osteogenic differentiation of the stem cells (16). Also, in this study, we demonstrated that saffron extract could differentiate BMSCs into osteoblast, however the greatest difference was observed in the groups treated with both saffron extract and PEMF compared to the control group. Once osteoblasts are active, they begin to produce huge amounts of ALP enzyme (14); hence, in this study ALP activity was measured to evaluate osteoblast differentiation and PEMF and saffron extract increased ALP activity. Saffron extract also could stimulate calcium deposition with BMSCs, which was higher in synergic group than the groups treated with either saffron extract or PEMF. Another study reported that PEMF increased ALP activity and mineralized nodule formation, and stimulated osteoblast-specific mRNA expression of RUNX2, ALP, BMP-2, DLX and bone sialoprotein genes (16). These data are consistent with our findings. Osteogenesis involving the mesenchymal cells differentiation happens throughout a multi-step molecular pathway which is regulated by various transcription factors and signaling proteins. The mineralized ECM is mainly composed of type I collagen and considerable amounts of matrix protein, osteopontin, bone sialoprotein, BMPs, TGF-β and the inorganic mineral hydroxylapatite (17). Analysis of bone cell-specific markers like OCN and OPN detection is vastly used to detect osteoblasts differentiation. In this study OCN and OPN genes expression were assessed by comparative semi-quantification RT-PCR. Densitometry analysis revealed that expression of OCN and OPN increased in the treatment groups compared to the control groups. Expression level of OPN was higher than OCN due to the fact that expression of the gene started in earlier stage of osteoblast differentiation. However, considerable up-regulation of OPN gene expression was seen after 14 days of treatment.

Conclusion

The results of this study indicate that saffron extract in combination with PMEF can promote osteogenesis at the initial stage (the commitment of undifferentiated MSCs into osteoblast). This method can be as a new approach in differentiation of stem cells into bone cells.

Acknowledgments

We thank all friends who help us to do this research.

Authors' contributions

JB designed the study, TR and MM did the laboratory works. MAS analyzed the results. All authors read and confirmed the manuscript for publication.

Conflict of interests

The authors declare no competing interests.

Ethical considerations

Ethical issues (including plagiarism, misconduct, data fabrication, falsification, double publication or submission, redundancy) have been completely observed by the authors.

Funding/Support

This research was financially supported by Islamic Azad University, Mashhad, Iran

References

1. Shekkeris AS, Jaiswal PK, Khan WK. Clinical applications of mesenchymal stem cells in the treatment of fracture non-union and bone defects. Curr Stem Cell Res Ther. 2012;7(2):127-33.
2. Potu BK, Bhat KM, Rao MS, et al. Petroleum ether extract of *Cissus quadrangularis* (Linn.) enhances bone marrow mesenchymal stem cell proliferation and facilitates osteoblastogenesis. Clinics (Sao Paulo). 2009;64(10):993-8.
3. Arinzeh TL. Mesenchymal stem cells for bone repair: preclinical studies and potential orthopedic applications. Foot Ankle Clin. 2005;10(4):651-65.
4. Undale AH, Westendorf JJ, Yaszemski MJ, Khosla S. Mesenchymal stem cells for bone repair and metabolic bone diseases. Mayo Clin Proc. 2009;84(10):893-902.
5. Kumar A, Salimath BP, Stark GB, Finkenzeller G. Platelet-derived growth factor receptor signaling is not involved in osteogenic differentiation of human mesenchymal stem cells. Tissue Engineering Part A. 2010;16(3):983-93.
6. Fan JJ, Cao LG, Wu T, et al. The dose-effect of icariin on the proliferation and osteogenic differentiation of human bone mesenchymal stem cells. Molecules. 2011;16(12):10123-33.
7. Ganesan K, Gengadharan AC, Balachandran C, Manohar BM, Puvanakrishnan R. Low frequency pulsed electromagnetic field--a viable alternative therapy for arthritis. Indian J Exp Biol. 2009;47(12):939-48.
8. Qu C, Qin QH, Kang Y. A hypothetical mechanism of bone remodeling and modeling under electromagnetic loads. Biomaterials. 2006;27(21):4050-7.
9. De Mattei M, Gagliano N, Moscheni C, et al. Changes in polyamines, c-myc and c-fos gene expression in osteoblast-like cells exposed to pulsed electromagnetic fields. Bioelectromagnetics. 2005;26(3):207-14.
10. Mayer-Wagner S, Passberger A, Sievers B, Aigner J, Summer B, Schiergens TS, et al. Effects of low frequency electromagnetic fields on the chondrogenic differentiation of human mesenchymal stem cells. Bioelectromagnetics. 2011;32(4):283-90.
11. Hosseinzadeh H, Modaghegh MH, Saffari Z. *Crocus sativus* L. (Saffron) extract and its active constituents (crocin and safranal) on ischemia-reperfusion in rat skeletal muscle. Evid Based Complement Alternat Med. 2009;6(3):343-50.
12. Bhargava V. Medicinal uses and pharmacological properties of *Crocus sativus* Linn (Saffron). Int J Pharm Pharm Sci. 2011;3(3):22-6.
13. Liu H, Xue WJ, Xie YF, Feng XS, Huo FQ. Tea polyphenol-induced neuron-like differentiation of mouse mesenchymal stem cells. Chin J Physiol. 2011;54(2):111-7.
14. Kalfas IH. Principles of bone healing. Neurosurg Focus. 2001;10(4):E1.
15. Cool SM, Nurcombe V. Substrate induction of osteogenesis from marrow-derived mesenchymal precursors. Stem Cells Dev. 2005;14(6):632-42.
16. Yang Y, Tao C, Zhao D, Li F, Zhao W, Wu H. EMF acts on rat bone marrow mesenchymal stem cells to promote differentiation to osteoblasts and to inhibit differentiation to adipocytes. Bioelectromagnetics. 2010;31(4):277-85.
17. Yamaguchi A, Komori T, Suda T. Regulation of osteoblast differentiation mediated by bone morphogenetic proteins, hedgehogs, and Cbfa1. Endocr Rev. 2000;21(4):393-411.

4

The effects of aerobic exercise with lavender essence use on cognitive state and serum brain-derived neurotrophic factor levels in elderly with mild cognitive impairment

Mohammad-Ali Kohanpour[1], Maghsoud Peeri[2*], Mohammad-Ali Azarbayjani[2]

[1]PhD Candidate, Department of Exercise Physiology, Islamic Azad University, Central Tehran Branch, Iran
[2]Professor, Department of Exercise Physiology, Islamic Azad University, Central Tehran Branch, Iran

ARTICLE INFO

Keywords:
Aerobic exercise
Lavender
Cognitive state
Brain-derived neurotrophic factor
Cognitive impairment
Elderly

ABSTRACT

Introduction: The aim of this study was to investigate the effects of 12-week aerobic exercise and lavender essence on cognitive states and brain-derived neurotrophic factor (BDNF) levels of elderly with mild cognitive impairment (MCI).
Methods: In this clinical study, 40 elderly whose scores for mini–mental state examination (MMSE) ranged 21 to 25 were purposively selected by simple sampling. They were randomly divided into 4 equal groups: aerobic exercise, lavender extract, aerobic-lavender. and placebo. They underwent their respective treatments for 12 weeks. The aerobic exercise consisted of 8-minute running session with intensity of 75%-85% HRR Max for the first session. One minute was added to the running span after each 2 sessions. Accordingly, the running span reached 26 minutes at the end of the 12-week exercise period. To conduct treatment with lavender, 2 drops of lavender essence were administered twice a day. Before and after the treatments, cognitive state was measured and blood samples collected to measure BDNF.
Results: BDNF levels of the exercise and exercise + lavender groups increased significantly compared to those of the other 2 groups ($P<0.05$). In addition, the cognitive states of the 3 intervention groups increased significantly compared to that of the placebo group ($P<0.05$).
Conclusion: Combination of 12-week aerobic exercise and lavender may decelerate or probably halt the progressive process of the impairment via improving the cognitive state in elderly with MCI.

Implication for health policy/practice/research/medical education:
Elderly with mild cognitive impairment (MCI) can be helped to improve their cognitive state via practicing aerobic exercise and using lavender.

Introduction

The population of over 60-year-old people of Iran will reach around 10 million up to 2020 and even will exceed 26 million (23% of the whole population) up to 2050 (1). Cognitive impairment is one of the common difficulties of the elderly such that around 35% of the elderly people suffer from various levels of cognitive impairment. Alzheimer disease is the progressive stage of cognitive impairment (2). Paying attention, recalling, orientation, actions, executive function, judgment, and problem solving become difficult due to cognitive impairment. Memory loss is the main cause of cognitive impairment (3). The normal functions of different systems of the brain are required for accurate cognitive performance. Cognitive impairments occur due to aging and depletion of the contributing factors in those systems. Hence, some interventions for progressive deceleration or even reverse of cognitive impairment seem essential.

Using herbs is one of the interventions that has attracted the attention of researchers in the recent years (4). Lavender is a shrub-like perennial plant with a height of about one meter and rectangular-shaped stalks that gradually become woody toward the lower part of the stem. This plant has pointed leaves that are placed on

***Corresponding author:** Maghsoud Peeri, Faculty of Physical Education and Exercise Sciences, Central Tehran Branch of Islamic Azad University, Iran Zamin Blvd., Shahrak-E Gharb, Tehran, Iran.
Email: m.peeri@iauctb.ac.ir

the stems in a bilateral manner. Volatile oil, flavonoids, tannins, coumarins, potassium, and calcium are the most prominent pharmaceutical components of lavender. Lavender is used in pharmaceutical products due to its medicinal properties including tranquilizing, anti-neuralgia, anti-depression, and anti-anxiety activities in the traditional medicine. In addition, its extract can serve as an anti-inflammatory one with inhibitory effects against acetylcholinesterase (AChE) to treat Alzheimer disease (5). However, no research has yet investigated the effects of lavender on elderly with mild cognitive impairment (MCI). Besides that, exercise (as an inexpensive therapeutic approach) can cause optimal effects on cognitive performance through neurotrophic factors (NTFs). Juncture studies have shown that active persons exhibit superior cognitive performance over their inactive peers (6). It has been suggested that use of antioxidants increases the effect of exercise. Measurement of the relevant post-intervention indices of neurological and cognitive states can help understand the effects of exercise and herbal supplements better. Accordingly, brain-derived neurotrophic factor (BDNF(is expressed as a secreted protein, consisting of 247 amino acid and with molecular weight of 27.8 kDa, that plays a role in neurological development, neuronal differentiation, synaptic plasticity, and cell death and exerts its effects inside the cells through 2 protein receptors, i.e. tyrosine kinase and low-affinity nerve growth factor receptor (LNGFR). BDNF has been reported to distribute in different brain regions especially hippocampus, which is responsible for learning and memory (7). To the best of our knowledge, no study has yet been conducted on the effects of lavender on BDNF levels; however, Kim et al reported that treadmill exercise would enhance cognitive performance through increasing the expression of the BDNF and tyrosine kinase B (8). In addition, Cho and Roh found that BDNF levels would significantly increase after aerobic exercise (9). In contrast, Schega et al study demonstrated that 4-week aerobic exercise would lead to enhancement of physical and cognitive performances without any significant increase in BDNF levels (10). Because MCI is one of the common problems of the elderly and is considered to lead ultimately to Alzheimer disease and death, and no definite treatment has yet been offered for Alzheimer disease, it seems essential to conduct preventative interventions that can decelerate, stop, or even reverse the progression of MCI. In addition, it is particularly important to use medicinal plants because of being natural and causing no or few side effects (4). Exercise and physical activity were reported to have definitely confirmed effects in improving cognitive function and neurological system (6).

Since no research has investigated the combination effects of aerobic exercise and lavender essence on cognitive state and BDNF levels in elderly with MCI, this study was conducted to investigate the effects of 12-week aerobic exercise and lavender essence on cognitive states and BDNF levels of elderly with MCI.

Materials and Methods

This clinical study was conducted with pretest and post-test on 4 groups of the elderly people. After we informed the societies of the elders of Shiraz about the purposes of the current study, 61 men aged 60-70 years volunteered to participate in this study. Then, the cognitive states of the participants were examined by using the mini–mental state examination (MMSE). The MMSE was developed by Folstein et al in 1975 and consists of 11 domains, including orientations to time and place, registration, attention and calculation, recall, language, ability to follow simple command, reading, writing, and ability to do delicate complex commands (11). The total score for the MMSE is 30 that represents absence of any problem in the above mentioned domains. Scores under 20 indicate severe (scores ≤9) and moderate (scores 10-19) cognitive impairment and scores 20-25 represent MCI. The consistency coefficient of the MMSE has been reported 0.87 by Cronbach α coefficient. In addition, its sensitivity and specificity were derived 90% and 84%, respectively (12). Forty people whose scores ranged from 21 to 25 were selected as the subjects. The participants' mean age was 67.85 ± 3.89 years, mean height 174.6 ± 6.007 cm, mean weight 78.30 ± 5.18 kg, and mean body mass index (BMI) 25.69 ± 0.54 kg/m^2. They were randomly divided into 4 groups: aerobic exercise, lavender, aerobic exercise + lavender, and placebo. The inclusion criteria were being male and over 60 years old, having sufficient general health to conduct aerobic exercise according to examinations conducted by a physician, attending at least 90% of the intervention sessions, attaining scores 21-25 for the MMSE, attaining scores under 10 for the Geriatric Depression Scale (GDS), and not being under treatment for cognitive impairments; the exclusion criteria were not attending more than 10% of the intervention sessions, being dependent on others in daily activities, suffering from other physical or mental illnesses, taking medication, being under treatment for cognitive impairments, and withdrawing from continuing participation in the study. The length of the interventions was determined to be 12 weeks. To prepare lavender essence, newly sprouted branches and flowers of this plant were used. The essence collection was conducted by distillation in Barij Essence Pharmaceutical Co. (Kashan, Iran). The essence was administrated at daily dose of 2 drops twice a day. The placebo was made by pharmacist at a concentration of 1/10 000 such that it did not possess any therapeutic effect. The 12-week aerobic exercise consisted of 3 weekly sessions. The first exercise session included 8-minute warm-up and 8-minute running with intensity of 75%-85% of HRR Max, and 5-minute cool down. After each 2 successive sessions, one minute was added to the very later session. Therefore, the running span reached 26 minutes at the end of the 12-week exercise period. Five milliliters blood samples were taken from the brachial vein of the subjects (as they were fasted for 12 hours) both 24 hours before and 48 hours after the interventions. In addition, the cognitive states of the subjects were examined by the MMSE. In order to isolate the blood serum, after coagulation, the samples were centrifuged at 2000 rpm for 10 minutes. The isolated serum samples were stored at -20°C until later use. The serum level of BDNF was gauged by Human BDNF PicoKine™ ELISA kit (Boster Biological Technology, China). Data were described by mean and standard deviation (SD). In order to compare variations in the variables, mixed analysis of variance (ANOVA) (within-subject and inter-subject) was conducted with Bonferroni post hoc correction at significance level of 0.05. Data analysis was conducted by SPSS 16.

Results

The results of descriptive statistics, mixed ANOVA (intra-subject and inter-subject), and Bonferroni post-hoc test are shown in Tables 1-3, respectively.

Statistically significant differences in weight variation, BMI, BDNF, and cognitive state were observed among the 4 groups ($P=0.001$). Differences in weight, BMI, and BDNF were significant between the exercise group and the lavender and placebo groups ($P<0.05$). In addition, differences in weight, BMI, and BDNF were significant between the exercise + lavender group and the lavender and placebo groups ($P<0.05$). In addition, differences in weight, BMI, and BDNF were not statistically significant between the exercise group and the exercise + lavender group ($P>0.05$). In addition, the differences in weight, BMI, and BDNF were not statistically significant between the lavender group and the placebo group ($P>0.05$). All differences in cognitive states between exercise + lavender and placebo groups, exercise and placebo groups, and lavender and placebo groups were statistically significant ($P=0.001$, 0.001, and 0.004, respectively). However, there were not any significant differences in cognitive state among the 3 intervention groups ($P>0.05$).

Discussion

In the current study, 12-week aerobic exercise, either alone or combined with lavender essence, led to significant increase in cognitive state and serum BDNF level in elderly with MCI. In addition, lavender essence usage led to significant enhancement of cognitive state. Although lavender use increased BDNF levels, such increment was not statistically significant. No significant difference was observed in cognitive state among the 3 intervention groups; however, variations in the BDNF levels of the 2 exercise groups were significantly higher than the corresponding changes in other 2 groups. Although adding lavender essence to aerobic exercise increased cognitive state score and BDNF level to some extent, these enhancements were not statistically significant. Perhaps, a longer-term intervention may lead to a significant interaction effect between the 2 interventions. As far as we searched, we found no study on the effect of lavender on cognitive state and serum BDNF levels. Lavender may help improve the cognitive state through other mechanisms.

Table 1. The mean (standard deviation) value of variables before and after intervention

Variables	Group	Before	After
Weight (kg)	Training + lavender	78.70±5.59	75.90±5.95
	Training	75.60±3.83	77.50±3.62
	Lavender	76.60±4.37	76.60±3.94
	Placebo	80.40±6.61	80.40±6.39
BMI (kg/m^2)	Training + lavender	25.50±0.44	24.58±0.48
	Training	25.74±0.42	25.11±0.58
	Lavender	25.62±0.62	25.63±0.50
	Placebo	25.90±0.63	25.93±0.80
BDNF (pg/mL)	Training + lavender	108.82±32.88	179.81±62.69
	Training	110.25±28.61	192.84±59.51
	Lavender	118.22±30.68	138.15±29.62
	Placebo	110.75±26.07	111.09±24.19
Cognitive state (MMSE)	Training + lavender	22.50±1.35	24.90±0.87
	Training	22.70±1.63	24.40±1.42
	Lavender	22.80±1.75	24.30±1.05
	Placebo	24.30±0.94	24.20±0.63

Abbreviations: BMI, Body mass index; BDNF, Brain-derived neutrophic factor; MMSE, mini–mental state examination.

Table 2. The results of mixed intra-subject and inter-subject ANOVA (time interaction in group)

Variables	*F* value	*P* value	Effect Magnitude
Weight	21.88	0.001*	0.64
BMI	20.33	0.001*	0.63
BDNF	9.94	0.001*	0.45
Cognitive state	11.85	0.001*	0.49

Abbreviations: BMI, Body mass index; BDNF, Brain-derived neutrophic factor.
*Significant at 0.05.

Table 3. Results of Bonferroni post hoc test to determine location of the significant difference

Pairwise Comparison	Weight	BMI	BDNF	Cognitive state
Training + Lavender/ Training	0.24	0.36	1	0.69
Training + Lavender/ Lavender	0.001*	0.001*	0.04*	0.27
Training + Lavender/ Placebo	0.001*	0.001*	0.002*	0.001*
Training/Lavender	0.001*	0.001*	0.007*	1
Training/Placebo	0.001*	0.001*	0.001*	0.001*
Lavender/Placebo	1	1	1	0.004*

Abbreviations: BMI, Body mass index; BDNF, Brain-derived neutrophic factor.
*Significant at 0.05.

Previous studies have shown the anti-inflammatory effect of lavender, which was attributed to the inhibitory effects of lavender on AChE (5). It has been confirmed the high level of AChE activity, and therefore reduction in acetylcholine (Ach) level and neurotransmission QWL can lead to Alzheimer disease and the loss of spatial memory (13). Cho and Roh reported consistent results with those of the present study regarding the effect of exercise on cognitive state and BDNF levels (9). In addition, Zembron-Lacny et al showed that the BDNF levels of active persons were higher than those of inactive ones (14). Different intensities of exercise are a prominent parameter to explain variations in various studies (15). It has been reported that serum BDNF level does not exhibit any significant increment after low-intensity (20% below VT1) exercise; however, BDNF level increased after 30-minute high-intensity (10% above VT1) exercise (15). Exercise increases BDNF level, which leads to generating more neurons in the brain, and consequently causes improvements in learning and memory (16). The enhancement of serum BDNF level is effective on the presynaptic and postsynaptic terminals through the TrkB receptor, which leads to regulating signaling transmission pathways, e.g. mitogen-activated protein kinase 1 and MAP kinase-activated protein kinase 2, at the presynaptic and postsynaptic terminals (17). In this regard, Miller et al reported the existence of a significant correlation between cognitive state and exercise (18). This correlation can be taken into account to explain decreases in oxidative stress and inflammation, enhancement of angiogenesis, secretions of neurotrophins and catecholamines, and neurogenesis especially in hippocampus anatomy (19). To the best of our knowledge, no study has yet been conducted on the combination effect of lavender use and aerobic exercise on cognitive state and BDNF levels; it is therefore difficult to interpret the findings of the current study with reference to other studies' findings. The effects of aerobic exercise alone and lavender alone on cognitive state were significant yet without any significant difference from their combination effect on cognitive state. However, the combination of lavender and aerobic exercise caused a slightly more marked effect compared to those caused by either of them. It is therefore necessary to conduct studies with larger number of subjects and longer-term interventions. In addition, because the BDNF levels increased significantly in both groups undergoing aerobic exercise but not in the group administered with lavender alone, other mechanisms are likely to play a role in the lavender-associated improvement of the cognitive states of the elderly with MCI. To argue for BDNF role in lavender-associated variations in cognitive state more definitely, we need to perform studies with larger sample size.

Conclusion

Combination of aerobic exercise and lavender essence may decelerate or probably halt the progressive process of the impairment in elderly with MCI through improving cognitive state. Aerobic exercise may cause such changes through BDNF mediation. However, lavender extract use did not lead to any significant increase in BDNF. Therefore, other mediators are likely to be involved in the improvement of cognitive state. This issue should be addressed in future studies. This study was first to investigate the combination effect of lavender and exercise. Although the effect of aerobic exercise combined with lavender increased the effects of either alone, this increase was not significant compared to that caused by either of the interventions alone. It is therefore necessary to conduct studies with larger number of subjects and longer-term interventions.

Acknowledgements

This research was derived from Mohammad-Ali Kohanpur doctoral thesis on exercise physiology. We gratefully thank the Research Office of the Islamic Azad University (Central Tehran Branch) for its priceless supports. At last but not least, the authors thank the people who kindly participated in this study.

Authors' contributions

All authors contributed to the study. MAK contributed to data collection and manuscript drafting and MAA made necessary corrections to the method especially data analysis. All read and confirmed the publication of the manuscript.

Conflict of interests

The authors declared no competing interests.

Ethical considerations

Ethical issues (including plagiarism, misconduct,

data fabrication, falsification, double publication or submission, redundancy) have been completely observed by the authors.

Funding/Support

This research was funded by the Islamic Azad University, Central Tehran Branch, Iran.

References

1. Sharif-zadeh QR, Moudi M, Akhbari H. Health situation of elderly supported by Imam Khomeini charity. Iran Elderly Mag. 2010;5(17):52-60.
2. Sohrabi MB, Zolfaghari P, Mahdizade F, et al. Evaluation and comparison of cognitive state and depression in elderly admitted in sanitarium with elderly sited in personal home. Knowledge & Health. 2008;3 (2):27. [Persian].
3. Torpy JM, Lynm C, Glass RM. JAMA patient page. Dementia. JAMA. 2010;304(17):972.
4. Karamian R, Mohammadian A, Hassanimoghadam E, et al. Identification and comparison of the yield and composition of essential oil constituents of 4 Eucalyptus species adapted to the climatic conditions of Khorramabad. J Herbmed Pharmacol. 2015;4(1):25-28.
5. Adsersen A, Minna A, Korolainen E, et al. Screening of plants used in Danish folk medicine to treat memory dysfunction for acetylcholiesterase inhibitory activity. J Ethnopharmacol. 2006;104:418-22.
6. Hillman CH, Motl RW, Pontifex MB, et al. Physical activity and cognitive function in a cross-section of younger and older community-dwelling individuals. Health Psychol. 2006;25:678-87.
7. Kuipers SD, Bramham CR. Brainderived neurotrophic factor mechanisms and function in adult synaptic plasticity:New insights and implications for therapy. Curr Opin Drug Discov Devel. 2006;9(5):580-586.
8. Kim TW, Choi HH, Chung YR. Treadmill exercise alleviates impairment of cognitive function by enhancing hippocampal neuroplasticity in the high-fat diet-induced obese mice. J Exerc Rehabil. 2016;12(3):156-62.
9. Cho SY, Roh HT. Effects of aerobic exercise training on peripheral brain-derived neurotrophic factor and eotaxin-1 levels in obese young men. J Phys Ther Sci. 2016;28 (4):1355-8.
10. Schega L, Peter B, Brigadski T, et al. Effect of intermittent normobaric hypoxia on aerobic capacity and cognitive function in older people. J Sci Med Sport. 2016;19(11):941-945.
11. Nillson J, Parker MG, Kabir ZN. Assessing health-related quality of life among older people in Rural Bangladesh. J Trans Cult Nurs. 2004;15(4):298-307.
12. Frooghian M, Jafari Z, Shirinbaiani P, et al. Standardization of brief examination of cognitive status of elderly in Tehran. Advanced Cognitive Science Journal. 2008;10 (2):29-37.
13. Kiyofumi Yamada TN. Animal models of Alzheimer's disease and evaluation of anti-dementia drugs. Pharmacol Ther. 2000;88:93-113.
14. Zembron-Lacny A, Dziubek W, Rynkiewicz M, et al. Peripheral brain-derived neurotrophic factor is related to cardiovascular risk factors in active and inactive elderly men. Braz J Med Biol Res. 2016;49(7). pii: S0100-879X2016000700603
15. Pour-Nemati P. Investigation of effects of two resistance and endurance trainings schedules on BDNF cortisol, IGF-I, IGFBP-3 on young male rats [PhD thesis]. Tehran: University of Tehran; 2012.
16. Goekint M, De Pauw K, Roelands B, et al. Strength training does not influence serum brain-derived neurotrophic factor. Eur J Appl Physiol. 2010;110(2):285-93.
17. Molteni R, Barnard RJ, Ying Z, et al. A high-fat, refined sugar diet reduces hippocampal brain-derived neurotrophic factor, neuronal plasticity, and learning. Neuroscience. 2002;112:803-14.
18. Miller I, Vanessa T, Patrick SR, et al. measuring the impact of exercise on cognitive aging:methodological issues. Neurobiol Aging. 2012;33:622-9.
19. Adlard PA, Perreau VM, Pop V, et al. Voluntary exercise decreases amyloid load in a transgenic model of Alzheimer's disease. J Neurosci. 2005;25:4217-21.

Phytochemical screening and antipyretic activities of dichloromethane-methanolic leaf and stem bark extracts of *Ximenia americana* in rat models

Daniel M. Gaichu*, **Amos M. Mawia, Godfrey M. Gitonga, Mathew P. Ngugi, David N. Mburu**

Department of Biochemistry and Biotechnology, School of Pure and Applied Sciences, Kenyatta University, P.O. Box 43844-00100, Nairobi, Kenya

ARTICLE INFO

Keywords:
Ximenia americana
DCM-MeOH
Antipyretic
Rectal temperature
Aspirin
Turpentine

ABSTRACT

Introduction: In most parts of Africa, *Ximenia americana* is used in folklore to treat various disorders such as oedema, pain, fever, helminthiasis, diarrhoea, burns among other diseases. This study tested the antipyretic activities of dichloromethane-methanolic (DCM-MeOH) stem bark and leaf extracts of *X. americana* in rats. Qualitative phytochemical screening was also done to evaluate the presence of alkaloids, flavonoids, steroids, saponins, cardiac glycosides, phenolics and terpenoids in the extract.
Methods: The plant materials were collected from Mbeere North sub-county, Embu county, Kenya. Methanol and dichloromethane in the ratio of 1:1 was used to extract the active compounds. Two to three months old male Wister rats were employed for the antipyretic studies. Animals were divided into six groups of five rats each: normal, negative, reference and three experimental groups (50, 100 and 150 mg/kg body weight). Pyrexia was induced experimentally using turpentine. The experimental groups were treated with predetermined dose quantities of prepared extracts. Aspirin was used as the reference drug. Data were analyzed using one-way analysis of variance (ANOVA).
Results: The extracts from the leaves lowered rectal temperature by 0.45% to 2.11% while the stem bark extracts lowered rectal temperature in the range of 0.71% to 2.13%. Aspirin lowered the rectal temperature in the range of 0.74% and 1.67%. Qualitative phytochemical screening showed presence of alkaloids, flavonoids, saponins, cardiac glycosides, phenolics and terpenoids in the extract.
Conclusion: DCM-MeOH leaf and stem bark extracts of *X. americana* is effective in management of fever and therefore it can be explored as a possible bio-resource in the development of herbal antipyretic medicines.

Implication for health policy/practice/research/medical education:
This study confirms the antipyretic potential of the leaf and stem bark of DCM-MeOH extracts of *X. americana* in experimental animals. Therefore, the DCM-MeOH leaf and stem bark extracts of *X. americana* might prove useful in managing pyrexia and thus serve as an alternative treatment bioresource.

Introduction

Conventional treatment of fever by synthetic drugs may cause side-effects and may not be universally affordable. Therefore, use of herbal medicines is more attractive in treatment because it is generally affordable, closely conforms to patient's ideology, arguably more tolerable than synthetic drugs and satisfies desire for more personalized healthcare (1).

***Corresponding author:** Gaichu Daniel Muthee,
Email: danielgaichu2016@gmail.com

Aqueous extracts of *Ximenia americana* have been traditionally used in fever management. However, there is no documented evidence on activities of organic extracts of *X. americana*. This study scientifically evaluated and provided preliminary information on organic leaf and stem bark extracts of *X. americana* as an alternative, arguably affordable and with less side effects in fever management. The study also tries to reveal the gaps for further research.

Fever is defined as elevation of the body temperature

above the normal range due to an increase in temperature regulatory set-point (2). It is caused by prostaglandin E_2 which is synthesized from arachidonic acid by the action of cyclooxygenase (COX) enzymes (3). Fever is part of acute-phase response to inflammatory response or an infection (4). it is induced by a class of inflammatory mediators known as cytokines. Examples of such cytokines are interleukin-1, interleukin-6 and tumor necrosis factor-α (TNFα) (5).

Turpentine induces fever in laboratory animals by increasing prostaglandins synthesis (6). This fever is better tolerated by animals than that induced by other exogenous pyrogens. Hence, turpentine was selected to be used in current study as a pyrogen (7).

Since pyrexia is a product of prostaglandins of the E series activities (8), blockade of prostaglandin E_2 synthesis helps alleviate fever. The synthesis of prostaglandin E_2 occurs in three steps: synthesis of arachidonic acid from cell membrane phospholipids, a process mediated by phospholipase A_2; synthesis of prostaglandin H_2 from arachidonic acid, a step catalyzed by COX and the last step is isomerization of prostaglandin H_2 into prostaglandin E_2 by the action of terminal prostaglandin E synthase (9). COX enzymes exist in two isoforms. The first is constitutive isoform, referred to as COX-1. COX-1 has clear physiologic functions. The second is inducible isoform, referred to as COX-2 (10). The non-steroidal anti-inflammatory drugs exert anti-inflammatory activities through COX-2 inhibition. The inhibition of COX-1 causes side-effects, such as erosion of gastric mucosa (10). The side effects associated with such synthetic drugs can be avoided by use of reliable naturally occurring agents which are effective with minimal side effects (11).

Medicinal plants are either directly or indirectly used. They are directly used as home remedies or indirectly in development of conventional drugs (12). Traditionally, *X. americana* is used in the treatment of a variety of disorders such as: pain, fever and inflammation (13,14), treatment of helminthiasis (15), diarrhea, wounds (16), headaches, skin ulcers, kidney and heart problems (17). Mbeere community (a community living upper eastern Kenya) use pounded stem bark and raw leaves of *X. americana* to treat stomach discomforts, fever, oedema, and pain. Despite the broad folklore use of *X. americana*, there is no scientific evaluation of its organic extracts. The current study was designed against this background to specifically bioscreen dichloromethane-methanolic (DCM-MeOH) stem bark and leaf extracts of *X. americana* for antipyretic potential.

Materials and Methods

Collection and preparation of plant samples

Leaves and stem barks of *X. americana* were collected with the help of local traditional herbalists from Mbeere-North in Embu county, Kenya. The plant materials were properly sorted, cleaned and packed in polythene bags and transported to Biochemistry and Biotechnology laboratories of Kenyatta University for further processing. The botanical authentication of the materials was done by a qualified taxonomist and the voucher specimen deposited in Kenyatta University Herbarium. The plant materials chopped, completely air dried at room temperature followed by grinding into fine homogenous powder with an electric mill and then sieved through mesh sieve.

Extraction

For each sample, 200 g of the powder was soaked in cold 1:1 mixture of methanol and DCM and stirred for six hours to extract the active compounds. This was followed by successive filtering of the extracts and the filtrate concentrated under reduced pressure and vacuum using rotary evaporator (Buchii R110). The concentrate was stored in airtight containers at -4°C before use in the bioassay studies (18).

Laboratory animals

Male Wister rats, *Rattus norvegicus,* aged 2-3 months and weighing between 140-180 g were used (19). The animals were acquired and bred at the animal breeding and experimentation laboratory in Kenyatta University, Department of Biochemistry and Biotechnology. The animals were kept in standard cages, under the conditions of a standard laboratory (ambient temperature of 25°C and 12-hour light followed by 12 hour dark cycle) throughout the experiments. The feeding was on standard pellets for rodents and water was supplied *ad libitum* (20). Throughout the study, all ethical guidelines and procedures on animal handling were followed (21).

Determination of antipyretic activities

The experimental animals (30 male Wistar albino rats) were divided into 6 groups of five rats each and treated as shown in the table (Table 1).

The digital thermometer was calibrated against mercury thermometer. The rectal temperature was recorded by inserting about 3 cm of the thermistor probe of the thermometer (model YB-009) into the rectum. The probe was well lubricated (22). For fever induction, turpentine 20% at a dose of 20 mL/kg body weight was injected intraperitoneally after recording of the initial basal rectal temperature. The animals were left for one hour. The fever magnitude response after one hour of intraperitoneal turpentine injection was defined as 100% fever response. The animals that recorded 0.8°C raise in rectal temperature were con-

Table 1. Treatment protocol for evaluation of antipyretic activities of DCM-MeOH leaf and stem bark extracts *Ximenia americana* in rats

Group	Status	Treatment
I	Normal control	DMSO
II	Negative control	Turpentine (20%) + DMSO (10%)
III	Positive control	Turpentine (20%) +100 mg/kg aspirin
IV	Experimental group A	Turpentine (20%) +50 mg/kg extract
V	Experimental group B	Turpentine (20%) +100 mg/kg extract
VI	Experimental group C	Turpentine (20%) +150 mg/kg extract

DMSO was used as a vehicle.

sidered pyretic and were employed in the study.
The rectal temperature was recorded at an hourly interval for four hours. The calculation of rectal temperature percentage change was done by comparing temperature before and after treatment as per the formulae below (23,24):

$$\frac{B-Cn}{B}\times 100$$

B: Temperature of the rectum, 1 hour after turpentine administration
C_n: Rectal temperature after drug administration.

Qualitative phytochemical screening
Qualitative phytochemical screening was done on the extracts by established methods to find out whether selected phytochemicals were present (25,26). The secondary metabolites tested were: alkaloids, tannins, steroids, saponins, cardiac glycosides, phenolics and terpenoids.

Management and statistical analysis of the data
The data on rectal temperature changes were recorded and tabulated in a spread sheet. The data was then imported to Minitab statistical software version 17 for descriptive statistical analysis. The results expressed as mean ± standard error of mean for analysis. One-way analysis of variance (ANOVA) was performed to compare the group means followed by Tukey's post hoc test for pair-wise mean separations and comparisons to obtain the specific significant differences among the different groups. Un-paired student *t* test was used to compare mean antipyretic activities between leaf and stem bark extracts of *X. americana*.
The statistical significance was considered at $P \leq 0.05$. The data on the percentage change in rectal temperature was presented using graphs.

Results

Antipyretic activity of DCM-MeOH leaf extract of *Ximenia americana* in rats
The DCM-MeOH leaf extracts of *X. americana* reduced rectal temperatures of turpentine-induced pyrexia in rats (Table 2; Figure 1).
The leaf extract of *X. americana* at three dose levels (50, 100 and 150 mg/kg body weight), reduced the elevated rectal temperatures by 0.98%, 0.93% and 1.27%, respectively, after one hour of the treatment (Figure 1). At all dose levels, antipyretic activities of the extract were significant in comparison to the normal and negative control groups ($P < 0.05$; Table 2) but there was no significant difference when compared to the positive group ($P > 0.05$, Table 2).
The DCM-MeOH leaf extract of *X. americana* at three dose levels (50, 100 and 150 mg/kg body weight) caused a reduction in elevated rectal temperature by 1.37%, 1.56% and 1.76%, respectively after the second hour of the treatment (Figure 1). The antipyretic effectiveness of the extracts was statistically significant compared to the normal and negative control groups ($P < 0.05$; Table 2), although there was no statistical significance when compared to positive group ($P > 0.05$, Table 2).
The leaf extract of *X. americana* at the three dose levels (50, 100 and 150 mg/kg body weight) was found to lower the elevated temperature by 0.9%, 1.45% and 2.05%, respectively in the third hour (Figure 1). After three hours, the antipyretic activities of the rats treated with 100 and 150 mg/kg body weight of the extract was comparable to the reference group ($P > 0.05$; Table 2.). At all dose levels

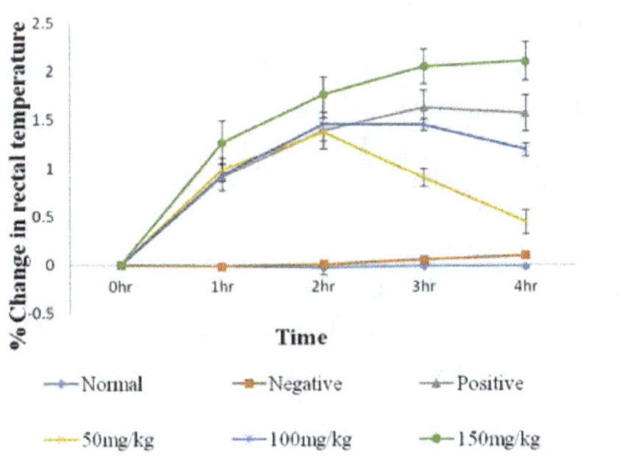

Figure 1. The change in percentage of rectal temperature caused by DCM-MeOH leaf extract of *Ximenia americana* on turpentine-induced pyretic rats

Table 2. Effects of intraperitoneal administration of DCM-MeOH leaf extract of *Ximenia americana* on turpentine induced pyrexia in rats

Group	Treatment	Percent change in rectal temperature (°C) after drug administration				
		0 h	1 h	2 h	3 h	4 h
Normal control	DMSO	100±0.00	100.01 ± 0.02^{a}	100.03 ± 0.07^{a}	100.02 ± 0.01^{a}	100.02 ± 0.01^{a}
Negative control	Turpentine	100±0.00	100.02 ± 0.02^{a}	99.995 ± 0.02^{a}	99.947 ± 0.01^{a}	99.900 ± 0.02^{a}
Positive control	Turpentine + aspirin (100 mg/kg b.w)	100±0.00	99.089 ± 0.14^{b}	98.610 ± 0.19^{b}	98.373 ± 0.18^{cd}	98.431 ± 0.19^{bc}
DCM: methanolic Leaf extract	Turpentine + 50 mg/kg	100±0.00	99.018 ± 0.12^{b}	98.626 ± 0.09^{b}	99.098 ± 0.09^{b}	99.554 ± 0.12^{a}
	Turpentine + 100 mg/kg	100±0.00	99.071 ± 0.04^{b}	98.544 ± 0.06^{b}	98.549 ± 0.06^{c}	98.808 ± 0.07^{b}
	Turpentine + 150 mg/kg	100±0.00	98.734 ± 0.23^{b}	98.239 ± 0.18^{b}	97.950 ± 0.18^{d}	97.892 ± 0.20^{c}

Values are expressed as mean ± SEM for five animals per group. Statistical comparison were made within a column and values with the same superscript are not significantly different by one-way ANOVA followed by Tukey's post hoc test ($P > 0.05$). Turpentine = 20%; DMSO = 10%;

of the extract, the antipyretic activities were significant in comparison to the normal group and the negative group ($P < 0.05$; Table 2).

The three dose levels of the leaf extract (50, 100 and 150 mg/kg body weight) were found to reduce pyrexia by 0.45%, 1.19% and 2.11%, respectively after the fourth hour (Figure 1). With the aspirin as standard drug, the antipyretic activity of the extract was comparable to the positive control at the dosages of 100 and 150 mg/kg body weight ($P > 0.05$; Table 2). There was significance in comparison to the negative group and normal group ($P < 0.05$; Table 2.). The dose level of 50 mg/kg body showed no significant difference from the negative group and the normal group ($P > 0.05$; Table 2).

Antipyretic activity of DCM-MeOH stem bark extract of *Ximenia americana* in rats

The DCM-MeOH stem bark extract of *X. americana* showed similar antipyretic activities (Table 3; Figure 2). The dichloromethane-MeOH stem bark extract of *X. americana* at three dose levels (50, 100 and 150 mg/kg body weight) decreased the elevated rectal temperature by 0.91%, 0.71% and 0.88%, respectively, after one hour of the treatment while aspirin reduced rectal temperature by 0.74% (Figure 2). At the three dose levels, the activity of the extracts was similar to that of aspirin ($P > 0.05$; Table 3). At the dose of 100 mg/kg body weight, the activity was not significantly different from the normal control group ($P > 0.05$; Table 3). This was as opposed to the dose levels of 50 and 150 mg/kg body weight of the extract that was significantly different from negative group and the normal group ($P < 0.05$; Table 3).

The dichloromethane-MeOH stem bark extract of *X. americana* at the dose levels of 50, 100 and 150 mg/kg body weight decreased the rats' elevated rectal temperature by 1.49%, 1.54% and 1.87%, respectively after the second hour of the treatment in a dose dependent manner (Figure 2). These effects were similar to that of aspirin ($P > 0.05$; Table 3).

Ximenia americana stem bark extract at the three dosages (50, 100 and 150) in mg/kg body weight, was found to reduce the elevated rectal temperature by 1.44%, 1.50% and 2.13% respectively in the third hour (Figure 2). The antipyretic activities at the three dose levels were not significant in comparison to positive group ($P > 0.05$; Table 3).

All the three dose levels (50, 100 and 150 mg/kg body weight), were found to reduce fever by 1.28%, 1.28% and 2.02%, respectively after the fourth hour (Figure 2). The antipyretic activities had no statistically significant difference from the positive group ($P > 0.05$; Table 3).

Comparison between the antipyretic activities of leaf and stem bark extract of *Ximenia americana*

In comparison, there was no significant difference in the antipyretic activities at the three dose levels (50, 100 and 150 mg/kg body weight), at the various test hour period of leaf and stem bark extract of *X. americana* (Figure 3). During the 4 hours of the test period, the level of significance was as follows: at the dosage of 50 mg/kg body weight ($P = 0.872$, 0.821, 0.307 and 0.176 respectively), at 100 mg/kg body weight ($P = 0.084$, 0.549, 0.769 and 0.501 respectively) and at 150 mg/kg body weight ($P = 0.205$, 0.608, 0.768 and 0.747 respectively).

Qualitative phytochemical screening

The qualitative phytochemical screening of DCM-MeOH leaf and stem bark extracts of *X. americana* showed the presence of alkaloids, cardiac glycosides, flavonoids, phenolics, saponins and terpenoids. However, alkaloids

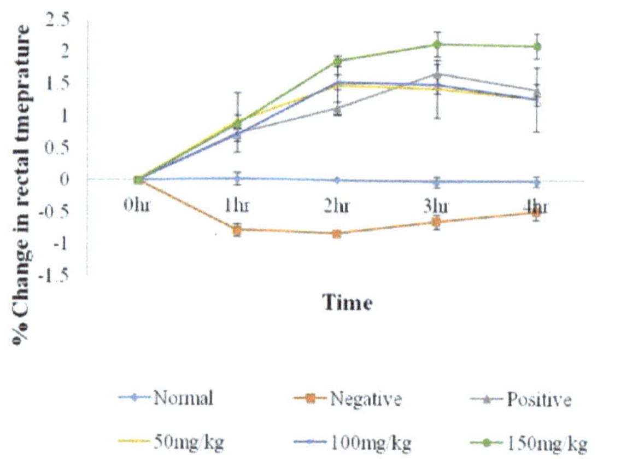

Figure 2. The change in percentage of rectal temperature caused by DCM-MeOH stem bark extract of *Ximenia* americana on turpentine-induced pyretic rats.

Table 3. Effects of intraperitoneal administration of DCM-MeOH stem bark extracts of *Ximenia americana* on turpentine-induced pyrexia in rats

Group	Treatment	Percent change in rectal temperature (°C) after drug administration				
		0 h	1 h	2 h	3 h	4 h
Normal control	DMSO	100±0.00	99.973 ± 0.09^{ab}	99.995 ± 0.01^{a}	100.02 ± 0.09^{a}	100.01 ± 0.09^{a}
Negative control	Turpentine + DMSO	100±0.00	100.77 ± 0.09^{a}	100.82 ± 0.06^{a}	100.64 ± 0.11^{a}	100.48 ± 0.13^{a}
Positive control	Turpentine + DMSO + aspirin	100±0.00	99.261 ± 0.08^{bc}	98.865 ± 0.09^{b}	98.329 ± 0.16^{b}	98.575 ± 0.09^{b}
DCM: Methanolic stem bark extracts	Turpentine + 50 mg/kg	100±0.00	99.088 ± 0.39^{c}	98.510± 0.47^{b}	98.562 ± 0.45^{b}	98.721 ± 0.49^{b}
	Turpentine + 100 mg/kg	100±0.00	99.288 ± 0.09^{bc}	98.459 ± 0.12^{b}	98.502 ± 0.14^{b}	98.723 ± 0.09^{b}
	Turpentine + 150 mg/kg	100±0.00	99.118 ± 0.15^{c}	98.131 ± 0.08^{b}	97.869 ± 0.19^{b}	97.984 ± 0.19^{b}

Values are expressed as Mean ± SEM for five animals per group. Statistical comparison were made within a column and values with the same superscript are not significantly different by one-way ANOVA followed by Tukey's post hoc test ($P > 0.05$). Turpentine = 20%; DMSO = 10%; Aspirin = 100 mg/kg.

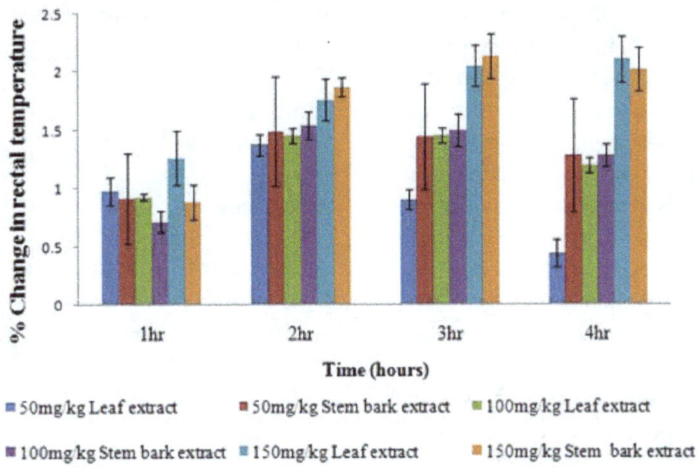

Figure 3. The percentage change comparison of rectal temperature caused by DCM-MeOH leaf and stem bark extracts of *Ximenia americana* on turpentine-induced pyrexia in rats.

and terpenoids were absent in the leaf extract of the *X. americana* while the steroids were absent in both leaf and stem bark extracts (Table 4).

Discussion

The present study was designed to evaluate the antipyretic activities of DCM-MeOH leaf and stem bark extracts of *X. americana* in rat models.

Pyrexia in rats was used to evaluate the antipyretic activity of steam distilled turpentine. Examples of other exogenous pyrogens which are used in fever induction in laboratory animals are: LPS, brewer's yeast, polyinosinic polycytidylic acid (poly I: C) and muramyl dipeptide (27,28).

Turpentine is injected intraperitoneally into the laboratory animals to induce fever. The turpentine-induced fever is through increase in prostaglandins synthesis (6). Different phytochemicals found in *X. americana* reduce fever by inhibition of these prostaglandins. Turpentine-induced fever is tolerated by the animals better than that induced by other exogenous pyrogens (7) and it is for this reason it was chosen for this study.

As shown in Tables 2 and 3, there was significant antipyretic activity in pyretic rats that was associated with administration of DCM-MeOH leaf and stem bark extracts of *X. americana*. The findings were consistent with other studies performed on some other herbal extracts in experimental animals. The aqueous stem bark extract of *X. americana* and its fractions showed the antipyretic properties (29). The study performed on *Solanum incanum* roots extract confirmed that there was antipyretic effect associated with the extract on pyrexia induced with lipopolysaccharide in male Wistar rats (30). Nonsteroidal anti-inflammatory drugs inhibit COX-2 expression and thus inhibiting PGE_2 biosynthesis leading to the reduction in elevated body temperature (31). The antipyretic activity of many antipyretic drugs is achieved through inhibition of COX-2 and the reduction of PGE_2 levels within the hypothalamus (32). Inhibitors of COX-2 are potent antipyretics and inhibit the transformation of arachidonic acid to PGE_2 (33). It is against this background that it was believed the extracts from *X. americana* used in this study conferred the antipyretic activities by inhibiting COX-2 that lead to reduced PGE_2 concentration.

Table 4. Qualitative phytochemical composition of DCM-MeOH leaf and stem bark extracts of *Ximenia* americana

Phytochemicals	*X. americana* leaf extract	*X. americana* stem bark extract
Alkaloids	-	+
Flavanoids	(+)	(+)
Steroids	-	-
Saponins	(+)	(+)
Cardiac glycosides	+	+
Phenolics	(+)	(+)
Terpernoids	-	+

Present phytochemical is denoted by (+) sign, absent phytochemical are denoted by (-) sign while + (trace) denotes slightly present phytochemical.

The dose levels of 50, 100 and 150 mg/kg body weight were used in this study for the evaluation of antipyretic activity of *X. americana* in turpentine-induced pyrexia in rats. Similar dose levels were used to evaluate antipyretic activity of organic extracts of *Carissa edulis* in rats (34). In addition, the same dose levels were used in evaluating the antipyretic effect of *Pseudocedrela kotschyi* ethanolic leaf extract in rats (35).

Dose dependent antipyretic activities were observed in the DCM-MeOH leaf and stem bark extracts of *X. americana*. The dose of 150 mg/kg produced the highest antipyretic activity (Tables 2 and 3). These dose dependent results were similar to the work performed on methanol extracts of *Costus speciosus* which had dose dependent antipyretic activities in the laboratory animals (36).

The antipyretic activities of DCM-MeOH leaf and stem bark extracts of *X. americana* were most efficient at 150 mg/kg dose level and least at 50mg/kg dose level (Tables 2 and 3).

Aspirin, the standard drug, exhibited optimum antipyretic effect during the third hour (Tables 2 and 3). Its activity declined after the third hour which might be attributed to its metabolism and excretion. The maximum antipyretic effect of the *X. americana* DCM-MeOH leaf and stem bark extracts was observed in the third hour which may be attributed to the transport of the bioactive molecules across the plasma membrane by passive diffusion from peritoneal cavity (37). There was better antipyretic activity at the dose level of 150 mg/kg body weight for both extracts of *X. americana* than that of aspirin (Tables 2 and 3). These findings indicated that probably there is a better inhibition of prostaglandin synthesis by the extracts than by the reference drug (aspirin).

The presence of several phytochemical constituents in the DCM-MeOH leaf and stem bark extracts of *X. americana* might be attributed to the extracts' antipyretic activities. Qualitative phytochemical screening confirmed the presence of various phytochemicals such as: alkaloids, flavonoids, saponins, terpenoids, cardiac glycosides and phenolics, in the extracts. Several of these phytochemicals have been shown to exhibit antipyretic effects in the experimental animals (38). Alkaloids have been reported to inhibit prostaglandin synthesis (39). The antipyretic effect observed by the DCM-MeOH leaf and stem bark extracts was believed to be due to the presence of the several phytochemicals.

Conclusion

In conclusion, the present study confirms the antipyretic potential of the leaf and stem bark DCM-MeOH extracts of *X. americana* in experimental animals. The significant reduction in rectal temperature which was comparable to the reference drug, showed that these extracts are endowed with significant antipyretic activities. Therefore, the DCM-MeOH leaf and stem bark extracts of *X. americana* might prove useful in managing fever and thus serve as an alternative treatment bioresource, which is more effective than the conventional synthetic drugs.

The present study showed that DCM-MeOH leaf and stem bark extracts of *X. americana* contain a class of phytochemicals attributable to antipyretic properties. Therefore, the study scientifically confirms and supports the use of *X. americana* in traditional management of fever.

Authors' contributions

GDM prepared the manuscript and was involved in execution of the work. MMA took care of the experimental animals and followed ethical issues. GGM collection and processing of plant materials. NMP performed experimental design development and literature review. MND performed data analysis and discussion. All read and confirmed publication of the article.

Conflict of interests

The authors declared no competing interests.

Ethical considerations

We confirm that our work is consistent with this Journal's guidelines and position on ethical publication issues.

Funding/Support

This research had no financial support.

References

1. Nasri H, Shirzad H. Toxicity and safety of medicinal plants. J Herbmed Plarmacol. 2013;2(2):21-22.
2. Axelrod YK, Diringer MN. Temperature management in acute neurologic disorders. Neurol Clin. 2008;26:585-603.
3. Purssell E, While AE. Does the use of antipyretics in children who have acute infections prolong febrile illness? A systematic review and meta-analysis. J Pediatr. 2013;163(3):822–827.
4. Roth J. Endogenous antipyretics. Clinica Chimica Acta. 2006;371:13-24.
5. Dinarello CA. Cytokines as endogenous pyrogens. J Infect Dis. 1999;179:S294-S304.
6. Soszynski D, Krajewska M. Lack of cross tolerance between pyrogenic effects of LPS and turpentine in rats. Journal of Thermal Biology. 2002;27:229-237.
7. Zhu ZZ, Ma KJ, Ran X, et al. Analgesic, anti-inflammatory and antipyretic activities of the petroleum ether fraction from the ethanol extract of *Desmodium podocarpum*. J Ethnopharmacol. 2011;133:1126-31.
8. Milton AS, Wendlandt S. A possible role for prostaglandin E1 as a modulator for temperature regulation in the central nervous system of the cat. J Physiol. 1970;207(2):76-7.
9. Ivanov AI, Romanovsky AA. Prostaglandin E2 as a mediator of fever: synthesis and catabolism. Front Biosci. 2004;9(1-3):1977-83.
10. Vane JR, Botting RM. Mechanism of action of aspirin-like drugs. InSeminars in arthritis and rheumatism. London: WB Saunders; 1997:2-10.
11. Borges R, Nascimento MV, de Carvalho AA, et al. Antinociceptive and anti-inflammatory activities of the ethanolic extract from *Synadenium umbellatum* Pax. (Euphorbiaceae) leaves and its fractions. Evid Based Complement Alternat Med. 2013;2013:715650.
12. Srinivasan D, Nathan S, Suresh T, Perumalsamy PL. Antimicrobial activity of certain Indian medicinal plants used in folkloric medicine. J Ethnopharmacol. 2001;74(3):217-220.
13. Tapsoba H, Deschamps JP. Use of medicinal plants for the treatment of oral diseases in Burkina Faso. J Ethnopharmacol. 2006;104(1):68-78.
14. Magassouba FB, Diallo A, Kouyaté M, et al. Ethnobotanical survey and antibacterial activity of some plants used in Guinean traditional medicine. J Ethnopharmacol. 2007;114(1):44-53.
15. Maikai VA, Kobo PI, Adau*di AO. Acute toxicity studies of aqueous stem bark extract of Ximenia americana*. Afr J Biotechnol. 2008;7(10):1600-1603.
16. Kone WM, Atindehou KK, Terreaux C, Hostettmann K, Traore D, Dosso M. Traditional medicine in North Côte-d'Ivoire: screening of 50 medicinal plants for antibacterial activity. J Ethnopharmacol. 2004;93(1):43-49.
17. Orwa C, Mutua A, Kindt R, Jamnadass R, Simons A. Agroforestree database: a tree species reference and selection guide version 4.0. Nairobi, KE: World Agroforestry Centre ICRAF; 2009.

18. Evans WC. Trease and Evans' Pharmacognosy. Elsevier Health Sciences; 2009.
19. Khan H, Saeed M, Gilani AH, et al. Antipyretic and anticonvulsant activity of Polygonatum verticillatum: comparison of rhizomes and aerial parts. Phytother Res. 2013;27(3):468-471.
20. Kirkham TC, Williams CM, Fezza F, Marzo VD. Endocannabinoid levels in rat limbic forebrain and hypothalamus in relation to fasting, feeding and satiation: stimulation of eating by 2-arachidonoyl glycerol. Br J Pharmacol. 2002;136(4):550-557.
21. Olfert ED, Cross BM, McWilliam AA, eds. Guide to the care and use of experimental animals. Ottawa: Canadian Council on Animal Care; 1993.
22. Grover JK. Experiments in pharmacy and pharmacology. Shahdara Delhi, India: CBS Publisher and Distributor; 1990.
23. Ray D, Sharatchandra KH, Thokchom IS. Antipyretic, antidiarrhoeal, hypoglycaemic and hepatoprotective activities of ethyl acetate extract of *Acacia catechu* Willd. in albino rats. Indian J Pharmacol. 2006;38(6):408.
24. Hukkeri VI, Nagathan CV, Karadi RV, Patil BS. Antipyretic and wound healing activities of Moringa oleifera Lam. in rats. Indian Journal of Pharmaceutical Sciences. 2006;68(1):124.
25. Kotake CK. Vallabh Prakashan, New Delhi, India. Practical Pharmacognosy. 2000;4:107–111.
26. Harbone JB. Phytochemical Methods: A Guide to Modern Techniques of Plant Analysis. London, UK: Chapman & Hal Publishers; 1998:60–66.
27. Soszynski D, Kozak W, Szewczenko M. Course of fever response to repeated administration of sublethal doses of lipopolysaccharides, polyinosinic: polycytidylic acid and muramyl dipeptide to rabbits. Experientia. 1991;47:43-47.
28. Tung K, Fujita H, Yamashita Y, Takagi Y. Effect of turpentine-induced fever during the enamel formation of rat incisor. Arch Oral Biol. 2006;51:464-470.
29. Soro TY, Zahoui OS, Néné-bi AS, Traoré F. Antipyretic activity of the fractions of the aqueous extract of *Ximenia americana* (Linnaeus) (Olacaceae). Int J Pharmacol Toxicol. 2015;5:104-108.
30. Mwonjoria JK, Kariuki HN, Waweru FN. The antinociceptive antipyretic effects of *Solanum incanum* (Linneaus) in animal models. Int J Phytopharmacol. 2011;2(1):22-26.
31. Weissmann G. Asprin. Scientific American Journal. 1991;264:84–90.
32. Biren NS, Avinash KS. Medicinal plants as a source of anti-pyretic agents – A review. Arch Appl Sci Res. 2010;2:188–195.
33. Chandrasekharan NV, Dai H, Roos KLT, Evanson NK, Tomsik J, Elton TS, et al. COX-3, a cyclooxygenase-1 variant inhibited by acetaminophen and other analgesic/antipyretic drugs: cloning, structure, and expression. Proceedings of the National Academy of Sciences. 2002;99:926-931.
34. Gitahi SM, Mwangi BM, Njagi JM, et al. Antipyretic properties of dichloromethane: Methanolic leaf and root Bark extracts of Carissa edulis in rats. Asian Journal of Biomedical and Pharmaceutical Sciences. 2015;5:12–20.
35. Akuodorl GC, Essien AD, Essiet GA, Essien DO, Akpan JL, Udoh, FV. Evaluation of antipyretic potential of pseudocedrela kotschyi schweint. harms (meliaceae). European J Med Plants. 2013;3:105-113.
36. Srivastava S, Singh P, Jha KK, Mishra G, Srivastava S, Khosa RL. Antiinflammatory, analgesic and antipyretic activities of aerial parts of costus speciosus koen. Indian J Pharm Sci. 2013;75(1):83-88.
37. Hossain E, Mandal SC, Gupta JK. Phytochemical screening and in-vivo antipyretic activity of the methanol leaf-extract of *Bombax malabaricum* DC (Bombacaceae). Tropical Journal of Pharmaceutical Research. 2011;10:55-60.
38. Okokon JE, Nwafor PA. Antiinflammatory, analgesic and antipyretic activities of ethanolic root extract of Croton zambesicus. Pak J Pharmaceut Sci. 2010;23:383-390.
39. Niazi J, Gupta V, Chakarborty P, Kumar P. Antiinflammatory and antipyretic activity of Aleuritis moluccana leaves. Asian Journal of Pharmaceutical Clinical Research. 2010;3: 35-37.

6

Haplophyllum tuberculatum

Abdolshakoor Raissi[1*], Mina Arbabi[2], Javad Roustakhiz[3], Masih Hosseini[4]

[1]Faculty of agriculture, Department of Horticulture, Velayat University, Iranshahr, Iran
[2]PhD Student of Medicinal Plant, Islamic Azad University, Science and Research Branch, Tehran, Iran
[3]Higher Educational Complex of Saravan, Saravan University, Saravan, Iran
[4]Medical Plants Research Center, Shahrekord University of Medical Sciences, Shahrekord, Iran

ARTICLE INFO

Keywords:
Haplophyllum tuberculatum
Medicinal plant
Sistan and Baloochestan

ABSTRACT

Introduction: *Haplophyllum tuberculatum*, belonging to the Rutaceae family, is distributed in south-eastern regions of Iran, particularly in Baloochestan. This study was aimed to investigate and collect scientific reports such as morphological characteristics, phytochemical compounds, ecology, biotechnology and evaluation of the therapeutic properties of this valuable medicinal plant.

Methods: In order to gather the information the keywords *Haplophyllum tuberculatum*, botany, genetic, biotechnology, therapeutic, and pharmacology were searched until 2016 from journals accessible in databases such as Scopus, EBSCO, Science Direct, Medline, PubMed, Embase, SID and Iran Medex.

Results: The results in this study revealed various pharmacological properties including anti-cancer, antioxidantant, uterus-relaxing, anti-bacterial and anti-HIV activities for this plant which are probably due to the presence of aromatic compounds such as two alkaloids named haplophytin-a and B, and essential oils.

Conclusion: *Haplophyllum tuberculatum* possesses various pharmacological properties and the bioactive molecules of this plant play an important role in human health, hence, it might be used for different drug productions.

Implication for health policy/practice/research/medical education:
The plant Haplophyllum tuberculatum in Sistan and Baluchistan province is an important medicinal plant that has many medicinal properties. The bioactive molecules of this plant play an important role in human health. Hence, it might be used for new drug preparation.

Introduction

Sistan and Baloochestan is extended in 187502 square kilometer and has dedicated equally 11.5% of the country's area to itself. This province is located between 25 degree and 3 minutes to 31 degree and 29 minutes of northern width and 58 degree and 20 minutes of eastern length, and 49 minutes to 36 degree. It is limited to Sothern Khorasan from the north, to Afghanistan and Pakistan from the east, to Oman sea from the south and to Kerman and Hormozgan provinces from the west (1).

The genus *Haplophyllum*, belonging to the Rutaceae family, comprises about 70 species distributed from the Mediterranean area to eastern Siberia (2). Haplophyllum is distributed from Morocco and Spain in the west to China in the east. It extends north to Romania and south to Somalia and in the east it extends north to the Lake Baikal region (3). Its range spans five different floristic regions: Mediterranean, Saharo-Arabian, Irano-Turanian, and Sudano-Zambezian regions (4). The main center of diversity is the Irano-Turanian region, Iran, Turkey, and Central Asia which harbours 60% of the species diversity. *Haplophyllum tuberculatum* is found in central and eastern areas of Asia.

This genus consists of 22 species in the Asia to N. Africa. Among the 18 species present in Iran, 9 species is endemic (5). The *Haplophyllum robustum* is distributed in central to south-eastern of Iran. The Persian name of this plant is "Sodaby" and its Baluchi name is "Sadaap". In Oman trivially refer to the plant as "shagarat al baootha", which means "plant of the mosquito" (6). In Sudan it is called "a plant of all disease". It is used in most of Sudanese homes as emergency medication and is mostly used by old Sudanese in the rural areas. The purpose of this study was to investigate and collect scientific reports such as mor-

***Corresponding author:** Abdolshakoor Raissi,
Email: Shakoorraissi@gmail.com

phological characteristics, phytochemical compounds, ecology, biotechnology and evaluation of the therapeutic properties of this valuable medicinal plant.

Methods

In order to gather the information the keywords *Haplophyllum tuberculatum*, botany, genetic, biotechnology, therapeutic, and pharmacology have been searched until 2016 from journals accessible in databases such as Scopus, EBSCO, Science Direct, Medline, PubMed, Embase, SID and Iran Medex.

Results

Genetic evaluations

The phylogenies established from DNA sequences and morphological as well as cytogenetic analyses support the separation of *Haplophyllum* species. The change in the number of chromosomes might be the main mechanism of speciation of the genus *Haplophyllum* (7). Phylogenetic analysis of the internal transcribed sequences of the ribosomal DNA was performed using neighbour-joining (NJ) and maximum-parsimony methods. Results showed that the *Haplophyllum bastetanumis* a diploid species (2n = 18) distinguished primarily for its non-trifoliate glabrous leaves, dark-green petals with a dorsal band of hairs, and a highly hairy ovary with round-apex locules. Another two Iberian species (*H. linifolium* and *H. rosmarinifolium*) are tetraploid (2n = 36) and have yellow petals. The species diversity in Haplophyllum in a phylogenetic and biogeographic context was evaluated. It was generated gene trees from DNA sequences of four regions of the chloroplast genome for 118 accessions, representing 66% of the species diversity. Additionally, Haplophyllum was examined morphologically. The phylogenetic analyses revealed that a number of species do not form reciprocally monophyletic groups. Optimization of morphological characters on the chloroplast DNA revealed that most of the species, in particular those with a widespread geographic distribution, might only be diagnosed by homoplasious character states. Homoplasy notwithstanding, the predominant characters used to classify the genus are consistent with the molecular phylogeny of Haplophyllum. The Mediterranean representatives of Haplophyllum were found to be embedded within a clade that include primarily Irano-Turanian species, suggesting multiple invasions of the Mediterranean basin from the east (8).

Botany

Synonyms: *Haplophyllum villosulum*

The mode of propagation: by seed or root suckers.

Life form: Hemicryptophyte

Floristic categories (Chorotype): IR-TR + SA-SI

Habit: Shrub

Habitat: Sandy soils and resistant to Swamp and Saline Habitats

Chromosome number: 2n = 18

Haplophyllum (5-locular ovary and dehiscent fruit).

Perennial herb, up to 40 cm tall, glabrous to short-hairy; stem usually much branched from the base, yellowish green to almost white; glands numerous on all parts; and very variable. Leaves alternate, strong smelling, variable in shape, from narrowly linear to short in size. Flowers are yellow and variable in size. Petiole short below, absent above; blade very variable, shortly obovate, elliptical, lanceolate or linear, sometimes deeply cut into 3 lobes. Inflorescence a lax corymbose cyme, upper leaf axils, 2–10 (–15) cm in diameter, many-flowered, but flowers well-separated; bracts small, green. The flowers are in loose corymbose terminal panicles, with five free ovate sepals. The stamens 10 are filamentous and hairy. The petals are five and bright yellow in color (9). Flowers bisexual, 5-merous, regular; sepals deltoid-ovate to broadly lanceolate, c. 1 mm long, free; petals elliptical-oblong, 3–5.5 mm long, boat-shaped, narrowed into a claw, bright yellow, glabrous; anthers twice as many as the petals; ovary almost round, 5-lobed, style 1.5–2.5 mm long. Fruit a 3–5-lobed capsule, 2.5–4.5 mm × 1.5–2 mm, hairy, with a lot of inconspicuous to warty glands, segments apically opening, 5–10-seeded. Seeds are kidney-shaped, dark brown or brownish-black, densely ridged.

Ecology

This common perennial herb is found wild even growing as a common weed among summer crops. *Haplophyllum tuberculatum* occurs in sandy desert, on a variety of soils, often on silt deposits, and also in dried watercourses, cultivated and ruderal localities, from sea-level up to 1330 m altitude. The psammophytic community inhabits the sand dunes of *Haplophyllum tuberculatum* on the upper positive part of axis 1 are correlated with species concentration of dominance. These combinations are typical of grass communities inhabiting the wadi bed and sand dunes (10). This genus distributed throughout temperate and subtropical zones of Eurasia and the northern tropical zone of eastern Africa (Somalia). The plant's chemical composition has been shown to vary as a function of geographic location and time of collection. It includes alkaloids, lignans, flavonoids and essential oils (11-13).

Traditional use

It is used in traditional medicine as a remedy for headaches and arthritis, skin discoloration, the juice is applied as a wart removal, and against parasitic diseases and other infections (12). It is also used to treat nervous system, infertility and fever (14). Decoctions of the plant are recommended by herbalists for preparations used as carminatives for children. In the north of Oman, the juice expressed from the leaves is used as a remedy for headaches and arthritis (15). In Saudi Arabia, *Haplophyllum tuberculatum* is used to treat malaria, rheumatoid arthritis and gynecological disorders (16). While, in Sudan the herb is used as an antispasmodic, to treat allergic rhinitis and gynecological disorders, asthma and breathing difficulties (17) and so on, indicating a large degree of variability in its traditional uses as a function of geographic and ecological location.

Phytochemical studies

Many studies have evaluated the medicinal properties and phytochemistry of some of these species, analyzing their contents for alkaloids, lignanes, glycosides and flavonoids, etc. During the phytochemical investigation of *Haplophyllum acutifolium*, two alkaloids named haplophytin-A and B have been obtained. In addition, some known constituents: flindersine, kusunokinin, β-sitosterol, cholesterol, oleanolic acid, and hexadecanoic acid, have also been obtained. Two new alkaloids, haplotubinone and haplotubine, were isolated from the aerial parts of *Haplophyllum tuberculatum* together with the known Lignan Diphyllin (18).

The chemical components of the *Haplophyllum tuberculatum* essential oil was analyzed by gas chromatography–mass spectral (GC–MS) as well as ^{13}C NMR spectroscopy. More than 30 compounds, constituting about 99.7% of the total oil, were identified. The most abundant oil components were β-phellandrene (23.3%), limonene (12.6%), (Z)-β-ocimene (12.3%), β-caryophyllene (11.6%), myrcene (11.3%), and α-phellandrene (10.9%) (9).

The GC-MS analyses on the essential oils from the aerial parts of *H. tuberculatum* led to the identification of 39 compounds, representing 91.3% of the whole oil. *H. tuberculatum* essentials oils were mainly composed by oxygenated monoterpenes (71.0 % of the whole oil). The major compounds of *H. tuberculatum* in essential oil of the plant were cis-*p*-menth-2-en-1-ol as well as *trans-p*-menth-2-en-1-ol (22.9 and 16.1 %, respectively) (19). In an investigation in Larestan, Iran, main components of *Haplophyllum tuberculatum* was borneol (25.73%). Other major compounds were α-Pinene (14%), Bornyl acetate (18.07%) and β-caryophyllene (7.43%) (20).

The main constituents were terpinene-4-ol (3.2.%) hexadec-1-ene (3.2%), -phellandrene (2.1%), -phellandrene (3.0%), p-cymene-8-ol (2.9%), piperitone (17.8), 2,4-bis(1,1-dimethylethyl)-phenol (28.3%), (1E,4E)-germacrene B (2.1%) and octadec-1-ene (2.1%), (63). The oil of this species from Oman revealed that the most abundant components were limonene (12.6%), α-phellandrene (23.3%), (Z)-β-ocimene (12.3%), β-caryophyllene (11.6%), myrcene (11.3%) and β-phellandrene (10.9%) (4). In other sample the major components were *cis-p*-menth-2-en-1-ol (13.2%), *trans-p*-menth-2-en-1-ol (19.2%), myrcene (10.1%), δ-3-carene (8.8%), β-phellandrene (6.9%), limonene (6.6%) and cis-piperitol (6.4%) (21).

Previous investigations on the essential oil of this species showed variable chemical compositions. Sample from Iran was found to contain limonene (27, 3%) and α-pinene (21, 9%) as major constituents (22). The air-dried aerial parts of *Haplophyllum robustum* growing in Iran and analyzed by gas chromatography (GC) and gas chromatography-mass spectrometry (GCMS) was poor in essential oil (yield = 0.5%). However, thirty constituents representing 99.23% of total essential oil were identified in it. The main constituents of the oil were found to be 1,8-cineole (38.1%), myrcene (10.69 %), α-pinene (8.46%), 4-terpineol (6.96%) and sabinene (6.15%). Other representative compounds were identified as methyl geranate (4.69%), γ-terpinen (4.3%) and α-terpinene (3.43%) (23). An earlier report shows the major components of *C. copticum* fruits essential oil as 1,8-cineole. But there is not any trace of sesquiterpenes in all samples of this work (24). These differences might have been derived both from harvest time and local, climatic and seasonal factors or we may hypothesize that this sample belongs to a different chemotype. However, further investigations are needed to elucidate this hypothesis.

Pharmacological aspects

Effect on skin diseases remedy

Natural products are considered as important source for new drug preparation. Many natural products, semi-synthetic or NP derived candidates are now in clinic or in clinical trials (25). This plant is a member of Rutaceae family, a family reported to be rich in furocoumarin (psoralen). These compounds are considered as one of the important class of natural compounds, widely used to treat dermatological conditions for different skin diseases. The available imported preparations of these compounds are very expensive. They have been prominent in the United States for phytochemotherapy of vitiligo, psoriasis, parapsoriasis, mycosis fungoides (26). Recently some other biological activities of Psoralens and related compounds have been reported, including anti-inflammatory, analgesic, antitumor, and calcium antagonist activities. Also these compounds show encouraging levels of phytochemicals against *Fusarium culmorum* and may have a potential use as phytoactive pesticides.

Anticancer effect

The extracts from *Haplophyllum tuberculatum* was toxic against the seven solid cancer cell lines studied with the highest IC_{50} values of 31.64 μg/mL (against Hep-G2 cells). *Haplophyllum tuberculatum* induced cell cycle arrest in G0/G1 and S phases. *Haplophyllum tuberculatum* extract caused apoptosis in CCRF-CEM cells by the alteration of the mitochondrial membrane potential (9).

Uterus-relaxing activity

The pharmacological profile of 6-MKG (6-Methoxykaempferol-3-O-glucoside) isolated from *Haplophyllum tuberculatum* was determined basis on its uterus-relaxing property, employing β_2-adrenoceptors as main target. It was tested on isolated pregnant or none-pregnant rats uteri, whilst docking studies were carried out modeling of the binding of 6-MKG to the rat β_2-adrenoceptorin. Studies have shown that 6-MKG was able to relax both the late-pregnant and the none-pregnant uterine contractility equalto 50% of the E_{max} of terbutaline, whilst the EC_{50} for 6-MKG was at least half of terbutaline result. A β_2-adrenoceptor antagonist 3-(isopropylamino)-1-[(7-methyl-4-indanyl) oxy]butan-2-ol (ICI118,551) antagonized competitively the relaxing effect of 6-MKG. Radioligand binding and cAMP studies confirmed the β2-adrenoceptors agonistic activity of this compound. In a study, 6-MKG bound to rat β_2-adrenoceptors with low ΔG_{bind} value interacted with four residues of the active site (Asp^{113}, Asn^{312}, Cys^{191} and Tyr^{316}). It is concluded that 6-MKG exerts weak β_2-adrenoceptor agonistic activity and might be considered as a natural compound with therapeutic effect in the field of premature pregnant uterine contractions and asthmatic problems (27). β_2-Adrenoceptor agonists have therapeutic potential due to their use for asthma (28) and to inhibit pre-term labour (19), which is still a medical challenge (29). A few β_2-adrenoceptor drugs are of a natural origin. The effects of a methanolic extract of *H. tuberculatum* and teflubenzuron on several reproductive variables and ecdysteroid titers were investigated. The test products were administered orally to newly emerged females at doses of 1500 and 10 µg/female of *Haplophyllum tuberculatum* and teflubenzuron, respectively. Both were able to delay the first oviposition and reduce fecundity and fertility. *Haplophyllum tuberculatum* and teflubenzuron also showed similar properties on ovarian growth, ecdysteroid titers and vitellogenesis. Both treatments induced a drop in hemolymph protein and reduced vitellogenin uptake by oocytes. This delay in oogenesis was accompanied by a resorption of terminal oocytes. However, whereas teflubenzuron completely blocked egg hatch, *Haplophyllum tuberculatum* had a modest preventive effect on this factor. Hemolymph and ovarian ecdysteroid titers, as measured by radioimmunoassay, were similarly low in control and treated females, except for a peak observed only in control females at the end of vitellogenesis. Assayed against various organisms, *H. tuberculatum* extracts have been observed to display insecticidal (5), nematicidal (30), antifungal and antibacterial (12,31) properties. The plant is used to cure scorpion stings. It is usually used to strengthen the children back muscles, chest pains, flatulence, stomach problems and has sedative effects (32).

Effect on nervous system

Four amides (veskamide, enferamide, becatamide, and oretamide) were investigated for their protective effects on H_2O_2-induced apoptosis in PC-12 cells. These compounds are Nphenylethylbenzoylamide-type phenolic amides, found in plants such as *Aniba riparia Begonia nantoensis, Haplophyllum tuberculatum*, and *Houttuynia cordata*. The decreasing order of the protective effects on H_2O_2-induced apoptosis was becatamide > enferamide ≥ oretamide > veskamide. Becatamide suppressed H_2O_2-induced mitochondrial membrane depolarization in a dose-dependent manner. At the concentration of 10 µM, becatamide maintained mitochondrial membrane depolarization at 16% compared to 51% in H_2O_2-treated PC-12 cells (33). Certain neurodegenerative diseases progressively deteriorate the structure and/or the function of neurons in the central nervous system, eventually leading to cell death (34,35). Neurodegenerative processes are very much responsible for several neuronal diseases such as Alzheimer's, Parkinson's, and Huntington's diseases (7,36). Although there are several mechanisms involved in neuronal cell death, a most common mechanism is through the well-known intrinsic mitochondrial apoptotic pathway (38). Depolarization of mitochondria membrane potential caused damage to outer membrane resulted in the loss of its dye from the mitochondria decreasing the intracellular fluorescence (39).

Anti-HIV effect

Anti-HIV agents from natural resources are belonged to various classes including terpenoids, coumarins, alkaloids, polyphenols, tannins and flavonoids (40). The buchapine, quinolone alkaloid, was isolated from methanolic extract of the epigeal part of *Haplophyllum bucharicum* (41), *Haplophyllum tuberculatum* (42). The natural products of this plant exhibit anti-HIV activity against HIV-1 in cultured human lymphoblastoid CEM-SS cells (EC_{50} 0.94 µM, IC_{50} 29.0 µM and EC_{50} 1.64 µM, IC_{50} 26.9 µM), respectively (43). Naturally occurring quinolone alkaloid buchapine was evaluated for anti-HIV activity on CEM-GFP (human CD4+ T cell line), infected with $HIV\text{-}1_{NL4.3}$ virus by p24 antigen capture ELISA assay. The compounds1and 2 revealed inhibitory activity with IC_{50} value of 2.99 and 3.80 µM, respectively (44). Further, 45 alkylated derivatives of a base compound, quinoline 2,4-diol were then synthesized and tested for anti-HIV potential in human CD_4^+ T cell line CEM-GFP. Among these, 13 derivatives have shown more than 60% inhibition. All active compounds showed higher CC_{50} values which indicate that they have better therapeutic indices. Bevirimat, a semi-synthetic derivative of betulinic acid, is in phase IIb trials in HIV-infected patients (25). Bevirimat blocks HIV maturation by inhibiting the final step of the HIV Gag protein processing. Batzelladines (45), harmine (46), michellamine B (47), calanolide A and B, calceolarioside B (48), mallotojaponin (49); and macrocarpals (50) are a few other examples of anti-HIV natural products.

Antimicrobial effect

Ten microlitres (25 mg) of pure oil of *Haplophyllum tuberculatum* partially inhibited the growth of *Escherichia coli, Salmonella choleraesuis*, and *Bacillus subtilis* to the same extent as 0.10 µg of gentamycin sulfate. The oil also affected the mycelial growth of *Curvularia lunata* and *Fusarium oxysporum* in a dose-dependent manner, however,it had not any effect on the germination of their spores (9). Antimicrobial testing of polyphenolic and alkaloid compounds, on solid medium, showed the presence of antibacterial properties of some tested strains including *Bacillus subtilis* ATCC 6633, *Staphylococcus aureus* ATCC 25923 and *Pseudomonas aeruginosa* ATCC 27953. Their MICs ranged from 0.625 mg/mL to 10 mg/mL for alkaloids and 5 mg/mL to 20 mg/mL for polyphenols (51).

Insecticidal effect

Haplophyllum tuberculatum is used to protect livestock from biting insects and flies (6). The ethanol extract of the aerial parts of *Haplophyllum tuberculatum* possess good insecticidal activity against *Culex quinquefasciatus* (52). The nematicidal properties of *Haplophyllum tuberculatum* against root-knot nematode were reported, which is due to the presence in the plant of three known alkaloids: fagarine, skimmianine and evoxine. The effects of *Plectranthus cylindraceus* and *Haplophyllum tuberculatum* oils to control *Meloidogyne javanica* were investigated. A mixture of plectranthus and haplophyllum oils (1:1) was highly toxic to *M. javanica* in vitro, as it killed all nematode juveniles and inhibited hatching of eggs at 12.5 mg/mL concentration after 24 hours exposure time. In the green-house, tomatoes grown in soil treated with a combination of the two essential oils caused fewer root galls than those grown in soil treated with higher doses of either oil. The oil mixture, at 2.5 and 5.0 mg/mL of soil, was not phytotoxic to tomato plant after 12 weeks exposure time, compared to treatment over the same period at lower effective doses (53). Nematicidal activities of the combined essential oils were suggested by the presence of C_{10} dienes, C_{10} trienes and C_{10} phenol (54). *Meloidogyne javanica* (Treub) Chitwood is one of the most common and widespread species of root-knot nematodes in world. This Meloidogyne species can cause severe yield losses on tomato, okra, eggplant, melon, onion, carrot, cabbage, pepper, sweet potato and lettuce in greenhouse (53). The major chemical components with nematicidal activities have been previously identified as thymol, carvacrol, pulegone, limonene, anethole, geranial and artemisia ketone (54).

Conclusion

Sistan and Baloochestan province is a rich center of medicinal plants. One of the important medicinal plants in this region, distributed in three locations of this province, is *Haplophyllum tuberculatum*. It is used in traditional medicine as a remedy for headaches and arthritis, the juice is applied as a wart removal, infections skin discoloration, and parasitic diseases. In Baloochestan, it is use by women for healing after childbirth ailments. It has many other medicinal properties and the bioactive molecules of this plant play an important role in human health, hence, it might be used for different drug productions. Because of importance of this plant, cultivation of it is very necessary.

Authors' contributions

All the authors wrote the manuscript equally.

Conflict of interests

The authors declared no competing interests.

Ethical considerations

Ethical issues (including plagiarism, misconduct, data fabrication, falsification, double publication or submission, redundancy) have been completely observed by the authors.

Funding/Support

None.

References

1. Raissi AH, Arbabi M, Rasoolizade MM. Cappariss pinosa L; An important medicinal plant from Sistanand Baloochestan province, Iran. Journal of Productivity and Development. 2016;2(3):90-101.
2. Willis JC. A Dictionary of Flowering Plants and Ferns. 8th ed. Cambridge: Cambridge University Press; 1980. p. 532.
3. Townsend CC. Taxonomic Revision of the Genus Haplophyllum (Rutaceae) (Hookers Icones Plantarum) Bentham-Moxon Trustees; 1986.
4. Takhtajan A. Floristic Regions of the World. Berkeley: University of California Press; 1986. p. 544.
5. Mohsen ZH, Jaffer HJ, Al-Saad M, Ali ZS. Insecticidal effects of Haplophyllum tuberculatum against Culex quinquefasciatus. Int J Crude Drug Res. 1989;27:17-21.
6. Miller AG, Morris M, Stuart S. Plants of Dhofar the Southern Region of Oman: Traditional, Economic and Medical Uses. Oman: The Office of the Adviser for Conservation of the Environment, Diwan of Royal Court, Sultanate of Oman; 1988.
7. Navarro FB, Suarez-Santiago VN, Blanca G. A new species of Haplophyllum A. Juss. (Rutaceae) from the Iberian peninsula: evidence from morphological, karyological and molecular analyses. Ann Bot (London). 2004;94;571-82.
8. Salvo G, Manafzade S, Ghahremaninejad F, Tojibaev K, Zeltner L, Conti E. Phylogeny, morphology, and biogeography of Haplophyllum (Rutaceae), a species-rich genus of the Irano-Turanian floristic region. International Journal of Taxonomy, Phylogeny and Evolution. 2011;1- 15.
9. Al-Burtamani SK, Fatope MO, Marwah RG, Onifade AK, Al-Saidi SH. Chemical composition, antibacterial and antifungal activities of the essential oil of Haplophyllum tuberculatum from Oman. J Ethnopharmacol. 2005;96(1-2):107-12.
10. Alatar AA, El-Sheikh M, Thomas J. Vegetation analysis of Wadi Al-Jufair, a hyper-arid region in Najd, Saudi Arabia. Saudi J Biol Sci. 2012;19:357-68.
11. Kashiwada Y, Hashimoto F, Cosentino LM, Chen CH, Garrett PE, Lee KH. Betulinic acid and dihydrobetulinic acid derivatives as potent anti-hiv agents. J Med Chem. 1996;39:1016-7
12. Al-Burtamani SK, Fatope MO, Marwah RG, Onifade AK, Al-Saidi SH. Chemical composition, antibacterial and antifungal activities of the essential oil of Haplophyllum buberculatum from Oman. J Ethnopharmacol. 2005;96:107-12.
13. Javidnia K, Miri R, Banani A. Volatile oil constituents of Haplophyllum tuberculatum (Forssk.) A. Juss. (Rutacae) from Iran. J Ess Oil Res. 2006;18:355-6.
14. Said O, Khalil K, Fulder S, Azaizeh H. Ethnopharmacological survey of medicinal herbs in Israel, the Golan Heights and the West Bank region. J Ethnopharmacol. 2002;83:251-65.
15. Mossa JS, Al-Yahya MA, Al-Meshal IA. Medical plants of Saudi Arabia. http://digital.library.ksu.edu.sa/ebook.
16. Al-Yahya MA, Al-Rehaily AJ, Mohammed SA, Mansourn S, Farouk S. New alkaloid from Haplophyllum tuberculatum. J Nat Prod. 1992;55:899–903.
17. Mohamed AH, Ali MB, Bashir AK, and Salih AM. Influence of Haplophyllum tuberculatum on the cardiovascular system. Pharm Biol. 1996;34:213-217.
18. Adnan J, Al-Rehailya, Tawfeq A. Alkaloids from Haplophyllum tuberculatum. Phytochemistry. 2001;57: 597-602.
19. Giles W, Bisits A. Preterm labour. The present and future of tocolysis. Best Pract Res Clin Obstet Gynaecol. 2007;21:857–868.
20. Vahdania M, Faridi P, Mohammad, Zarshenas M,

Javadpour S, Abolhassanzadeh Z, et al. Major compounds and antimicrobial activity of essential oils from five iranian endemic medicinal plants. Pharmacognosy. 2011;3(22):1-4

21. Al-Rehaily AJ, Alqasoumi SI, Yusufoglu HS, et al. Chemical composition and biological activity of Haplophyllum tuberculatum Juss. essential oil. Journal of Essential Oil Bearing Plants. 2014;17(4):452-9.
22. Yari M, Masoudi S, Rustaiyan A. Essential oil of Haplophyllum tuberculatum (Forssk.) A. Juss. grown wild in Iran. J Ess Oil Res. 2000;12:69-70.
23. Rahimi-Nasrabadi M, Gholivand MB, Batooli H. Chemical composition of the essential oil from leaves and flowering aerial parts of Haplophyllum robustumbge. (Rutaceae). Dig J Nanomater Biostruct. 2009;4(4):819-22.
24. Bamonieri A, Safaei-Ghomi J, Asadi H, Batooli H. Essential oils from leaves, stems, flowers and fruits of haplophyllum robustum bge. (rutaceae) grown in Iran. J Ess Oil Res. 2006; 379(18): 1-4
25. Butler M, Nat S. Natural products to drugs: natural product-derived compounds in clinical trials. Nat Prod Rep. 2008;25:475.
26. Arif D, Jawad E, Al-Khateeb E, Al-Shamma A. Qualitative and quantitative investigations of furocoumarin derivatives (Psoralens) of Haplophyllum tuberculatum (Rutaceae). AJPS. 2005;2(2):1-4.
27. Aimun AE, Arpad M, Robert G, et al. β_2-Adrenergic activity of 6-methoxykaempferol-3-O-glucoside on rat uterus: In vitro and in silico studies. Eur J Pharmacol. 2011;667(1-3):348-54.
28. D'Urzo AD, Pieter J, Bouchard J, Jhirad R, Tamari, I. Safety of longacting beta2-agonists in the management of asthma: a Primary Care Respiratory Alliance of Canada perspective. Can Fam Physician. 2010;56(119–120):123-4.
29. Clouse AK, Riedel E, Hieble JP, Westfall TD. The effects and selectivity of beta adrenoceptor agonists in rat myometrium and urinary bladder. Eur J Pharmacol. 2007;573:184-9.
30. Onifade AK, Fatope MO, Deadman ML, Al-Kindy SMZ. Nematicidal activity of Haplophyllum tuberculatum and Plectranthuscy lindraceus oils against Meloidogyne javanica. Biochem Syst Ecol. 2008;36:679-83.
31. Sheriha GM, Abouamer K, Elshtaiwi BZ. An alkaloid from Haplophyllum tuberculatum. Phytochemistry. 1985;24:884-6.
32. Phondani PC, Bhatt A, Elsarrag E, Horr YA. Ethnobotanical magnitude towards sustainable utilization of wild foliage in Arabian Desert. J Tradit Complement Med. 2015;6(3):209-18.
33. Park JB. Protective effects of veskamide, enferamide, becatamide, and oretamide on H_2O_2-induced apoptosis of PC-12 cells. Phytomedicine. 2011;18(10):843-7.
34. Martinelli P, Rugarli EI. Emerging roles of mitochondrial proteases in neuro degeneration. Biochim Biophys Acta. 2010;1797:1-10.
35. Glass CK, Saijo K, Winner B, Marchetto MC, Gage FH. Mechanisms underlying inflammation in neuro degeneration. Daru. 2010;140:918-34.
36. Duyckaerts C, Delatour B, Potier MC. Classification and basic pathology of Alzheimer disease. Acta Neuropathol. 2009;118:5-36.
37. Winklhofer KF, Haass C. Mitochondrial dysfunction in Parkinson's disease. Biochim Biophys Acta. 2010;1802:29-44.
38. Rohn TT, Head E. Caspase activation in Alzheimer's disease: early to rise and late to bed. Rev Neurosci. 2008;19:383-393.
39. Lemasters JJ, Nieminen AL, Qian T, Trost LC, Elmore SP, Nishimura Y, et al. The mitochondrial permeability transition in cell death: a common mechanism in necrosis, apoptosis and autophagy. Biochim Biophys Acta. 1998;1366(1-2):177-96.
40. Singh IP, Bharate SB, Bhutani KK. Anti-HIV natural products. Curr Sci. 2005;89:269-290.
41. Nesmelova EF, Bessonova IA, Yunusov SU, Khim PS. Buchapine - a new alkaloid from haplophyllum bucharicum. Chemistry of Natural Compounds. 1982;4:532.
42. Giuma MS, Karima A, Bahlul ZE, Aziza SA, Fatma AA, Hala HA. Quinoline alkaloids and cytotoxic lignans from Haplophyllum tuberculatum. Phytochemistry. 1987;26:33-9.
43. McCormick JL, McKee TC, Cardellina JH, Boyd MR. Cytotoxic triterpenes from a marine sponge, Stelletta sp. J Nat Prod. 1996;59:469.
44. Nafees A, Keyur G, Brahmbhatt SS, Debashis M, Inder PS, Kamlesh KB. Synthesis and anti-HIV activity of alkylated quinoline 2,4-diols. Bioorg Med Chem. 2010;18:2872-9.
45. Patil AD, Kumar NV, Kokke WC. Novel alkaloids from the Sponge Batzella Sp - Inhibitors of HIV GP120-Human CD4 binding. Journal of Organic Chemistery. 1995;60:1182.
46. Ishida J, Wang HK, Oyama M, Cosentino ML, Hu CQ, Lee KH. Anti-AIDS agents. Anti-HIV activity of harman, an anti-HIV principle from Symplocos setchuensis, and its derivatives. J Nat Prod. 2001 Jul;64(7):958-60.
47. Manfredi KP, Blunt JW, Cardellina JH 2nd, McMahon JB, Pannell LL, Cragg GM, et al. Novel alkaloids from the tropical plant Ancistrocladus abbreviatus inhibit cell killing by HIV-1 and HIV-2. J Med Chem. 1991;34(12):3402-5.
48. Kim HJ, Yu YG, Park H, Lee YS. Inhibitory effect of tumor cell proliferation and induction of G2/M cell cycle arrest by panaxytriol. Planta Med. 2002;68:1034.
49. Nakane H, Arisawa M, Fujita A, Koshimura S, Ono K. Inhibition of HIV-reverse transcriptase activity by some phloroglucinol derivatives. FEBS Lett. 1991;286(1-2):83-5.
50. Nishizawa M, Emura M, Kan Y, Yamada H, Ogawa K, Hamanaka N. Macrocapals: HIV-RTase inhibitors of Eucalpytus globules. Tetrahedron Lett. 1992;33:2983.
51. Acheuk F, Djouahra-Fahem J, Ait Kaci K, Fazouane F. Antibacterial effect of alkaloids and polyphenols of algerian medicinal plant: Haplophyllum tuberculatum (fORSSK.) A. JUSS. 11th International Symposium on the Chemistry of Natural Compounds (SCNC 2015) October 1-4, 2015; Antalya, Turkey.
52. Zohair HM, Hamed JJ, May A, Ali ZS. Insecticidal effects of Haplophyllum tuberculatum against Cluexquinquefasciatus. Journal of Crude Drug Research. 1989;27:17–21.
53. Stephan ZA, AI-Askari AA. Effect of Hoplophyllum tuberculum plant extract on root knot nematode. International Nematology Network Newsletter (USA). 1989;6:31-2.
54. Onifade AK, Fatope MO, Deadman ML, Al-Kindy SMZ. Nematicidal activity of Haplophyllum tuberculatum and Plectranthus cylindraceus oils against Meloidogyne javanica. Biochem Syst Ecol. 2008;36:679-83.

7

Aegle marmelos (L.) Correa as a potential candidate for treatment of diabetes mellitus

L.D.A. Menuka Arawwawala[1*] and D.L.S. Madushani Jayaratne[1]

[1]Industrial Technology Institute, Bauddhaloka Mawatha, Colombo7, Sri Lanka

ARTICLE INFO

Keywords:
Aegle marmelos
Diabetes mellitus
Clinical
Toxicity

ABSTRACT

Introduction: *Aegle marmelos* (L.) Correa is an important medicinal plant, commonly known as Bael which is belonged to family Rutaceae. It is widely distributed in Asian countries. According to the literature, various chemical constituents and pharmacological effects have been reported for this plant. In Ayurvedic and traditional medicinal systems, different parts of *A. marmelos* are used for diabetes mellitus. In the present review, an attempt was made to summarize the in vivo and in vitro studies and clinical trials conducted to evaluate or validate the anti-diabetic activity and toxicity of *A. marmelos*.
Methods: PubMed, Science Direct, Google Scholar, Directory of open access journals (DOAJ), EMBASE, and Web of Science were searched using the keywords *Aegle marmelos* and diabetes.
Results: Anti-diabetic potential, clinical applications of different parts of *A. marmelos* and possible toxic effects have been revealed in *A. marmelos* extract.
Conclusion: *Aegle marmelos* can be used as a potential candidate for diabetes mellitus.

Implication for health policy/practice/research/medical education:
Different parts of *A. marmelos* are used to control diabetes mellitus. Therefore, isolation of active compounds which exhibit anti-diabetic activity may lead to development of new anti-diabetic drugs.

Introduction

Diabetes mellitus has been recognized as one of the emerging health problems worldwide because of its high prevalence, adverse clinical outcomes, marked reduction in the quality of life of patients and high healthcare costs (1-3). It is characterized by abnormalities in carbohydrate, lipid and lipoprotein metabolism. The disease not only leads to hyperglycemia but also causes many complications such as hyperlipidemia, hyperinsulinemia, hypertension and atherosclerosis (4,5). Global projections suggest that more than 350 million people will have diabetes by 2030 and the cost of treating diabetes and its complications could reach more than trillion dollars annually. Accordingly, it has become an adverse public health crisis in most of the South Asian countries including Sri Lanka with a prevalence of 8.5% in the general population (6,7). Before the discovery of insulin in 1922, the only treatment options for diabetes were those based on the traditional practices. Ethno-botanical knowledge has played a particularly important role in historical diabetes therapies, with over 1200 species of medicinal plants recognized throughout the world for their ability to treat diabetic indications (8,9). *Aegle marmelos* (L.) Correa (Figure 1) is one of the medicinal plants used in Asian countries to treat diabetes mellitus. This article aimed to review (*a*) chemical composition (*b*) the anti-diabetic properties (in vivo, in vitro experiments and clinical trials) and (*c*) toxicities of different parts of *A. marmelos*.

*Corresponding author: L.D.A.M. Arawwawala, Ph.D, Industrial Technology Institute, Bauddhaloka Mawatha, Colombo 07, Sri Lanka. Email: menuka@iti.lk

Taxonomy of *Aegle marmelos* L.

Kingdom: Plantae
Order: Sapindales
Family: Rutaceae
Sub family: Aurantioideae

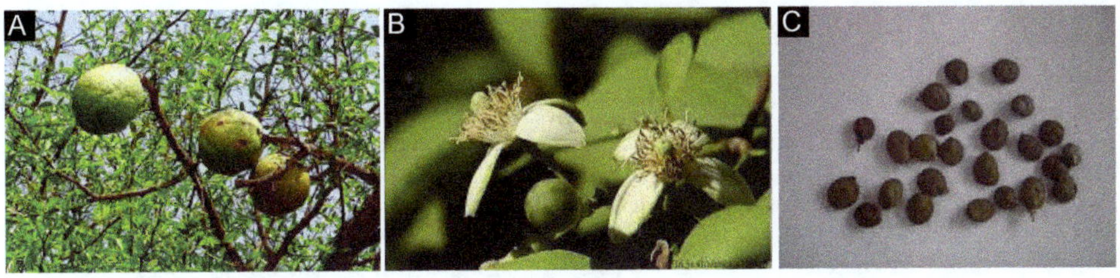

Figure 1. Fruits (A), flowers (B) and seeds (C) of *Aegle marmelos* L.

Genus: *Aegle*
Species: *A. marmelos*

Morphology

Aegle marmelos tree is a slow-growing of medium size up to 25 or 30 feet tall with short trunk, thick, soft, flaking bark, and spreading, sometimes spiny branches, the lower ones drooping. Young suckers bear many stiff, straight spines. There are sharp, axial one inch long spikes on this tree. The leaflets are oval or lancet shaped 4-10 cm long, 2-5 cm wide. Leaves composed of 3 to 5 leaflet in it. The lateral leaflets are without petiole and the terminal one has a long one. The petiole is 1 to 2.5 inch long. Mature leaves emit a peculiar fragrance when bruised. Flowers occurs in clusters of 4 to 7 along the young branchlets, have 4 recurved, fleshy petals. The flowers are greenish white in color with a peculiar fragrant. Flowering occurs during the month of May and June (10). Fruit is spherical or oval in shape with a diameter of 2 to 4 inch. Shell is thin, hard and woody in nature. It is greenish when unripe and upon ripening it turns into yellowish color. The pulp of the fruit has 8 to 15 segments. The pulp is yellow, soft, pasty, sweet, resinous and fragrant. Fruition occurs in the month of May and June. The seeds are embedded in the pulp. The seeds are small (nearly 1 cm in length), hard, flattened-oblong, bearing woolly hairs and each enclosed in a sac of adhesive (10,11).

Distribution

Aegle marmelos is a subtropical plant growing well in the dry forests on hilly and plain regions. It is a widely distributed plant and found in India, China, Nepal, Sri Lanka, Myanmar, Vietnam, Laos, Cambodia, Pakistan, Bangladesh, Thailand, Indonesia, Java, Philippines Malaysia, Tibet, and Fiji. In India it found in sub-Himalayan tracts from Jhelum eastwards to West Bengal, in central and south India (10-12). *A. marmelos* is known by different names in different parts of world, some of them are mentioned in Table 1 (13).

Table 1. Names of *Aegle marmelos* L. in different languages

Name	Language
Aegle marmelos	Latin
Wood/Stone apple, Bengal Quince, Indian Quince	English
MbauNau, Trai Mam	Vietnamese
Bel, Gudu	Nepali
Toum	Lao (Sino-Tibetan)
Bnau	Khmer
Modjo	Javanese
Oranger du Malabar	French
Ohshit, opesheet	Burmese
Mojo tree	Indonesian
PokokMajaBatu	Malay
Mapin, Matum, Tum	Thai
Shreephal, Bilva, Bilwa	Sanskrit
Sir Phal	Old Hindi
Bel, Shreefal	Bengali
Kaveeth	Marathi
VilvaMaram, VilvaPazham	Tamil
Maredu	Telugu
Bel	Urdu
Belli	Sinhala

Propagation

Usually seeds are used for propagation. At first, ripe fruits are collected. Then seeds are squeezed out, washed thoroughly, dried in shade and stored in airtight containers. Seeds are pretreated by soaking in cold water for 24 hours and sown on sandy beds. The beds should be regularly watered. Germination commences on the ninth day onwards and completed within 20 days. The percentage of germination is around 90%. Four leaved seedlings are transplanted to containers.

Sprouted root cuttings are also used for propagation. These are obtained by making incision on lateral roots and taking root cuttings with sprouted portions, usually 9-12 months after making incision (14).

Phytochemical constituents

Several research groups have isolated and identified various chemical constituents present in different parts of *A. marmelos* (Table 2).

Anti-diabetic activity

In vivo experiments

In vivo experiments on anti-diabetic activity of *A. marmelos* are summarized in Table 3.

Table 2. Phytochemical constituents of different parts of *Aegle marmelos* L.

Type of the part plant	Chemical constituents	References
Fruit	Hexanal, isoamyl acetate, limonene, β-phellandrene, p-cymene, acetoin, (E)-2-octenal, (E,E)-2,4-heptadienal, dehydro-p-cymene, linalool, 3,5-octadiene-2-one, α-cubebene, trans-p-mentha-2,8-dienol, citronellal, cineole, p-cymene, citronella, citral, cuminaldehyde, β-cubebene, β-caryophyl-lene, hexadecane, pulegone, α-humulene, verbenone, carvone, carvylacetate, dihydro-β-ionone, (E)-6,10-dimethyl-5,9-undecadien-2-one, β-ionone, caryophyllene oxide, humulene oxide and hexadecanoic acid	(15)
Fruit	Coumarins like aegeline, aegelenine, marmelin, o-mtheylhalfordinol, alloimperatorin, furocoumarins, psoralen, o-isopentenylhalfordinol, marmelosin, tartaric acid, linoleic acid, tannins, phlobatannins, leucoanthocyanins, anthocyanins, flavonoid glycosides	(16-19)
Fruit Pulp	Carotenoids, phenolics, alkaloids, pectins, tannins, coumarins, flavonoids, terpenoids	(15,17-19)
Bark	Isomeric lignan-glucosides: glucoside, (-) – lyoniresinol 2α-O-β-D glucopyranoside, (-) 4 - epi-lyoniresinol, 3α -O -β -D-glucopyranoside, glucosides, (+)- lyoniresinol. 3α-O-β-D-glucopyranoside, (-)-lyoniresinol 3α-O-β-D-D-glucopyranoside	(20)
Stem Bark	Marmesin – 1''- α -L – rhamnopyranoside, 1,5 -dihydroxy - 6 - methoxy -2 -methyl anthraquinone, lupeol, β-sitosterol	(21)
Leaves	Aegeline, lupeol, rutin, marmesinine, β-sitosterol, flavone, glycoside, oisopentenyl halforidol and phenylethyl cinnamamides, N-2-[4-(3', 3'-dimethylallyloxy) phenyl] ethylcinnamide,N-2-hydroxy-2-(4-hydroxyphenyl) ethylcinnamide, marceline, shahidine	(22-24)

In vitro experiments

In an experiment lectin extract of *A. marmelos* increased the glucose uptake in yeast cell by 71.1% at the highest concentration (5 μg/mL) and 2.6% at the lowest concentration used (0.313 μg/mL) whereas the standard drug, metformin increased the glucose uptake in yeast cell by 4.6 % at the highest concentration (5 μg/mL). This result indicates that lectin extract of *A. marmelos* has high efficiency in increasing the glucose uptake by yeast cells as compared to standard drug i.e. metformin.

Two groups of researchers have carried out alpha amylase inhibition assay to evaluate in vitro anti-diabetic activity of *A. marmelos*. According to Saha and Verma (35), aqueous methanol extracts (50% and 100%) were prepared using leaves of *A. marmelos*.

Both extracts obtained were subjected to an in vitro amylase inhibitory assay using starch as a substrate and pancreatic amylase as the enzyme. The plant leaves methanol extract (50%) at doses of 50 to 500 μg/mL decreased amylase activity. However, the 100% methanol extract showed the least inhibitory activity. According to Soneji et al (36), petroleum ether and ethanol extracts were prepared using leaves of *A. marmelos*. Petroleum ether and ethanol extracts of *A. marmelos* revealed a significant inhibitory action of alpha amylase enzyme (36). As a concentration of 20 ug/mL of *A. marmelos* petroleum ether and ethanol extracts showed a 90.3% and 96.6% inhibition respectively and for 100 ug/mL extracts showed 94.5% and 99.3% inhibition respectively.

In a non-enzymatic glycosylation of hemoglobin (Hb) assay the petroleum ether and ethanol extracts of *A. marmelos* showed higher inhibition of glycosylation for the concentrations of 20 ug/mL and 40 ug/mL as compared to the reference drug (36).

Clinical trials on anti-diabetic activity of different parts of *Aegle marmelos L.*

A study was conducted to evaluate the hypoglycemic effect of the *A. marmelos* flower extract in diabetic patients (37). In diabetic patients, daily administration of *A. marmelos* flower extract significantly reduced the fasting glucose levels and oral glucose tolerance test (OGTT) values, while the post glucose load plasma insulin levels were significantly increased by 62%. Serum levels of tested enzymes, creatinine and Glycated hemoglobin (HbA1c) were not significantly altered at the end of one month. The *A. marmelos* flower extract exerted a significant hypoglycemic effect and increased insulin secretion in type II diabetic patients with no adverse effects.

In another study *A. marmelos* leaves were evaluated on non-insulin dependent diabetes mellitus patients. It caused significant changes in postprandial blood glucose level (PPBGL) of patients who were receiving *A. marmelos* leaves in comparison to patients who were on their standard oral hypoglycemic therapy (38).

Toxicity on different parts of *Aegle marmelos L.*

Herbal medicines are regarded by the public and some health care providers to be gentle and safe, but there is no scientific basis for this belief. The active components of plants have potential to cause serious adverse effects (39). The usefulness of drugs depends greatly on their lack of toxicities or adverse side effects. Therefore, many attempts have been taken by researches to assess any toxic effects of *A. marmelos* using different parts of the plant.

A single dose of 500 mg/kg *A. marmelos* flower extract was used for 42 consecutive days to evaluate any toxic effects on the levels of blood aspartate aminotransferase (AST), alanine aminotransferase (ALT), alkaline phosphatase (ALP), Hb, creatinine and gamma GT on rats (40).

Table 3. In vivo experiments on anti-diabetic activity of different parts *Aegle marmelos* L.

Preparation of the extract	Experimental procedure	Results	Ref
Seeds were extracted with boiling water for 10 h and filtered. The filtrate was evaporated in a vacuum to give a residue.	The anti-diabetic property was evaluated in diabetic rats by following methods: (*a*) Evaluating the effect of different doses of *A. marmelos* seed extract on blood glucose levels in rat. (*b*) Evaluating by giving the most effective dose of the extract (250 mg/kg) once a day for 14 consecutive days and observing the changes in FBG level, body weight, urine sugar and lipid profile.	A significant ($P \leq 0.05$) reduction in blood glucose level was observed after 6 h of administration. Highest hypoglycemic activity was observed with 250 mg/kg. The mid dose (250 mg/kg) of *A. marmelos* produced a maximum anti-diabetic activity after 2 h of glucose administration. The FBG levels of rats were decreased by 37.4% and 60.8% respectively, after 1 h and 2 weeks of treatment. Furthermore, decreased the levels of TC (by 25.4%), LDL (by 53.9%), TG (by 45.7%) and urine sugar levels (75%) while increased the levels of HDL (by 33.3%) and body weights after continuous treatment of 14 days.	(25)
Aqueous fruit extract (brown dry powder) was suspended in distilled water	Evaluating by giving 125, 250 mg/kg doses twice a day for 28 consecutive days to STZ-induced diabetic rats	A significant reductions in blood glucose, plasma thiobarbituric acid, hydroperoxides α-tocopherol and ceruloplasmin as well as an elevation in plasma glutathione and vitamin C in diabetic rats. At dose of 250 mg/kg was more effective than the reference drug, glibenclamide in restoring the values of these parameters.	(26)
Aqueous fruit extract was suspended in distilled water	Experimentation design was similar to the previous study (25). After 30 days of treatment blood was collected to determine FBG level and removed the heart and pancreas (to assess the antioxidant activities) after the rats were sacrificed.	A significant reduction blood glucose was observed in rats treated with extracts The lowered glutathione content in the heart and pancreas of diabetic rats was found to increase on treatment with extracts. The effect of 250 mg/kg dose was more than that of the reference drug, glibenclamide.	(27)
Aqueous fruit extract was suspended in distilled water	By evaluating anti-lipid peroxidative activity in hepatic and renal tissues in diabetic rats. Experimentation design was similar to the previous study (26).	*A. marmelos* fruit extracts prevented STZ-induced hyperglycaemia and hypoinsulinemia. A significant decrease in peroxidation products and hydroperoxides in diabetic rats. Antioxidant enzymes such as superoxide dismutase, catalase and glutathione peroxidase increased in the hepatic and renal tissues of diabetic animals treated with extracts. *A. marmelos* fruit extract at a dose of 250 mg/kg, was more effective than glibenclamide.	(28)
Aqueous fruit extract was suspended in distilled water	Positive effects on heart and pancreas antioxidants in STZ-induced diabetic rats. Experimentation design was similar to the previous study (25).	A significant reduction was observed in rats treated in the elevated levels of peroxidation products, viz. thiobarbituric acid reactive substances and hydroperoxides in the tissues of diabetic rats. The depressed activities of superoxide dismutase, catalase and glutathione peroxidase and lowered glutathione content in the heart and pancreas of diabetic rats increased. However, effect of 250 mg/kg dose of *A. marmelos* on tested parameters was found to be more than that of the reference drug, glibenclamide.	(27)
Aqueous fruit extract was suspended in distilled water	Effects in normal and STZ- induced diabetic rats and anti-lipid peroxidative activity was studied in hepatic and renal tissues in diabetic rats (26)	The fruit extracts prevented STZ-induced hyperglycemia and hypoinsulinemia and produced significant decrease in peroxidation products and hydroperoxides in diabetic rats. The activity of antioxidant enzymes such as superoxide dismutase, catalase and glutathione peroxidase increased in the hepatic and renal tissues of diabetic animals treated with extracts. However, *A. marmelos* fruit extract at a dose of 250 mg/kg, was more effective than glibenclamide.	(28)
Aqueous fruit extract was suspended in distilled water	Effects in normal and STZ- induced diabetic rats and serum and tissue (e.g. Liver, kidney and heart) lipids such as total cholesterol, triglycerides, free fatty acids and phospholipids were evaluated	The fruit extract at doses of 125 and 250 mg/kg to diabetic rats twice daily for 1 month significant lowered these lipids in diabetic rats. The fruit extract at a dose of 250 mg/kg had greater effect than that of glibenclamide (300 μg/kg). The results of this study demonstrate that an aqueous *A. marmelos* fruit extract exhibits an antihyperlipidemic effect in STZ-induced diabetic rats.	(29)

Table 3. Continued.

Aqueous fruit extract was suspended in distilled water	Effects in histopathological examinations of the pancreas of STZ- induced diabetic rats	*A. marmelos* fruit extract improved functional state of the pancreatic β-cells and partially reversed the damage caused by STZ to the pancreatic islets.	(30)
Methanolic extract of the bark	Effects in hypoglycemic and β-cells regenerative effects of STZ- induced diabetic rats	At 200 and 400 mg/kg doses showed significant reduction in blood glucose level by 19.1% and 47.3%, respectively in diabetic rats. *A. marmelos* bark extract treatment significantly increased insulin level, and produced similar effects on other biochemical parameters. Histological studies showed the regenerative effect of *A. marmelos* bark extract on the β-cells of diabetic rats. The extract increased insulin immunoreactive β-cells.	(31)
Hot aqueous flower extract	Effects in hypoglycemic effects of alloxan monohydrate - induced diabetic rats	500 mg/kg for continuous 42 days increased hypoglycemic effect and decreased the HbA1c level in diabetic rats.	(32)
Methanolic extract of the leaves	Hypoglycemic effects and antioxidant activity of alloxan monohydrate - induced diabetic rats	Reduce blood sugar in alloxan diabetic rats. Decrease the lipid peroxidation, conjugated diene and hydroperoxide levels in serum as well as in liver induced by alloxan. Catalase and glutathione peroxidase activities in blood and liver were found to be increased from 9th day onwards after drug administration. Superoxide dismutase and glutathione levels were found to be increased only on 12th day.	(33)

Abbreviations: FBG, fasting blood glucose; $HbA1_c$, glycated hemoglobin; Hb, hemoglobin; HDL, high density lipoprotein; LDL, low density lipoprotein; TC, total cholesterol; TG, triglyceride; STZ, streptozotocin.

There was no statistically significant ($P > 0.05$) difference between the values of above parameters of test group compared to the control group. The results of the present study showed that the water extract of dried flowers of *A. marmelos* does not exert any adverse effects as judged by the parameters studied (40).

Acute, sub acute toxicities and LD_{50} values of total alcoholic, total aqueous and methanolic extracts prepared from leaves of *A. marmelos* were evaluated. There were no remarkable changes noticed in the histopathological studies after 50 mg/kg body weight of the extracts of *A. marmelos* when administered intraperitoneally for 14 days successively. Pathologically, neither gross abnormalities nor histopathological changes were observed. After calculation of LD_{50} values using graphical methods, we found a broad therapeutic window and a high therapeutic index value for *A. marmelos* extracts. Intraperitoneal administration of different doses of the leaves extracts of the plant (50, 70, 90 and 100 mg/kg for 14 consecutive days) to male and female Wistar rats did not induce any short term toxicity (41).

Conclusion

Aegle marmelos has been evaluated for its anti-diabetic activity by using in vivo, in vitro and clinical researches. According to the promising anti-diabetic properties and non toxicity, *A. marmelos* can be used as a potential candidate for treatment of diabetes mellitus. Therefore, necessary researches should be undertaken for the development of functional foods, nutraceuticals and herbal medicine for better therapeutic utilization of the plant.

Authors' contributions

All the authors contributed to data collection and preparation of the manuscript equally. All read the final version and confirmed for publication.

Conflict of interests

The authors declared no competing interests.

Ethical considerations

Ethical issues have been completely observed by the authors.

Funding/Support

None.

References

1. Chen L, Magliano DJ, Zimmet PZ. The worldwide epidemiology of type 2 diabetes mellitus--present and future perspectives. Nat Rev Endocrinol. 2011;8(4):228-36.
2. Guariguata L, Whiting DR, Hambleton I, Beagley J, Linnenkamp U, Shaw JE. Global estimates of diabetes prevalence for 2013 and projections for 2035. Diabetes Res Clin Pract. 2014;103(2):137-49.
3. Ramachandran A, Snehalatha C, Ma RC. Diabetes in South-East Asia: an update. Diabetes Res Clin Pract. 2014;103(2):231-7.
4. Chait A, Brunzell JD. Diabetes, lipids and atherosclerosis. In: LeRoith D, Taylor SI, Olefsky JM, eds. Diabetes Mellitus. Philadelphia: Lippincott - Raven; 1996:467-9.
5. Watkins PJ. ABC of Diabetes. 5th ed. Tavistock Squre, UK; BMJ Publishing Group Ltd; 2003.
6. Forouhi NG, Wareham NJ. Epidemiology of diabetes. Medicine (Abingdon). 2014;42(12):698-702.
7. Somani R, Kasture S, Singhai AK. Antidiabetic potential of *Butea monosperma* in rats. Fitoterapia. 2006;77(2):86-90.
8. Marles RJ, Farnsworth NR. Antidiabetic plants and their active constituents. Phytomedicine. 1995;2(2):137-89.
9. Kim SH, Hyun SH, Choung SY. Anti-diabetic effect of cinnamon extract on blood glucose in db/db mice. J Ethnopharmacol. 2006;104(1-2):119-23.
10. Jayaweera DMA. Medicinal Plants (Indigenous and Exotic) Used in Ceylon. Colombo, Sri Lanka: National Science Council; 1980.
11. Lambole VB, Murti K, Kumar U, Sandipkumar PB, Gajera V. Phytopharmacological properties of *Aegle marmelos* as a potential medicinal tree: An Overview. Int J Pharm Sci Rev Rese. 2010;5(2):67-72.
12. Dhankhar S, Ruhil S, Balhara M, Dhankhar S, Chhillar AK. *Aegle marmelos* (Linn.) Correa: a potential source of phytomedicine. J Med Plants Res. 2011; 5(9): 1497-1507.
13. The Ayurvedic Pharmacopoeia of India Part 1, Vol 1. India: Government of India, Ministry of Health and Family Welfare, Department of Ayush; 1999:35-6.
14. Warrier PK, Nambiar VPK, Ganaoathy PM. Some Important Medicinal Plants of the Western Ghats, India: A Profile. India: Medicinal and Aromatic Plants Program in Asia (MAPPA); 2001.
15. Charoensiddhi S, Anprung P. Bioactive compounds and volatile compounds of Thai bael fruit (*Aegle marmelos* (L.) Correa) as a valuable source for functional food ingredients. Int Food Res J. 2008;15(3):287-295.
16. Rastogi RP, Mehrotra BN. Compendium of Indian medicinal plants. Lucknow India: Central Drug Research Institute; 1990.
17. Parmar C, Kaushal MK. Wild Fruits of the Sub-Himalayan Region. New Delhi, India: Kalyani; 1982.
18. Roy SK, Khurdiya DS. Other subtropical fruit. In: Alunkhe DK, Kadam SS, eds. Handbook of Fruit Science and Technology: Production, Composition, Storage and Processing. New York: Marcel Dekker; 1995.
19. Maity P, Hansda D, Bandyopadhyay U, Mishra DK. Biological activities of crude extracts and chemical constituents of Bael, *Aegle marmelos* (L.) Corr. Indian J Exp Biol. 2009;47(11):849-61.
20. Ohashi K. Isolation of some isomeric lignin glycosides from the bark of *A. marmelos*. Chem Lett. 1995; 10: 881-910.
21. Nema D, Srivastava SK. Isolation some pigment from stem bark of the *A. marmelos*. Physical Sci J. 1991;61:452-67.
22. Govindachari TR, Premila MS. Some alkaloids from aegle marmelos. Phytochemistry. 1983;22(3):755-7.
23. Pattnaik S, Subramanyam VR, Kole C. Antibacterial and antifungal activity of ten essential oils in vitro. Microbios. 1996;86(349):237-46.

24. Baslas KK, Deshpandey SS. Edible Medicinal and Non-Medicinal Plants. Fruits J Indian Chem Soc. 1951;28:19-22.
25. Kesari AN, Gupta RK, Singh SK, Diwakar S, Watal G. Hypoglycemic and antihyperglycemic activity of *Aegle marmelos* seed extract in normal and diabetic rats. J Ethnopharmacol. 2006;107(3):374-9.
26. Kamalakkannan N, Prince PS. Hypoglycaemic effect of water extracts of *Aegle marmelos* fruits in streptozotocin diabetic rats. J Ethnopharmacol. 2003;87(2-3):207-10.
27. Kamalakkannan N, Stanely Mainzen Prince P. Effect of *Aegle marmelos* Correa. (Bael) fruit extract on tissue antioxidants in streptozotocin diabetic rats. Indian J Exp Biol. 2003;41(11):1285-8.
28. Kamalakkannan N, Prince PS. Antidiabetic and anti-oxidant activity of *Aegle marmelos* extract in streptozotocin-induced diabetic rats. Pharm Biol. 2004;42(2):125-30.
29. Kamalakkannan N, Prince PS. Antihyperlipidaemic effect of *Aegle marmelos* fruit extract in streptozotocin-induced diabetes in rats. J Sci Food Agric. 2005;85(4):569-73.
30. Kamalakkannan N, Prince PS. The effect of *Aegle marmelos* fruit extract in streptozotocin diabetes: a histopathological study. J Herb Pharmacother. 2005;5(3):87-96.
31. Gandhi GR, Ignacimuthu S, Paulraj MG. Hypoglycemic and beta-cells regenerative effects of *Aegle marmelos* (L.) Corr. bark extract in streptozotocin-induced diabetic rats. Food Chem Toxicol. 2012;50(5):1667-74.
32. Kumari KDKP, Samarasinghe K, Suresh TS. Hypoglycemic effect of the traditional drink, the water extract of dried flowers of *Aegle marmelos* (L) Correa (bael fruit) in Wister rats. Indian Journal of Traditional Knowledge. 2013;12(3):384-9.
33. Sabu MC, Kuttan R. Antidiabetic activity of *Aegle marmelos* and its relationship with its antioxidant properties. Indian J Physiol Pharmacol. 2004;48(1):81-8.
34. Saha RK, Nesa A, Nahar K, Akter M. Antidiabetic activities of the fruit *Aegle marmelos*. J Mol Biomark Diagn. 2016;7(2):272.
35. Saha S, Verma R. Inhibitory potential of traditional herbs on alpha-amylase activity. Pharm Biol. 2012;50(3):326-31.
36. Soneji IB, Thokal VN, Khan ZH. In vitro antidiabetic activity of *Aegle marmelos* leaves. Eur J Biom Pharm Sci. 2016;3(5):530-2.
37. Kumari KDKP, Suresh TS, Samarasinghe K, Handunnetti SM, Samaranayake TSP. Evaluation of a traditional Sri Lankan herbal beverage (water extract of dried flowers of *Aegle marmelos*, Bael fruit) in type II diabetic patients. 4th World Congress on Diabetes Metabolism; Holiday Inn, USA; August 14-16, 2013.
38. Yaheya M, Ismail M. Clinical evaluation of antidiabetic activity of *Trigonella* seeds and *Aegle marmelos* leaves. World Applied Sciences Journal. 2009;7(10):1231-4.
39. De Smet PA. Health risks of herbal remedies: an update. Clin Pharmacol Ther. 2004;76(1):1-17.
40. Kumari KD, Suresh TS, Samarasinghe K. Effect of long term feeding of the water extract of dried flowers on *Aegel marmelos* in Wistar rats. Planta Med. 2012;78:121.
41. Veerappan A, Miyazaki S, Kadarkaraisamy M, Ranganathan D. Acute and subacute toxicity studies of Aegle marmelos Corr., an Indian medicinal plant. Phytomedicine. 2007;14(2-3):209-15.

8

Phytochemical analysis, analgesic and antipyretic properties of ethanolic leaf extract of *Vernonia amygdalina* Del.

Mustapha A Tijjani[1*], Garba T Mohammed[2], Yagana T Alkali[3], Thiza B Adamu[1], Fanna I Abdurahaman[1]

[1]Department of Chemistry, Faculty of Science, University of Maiduguri, P.M.B 1069, Maiduguri, Borno State, Nigeria
[2]Department of Pharmaceutical Chemistry, Faculty of Pharmacy, University of Maiduguri, P.M.B 1069, Maiduguri, Borno State, Nigeria
[3]Department of Biological Sciences, Faculty of Sciences, University of Maiduguri, P.M.B 1069, Maiduguri, Borno State, Nigeria

ARTICLE INFO

Keywords:
Vernonia amygdalina
Phytochemicals
Analgesic
Antipyretic agent extracts

ABSTRACT

Introduction: *Vernonia amygdalina* Del. has been traditionally used in relieving pain and inflammatory conditions as well as in treatment of feverish conditions by local people of the North-east Nigeria. Consequently this study aims at evaluating the phytochemical content, antipyretic and analgesic properties of *V. amygdalina* (biter leaf).
Methods: The leaf of *V. amygdalina* was soxhlet extracted with ethanol and sequentially partitioned using solvent of different polarities. Phytochemical test was conducted to ascertain the secondary metabolites present in the extract using standard procedures. Acute toxicity (LD_{50}) of the extract on laboratory rats was estimated by following protocols of Lorke. The antinociceptive activity of the ethanolic extract was also evaluated using acetic acid induced pain and hot plate method.
Results: The results revealed the presence of tannins, phlobatannins, saponins, carbohydrates, cardioactive glycoside, flavonoids, alkaloids, steroids and terpenes. Anthraquinones were absent in the extract. The intraperitoneal LD_{50} was found to be 3721 mg/kg. On administration of 5000 mg/kg dose of the extract via oral route, there was no dead. The extract demonstrated significant antinociceptive activities as 36.0±0.81, 43.8±0.11 and 52.8±0.37 (Mean number of writhings) respectively for the doses 600, 400 and 200 mg/kg i.p.) as compared to the control (60.0 ± 0.11). High dose of 400 mg/kg significantly reduced rectal temperature ($P<0.05$)
Conclusion: These results demonstrated the medicinal potentiality of *V. amygdalina* and might be used as analgesic, and antipyretic agent. Phytochemicals found in such as flavonoids, tannins, alkaloids and steroids seem to be implicated in having such pharmacological activities.

Implication for health policy/practice/research/medical education:
The ethanolic extract from *V. amygdalina* has phytochemicals such as flavonoids, tannins, alkaloids and steroids and the extract is non-toxic. It has pharmacological properties such as analgesic and antipyretic activities which could be due to the presence of secondary metabolites.

Introduction

For long, plants have been utilized by man in treatment of various ailments and diseases. Medicinal plants are important source of pharmacological and toxicological value. Furthermore, an increasing reliance on the use of medicinal plants in the industrialized societies has been traced to the extraction and development of several drugs and chemotherapeutics from these plants as well as from traditionally used rural herbal remedies (1). Biter leaf (*Vernonia amygdalina*) is an indigenous African plant species, which grows in most parts of sub-Saharan Africa. *Vernonia* is a genus of about 1000 species of forbs and shrubs of which *V. amygdalina* is the most prominent specie and one of the pantropical tribes of the family Asteraceae (2). It grows predominantly in tropical areas of Africa, especially in Nigeria, Zimbabwe and South Africa and it is domesticated in parts of West Africa (3). Traditional medicinal plants play an important role in the medical system in Nigeria; however, plant materials remain an important resource to combat serious diseases in the world. It has been reported that *V. amygdalina* has many medicinal properties such as antihelminth and laxative properties and possess cytotoxic effects towards human carcinoma cells, it is effective against

***Corresponding author:** Mustapha A Tijjani, mustaphatijjani22@yahoo.com

gastrointestinal disorders and has antimicrobial and antiparasitic activities.

Vernonia amygdalina has been reported to be effective against amoebic dysentery, gastrointestinal disorders, hepatotoxicities and diabetes mellitus (4). The reported bioactive compounds of *V. amygdalina* are saponins, alkaloids, terpenes, steroids, coumarins, flavonoids, phenolic acids, lignans, xanthones, anthraquinones (5), edotides (4), tannins (6) and sesquiterpene lactone (7). These compounds have been shown to be responsible for the observed biological activities. For example, the antiplasmodial (antimalarial) activity of its extracts has been related to the presence of flavonoids, saponins and alkaloids (7).

Also, there has been report that *V. amygdalina* was used in relieving pain and inflammatory conditions as well as in treatment of feverish conditions by the local people, Numan in Adamawa state and Bali in Taraba state of the North-east Nigeria. Consequently, scientific basis for the folkloric claimed is needed to be established. So the aim of this research was to verify some pharmacological properties of *V. amygdalina* (obtained from Adamawa state of Nigeria), such as analgesic and antipyretic activities as well evaluating its phytochemical composition.

Materials and Methods

Sample collection and identification

The leaves of *V. amygdalina* (biter leaf) was collected in Numan Local Government Area of Borno state of Nigeria. The plant specimen was identified and authenticated by a Plant Taxonomist, Prof. S. S. Sanusi of the Department of Biological Sciences, Faculty of Science, University of Maiduguri. The herbarium specimen with a voucher number 666b was deposited at the Post Graduate Research Laboratory, Department of Chemistry, University of Maiduguri, Nigeria. The leaf of *V. amygdalina* (biter leaf) was cleaned and air-dried in the laboratory. 800 g of the sample was pulverized into a coarse powder using mortar and pestle.

Extraction and phytochemical analysis

The weighed powdered air-dried sample (800 g) was soxhlet extracted with ethanol and partitioned sequentially with chloroform, ethyl acetate, and n-butanol. The extract obtained was concentrated to dryness in vacuo at 40°C using a rotary evaporator. The extract concentrate was labeled and the percentage yields were calculated in $^{w}/_{w}$. The ethanolic extract was subjected to qualitative chemical screening for identification of phytochemicals such as flavonoids, alkaloids, sterols, triterpenes, saponins, anthracenosides, tannins, polyuronides, emodol, etc as described by previous studies (8-10).

Pharmacological evaluations

Animals

Eighty Albino rats of both sexes weighing 100-150 g, thirty mice of both sexes weighing 20-30 g, and 2 male rabbits were used for the experiments. They were obtained from a colony of rats maintained at the animal house of the Institute of Trypanosomiasis Research Vom, Nigeria. They were housed in clean cages and had access to feeds (ECWA Feeds) and water *ad libitum*. They were allowed to acclimatize for 2 weeks in the Veterinary Physiology, Pharmacology and Biochemistry Laboratory before the commencement of the study. All the animals were handled according to the guiding principles of biomedical research involving animals (11) as certified (VPPB, 069) by the ethics committee of Faculty of Veterinary Medicine, University of Maiduguri.

Acute toxicity evaluation (LD_{50})

The acute toxicity (LD_{50}) value of the crude ethanolic leaf extract was determined using standard procedures (12). In this study two different routes of administration were considered, that were oral and intra-peritoneal. In phase I the rats were divided into 3 groups of three rats for each route and then treated with crude ethanolic extract at doses of 10, 100 and 1000 mg/kg body weight intraperitoneally and orally and observed for 24 hours for mortality. In the phase II, 4 rats for each route were divided into 4 groups of one rat each and the ethanolic extract was administered at various doses to be determined after the phase one. The final LD_{50} value was calculated as the geometric mean of the surviving group and the death group in the second phase.

Effect of extract on acetic acid-induced writhing in Mice

Adult mice weighing 20-30 g were used for the experiment. The abdominal constriction resulting from i.p. injection of acetic acid (0.6% v/v) consisting of a contraction of abdominal muscle, together with a stretching of hind limbs, was carried out according to the procedure previously described (13-16). The animals were divided into 4 groups of 6 mice per cage. Group was served as control while the groups 2-4 were pretreated with graded doses (mg/kg) of the extract (i.p.). Thirty minutes later, acetic acid was administered. The number of writhing movements was counted for 30 minutes.

Effect of extract on thermally-induced pain in mice

The effect of the extract on hot plate-induced test was investigated in mice (20-30 g). In this experiment, the electric hot plate was maintained at 45±1°C (as it was connected to the thermostatically controlled water bath). Animals were placed into a glass beaker of 50 cm^3 diameter on the heated surface and the time(s) between placement and the shaking or licking of the paws or jumping was recorded as the index of response latency. An automatic 30 seconds cut-off was used to prevent tissue damage. The animals were divided into 4 groups of 5 mice per cage. Group I was served as control and received only water. Groups 2-4 were pretreated with graded doses (g/kg) (i.p.) of the extract. Ten minutes prior to their being placed on the hot plate (13,14)

Antipyretic evaluation

The procedure described by Besra et al (17) was

adopted. Thirty-five rats of both sexes were used for this experiment. The rats were given a solution of 20% Brewer's yeast (1 mL) subcutaneously at the neck region and fasted to induce fever. About 18 hours thereafter, their body weight and temperature were recorded. Twenty rats with elevated temperature were selected and divided into 4 groups of 5 rats each. Group A served as the control and was given distilled water only; while groups B, C and D were given various doses of 100 mg/kg, 200 mg/kg and 300 mg/kg of the methanolic extract. The body temperature of the rats in various groups was determined at 1 hour interval following the administration of the ethanolic extract using a probe thermometer.

Statistical analysis

Data were expressed as mean ± SD and mean ± SEM. Test of significance between control and treatment means was carried out by analysis of variance (ANOVA) using GraphPad software.

Results

The extracts concentrate yield of ethanol was 17% $^{w}/_{w}$. Phytochemical analysis of the ethanolic leaves extract of *V. amygdalina* (biter leaf) revealed the presence of tannins, phlobatannins, saponins, carbohydrates, cardioactive glycoside, flavonoids, alkaloids, steroids and terpenes. Anthraquinones were absent in the extract (Table 1).

Acute toxicity

The intraperitoneal LD_{50} was found to be 3721 mg/kg. On administration of 5000 mg/kg dose of the extract via oral route, there was no dead, hence the extract was considered safe to be administered.

Analgesic evaluations

All the doses were found to show significant ($P<0.05$) analgesic activities (Table 2). The ethanolic extract demonstrated significant antinociceptive activities as 36.0±0.81, 43.8±0.11 and 52.8±0.37°C (Mean number of writhings) respectively for the doses of 600, 400 and 200 mg/kg i.p. as compared to the control (60.0±0.12) ($P<0.05$). The activity was more pronounced at a high dose of 600 mg/kg which give the highness percentage of 43.2% inhibition of the abdominal constriction induced by acetic. Also, the extract appeared to induce an increase in pain threshold to Eddy's hot plate when compared to control (Table 3) ($P<0.05$).

Antipyretic evaluations

The ethanolic leaf extract of *V. amygdalina* possessed antipyretic properties (Table 4). High dose of 400 mg/kg significantly reduced rectal temperature from 40.22±0.03°C after 18 hours of induction of fever by yeast to 38.10±0.12°C after one hour on administration of the extract. Four hours later the rectal temperature reduced to 37.21±0.23°C. Also aspirin (60 mg/kg) reduced the rectal temperature from 40.80±0.13 on 18 hours of fever induction to 38.09±0.10°C after just one hour and subsequently to 37.20±0.21 after 5 hours. The effects of the aspirin (60 mg/kg) was high as compared to the extract.

Table 1. Phytochemical analysis of ethanolic leaf extract of *Vernonia amygdalina*

Class of chemical components	Results
Test of Alkaloids	
Dragendorff reagent	+
Mayer's reagent	+
Test for flavonoid	
Shinoda test	+
Lead acetate test	+
Sodium hydroxide test	+
Ferric chlorides test	+
Test for carbohydrate	
General Test (Molish test)	+
Test of monosaccharide	–
Test for reducing sugar (Fehling test)	+
Combine reducing sugar test	+
Test for ketoses	+
Test for pentose	–
Test for tannins	
Ferric chloride	+
Lead acetate	+
Hydrochloric acid test	+
Test for free Anthraquinones (Bontrase)	–
Test for combined anthraquinone	–
Test for cardio active glycoside	
Salkowski test	+
Liebermann Burchard test	+
Terpenoid test	+
Test for soluble starch	+
Test for phlobatannins	+
Test for saponins	
Frothing test	+
Fehling test	+

– Absen; + Present in low concentration.

Table 2. Effects of stem bark ethanolic extract of *Vernonia amygdalina* of acetic acid (0.6 %) induced writhes in mice

Treatment	Dose (mg/kg)	No. of Writhes Mean ± SEM	Protection (%)
Control (DW)		52.8 ± 0.37	0.00
Extract + AA	200	55.8 ± 0.37*	15.0
Extract + AA	400	43.8 ± 0.11*	30.1
Extract + AA	600	36.0 ±0.81*	40.9
Pentazocine + AA	60	4.60 ± 0.40*	93.0

Abbreviations: DW, distilled water; AA, acetic acid.
*$P<0.05$ is significantly different from the control.

Discussion

The presence of the phytochemicals or phytonutrients or secondary metabolites such as tannins, phlobatannins, saponins, carbohydrates, cardioactive glycoside,

Table 3. Effects of ethanolic extract of *Vernonia amygdalina* of thermal nociception in mice

Treatment	Dose (mg/kg)	Time of pad licking or jumping (s)	No. of rats used
Control (DW)		1.90 ± 0.09	5
Extract	100	4.40 ± 0.55*	5
Extract	200	6.80 ± 0.44*	5
Extract	400	8.60 ± 0.55**	5
Pentazocine	20	10.0 ±0.54**	5

Abbreviation: DW, distilled water.
*$P < 0.05$ is significantly different from the control.
**$P < 0.001$ is significantly different from the control.

flavonoids, alkaloids, steroids and terpenes could be the reason why *V. amygdalina* leaf has pharmacological activities. These chemical agents have been implicated in so many literatures of having medicinal relevance and properties such and reducing or relieving fever or pyrexia, blocking inflammatory acting on pain or analgesia, having antioxidant properties, antimicrobial activities, etc (13). As shown in Table 1, *V. amygdalina* has all the phytochemicals that have such activities listed and this might be the reason why it is used in local pharmacopoeia. According the classification of Clarke and Clarke (18), substances that have an intraperitoneal LD_{50} between 50 and 500 mg/kg are considered toxic. The fact that no dead was obtained with high doses tested and hence we could not get LD_{50}, is might be indicated that the extract could be administered with some degree of safety both on the oral and intraperitoneal routes.

The ethanolic extract demonstrated significant antinociceptive activities as 36.0±0.81, 43.8±0.11 and 52.8±0.37 (Mean number of writhings), respectively for the doses 600, 400 and 200 mg/kg i.p. as compared to the control (60.0±0.12). The activity was more pronounced at a high dose of 600 mg/kg which give the highness percentage of 43.2% inhibition of the abdominal constriction induced by acetic acid. This was found to be significantly lower than pentazocine (20 mg/kg) in the extent to which the writhing or stretching induced by acetic acid was reduced.

All the doses were found to show significant ($P<0.05$) analgesic activity. The analgesic activity may be due to presence of bioactive compounds such as flavonoids and tannins that are present in the extract. Flavonoids and tannins possessed analgesic and/or anti-inflammatory activities (19). Also, the extract appeared to induce an increase in pain threshold to Eddy's hot plate when compared to control group. The various extract doses (200, 400 and 600 mg/kg) significantly increased the time of pad licking. Also pentazocine significantly increased the time of pad licking with superior effect compared to the extract.

The ethanolic leaf extract of *V. amygdalina* possessed antipyretic properties. Also aspirin (60 mg/kg) reduced the rectal temperature. Also, the extract efficacy in rectal temperature reduction was higher than the control. This observation supports the claim of local people in folkloric treatment of fever. Fever may be a result of infection or one of the consequence of tissue damage or other diseases state (16). Reduction of elevated body temperature may be due to presence of flavonoid compounds in the extract as some flavonoidal compounds are predominant inhibitors of cyclooxygenase and lipoxygenase (10).

Conclusion

Extraction of *V. amygdalina* yielded 17% $^{w}/_{w}$ which is relatively high. Phytochemical analysis of the ethanolic leaf extract of revealed the presence of tannins, phlobatannins, saponins, carbohydrates, cardioactive glycoside, flavonoids, alkaloids, steroids and terpenes. The LD_{50} showed that the extract could be administered with some degree of safety. The extract has analgesic and antipyretic activities when tested on laboratory animals. These pharmacological properties observed could be due the presence of the secondary metabolites present in the extract and thus *V. amygdalina* leaf might be used as an analgesic and antipyretic remedy.

Acknowledgements

The authors wish to acknowledge the technical assistance of Mr. Fine Akawo of the Research Laboratory of Department of Chemistry and Mr. Bitrus Wampana of Department of Veterinary Physiology, Pharmacology and Biochemistry, University of Maiduguri, Nigeria.

Table 4. Effect of ethanolic extract of *Vernonia amygdalina* against Brewer's yeast induced hyperpyrexia in rats

Treatment groups (mg/kg)	Rectal temperature (man ±SD)					
	After yeast injection		After drugs administration			
i.p.	0 (min)		60 (min)	120 (min)	180 (min)	240 (min)
Control (DW)	37.0	39.3 ± 0.11	39.4 ± 0.12	38.1 ± 0.44	38.00 ± 0.22	37.9 ± 0.01
100	37.1	40.81 ± 0.34	40.11 ± 0.42	39.72 ± 0.12	38.90 ± 0.11	37.7 ± 0.24*
200	37.5	40.47 ± 0.55	39.12 ± 0.19*	38.80 ± 0.13	37.92 ± 0.12	37.50 ± 0.15*
300	37.5	39.91 ± 0.23	38.56 ± 0.17*	37.11 ± 0.24 *	37.14 ± 21*	37.0 2 ± 0.10*
400	37.5	40.22 ± 0.03	38.10 ± 0.13	38.00 ± 0.80*	37.9 ± 0.23 *	37.2 ± 0.23*
Aspirin (60 mg/kg)	37.5	40.80 ± 0.13	38.09 ± 0.10*	37.82 ± 0.14*	37.52 ± 0.67*	37.21 ± 0.23*

*$P < 0.05$ significant compared to control.

Authors' contributions

This research was carried out in collaboration with four authors. MAT is the principal author, conceived the idea, designed the methodology and the literature. GTM and YTA assisted in carrying out the pharmacological evaluations. TBA collected the sample, played key role in extraction of the samples and the phytochemical test. FIA assisted in interpretation of results and supervision of the research. All the authors have gone through the manuscript and approved it.

Conflict of interests

None.

Ethical considerations

Ethical issues such as plagiarism, falsification and fabrication of results, double publication etc were observed and strictly adhered to government.

Funding/Support

This study/ research was funded by the authors.

References

1. Ansari AA. Threatened medicinal plants from Madhali forest of Garakhpur. Journal of Economic and Taxonomic Botany. 1993;17(10):241-245.
2. Igile GO, Oleszek W, Jurzysta M. Vernoniosides DE. Two novel saponins from *Vernonia amygdalina.* J Nat Prod. 1995;58(4):1438–1443.
3. Farombi EO. African indigenous plants with chemotherapeutic potentials and biotechnological approach to the production of bioactiveprophylactic agents. Afr J Biotech. 2003;2(5):662–671.
4. Izevbigie EB. Discovery of water soluble anticancer agents (Edotides) from vegetables found in Benin City, Nigeria. Exp Biol Med. 2003;228:293-298.
5. Cimanga RK, Tona L, Mesia K, et al. In vitro antiplasmodial activity of extracts and fractions of seven medicinal plants used in the Democratic Republic of Congo. J Ethnopharmocol. 2004;93:27-32.
6. Harborne JB. Phytochemical Methods. London: Chapman and Hall; 1973:278.
7. Kupchan SM, Hemingway RJ, Karim A, Wemer D. Tumor inhibitors. Vernodaline and Vernomygdine, two new cytotoxic sesquiterpene lactone from *Vernonia amygdalina* Del. J Org Chem. 1969;34:3908-3911.
8. Sofowora A. Recent Trends in Research into African Medicinal plants. J Ethnopharmacol. 1993;38:209-214.
9. Sofowora A. Medicinal Plant and Traditional Medicine in Africa. 2nd ed. Ibadan, Nigeria: Spectrum Books; 1993.
10. Trease and Evans Pharmcognosy. 15th edition. Harcourt Publishers; 2002.
11. Council for International Organisations of Medical Sessions (CIOMS). International Guiding Principles for Biomedical Research Involving Animals. Geneva, Switzerland: WHO; 1985.
12. Lorke D. Approach to scute toxicity testing. Arch Toxicol. 1983;54:275-87.
13. Santos A, Cechinel RS, Filho V, et al. Analgesic effects of Callus culture from selected species of phyllantus. J Pharm Pharmacol. 1994;46:755-759.
14. Correa CR, Calixto JB. Evidence of participation of B_1 and B_2 Kinin receptors in formalin-induced nociceptive response in mouse. Br J Pharmacology. 1993;110:193-198.
15. Nwafor PA. Anticoceptive and other pharmacological effects of Asparagus pubescent bark root and Cassia nigricans leaves [Ph.D thesis]. Nigeria: University of Jos; 1998:38.
16. Abdurrahman FI. Studies on the chemical contents and pharmacological activities of the root-bark extract of *Vitex doniana* (Black Plum) [Ph.D. Thesis]. Maiduguri, Nigeria: University of Maiduguri; 2004: 34.
17. Besra SE, Sharma RM, Gomis A. Anti-inflammatory effect of petroleum ether extract of leaves of *Lichi chinesis* Gearten (Sapiindaceae). J Ethnopharrn. 1996;3:234-235.
18. Clarke EG, Clarke ML. Veterinary Toxicology. London: Cassel and Collier; 1997:268-277.
19. Ahmadiani A, Fereidon M, Semnanian S, Kamalinejad M, Sereni S. Anti-nociceptive and anti-inflammatory effects of sambucus ebulus rihzome extracts in rats. J Ethnopharmacol. 1998;61:229-235.

9

Antimicrobial and anti-inflammatory activity of aqueous extract of *Carica papaya*

Amit Gupta[1,2*], **Samrat S Patil**[2], **Nilima Pendharkar**[2]

[1]School of Sciences, P.P. Savani University, Kosamba, Surat, Gujarat, India
[2]Department of Microbiology, Vidya Pratishthan's, Arts, Science and Commerce College, Baramati, Maharashtra, India

ARTICLE INFO

Keywords:
Carica papaya
Ovalbumin
Antimicrobial activity
Anti-inflammatory activity

ABSTRACT

Introduction: Over centuries, *Carica papaya* (papaya) has been used as a nutritious and medicinal plant. In view of its medicinal uses, our group focused on aqueous leaves extract of papaya and tried to determine its antimicrobial (using bacterial strains i.e. gram positive and gram negative ones) and anti-inflammatory (virally infected human whole blood) activities. The protein content of the plant and its secondary metabolites were also analysed qualitatively.
Methods: The protein content from aqueous leaves extract of *C. papaya* was quantified using Nanodrop method. ELISA studies were conducted in order to determine the antibody production against ovalbumin (OVA) using papaya aqueous leaves extract. Also, its antigen specific proliferation in virally infected human whole blood samples was determined through MTT assay. In addition, antimicrobial studies (using gram positive and gram negative strains) and cytotoxicity were also studied.
Results: The aqueous leaves extract of papaya showed enhancement in protein content and also raised antibody production against OVA. In addition, aqueous extract also showed decline in bacterial population and proliferation rate at higher doses as compared to control group. In contrast, aqueous extract showed anti-inflammatory and antimicrobial activities at higher doses.
Conclusion: The aqueous leaves extract of papaya plant showed anti-inflammatory and antimicrobial activities. Hence, it might be used for preparation of a new drug for these purposes.

Implication for health policy/practice/research/medical education:
Aqueous leaves extracts of papaya plant showed some inhibition in bacterial population along with proliferation rate in virally infected human whole blood samples. So, this aqueous extract might be used as anti-inflammatory and antimicrobial agent.

Introduction

Since time immemorial, the bulk of the people particularly villagers have been totally relied upon medicinal plants as phyto-therapeutic agents in order to prevent/heal several ailments (1). Recently, pharmaceutical industries have adopted modern as well as scientific techniques and novel biotechnological methods including bioinformatics tools to develop life-saving drugs (2). In this regard, scientists have focused on medicinal plant parts, like leaves, stems and roots to prepare new drugs with minimal side effects (3). This research studied medicinal properties of *Carica papaya* leaves and tried to determine its immunopharmacological and antimicrobial activities.

Carica papaya (papaya; family *Caricaceae*) is one of the laticiferous plants which grows best in a well aerated and rich organic matter soil (pH 5.5–6.7). The plant is considered as one of the most valuable medicinal plants with respect to human health (4,5). Generally, leaves, fruits and seeds of this plant are used as ethno-medicine. The leaves of papaya have been shown to contain alkaloids (i.e. carpaine and pseudocarpine) with some positive specific effects on heart and respiratory rates. In addition, aqueous extract of papaya leaves exhibits anti-tumoral activity. Most biologically active components are abundantly

***Corresponding author**: Dr Amit Gupta, Assistant Professor,
Email: amit.gupta@ppsuni.ac.in

found in papaya leaves such as alkaloids (carpaine, pseudocarpaine, dehydrocarpaine); phenolic compounds (caffeic acid, chlorogenic acid, quercetin, kaempferol) and minerals (calcium, potassium, sodium, magnesium, iron, manganese) (4-7). These compounds have been used as antispasmodic, analgesic, antibacterial, antioxidant and as a remedy for digestive disorders.

As per the literature, numerous studies were conducted related to papaya fruits and seeds which were published and mentioning about its macro and micro mineral contents (4-7). In short, papaya is also considered as a good source of carotenoids, vitamin C, thiamine, riboflavin, niacin, vitamin B6 and vitamin K (6,7). Many studies have proved that papaya leaves (in the form of juice or extract) are used as traditional medicine for curing dengue fever without showing any side effects (8,9). In this regard our group focused on aqueous leaves extract and tried to determine its antimicrobial (bacterial population) and anti-inflammatory (virally infected human blood samples) activities.

Materials and methods

Plant material

Papaya plant was collected from Nakshatra udyan, Baramati, Maharashtra, India. The papaya leaves were washed thoroughly under tap water and then with distilled water. Thereafter, papaya leaves were shade dried and powdered with a mortar and pestle. The powder was added to phosphate-buffered saline (PBS) to determine its protein content and secondary metabolites qualitatively.

Estimation of primary and secondary metabolites

Fresh leaves of papaya plant (5 g lot) were macerated in liquid nitrogen and dissolved in phosphate buffered saline (PBS; 50 mL; pH 7.4). Aqueous leaves extract of papaya plant was filtered and the supernatant collected for estimation of primary and secondary metabolites. In order to analyse both primary and secondary metabolites including protein content (Nanodrop method), flavonoids (lead acetate test), saponins (foam test), tannins (ferric chloride test), terpenoids (using chloroform, sulphuric acid) and alkaloids (Mayers test) various assays or tests were accomplished.

Antimicrobial and anti-inflammatory activity

In this study, we determined antimicrobial activity using various concentrations of aqueous leaves extract of papaya plant against Gram-positive bacteria (*Bacillus subtilis*) and gram-negative bacteria (*Pseudomonas fluorescens, Escherichia coli, Salmonella typhi*).

For these studies, bacterial samples were collected from soil sample, Vidya Pratishthan except *Salmonella typhi* (ATCC strain). The bacterial samples were identified and screened on the basis of Gram staining method (10). All these antimicrobial studies were conducted under CLSI guidelines. The bacterial samples (gram positive and gram negative) were normally grown in nutritive rich media containing glucose, yeast extract, sodium chloride, agar and other trace elements with pH 7.4 and maintained in the incubator for 24 hours. After incubation, all bacterial colonies were identified according to Bergey's manual of determinative bacteriology. One colony of each strain of bacteria was diluted in phosphate buffered saline (PBS, pH 7.4) to reach the final concentration of 10^6 CFU/mL. Bacterial strains, gram positive and gram negative bacteria (10^6 CFU/mL; 50 μL) were taken in 96 well flat bottom tissue culture plates and then exposed to lysed human non-infected whole blood (100 μL). Finally they were treated with variable concentrations of aqueous leaves extract of papaya plant (0.625- 2.5 mg/mL, 50 μL) for determining the antimicrobial activity (10).

Infected human EDTA blood samples were collected from Mangal Pathology laboratory, Baramati region, District Pune, Maharashtra, India. In this study, we evaluated its antigen specific proliferation in virally infected human whole blood samples using aqueous leaves extract of papaya. The lysed human whole blood (2×10^6 cell/mL, 100 μL) was pipetted into 96 well flat bottom tissue culture plates and treated with various concentrations of aqueous leaves extract of papaya (0.625–2.5 mg/mL; 50 μL).

Both plates were incubated for 48 hours and then centrifuged to remove the supernatant and added fresh medium containing 10 % FBS. Finally, MTT (5 mg/mL; 10 μL) solution was added in 96 well plates and incubated it for another 4 hours. After incubation, formazan crystals were appeared and settled at the bottom. The supernatant was removed after centrifuging and then dissolved in dimethyl sulphoxide (DMSO). The optical density was measured at 570 nm (11,12).

ELISA

Indirect ELISA was performed using Ovalbumin (OVA, 50 μg/well) as coating antigen in high protein binding 96-well plates (Himedia). Variable doses (0.6253–2.5 mg/mL) of aqueous extract of papaya leaves were used with anti-OVA as standard, for the estimation of IgG antibody titre. Horse anti-serum was used as secondary antibody and optical density was measured at 450 nm (13).

Statistical analysis

Data were reported as mean ± standard error (SE). The difference between the control and treated samples of aqueous extract of papaya leaves was determined by one-way analysis of variance (ANOVA) test (Bonferroni multiple comparison test). $P<0.05$ was considered as statistically significant.

Results

Evaluation of protein content

Estimation of protein content in aqueous extract of papaya

leaves using Nanodrop method is illustrated in Figure 1. The results showed the presence of protein (0.836 mg/mL) in papaya leaves extract.

Antimicrobial activity

The effect of aqueous leaves extract of papaya for determining its antimicrobial activity using bacterial strains in lysed non-infected human whole blood is shown in Figure 2. Aqueous leaves extract at higher doses showed a decline in bacterial population as compared to control group. Overall, this study indicated the extract antimicrobial activity.

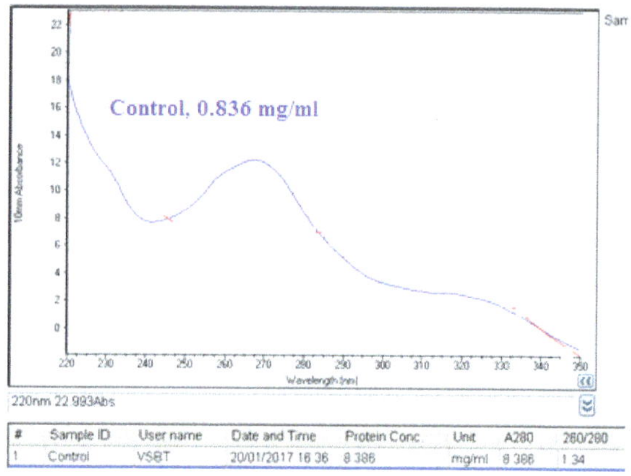

Figure 1. Estimation of protein content in aqueous leaves extract of papaya plant using Nanodrop method. In this figure, line indicates the presence of protein content using PBS as blank. This protein is extracted from leaves using Tris HCl and ice cold acetone.

Anti-inflammatory activity

Anti-inflammatory activity was evaluated using various concentrations of papaya leaves extract in lysed infected human whole blood (Figure 3). Aqueous leaves extract showed decline in cell population at higher doses. Overall, this study indicated the plant anti-inflammatory activity.

ELISA

The effect of aqueous leaves extract of papaya for determining its antibody production against OVA is shown in Figure 4. Higher doses of aqueous leaves extract enhanced antibody production as compared to control group.

Discussion

Numerous studies have been conducted extracting secondary metabolites from papaya leaves (14,15). In the present study, we determined the antimicrobial and anti-inflammatory activities of aqueous leaves extract of papaya plant. The use of these medicinal plant extracts with well-known antimicrobial properties is of great significance for the therapeutic treatments. In view of this, the aqueous extract showed considerably inhibition with respect to the growth of gram positive and gram negative bacteria as compared to control group. Maximum inhibition of these bacterial strains was observed at higher doses and this could be due to the presence of primary and secondary metabolites. In other words, this study may lead to the establishment of some valuable herbal medicines derived from aqueous leaves extract of papaya plant (11). Further antimicrobial studies are needed to identify the most active biological compounds and to evaluate the efficiency of the active constituents against pathogenic microorganisms associated with various human diseases.

In this study, the results also showed that papaya aqueous leaves extract possessed anti-inflammatory properties. This activity could be due to decline in proliferation rate in case of virally infected human whole blood after treating with variable doses of aqueous leaves extract of papaya plant. These studies suggest that aqueous leaves extract has a suppressive effect on lymphocyte activation

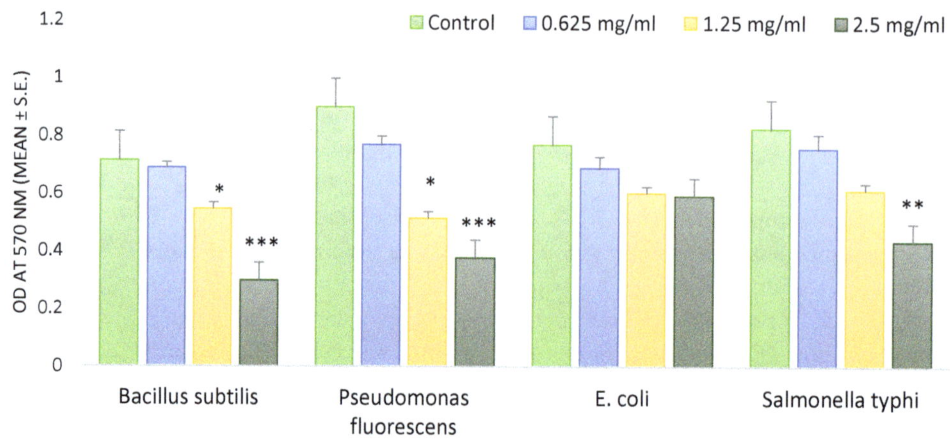

Figure 2. Antimicrobial activity of *Carica papaya*. To determine the effect of variable doses of papaya leaves extract (0.625–2.5 mg/mL, 50 μL) on different strains of bacterial pathogens in lysed human whole blood. Values are expressed as mean ± SE. The difference between the controls versus variable doses of terpenoid is determined by one-way ANOVA test (Bonferroni multiple comparison test). *$P < 0.05$; **$P < 0.01$, ***$P < 0.001$.

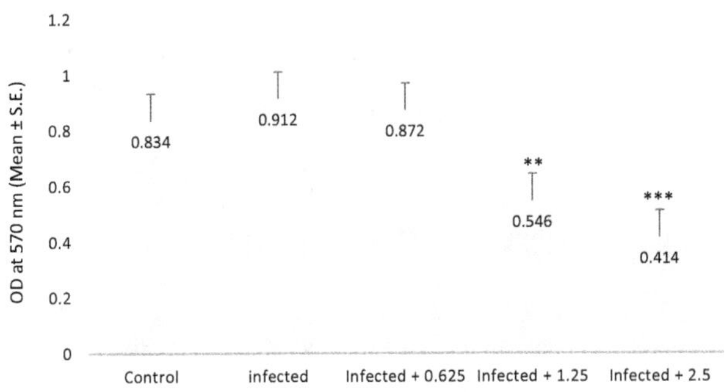

Figure 3. Anti-inflammatory activity of Carica papaya. To determine the effect of variable doses of papaya leaves extract (0.625 – 2.5 mg/mL, 50 µL) on virally infected lysed human whole blood. Values are expressed as mean ± SE. The difference between the controls versus variable doses of terpenoid is determined by one way ANOVA test (Bonferroni multiple comparison test). **P* < 0.05; ***P* < 0.01, ****P* < 0.001.

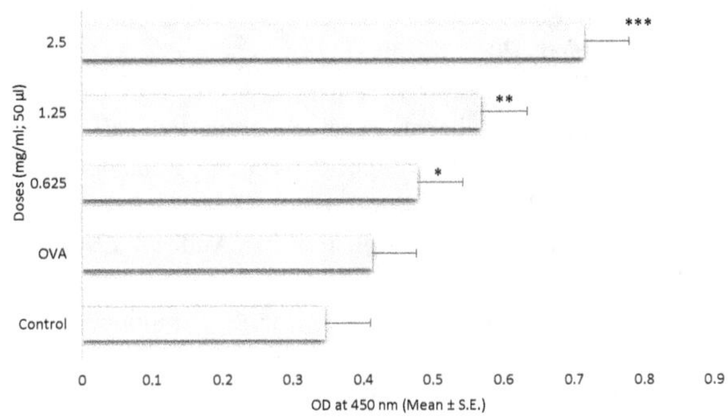

Figure 4. ELISA assay. To determine its antibody production against OVA using variable doses of papaya leaves extract (0.625–2.5 mg/mL, 50 µL). Values are expressed as mean ± SE. The difference between the controls versus variable doses of terpenoid is determined by one way ANOVA test (Bonferroni multiple comparison test). **P* < 0.05; ***P* < 0.01, ****P* < 0.001.

in case of virally infected blood samples even at non-toxic concentrations. In other words, lymphocytes activation is usually modulated (stimulatory or suppressive) by expression of co-stimulatory molecules present in the cell membrane and also through the action of several cytokines. So, cytokines depending upon lymphocyte proliferation play a crucial role in controlling the expansion of T cells during immune response to pathogenic antigens (16-18). Similarly, various immunoassay methods have been developed related to medicinal plants on the basis of antibody production against weak antigen i.e. OVA. In this study, there was an enhancement in antibody production with respect to papaya leaves extract against OVA at higher doses. This technique related to medicinal plants can be developed into a novel technique for detecting antibody production (13).

Conclusion

This study suggests anti-microbial and anti-inflammatory activities of papaya aqueous leaves extract. Further investigations on the aqueous leaves extract of papaya plant should be done through in vivo assessment of immune-pharmacological relevance to identify the major active components responsible for anti-microbial and anti-inflammatory activities.

Authors' contributions

This work was carried out in collaboration of three authors. AG designed the study, wrote the protocol and interpreted the data where SSP anchored the field study, gathered the initial data related to his MSc degree. Preliminary data analysis and microbiology dissertation work were done under AG supervision. NP managed the literature searches whereas AG produced the initial draft. The final manuscript was read and approved by all authors.

Conflict of interests

The authors declared no competing interests.

Ethical considerations

Not applicable.

Funding/Support

This research was financially supported by our organization (In-house project).

References

1. Gupta A, Khamkar PR, Chaphalkar SR. Applications and uses of active ingredients from medicinal plants. Indian Journal of Novel Drug Delivery. 2014;6(2):106-11.
2. Bortoli MD, Biglia N. Gene expression profiling with DNA microarrays: Revolutionary tools to help diagnosis, prognosis, treatment guidance, and drug discovery. In: Gasparini G, Hayes DF, eds. Biomarkers in Breast Cancer: Molecular Diagnostics for Predicting and Monitoring Therapeutic Effect. Totowa, NJ: Humana Press Inc; 2006:47-61.
3. Gupta A, Khamkar PR, Chaphalkar SR. Immunomodulatory and anti-inflammatory activity of aqueous extract of leaf, stem and root of *Ficus religiosa* on human whole blood and peripheral blood mononuclear cells. Int J Med Pharm Res. 2014;-2(4):-732-9.
4. Otsuki N, Dang NH, Kumagai E, Kondo A, Iwata S, Morimoto C. Aqueous extract of *Carica papaya* leaves exhibits anti-tumor activity and immunomodulatory effects. J Ethnopharmacol. 2010;127(3):760-7.
5. Imaga NA, Gbenle GO, Okochi VI, Adenekan S, Duro-Emmanuel T, Oyeniyi B, et al. Phytochemical and antioxidant nutrient constituents of *Carica papaya* and *Parquetina nigrescens* extracts. Scientific Research and Essays. 2010;5(16):2201-5.
6. Somanah J, Aruoma OI, Gunness TK, Kowelssur S, Dambala V, Murad F, et al. Effects of a short term supplementation of a fermented papaya preparation on biomarkers of diabetes mellitus in a randomized Mauritian population. Prev Med. 2012;54 Suppl:S90-7.
7. Juarez-Rojop IE, Diaz-Zagoya JC, Ble-Castillo JL, Miranda-Osorio PH, Castell-Rodriguez AE, Tovilla-Zarate CA, et al. Hypoglycemic effect of Carica papaya leaves in

streptozotocin-induced diabetic rats. BMC Complement Altern Med. 2012;12:236.

8. Karishna KL, Paridhavi M, Patel JA. Review on nutritional, medicinal and pharmacological properties of papaya (*Carica papaya* Linn.). Natural Product Radiance. 2008; 7(4):364-373.
9. Hampilos KE, Corn J, Hodsdon W, Anderes EN, Roop RP, Wagner P, et al. Effect of *Carica papaya* leaf extract on platelet count in chronic immune thrombocytopenic purpura: A case series. Blood. 2015;126(23):4660.
10. Gupta A, Potdar J, Chaphalkar SR. Evaluation of antibacterial activity of medicinal plants against *Pseudomonas fluorescens* and *Bacillus subtillis*. World J Pharm Med Res. 2016;2(4):142-5.
11. Gupta A, Chaphalkar SR. Anti-inflammatory and immunosuppressive activities of flavonoids from medicinal plants. J Herbmed Pharmacol. 2016;5(3):121-4.
12. Gupta A, Chaphalkar SR. Potential immunosuppressive and anti-inflammatory activity of aqueous extract of *Mangifera indica*. Adv Herb Med. 2015;1(4):47-54.
13. Gupta A, Chaphalkar SR. Immunoadjuvant potential of *Azadirachta indica* against rabies, hepatitis and DPT vaccine antigen. Int J Med Pharm Sci. 2015;5(7):1-5.
14. Chandra M. Antimicrobial activity of medicinal plants against human pathogenic bacteria. Int J Biotechnol Bioeng Res. 2013;4(7):653-8.
15. Selvamohan T, Ramadas V, Kishore SSS. Antimicrobial activity of selected medicinal plants against some selected human pathogenic bacteria. Adv Appl Sci Res. 2012;3(5): 3374-81.
16. Karttunen R. Blood lymphocyte proliferation, cytokine secretion and appearance of T cells with activation surface markers in cultures with *Helicobacter pylori*. Comparison of the responses of subjects with and without antibodies to *H. pylori*. Clin Exp Immunol. 1991;83(3):396-400.
17. Trinchieri G, Kubin M, Bellone G, Cassatella MA. Cytokine cross-talk between phagocytic cells and lymphocytes: relevance for differentiation/activation of phagocytic cells and regulation of adaptive immunity. J Cell Biochem. 1993;53(4):301-8.
18. Ramanathan S, Gagnon J, Ilangumaran S. Antigen-nonspecific activation of CD8+ T lymphocytes by cytokines: relevance to immunity, autoimmunity, and cancer. Arch Immunol Ther Exp (Warsz). 2008;56(5):311-23.

Haemolytic and immunoadjuvant effect of *Butea frondosa* on the immune response to hepatitis B vaccine containing surface antigen in mice

Amit Gupta* **and Sushama R Chaphalkar**

Vidya Pratishthan's School of Biotechnology (VSBT, Research centre affiliated to Savitribai Phule Pune University), Baramati-413133,Maharashtra, India

ARTICLE INFO

Keywords:
Adjuvants
Butea frondosa
Hepatitis B vaccine
ELISA
Haemolytic

ABSTRACT

Introduction: Immunological adjuvants derived from various synthetic micro-organisms or from medicinal plant products enhance specific immune responses against vaccine antigens. Immunological studies have already done pertaining to identify compounds from medicinal plant metabolites that are suitable for vaccine formulation. In this study, aqueous leave extracts of *Butea frondosa* were selected to evaluate their haemolytic activity and immunoadjuvant effects.

Methods: For this study, immunoadjuvant activity was investigated *ex vivo* in mice model based studies using splenocyte proliferation assay and also measured IgG titre in cell culture supernatant (using indirect ELISA). Swiss mice were immunized subcutaneously with specific protein antigen i.e. hepatitis B vaccine containing surface antigen (HBsAg, 20 μg/mL; 10 μl) on day 0 and collected the spleen cells on day 4 and proceeded for proliferation assay of variable doses of aqueous leaves extracts of *Butea frondosa* (0.5–30 mg/ml; 50 μl) along with hepatitis B surface antigen (HBsAg) (challenging dose; 20 μg/mL; 10 μl) and also estimated the antibody (IgG) titre in splenocyte cell culture supernatant including determination of its haemolytic activity in human whole blood samples.

Results: The results demonstrated that aqueous leave extracts stimulated HBsAg population at lower doses (0.5 mg/mL) and also enhanced IgG titre as compared with control and HBsAg treated group. In addition, aqueous leaves extracts of *Butea frondosa* showed anti-HBsAg titre at higher doses and also showed slightly haemolytic effect in human whole blood.

Conclusion: These results suggested that aqueous extract of *Butea frondosa* may represent viable candidate for effective vaccine adjuvants due to their higher immune response (with respect to IgG titre and proliferation assay) and lower or non-haemolytic effects.

Implication for health policy/practice/research/medical education:
Butea frondosa aqueous leaves extracts are capable of enhancing both antibody and cell mediated immune responses against hepatitis B surface antigen (HBsAg) in mice. Furthermore, they expressed a lower haemolytic effect and might be safely used as an adjuvant.

Introduction

Medicinal plants are normally used as raw material for separating the active ingredients which are generally used for the synthesis of compounds (simple or complex). In contrast, these medicinal plant products (stem, root, leaves, flowers, etc.) showed many immunopharmacological properties e.g. anti-arthritic, anti-inflammatory, adjuvant, immunomodulation, anti-tumor, etc (1-5). Lots of research works have already been done related to those medicinal plant products which proved that metabolites (primary or secondary) have their ability to prevent the appearance or burden of some diseases e.g. glycosides from *Picrorhiza kurroa* (6), polysaccharides (7) fraction from *Boswellia serrata*, aqueous extract of *Azadirachta indica*, etc (8). These medicinal plants have their ability to reduce the burden of disease and used as adjuvants for vaccine antigen.

Adjuvants have been used in vaccines for many years pertaining to increase the immunogenicity of vaccine antigen. Only one adjuvant approved for human use i.e.

***Corresponding author:** Dr. Amit Gupta, Assistant Professor/Scientist, Department of Immunology and Virology.
Email: amitgupta@vsbt.res.in

alum which increased only humoral response and poorly elicited cell mediated immunity (9). Recently, synthetic formulation or plant derived adjuvants (e.g. oil in water emulsion, water in oil emulsion, liposomes, cytokines, lipid A, bacterial toxins, carbohydrate polymers and saponins) have been categorized into two major subtypes i.e. particulate and non-particulate (9). Thus, immunological efforts have been made pertaining to identify the ideal adjuvant for vaccine antigen (9,10). As per the literature, metabolites (primary or secondary) extracted from various medicinal plants showed some adjuvant effects against s vaccine antigens. For example, saponins showed highly cytotoxic effects and induced both Th1 and Th2 type of immune response (2-4). Thus, researchers focused only on those medicinal plant metabolites with high immune activity with respect to antibody and cell mediated immune response with low haemolytic effect.

Among medicinal plants, *Butea frondosa* (commonly known as palas; family Fabaceae), grows all over India especially central and western India (11,12). As per the literature, seeds, flowers, leaves, bark etc. have great medicinal value and showed various medicinal properties or uses (11,12). In addition, these medicinal plant parts including leaves have shown anti-inflammatory as well as anti-microbial activities, as well. In this study, our group focused on *Butea frondosa* in order to analyse its haemolytic activity on red blood cells and compared their immunobiological effect to those adjuvants e.g. alum which are commonly used in animal and human vaccination.

Materials and methods

Plant material and phytochemical investigation

Fresh healthy plant leaves of *Butea frondosa* were collected from Vidya Pratishthan's School of Biotechnology garden during the month of January 2016. The plant materials were dried in a shady area and prepared in finely powdered form. For phytochemical investigation, three grams of leaves powder (*Butea frondosa*) were macerated in liquid nitrogen with mortar and pestle and then dissolved in phosphate buffered saline (PBS) (pH 7.2; 30 mL). The aqueous extracts were filtered and used to determine the presence of secondary metabolites. The phytochemical investigation of the aqueous extracts was carried out as per standard methods and evaluated for the presence of phenolic compounds, flavonoids (by alkaline reagent test), saponin (by foam test), terpenoids (by acetic anhydride test) and glycosides. In addition, thin layer chromatography of the aqueous extract was performed using n butanol: acetic acid: water (5:3:2). The observed spots were then visualized using anisaldehyde-sulphuric acid reagent (11).

Immunization

Swiss mice (n = 5) were immunized subcutaneously on day 0 with HBsAg (10 μg) in a final volume of 0.2 mL containing PBS. For this study, PBS was used as negative control.

Splenocyte proliferation assay (ex-vivo)

Splenocyte proliferation was done as per the guidelines of animal ethics committee, CPCSEA. On day 7, Swiss mice were sacrificed by cervical dislocation and the splenocytes were seeded in triplicates at a concentration of 106 cells/mL, 0.1 mL along with variable concentration of aqueous leaves extract of *Butea frondosa* (0.5-30 mg/mL; 50 μl) in flat bottom tissue culture 96 well plate in a final volume of 0.2 mL. hepatitis B surface antigen (HBsAg) (Serum Institute of India; 20 μg/mL; 10 μl) was added to all the wells with or without aqueous extract in a volume of 0.2 mL. After the addition, the samples were incubated for 48 hours at carbon dioxide incubator and then supernatant were collected after centrifugation for IgG titre. After adding fresh medium in 96-well plate, the plate was incubated for another 2 hours. After incubation, MTT solution (2.5 mg/mL; 10 μl) was added. These samples were incubated for another 3 hours at carbon dioxide incubator and then the formazan crystals were observed and dissolved in dimethyl sulphoxide (DMSO). Finally, optical densities (ODs) of each well were evaluated using an ELISA reader at 570 nm (10,11).

ELISA performance

Indirect ELISA was performed using hepatitis B vaccine (HBsAg; 2 μg/mL) as coating antigen. Aqueous leaves extracts of *Butea frondosa* were prepared and the culture supernatants were collected after 48 hours from splenocyte proliferation assay for the estimation of IgG antibody titre. Horse anti-mouse serum was used as secondary antibody, and the OD was measured at 450 nm (8).

Haemolytic activity assay

The haemolytic activity in human whole blood was determined using aqueous extract of *Butea frondosa*. Distilled water was used as positive control for the study. In this study, human whole blood suspension was collected from Mangal Pathology Laboratory, Baramati, and these samples were prepared by diluting the pellet to 0.5% with PBS along with variable concentrations of aqueous leaves extracts of *Butea frondosa*. The samples were incubated for 2 hours at carbon dioxide incubator. After incubation, the samples were centrifuged and the supernatants were collect and estimated the free haemoglobin in the supernatants using spectrophotometer. The OD was measured at 405 nm (13).

Statistical analysis

The difference between control and treated groups of *Butea frondosa* was determined by one-way analysis of variance (ANOVA) test (Bonferroni multiple comparison test). Values were expressed as mean ± standard error of mean (SE).

Results

Splenocyte proliferation assay

The effects of variable doses of aqueous leaves extracts of *Butea frondosa* on splenocyte proliferation assay in mice model are shown in Figure 1. The results showed that there was enhancement in proliferation with respect to

HBsAg using aqueous leaves extracts at lower doses. HB-sAg was used as standard and there was enhancement in proliferation as compared to control.

ELISA results

The effects of variable doses of aqueous leaves extracts on IgG antibody titre are as shown in Figure 2. The aqueous leaves extract showed IgG antibody titre at higher doses whereas cell culture supernatant of spleen cells collected after 48 hours showed enhancement of IgG antibody titre at lower doses as compared to control.

Haemolytic activity

The effects of variable doses of aqueous leaves extracts of *Butea frondosa* on haemolytic activity are shown in Figure 3. The aqueous leaves extract did not show any haemolytic activity at higher doses whereas distilled water was used as positive control and showed high haemolytic activity as compared to control.

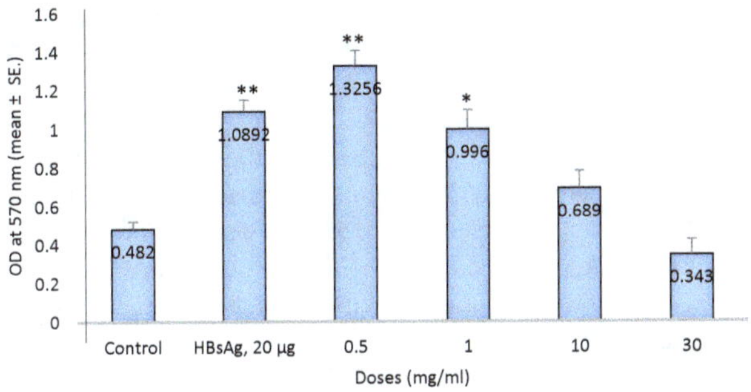

Figure 1. Splenocyte proliferation assay (*ex vivo*). Splenocytes of Swiss mice were prepared on day 4 after immunization with HBsAg, 10 µg on day 0 and cultured with HBsAg or together with variable concentration of aqueous leaves extract (0.5–30 mg/ml; 50 µl) for 48 hours. Splenocyte proliferation was measured using MTT assay as described in materials and methods section. The values are presented as the mean ± SE (n = 6). Significant differences with control groups (samples blank) were designated as $^{*}P < 0.05$ and $^{**}P < 0.01$.

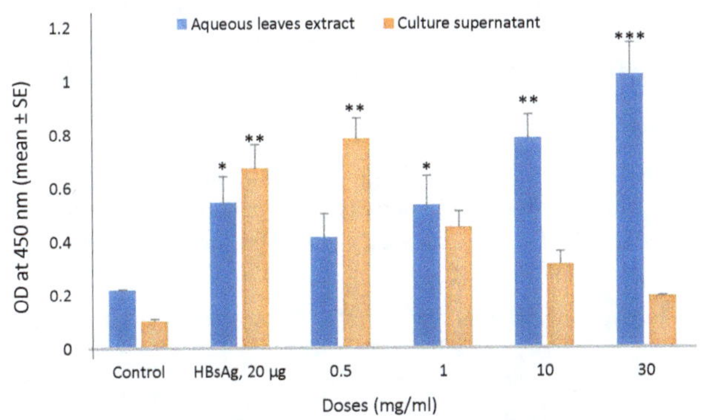

Figure 2. Indirect ELISA (IgG titre). Indirect Elisa was performed using standard HBsAg (1:1000 dilution) vaccine as coating antigen. For IgG titre, aqueous leaves extract of Butea frondosa were prepared and also collect the splenocyte cell culture supernatant were used for the estimation of anti-HBsAg antibody titre. Horse anti-serum used as secondary antibody and optical density measured at 450 nm. The values are presented as the mean ± SE (n = 6). Significant differences with control groups (samples blank) were designated as $^{*}P < 0.05$ and $^{**}P < 0.01$.

Discussion

Immunomodulation means to modulate the immune system either stimulatory or suppressive showed some adjuvant effects against specific (e.g. protein) as well as non-specific (e.g. sheep red blood corpuscles; sub-immunogenic dose) antigens (14). For many years, immunopharmacologists have focused on various medicinal plant products in order to carry out their various immunobiological activities e.g. anti-viral, anti-bacteria, anti-inflammatory with respect to antibody and cell mediated immune response (2-5). According to the literature, lots of research works has already been done with respect to medicinal plants that are responsible for curing immunological disorders. In addition, these medicinal plants also played a vital role in the promotion of health by strengthening host defence mechanisms against various diseases (10,11). In order to achieve this objective, our group focused on its haemolytic as well as immunoadjuvant activity of aqueous leaves extract of *Butea frondosa.*

In Asian countries especially India, people believe on various medicinal plants including *Butea frondosa* that have been used in traditional system of medicine for several thousand years and these plants constituted to be an important and basic resource for ethnobotanical research in many ways. In the present study, our group focused on immunoadjuvant activity of *Butea frondosa* using HB-sAg as specific protein antigen pertaining to determined its T cell-mediated immunity (i.e. complex interactions between the lymphoid and phagocytic cells) that played an important role in eliminating intracellular infections and was responsible for enhancing the lymphocyte proliferative response (10,11). In this study, HBsAg was used as standard for the study and enhanced the lymphocyte proliferation as compared to control. As shown in Figure 1. Our data showed that aqueous leaves extract of *Butea frondosa* at lower doses enhanced proliferative response as compared to HBsAg and control. Overall, the data showed

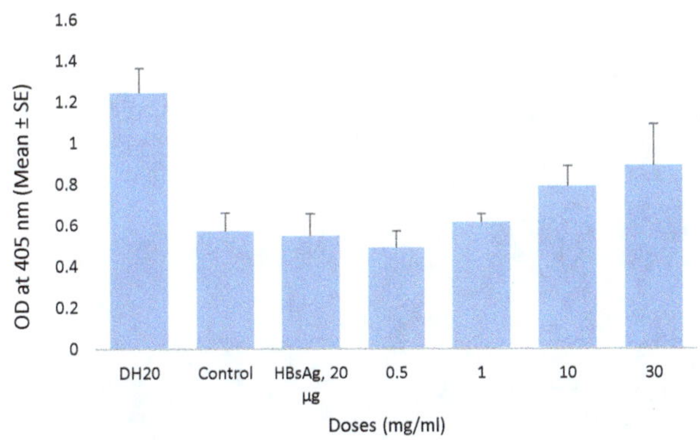

Figure 3. Haemolytic activity. Human whole blood samples were prepared by diluting the pellet in PBS along with variable concentration of aqueous leaves extract of *Butea frondosa.* Haemolytic percentages of PBS and distilled water were included as minimal and maximal haemolytic controls. All values represent the mean ± SE (n = 6). The optical density (OD) was measured at 405 nm.

that the aqueous leaves extract could significantly enhance the T cell response i.e. cell mediated immunity.

The results also showed that aqueous leaves extracts caused enhancement in antibody titre at higher doses whereas splenocyte cell culture supernatant showed some enhancement at lower doses as compared to control. HBsAg containing alum was used as standard for the study and enhanced the production of IgG titre as compared to control. Overall this study claimed that aqueous leaves extract of *Butea frondosa* were effective on antibody and cell mediated immune response with respect to IgG titre and lymphocyte proliferative response using HBsAg containing alum. In addition, aqueous leaves extracts showed slightly haemolytic effect as compared to control. In short, ex vivo experimental results indicated the adjuvant activity of *Butea frondosa* against specific antigen i.e. HBsAg.

Conclusion

Butea frondosa, aqueous leaves extract are capable of enhancing both antibody and cell mediated immune responses against HBsAg in mice. Furthermore, they expressed a lower haemolytic effect and could be safely used as an adjuvant.

Authors' contributions

This work was carried out in collaboration between two authors. AG designed the study, wrote the protocol and interpreted the data. AG and SRC anchored the field study, gathered the initial data and performed preliminary data analysis. AG and SRC managed the literature searches and produced the initial draft. Both the authors read and approved the final manuscript.

Conflict of interests

The authors declared no competing interests.

Ethical considerations

These studies were conducted under ethical guidelines with registration no. 1814/PO/ERE/S/15/CPCSEA.

Funding/Support

This research was financially supported by our organization (in house project).

References

1. Saluja PK, Shukla K, Yadav H. Antiarthritic activity of ethano-medicinal herbal plants. IOSR Journal of environmental Science, Toxicology and Food Technology. 2015;1(5):12–23.
2. Gupta A, Chaphalkar SR. Flow cytometric analysis of crude saponin from the leaves of Mangifera indica and Anthocephalus cadamba for its anti-inflammatory activity. European Journal of Biomedical and Pharmaceutical Sciences. 2015;2(2):163-173.
3. Gupta A, Chaphalkar SR. Flow cytometric analysis of immunoadjuvant activity of Emblica officinalis on human whole blood. World J Pharm Res 2015;4(2):1063-71.
4. Khajuria A, Gupta A, Garai S, Wakhloo BP. Immunomodulatory effects of two Sapogenins 1 and 2 isolated from Luffa cylindrica in Balb/C mice. Bioorg Med Chem Lett. 2007;17(6):1608-1612.
5. de Melo JG, Santos AG, de Amorim EL, do Nascimento SC, de Albuquerque UP. Medicinal plants used as antitumor agents in Brazil: an ethnobotanical approach. Evid Based Complement Alternat Med. 2011;2011:365359.
6. Khajuria A, Gupta A, Singh S, Malik F, Singh J, Suri KA, Satti NK, Qazi GN, Srinivas VK, Gopinathan and Ella K. RLJ-NE-299A: A new plant based vaccine adjuvant. Vaccine. 2007;25(14):2706-2715.
7. Khajuria A, Gupta A, Singh S, Suden P, Singh J, Gupta BD, et al. Immunomodulatory activity of biopolymeric fraction BOS 2000 from Boswellia serrata. Phytother Res. 2007;22(3):340-348.
8. Gupta A, Chaphalkar SR. Immunoadjuvant potential of Azadirachta indica against rabies, hepatitis and DPT vaccine antigen. International Journal of Medical and Pharmaceutical Sciences. 2015;5(7):1-5.
9. Gupta A, Chaphalkar SR. Vaccine adjuvants: Current necessity of life. Shiraz E Medical Journal (Iranian Medical Health Sciences) 2015;16 (7):1-11.
10. Gupta A, Khajuria A, Singh J, Suri KA. Adjuvant effect of biopolymeric fraction from Picrorhiza kurroa to promote both Th1 and Th2 immune responses. Journal of Progressive Research in Biology 2015;1(1):7-16.
11. Gupta A, Chaphalkar SR. Anti-inflammatory and anti-microbial activity of aqueous leaves extract of Butea frondosa. J Herbmed Pharmacol. 2016;5(2):85-88.
12. Soman I, Mengi SA, Kasture SB. Effect of leaves of Butea frondosa on stress, anxiety and cognition in rats. Pharmacol Biochem Behav. 2004;79(1):11-16.
13. Gupta A, Khamkar PR, Chaphalkar SR. Immunomodulatory and anti-inflammatory activity of aqueous extract of leaf, stem and root of Ficus religiosa on human whole blood and peripheral blood mononuclear cells. International Journal of Medicine and Pharmaceutical Research. 2014;2(4):732-739.
14. Gupta A, Khajuria A, Singh J, Bedi KL, Satti NK, Dutt P, et al. Immunomodulatory activity of biopolymeric fraction RLJ-NE-205 from Picrorhiza kurroa. Int Immunopharmacol. 2006;6(10):1543-1549.

11

Antiplasmodial and antioxidant activities of methanolic leaf extract and fractions of *Alchornea cordifolia*

Anosike Nnamdi[1], Ette Ettebong[2*], Koofreh Davis[3]

[1]Department of Pharmacology and Toxicology, Faculty of Pharmacy, University of Uyo, Uyo, Nigeria
[2]Department of Clinical Pharmacology and Therapeutics, Faculty of Clinical Sciences, University of Uyo, Uyo, Nigeria
[3]Department of Physiology, Faculty of Basic Medical Sciences, University of Uyo, Uyo, Nigeria

ARTICLE INFO

Keywords:
Antiplasmodial
Alchornea cordifolia
Plasmodium berghei
Antioxidant

ABSTRACT

Introduction: *Alchornea cordifolia* is widely used in Nigeria for the treatment of malaria. This study was aimed at assessing the in vivo antimalarial activities of the extract and fractions (n-hexane, chloroform, ethylacetate, butanol, aqueous) of the *A. cordifolia* in *Plasmodium berghei* infected mice as well as the antioxidant potentials of the crude extract and its fractions.
Methods: Antioxidant activity was assessed by 1,1-diphenyl-2-picryl-hydrazyl (DPPH), nitric oxide scavenging, reducing power and hydrogen peroxide assays. By orally administering the extract (120 mg/kg, 240 mg/kg and 360 mg/kg) and fractions (240 mg/kg), antimalarial activities were evaluated using suppressive, prophylactic and curative tests. Chloroquine (5 mg/kg), pyrimethamine (1.2 mg/kg) and artesunate (5 mg/kg) were used as positive controls.
Results: The crude extract showed a significant ($P<0.05$–0.001) dose-dependent antimalarial activity in the suppressive, prophylactic and curative tests and increased animal survival time. All fractions caused significant reduction in parasitaemia with the ethylacetate fraction showing the highest activity. The extract and the fractions showed a significant ($P<0.05$–0.001) dose-dependent antioxidant activity.
Conclusion: *Alchornea cordifolia* exhibited significant antimalarial and antioxidant potentials, which may be useful in the on-going fight against malaria.

Implication for health policy/practice/research/medical education:
Alchornea cordifolia possesses antiplasmodial and antioxidant properties which may be beneficial in combating malaria in the future.

Introduction

Malaria is a mosquito-borne infectious disease that affects humans and animals. It is caused by protozoans belonging to the genus *Plasmodium* (1). It is one of the most dangerous diseases in the world and is among the most prevalent communicable diseases globally (1). Apart from being a major public health problem with high morbidity and mortality, it has caused major socio-economic problems including global instability and poverty. Malaria is occurred in Africa and Asia and continues to constitute a major threat to mankind (3). *Alchornea cordifolia* is a sprawling, much-branched scandent shrub or tree that grows to about 8 m in height, especially where it is near sea and fresh-water. It is dispersed throughout all countries of the Region and widespread across tropical Africa (4)· The English people call it *chrismas bush*, the Igbos (*Ubebe*), the Efiks and Ibibios of southern Nigeria, *mbom*. It is commonly used as a medicinal plant throughout its area of distribution for treatment of malaria. The leaves or leafy stems are used to treat a variety of respiratory conditions such as sore throat, cough and bronchitis, genital-urinary problems including venereal diseases, female sterility, and gastric ulcers, diarrhoea, amoebic dysentery and helminthic infections. It is used as purgative, enema and emetic in high doses when taken orally (4). It is also taken as a blood purifier, as a tonic and to treat anaemia and epilepsy. In Senegal the leaf decoction is taken to treat tachycardia (5).

The phytochemical constituents of the leaf extract include anthraquinones, saponins, flavonoids, tannins,

*Corresponding author: Ette Ettebong, Email: ettebong@yahoo.com

steroidal and cardiac glycosides (6). The roots and stem bark have been reported to contain terpenoids, steroid glycosides, flavonoids, tannins, saponins, carbohydrates and the imidazopyrimidine alkaloids such as alchorneine, alchornidine and several guanidine alkaloids (7). The results of tests on anti-HIV activities of the seed extract are inconclusive. Tests done in Africa have shown that HIV-1 strains were sensitive to the seed extract whereas American tests seemed inconclusive. Methanol or ethanol extracts of leaf and root at a concentration of 100 μg/mL did not show cytotoxic activity against 60 different tumor cell lines from 8 organs (8). The ethanol extracts of the leaf and fruit have trypanocidal, anthelminthic and amoebicidal activities. The amoebicidal activity of the root bark was even much higher (9). The ethanol extract of the leaf produced mild in-vitro properties against *Plasmodium falciparum*, whereas chloroform and ether extracts were inactive (10). There is little or no scientific literature on the in vivo antimalarial activities of this plant. This study was therefore embarked upon so as to find out if this plant has in vivo antimalarial potential and hence lend support for its ethnobotanical use.

Materials and Methods

Plant preparation

Leaves of *A. cordifolia* were collected during the month of November, 2015 at Ibiono, Akwa Ibom state, Nigeria. It was identified and authenticated by Prof. Margret Bassey, a taxonomist in the Department of Botany and Ecological Studies, University of Uyo, where a voucher specimen (UUH3501) was deposited. The fresh leaves of *A. cordifolia* were collected and air-dried at room temperature. The dried leaves were then pulverized using a manual blender and 1.8 kg of powder-dried plant was cold-macerated in 12 L methanol at room temperature for 72 hours and thereafter filtered. The filtrate was dried *in vacuo* using rotary evaporator to obtain 215.7 g of dried extract. One hundred grams of the dried extract was partitioned using various solvents: n-hexane, chloroform, ethyl acetate, butanol and water to obtain their fractions (20.5 g, 18.3 g, 15.2 g, 12.4 g and 27 g). The crude extract and its fractions were stored in refrigerator at -4°C until needed.

Phytochemical screening

The extract was screened for phytochemical constituents such as saponins, alkaloids, flavonoids, anthraquinones, phlobotannins and cardiac glycosides using standard procedures (11,12).

Animal stock

Adult albino mice were obtained from the Animal House University of Jos and were maintained in the University of Uyo Animal House and fed with grower pellet feed. Water was given as needed. Ethical approval for the use of animals was obtained from the Animal Ethics Committee of the Faculty of Pharmacy, University of Uyo.

Micro-organisms

A chloroquine-sensitive strain of *Plasmodium berghei* was obtained from National Institute of Medical Research (NIMER) in Lagos and maintained by sub-passage in mice.

Inoculum preparation

The mice were inoculated intraperitoneally with 0.2 mL of infected blood containing about 1×10^7 *P. berghei* parasitized erythrocytes. This was prepared by determining both the percentage of parasitaemia and the erythrocytes count of the donor mouse, and the blood was diluted with isotonic saline in proportions according to both determinations.

Drug administration

Artesunate, chloroquine and pyrimethamine, extract and fractions used in the antiplasmodial study were orally administered using a stainless metallic feeding cannula.

Acute toxicity test

This was carried out to ascertain the median lethal dose using Lorke's method (13). Adult albino mice were fasted overnight and thereafter administered with different doses of the crude extract and observed for 2 hours and the mortality was recorded for 24 hours. Mortality, body weight changes and spontaneous motor activity were assessed in mice.

Antimalarial activities of the extract

Evaluation of suppressive activity of the crude extract (4-day test)

A 4-day suppressive test was determined as described by Knight and Peters and modified by Ettebong et al (14). On the first day (D_0), 36 mice were inoculated with the parasite and randomly divided into 6 groups of 6 mice in each group. Ten minutes later, the mice in group one were orally administered with 10 mL/kg of distilled water and served as control group. Group 2-4 received 120 mg/kg, 240 mg/kg and 360 mg/kg of crude extract, respectively. Group 5 and 6 recieved chloroquine and artesunate (standard drugs at 5 mg/kg each) as positive controls. The administration of the extract and drug was continued for 4 consecutive days.

On the fifth day, thin blood film was made from tail blood of each mouse and stained with Leishman stain to reveal parasitized erythrocytes. The percentage of parasitaemia was calculated by counting the number of parasitized red blood cells out of 500 erythrocytes in random fields of microscope using Neubaure counting chamber.

$$\%\ Parasitaemia = \frac{No. of\ parasitized\ erythrocyte}{Total\ No. of\ RBC\ counted} \times 100$$

Average percentage of chemo-suppression was calculated

as $100(\frac{A-B}{A})$

Where, A is the average percentage of parasitaemia in negative control group and B, average percentage of parasitaemia in the test group.

Evaluation of prophylactic or repository activities of extract
The prophylactic property of the extract was evaluated using the method described by Peters and modified by Ettebong et al (14,15). Mice were randomly divided into 5 groups of 6 mice each. Group one was orally administered with 10 mL/kg of distilled water and served as control. Group 2-4 recieved 120 mg/kg, 240 mg/kg and 360 mg/kg of crude extract respectively. Group 5 received pyrimethamine (1.2 mg/kg) each as positive control. Administration of the extract/drug was continued for 3 consecutive days (D_0-D_2). On the fourth day (D_3) the mice were inoculated with *P. berghei* infected red blood cells. The level of parasitaemia was assessed using blood smears 72 hours later. Percentage parasitaemia and average chemosuppression were calculated as stated above.

Evaluation of curative activities of the crude extract (Rane's test)
The antiplasmodial activity of the extract in established infection was done using the method of Ryley and Peters and modified by Ettebong et al (14,16). *P. berghei* infected red blood cells was injected into another 36 mice (i.p) on the first day. Seventy-two hours later, the mice were randomly divided into 6 groups of 6 mice each. Group 1 was orally administered with 10 ml/kg of distilled water as negative control. Group 2-4 recieved 120 mg/kg, 240 mg/kg and 360 mg/kg of crude extract respectively. Groups 5 and 6 recieved chloroquine and artesunate (5 mg/kg each) and served as positive controls. The extracts and drugs were administered once daily for 5 days. Tail blood sample from each mouse was collected daily for 5 days. Leishman's stain and thin smears were then prepared from tail blood samples collected daily to monitor parasitaemia level. The mean survival time (MST) of each group was determined over a period of 30days (D_0-D_{30}).

$$MST = \frac{No.of\ days\ survived}{Total\ No.of\ days\ (30)} \times 100$$

Evaluation of suppressive activity of the fractions (4-day test)
The method of Ettebong et al (14) and Knight and Peters (17) was used to evaluate the suppressive effect of the fractions. Forty-two mice were each inoculated on the first day (day 0), intraperitoneally with 0.2 mL of infected blood and randomly divided into 7 groups of 6 mice each. Group 1 was orally administered with 10 mL/kg of distilled water and served as control group. The mice in groups 2, 3, 4 and 5 were administered with n-hexane, chloroform, ethyl acetate, butanol or aqueous fraction of the extract, respectively while groups 6 and 7 were administered with chloroquine and artesunate (5 mg/kg respectively). On the fifth day, thin blood film was made and stained with Leishman's stain to reveal parasitized erythrocytes. The average percentage suppression of parasitaemia was calculated.

In vitro antioxidant activity
Reducing power assay
The reducing power of n-hexane, ethyl acetate, chloroform, and aqueous extract of *Alchornea cordifolia* was determined using various concentrations of the plant extract and fractions. To 1.0 mL of deionized water was added phosphate buffer (2.5 mL) and 2.5 mL of potassium ferricyanide (30 mM) and incubated at 50°C for 20 minutes. Then 2.5 mL of trichloroacetic acid of the solution was mixed with 2.5 mL of distilled water and 0.5 mL of $FeCl_3$ and its absorbance was recorded at 700 nm (18).

Nitric oxide scavenging assay
In this model, 3.0 mL of 10 mM sodium nitroprusside in phosphate buffer was added to 2.0 mL of extract/fractions and reference compound at different concentrations (20-100 ug/mL). The solution obtained was thereafter incubated at 25°C for 60 minutes. The procedure was repeated with methanol as blank, serving as control. To 5.0 mL of the incubated sample, 5.0 mL of Griess reagent (1% sulphanilamide, 0.1% naphthyethylene diamide dihydrochloride in 2% of H_3PO_3) was added and the absorbance of the chromophore formed was read at 540 nm (19.)

Hydrogen peroxide radical scavenging (H2O2) assay
The radical scavenging property of the extracts to hydrogen peroxide (H_2O_2) was determined using a solution of hydrogen peroxide (40 mM) prepared in phosphate buffer, pH 7.4. The concentration of hydrogen peroxide was assayed by absorption at 230 nm using a spectrophotometer. The extracts (0.5-2.5 µg/mL) in distilled water were added to a hydrogen peroxide solution and the absorbance was read at 230 nm after ten minutes against a blank solution containing phosphate buffer without hydrogen peroxide. Ascorbic acid was used as the standard (19).

Determination of DPPH radical scavenging activity
A dose of 0.2 mL of the crude extract and fractions was added to 3.8 mL of ethanol solution of DPPH radical until a final concentration of 0.1 mM was obtained (20). The mixture was agitated vigorously for 1 minute and left to stand at room temperature for 30 minutes. The absorbance of each of the samples (As) was read at 517 nm against ethanol as blank. Negative control (A) was taken after adding DPPH solution to 0.2 mL of the respective

extracts. The percentage of DPPH discolouration of the sample was calculated according to the equation.

$$\% \text{ inhibition} = A - \frac{A_s}{A} \times 100$$

Where A is the absorbance for control and As is the absorbance for test.

Statistical analysis

Results were expressed as multiple comparisons of mean ± SEM. Significance was determined using One-way analysis of variance (ANOVA) followed by Tukey-Kramer multiple comparison post-test. A probability level of 5% or less was considered significant.

Results

The median lethal dose (LD_{50}) was calculated to be 1200 mg/kg. The phytochemical screening of the extract showed the presence of alkaloids, flavonoids, saponins, tannins, terpenes, cardiac glycosides and carbohydrates. In the suppressive test (Table 1), there was a dose-dependent decrease in the level of parasitaemia following administration of the extract compared to control group. This decrease was statistically significant (P<0.05-0.001). However, the suppressive effect was less compared with the standard drugs chloroquine and artesunate. The ethyl acetate fraction had the highest chemo-suppressive effect followed by n-hexane, aqueous, butanol and chloroform fractions, respectively as shown in Table 2. In the repository test, the methanol extract of *A. cordifolia* exerted a dose-dependent prophylactic activity at the various doses employed, resulting in significant (P<0.05-0.001) reduction of parasitaemia in extract treated groups when compared to control as shown in Table 3. The extract showed a dose-dependent effect on the parasitaemia. In the curative test, there was a significant dose-dependent antiplasmodial activity of the extract when tested on established infection, which was comparable to chloroquine and artesunate-treated group (Figure 1). The negative control group showed daily increase in parasitaemia. The MSTs of the extract treated groups of mice increased dose-dependently and significantly. The extract increased the MST from 5 to 15 days when compared to control group. However, when compared to standard drug (chloroquine and artesunate), the MSTs were shorter (Table 4).

The antioxidant activity of the extract was demonstrated using Nitric oxide, DPPH, Hydrogen peroxide and reducing power assays. In the nitric oxide scavenging test, the extract and fractions effectively reduced the generation of nitric oxide. When compared with the standard drug, aqueous fraction had more inhibitory effect, followed by crude extract and ethyl acetate fractions (Figure 2).

In the DPPH quenching capacity, the extract and fractions of *A. cordifolia* were capable of neutralizing the DPPH free radicals via hydrogen donating activity at different concentrations. Scavenging activity was increased in a concentration dependent manner. However, ethyl acetate had the highest inhibitory activity when compared with the control, vitamin C (Figure 3).

Table 1. Suppressive antiplasmodial activity of methanol extract of *Alchornea cordifolia*

Drug/extract	Dose (mg/kg)	Parasitaemia (×10^7)	% Chemosuppression
Distilled water	10 mL/kg	50.00 ± 1.00	-
Extract	120	12.00 ± 0.50^a	76.00
	240	4.80 ± 0.50^a	90.40
	360	4.20 ± 0.08^a	91.60
Artesunate	5.0	0.66 ± 0.05^a	98.80
Chloroquine	5.0	0.30 ± 0.50^a	99.40

Values are expressed as mean ± SEM.

Significance relative to control: $^a P$ < 0.001; n = 6.

Table 2. Suppressive antiplasmodial activity of fractions of *Alchornea cordifolia*

Drug/extract	Dose (mg/kg)	Parasitaemia (×10^7)	% Chemosuppression
Distilled water	10 mL/kg	35.50 ± 0.40	-
Ethylacetate fraction	240	8.50 ± 0.66^a	76.20
N-hexane fraction	240	14.00 ± 0.15^a	60.50
Aqeous fraction	240	16.30 ± 0.66^a	54.00
Butanol fraction	240	22.70 ± 0.20^a	36.00
Chloroform fraction	240	24.40 ± 0.54^a	31.30
Chloroquine	5.0	0.20 ± 0.00^a	99.40

Values are expressed as mean ± SEM.

Significance relative to control: $^a P$ < 0.001; n = 6.

Table 3. Prophylactic antiplasmodial activity of methanolic extract of *Alchornea cordifolia*

Drug/extract	Dose (mg/kg)	Parasitaemia (×10^7)	% Chemosuppression
Distilled water	10 mL/kg	35.20 ± 0.80	-
Extract	120	20.60 ± 0.50^a	27.30
	240	12.10 ± 0.57^a	65.60
	360	6.80 ± 0.70^a	80.00
Pyramethamine	5.0	2.00 ± 0.15^a	94.30

Values are expressed as mean ± SEM.

Significance relative to control: $^a P$ < 0.001; n = 6.

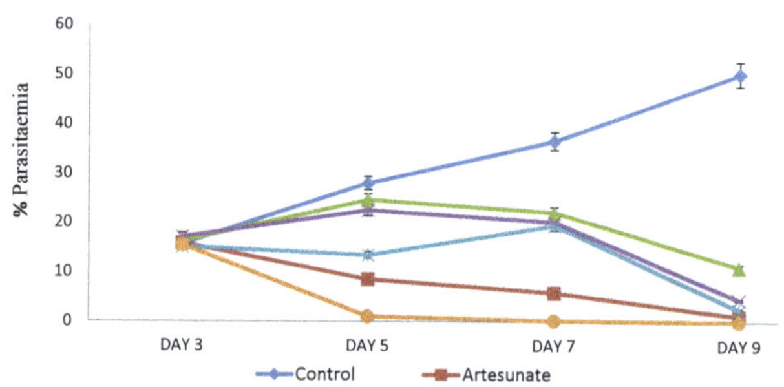

Figure 1. Antiplasmodial activity of methanolic extract *Alchornea cordifolia* during established infection (curative test).

Table 4. Mean survival time of mice receiving various doses of methanol extract of *Alchornea cordifolia*

Drug/extract	Doses (mg/kg)	MST (days)
Distilled water	10 (mL/kg)	12.67 ± 0.66
Extract	120	17.70 ± 0.66[a]
	240	23.67 ± 0.33[a]
	360	27.71 ± 0.66[a]
Artesunate	5.00	20.67 ± 0.33[a]
Chloroquine	5.00	29.33 ± 0.66[a]

Values are expressed as mean ± SEM.
Significance relative to control: [a] $P < 0.001$; n = 6.

On reducing power, the reducing power activity of methanol leaf extracts and fractions of *A. cordifolia* increased consistently with the increase in the volume of extract from 20 µg to 100 µg. The aqueous fraction showed the highest scavenging activity, but was less when compared with the standard drug, vitamin C (Figure 4). In the hydrogen peroxide test, the result showed that hydrogen peroxide scavenging activity of methanol leave extract and fractions of *A. cordifolia* increased consistently with increase in concentration of extract. It was observed that chloroform and ethyl acetate fractions showed the highest scavenging activity even more than the standard drug (Figure 5).

Discussion

In this study, the acute toxicity evaluation of the extract revealed that LD_{50} was 1200 mg/kg, which makes it slightly toxic (21). The phytochemical screening carried out on the leave extract of *A. cordifolia* revealed the presence of alkaloids, saponins, tanins, glycosides, flavonoids, terpenes and carbohydrates which likely contributed to the observed pharmacological effects. This finding confirmed the phytochemical study of the leave extract carried out by Osadebe and Okoye (6). The antimalarial activity of the crude extract and fractions of *A. cordifolia* was investigated to establish the antimalarial potentials of the plant. The results obtained show that the leaves of *A. cordifolia* significantly depicted antimalarial activity in a dose-dependent manner which is comparable to that of standard drug used. This antiplasmodial action could be as a result of various phytochemicals present in the leaf of the plant, which may be acting alone or in combination with one another to exert the observed antiplamodial effect (22).

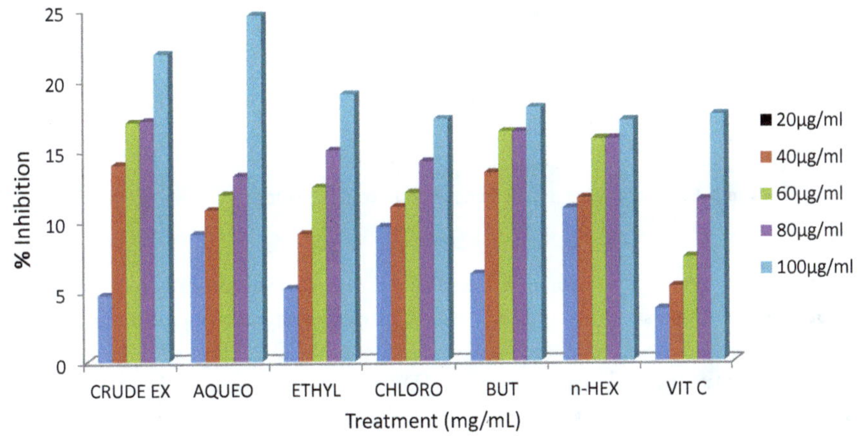

Figure 2. Effect of extract and its fractions on nitrogen oxide assay.

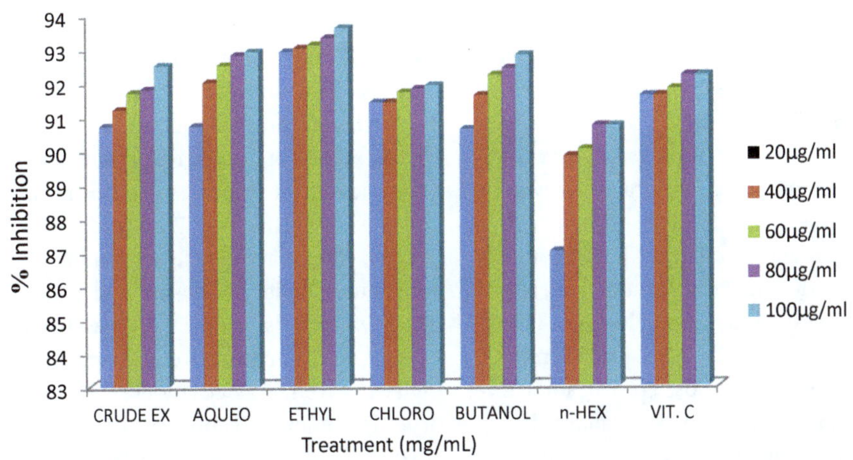

Figure 3. Effect of extract and its fractions on 1,1-diphenyl-2-picrylhydrazyl (DPPH).

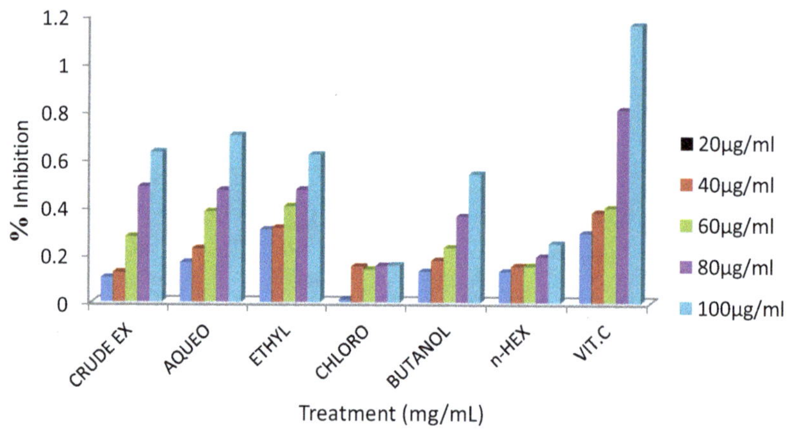

Figure 4. Effect of extract and its fractions on reducing power assay.

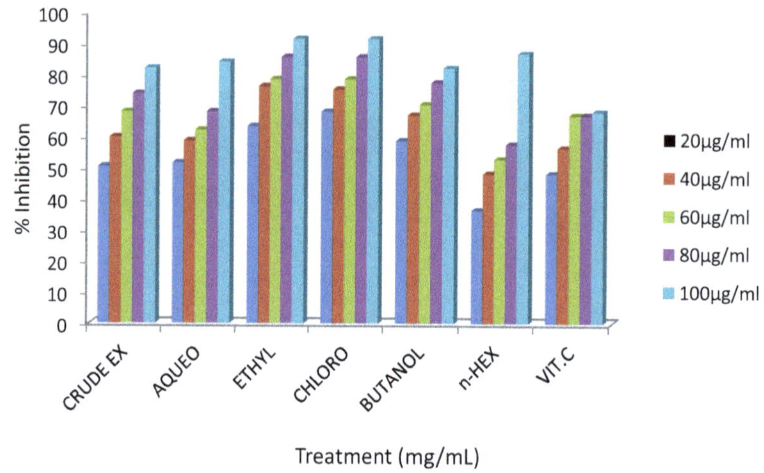

Figure 5. Effect of extract and its fractions on hydrogen peroxide.

Alkaloids have been shown to have in vitro antimalarial activity by blocking protein synthesis in *P. falciparum* (23). Flavonoids have also been reported to exert their antiplasmodial activity through chelating the nucleic acid base pairs of the malarial parasite (13). The presence of flavonoids in the leave extract of *A. cordifolia* may contribute to its antiplasmodial activity. Flavonoids may be acting in synergy with alkaloids to exhibit antimalarial effect. Flavonoids are known to inhibit the intra-erythrocytic growth of certain strains of *P. falciparum* (24,25) Tannins are reported to possess antioxidant activity (26). This could be one of the mechanisms of action against malarial parasite observed in the leave extract of *A. cordifolia*. The fractions were tested for antiplasmodial activity to determine which of the fractions has the highest activity. The fractions exhibited good antiplasmodial activity with ethyl acetate fraction exhibiting the highest antiplasmodial action. This suggests that the bioactive compounds in the plant extract are most probably non-polar compounds. The free radical scavenging potential of leave extract of *A. cordifolia* and its fractions was studied using different antioxidant models; the in vitro antioxidant activity of methanol leave extract of *A. cordifolia* was investigated for the scavenging activity of nitric oxide radical, reducing power assay, hydrogen peroxide (H_2O_2) assay and 1,1-diphenyl-2picryhydrazyl (DPPH) radical assay. From the results, a significant correlation existed between concentrations of the extract and percentage inhibition of free radicals, reducing power or inhibition of lipid peroxidation. These results suggest that the polyphenolic compounds of *A. cordifolia* play an important role in reducing ferric ions to ferrous ions and capable of donating electrons that scavenge the free radicals. The antioxidant and free radical scavenging properties of iron chelators are based on their capacities to chelate metal ions, cause reduction of ferric to ferrous ion, scavenge non-biological stable free radical such as DPPH and scavenge active biological oxidants like H_2O_2 and •OH (27,28). This may represent yet another mechanism that contributes to its antiplasmodial activity. The fractions of the extract also showed a dose-dependent scavenging activity with ethyl acetate and aqueous fractions having highest scavenging activity even more than the standard drug. This is an indication that the fractions of *A. cordifolia* are capable of reducing oxidative stress by scavenging ROS which is implicated in the pathogenesis of malaria.

Conclusion

The results of this study show that the extract of *A. cordifolia* has suppressive, repository and curative antiplasmodial properties. The fractions exhibited good antiplasmodial activity with ethyl acetate fraction exhibiting the highest antiplasmodial action. The fractions also showed a dose-dependent scavenging activity with ethyl acetate and aqueous fractions having the highest scavenging activity.

Acknowledgements

We acknowledge the technical assistance of Mr. Aniefiok Ukpong, the Department of Pharmacology and Toxicology, University of Uyo, Uyo.

Author's Contributions

EE designed the study, interpreted the results, and wrote the manuscript. AN and KD did the experiments and assisted in the writing of the manuscript.

Conflict of interests

None.

Ethical considerations

All experimental procedures involving animals were conducted in accordance to Organization for Economic Co-operation and Development guidelines and approved by Animal Ethics Committee, Faculty of Pharmacy, University of Uyo, Nigeria.

Funding/Support

Education Trust Fund (ETF) of the University of Uyo supported the study.

References

1. World Health Organization. Malaria, 1982–1997. Weekly Epidemiology Record. 2016;4:265-270.
2. Snow RW, Guerra CA, Noor AM, Myint HY, Hay SI. The global distribution of clinical episodes of Plasmodium falciparum malaria. Nature. 2005;434(7030):214-7.
3. Gallup JL, Sachs JD. The economic burden of malaria. Am J Trop Med Hyg. 2001;64(1-2 Suppl):85-96.
4. Kamara AY, Akobundu IO, Sanginga N, Jutzi SC. Effect of mulch from 14 selected multipurpose trees (mpts) on growth, nitrogen nutrition and yield of Maize (*Zea mays* L.). Journal of Agronomy and Crop Science. 2000;184(2):73–80.
5. Latham P. Useful plants of Bas-Congo Province, Democratic Republic of the Congo. London: DFID; 2004:320.
6. Osadebe PO, Okoye FB. Anti-inflammatory effects of crude methanolic extract and fractions of *Alchornea cordifolia* leaves. J Ethnopharmacol. 2003;89(1):19-24.
7. Obadoni BO, Ochuko PO. Phytochemical studies and comparative efficacy of the crude extracts of some haemostatic plants in Edo and delta states of Nigeria. Global Journal of Pure and Applied Sciences. 2002;8(2):203-8.
8. Ayisi NK, Nyadedzor C. Comparative in vitro effects of AZT and extracts of *Ocimum gratissimum, Ficus polita, Clausena anisata, Alchornea cordifolia,* and *Elaeophorbia drupifera* against HIV-1 and HIV-2 infections. Antiviral Res. 2003;58(1):25-33.
9. Adewunmi CO, Agbedahunsi JM, Adebajo AC, Aladesanmi AJ, Murphy N, Wando J. Ethno-veterinary medicine: screening of Nigerian medicinal plants for trypanocidal properties. J Ethnopharmacol. 2001;77(1):19-24.
10. Banzouzi JT, Prado R, Menan H, Valentin A, Roumestan C, Mallie M, et al. In vitro antiplasmodial activity of extracts of *Alchornea cordifolia* and identification of an active constituent: ellagic acid. J Ethnopharmacol. 2002;81(3):399-401.
11. Harborne JB. Phenolic compounds. In phytochemical methods. Netherlands: Springer; 1973:33-88.
12. Lorke D. A new approach to practical acute toxicity testing. Arch Toxicol. 1983;54(4):275-87.
13. Sofowora A. Medicinal Plants and Traditional Medicine in Africa. 24th Ed. New York: John Wiley and Sons; 1992:8.
14. Ettebong EO, Nwafor PA, Okokon JE. In vivo antiplasmodial activities of ethanolic extract and fractions of *Eleucine indica.* Asian Pac J Trop Med. 2012;5(9):673-6.
15. Peters W. Drug resistance in *Plasmodium berghei* Vincke and Lips, 1948. II. Triazine resistance. Exp Parasitol. 1965;17(1):90-6.
16. Ryley JF, Peters W. The antimalarial activity of some quinolone esters. Ann Trop Med Parasitol. 1970;64(2):209-22.
17. Knight DJ, Peters W. The antimalarial activity of N-benzyloxydihydrotriazines. Ann Trop Med Parasitol. 1980;74(4):393-404.
18. Oyaizu M. Studies on products of browning reaction-antioxidative activities of products of browning reaction prepared from glucosamine. Japanese Journal of Nutrition. 1986;44:307-15.
19. Awah FM, Verla Aw. Antioxidant activity, nitric oxide scavenging activity and phenolic contents of *Ocimum gratissimum* leaf extract. J Med Plant Res. 2010;4(23): 2479-87.
20. Nabavi SM, Ebrahimzadeh MA, Nabavi SF, Jafari M. Free radical scavenging activity and antioxidant capacity of *Eryngium caucasicum* Trautv and Froripia subpinnata. Pharmacologyonline. 2008;3:19-25.
21. Loomis JA. Essentials of Toxicology. 3rd ed. Philadelphia: Lea and Febiger; 1979:241.
22. Nergiz C, Ötleş S. Chemical composition of *Nigella sativa* L. seeds. Food Chem. 1993;48(3):259-61.
23. Liu KC, Yang SL, Roberts MF, Elford BC, Phillipson JD. Antimalarial activity of *Artemisia annua* flavonoids from whole plants and cell cultures. Plant Cell Rep. 1992;11(12):637-40.
24. Lehane AM, Saliba KJ. Common dietary flavonoids inhibit the growth of the intraerythrocytic malaria parasite. BMC Res Notes. 2008;1:26.
25. Ferreira JF, Luthria DL, Sasaki T, Heyerick A. Flavonoids from *Artemisia annua* L. as antioxidants and their potential synergism with artemisinin against malaria and cancer. Molecules. 2010;15(5):3135-70.
26. Builders MI, Tarfa F, Aguiyi JC. The potency of African Locust Bean tree as antimalarial. J Pharmacol Toxicol. 2012;7(6):274-287.
27. Adjimani JP, Asare P. Antioxidant and free radical scavenging activity of iron chelators. Toxicol Rep. 2015;2:721-8.
28. Loganayaki N, Siddhuraju P, Manian S. Antioxidant activity and free radical scavenging capacity of phenolic extracts from *Helicteres isora* L. and *Ceiba pentandra* L. J Food Sci Technol. 2013;50(4):687-95.

Ethanolic extract of anise (*Pimpinella anisum* L.) attenuates morphine physical dependence in mice

Dara Shirzadi[1], Saeid Abbasi-Maleki[2*], Ali Zanbouri[1]

[1]Physiology Department, Maragheh Branch, Islamic Azad University, Maragheh, Iran
[2]Pharmacology & Toxicology Department, Urmia Branch, Islamic Azad University, Urmia, Iran

ARTICLE INFO

Keywords:
Pimpinella anisum L.
Addiction
Morphine
Physical dependence
Mice

ABSTRACT

Introduction: Previous studies revealed that anise (*Pimpinella anisum* L.) has several pharmacological effects including analgesic, antidepressant, anxiolytic, anti-inflammatory and antispasmodic activities. This study aimed to evaluate its effect on morphine physical dependence in mice.

Methods: In this experimental study, 40 male NMRI mice (25-30 g) were randomly divided into 5 groups of 8. Control group received morphine and normal saline (10 mL/kg, i.p.) and other groups received diazepam (5 mg/kg) plus one of three doses of *P. anisum* (50,100 or 200 mg/kg, i.p.). Dependence was induced by administration of increasing doses (50-75 mg/kg, i.p.) of morphine. A time of 30 minutes after naloxone injection was considered for the critical period of the withdrawal syndrome. The number of jumps and scores of 0 to 3 were given for incidences of wet dog shakes, teeth chattering, climbing, writing, diarrhea, grooming, and rearing during a 30-minute period.

Results: All doses of *P. anisum* ($P<0.01$) reduced the number of jumps. Additionally, all doses of the extract reduced the behaviors of grooming ($P<0.05$, $P<0.01$ and $P<0.01$, respectively) and writhing ($P<0.05$, $P<0.001$and $P<0.001$, respectively). None doses of the extract could reduce diarrhea ($P>0.05$). Climbing, rearing and wet dog shakes reduced only by the high dose of the extract ($P<0.05$). Teeth chattering reduced by 100 and 200 mg/kg of the extract ($P<0.05$).

Conclusion: These results obviously show that *P. anisum* ethanolic extract is effective in suppression of morphine physical dependence and further studies are needed to find out the responsible constituents and also the exact mechanisms of actions.

Implication for health policy/practice/research/medical education:
Opioid dependence is a major health problem in worldwide. The present study findings suggest that the plant anise (*Pimpinella anisum* L) is effective in suppression of some aspects of opioid (e.g. morphine) physical dependence in addicts related to morphine withdrawal and might be beneficial in these patients.

Introduction

Opioid dependence is a major health problem worldwide that often requires long-term treatment and care. Morphine is one of the major opioid analgesics mainly used for alleviating pain and chronic diarrhea. But, its repeated use leads to physical dependence and tolerance (1). Furthermore, after abrupt cessation of morphine or an administration of opioid antagonist (e.g. naloxone), withdrawal signs will appear (2). Today, pharmacotherapies for opioid addiction include administration of opioid agonists (e.g. methadone), partial agonists (e.g. buprenorphine), opioid antagonists (e.g. naltrexone), and alpha-2-adrenergic agonists (e.g. clonidine), which are targeted toward either detoxification or long-term agonist maintenance (3). Several medicinal herbs including *Cymbopogon citratus, Avena sativa, Carthamus tinctorius, Rosa damascena, Otostegia percica, Carum copticum,* and *Rodmarinus officinalis* have been investigated for the treatment of some aspects of morphine dependence in animal models of drug dependence (4-11).

Pimpinella anisum L. form Apiaceae (Umbelliferae) family grows in different parts of Mediterranean countries and Iran. In Iranian traditional medicine, *P. anisum* is used for treating gastrointestinal and nervous system disorders. Previous phytochemical studies revealed that the prominent component of *P. anisum* is 1.5%–6.0% essential oil consisting primarily of *trans*-anethole. Other studies demonstrated the presence of eugenol,

***Corresponding author:** Saeid Abbasi-Maleki,
Email: s.abbasi@iaurmia.ac.ir

trans-anethole, methyl chavicol, anisaldehyde, estragole, coumarins, scopoletin, umbelliferone, estrols, terpene hydrocarbons, polyenes, and polyacetylenes as the other major components of the essential oil (12,13). *P. anisum* L. extract and essential oil showed different biological and pharmacological activities including antispasmodic, analgesic, anticonvulsant, antibacterial and laxative effects, as well as alleviating morphine dependence property (14-18). Furthermore, our recent study revealed the antidepressant - like effects of *P. anisum* in animal models of depression (19). Hence, the aim of the present study was to investigate the effect of *P. anisum* ethanolic extract on morphine physical dependence in mice.

Materials and Methods

Preparation of extract

Fruits of *P. anisum* were obtained from a local market in Urmia, Iran. *P. anisum* authenticated in the herbarium unit of the school of pharmacy, Tehran University of Medical Science, Tehran, Iran (Voucher No. 723.2). The fruits were dried in shadow and pulverized using a grinder-mixer. Then, 50 g dried fruits powder was macerated separately for 48 hours in 200 mL 70% (v/v) ethanol for extraction. The solvent of the extracts was removed at room temperature to be dried, and the dried extract was kept in clean vials in cool conditions.

Animals

Male NMRI mice 25-30 g were used for the study. They had free access to food and water and maintained at 25 ± 1°C with a 12-h light/12-h dark cycle. All experiments were carried out in accordance with guidelines of National Institutes of Health guide for the care and use of Laboratory animals (NIH Publications No. 8023, revised 1978).

Induction of morphine physical dependence

Morphine was injected i.p. into mice at doses of 50, 50 and 75 mg/kg three times daily (9:00 AM, 13:00 and 17:00 PM, respectively) for 3 days. On the fourth day, a single dose of morphine (50 mg/kg) was injected 2 hours before naloxone treatment (20).

Naloxone-precipitated withdrawal syndrome

Two hours after the last injection of morphine (50 mg/kg), withdrawal signs were elicited by i.p. injection of naloxone hydrochloride (5 mg/kg). The signs were recorded during a 30-minute period starting immediately after naloxone injection. Jumping's were counted, but other checked signs including grooming, rearing, diarrhea, climbing, teeth chattering, writing and wet dog shakes were evaluated with one point given for the presence of each sign during each period (range of scores: 0-3) (7,21).

Experimental design and animal grouping

Mice were randomly divided into 5 groups (8 mice per group):

1- One chronically i.p. injected morphine (as a negative control group): In this group normal saline (10 mL/kg) was administered i.p. Thirty minutes after the last dose of morphine and 30 minutes later, naloxone was injected.

2- One chronically i.p. injected morphine (as a positive control group): In this group diazepam (5 mg/kg) was administered i.p. Thirty min after the last dose of morphine and 30 minutes later, naloxone was injected.

3- Three chronically i.p. injected morphine (as a treatment group): In this group, different doses of *P. anisum* L. (50, 100 or 200 mg/kg, i.p.) ethanolic extract were administered i.p. Thirty minutes after the last dose of morphine and 30 minutes later, naloxone was injected (19).

Statistical analysis

Statistical analysis was performed using SPSS version 19 software for Windows. The results were expressed as mean ± standard error of the mean (SEM). One-way analysis of variance (ANOVA) followed by Tukey test was used for comparison of data and *P* values less than 0.05 were considered significant. The Mann-Whitney U test was used for comparison of checked signs data.

Results

The results demonstrated that acute administration of *P. anisum* hydro-ethanolic extract at doses of 50, 100 and 200 mg/kg significantly reduced the number of jumping episodes compared to control group ($P<0.01$) (Figure 1). Diazepam, as a standard drug, significantly reduced the number of jumping episodes ($P<0.01$) (Table 1). All doses of the extract significantly decreased grooming ($P<0.05$, $P<0.01$ and $P<0.01$, respectively) and writhing ($P<0.05$). Only 100 and 200 mg/kg of the extract significantly reduced teeth chattering behavior ($P<0.05$). Diazepam group compared to control group significantly reduced other signs such as grooming ($P<0.01$), teeth chattering ($P<0.05$), climbing ($P<0.05$), rearing ($P<0.05$), writhing ($P<0.05$), wet dog shakes and diarrhea ($P<0.01$) (Table 1).

Discussion

The aim of the present study was to evaluate the effect of the *P. anisum* hydro-alcoholic extract on morphine

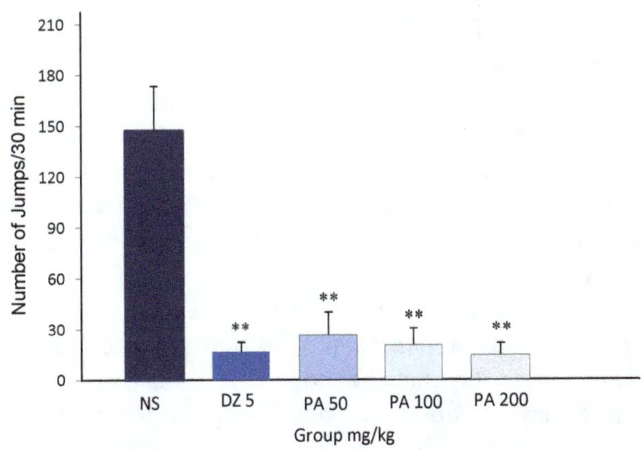

Figure 1. The effect of different doses of *Pimpinella anisum* on number of jumping during 30 min. Normal Saline: NS (10 mL/kg, i.p.); DZ: Diazepam (5 mg/kg, i.p.); *P. anisum*: PA (50-200 mg/kg, i.p.) (n = 8, mean ± SEM, ** $P<0.01$ compared to NS group, Tukey test).

Table 1. The effect of different doses of *Pimpinella anisum* on morphine withdrawal signs

Treatment/Group	Grooming	Teeth chattering	Climbing	Rearing	Wet dog shakes	Writhing	Diarrhea
Control (NS)	2 ± (2-3)	2 ± (1.5-3)	2 ± (1-2.5)	3 ± (1-3)	1 ± (1-2)	2 ± (1.5-3)	3 ± (2-3)
Diazepam 5 mg/kg	1 ± (0-1)**	1 ± (0.5-1)*	1 ± (0-1)*	1 ± (0-1)*	1 ± (0-1.5)	0 ± (0-1)*	1 ± (0-1)**
Mann-Whitney U	0.0	2.0	3	3.0	6.5	1	0
PA 50 mg/kg	1 ± (0.5-1.5)*	1 ± (1-2)	1 ± (1-2)	1 ± (1-2)	1 ± (0.5-2)	1 ± (0-1.5)*	2 ± (2-2.5)
Mann-Whitney U	0	7	9	7	10	3	7.5
PA 100 mg/kg	1 ± (0.5-1)**	0 ± (0-1.5)*	1 ± (1-1)	1 ± (1-1)	1 ± (0.5-1)	1 ± (0-1.5)*	2 ± (1.5-2.5)
Mann-Whitney U	1.5	2.5	5	5	6	3	6.5
PA 200 mg/kg	1 ± (1-1)**	1 ± (0-1.75)*	1 ± (0.5-1)*	1 ± (0.5-1)*	1 ± (0.5-1)*	1 ± (0.5-1.5)*	2 ± (2-2.5)
Mann-Whitney U	0	3	4	4	4	3.5	7.5

The upper numbers show the median, and the numbers in the parenthesis show the range of scores (n = 8, Median, *$P < 0.05$ and **$P < 0.01$; statistically significant between test groups and NS group, respectively).
NS, normal saline; PA, *Pimpinella anisum*: PA

physical dependence in mice. In the present study, the increasing doses of morphine over a four-day schedule followed by naloxone injection produced full-blown withdrawal signs. This method was used to evaluate the ability of the essential oil to inhibit morphine withdrawal signs such as jumping, grooming, teeth chattering, climbing, wet dog shakes, writing and diarrhea. In the naloxone-precipitated withdrawal signs, acute injection of *P. anisum*, 1 hour after the last injection of morphine significantly reduced withdrawal signs. Jumping is one of the main opioid dependence signs. The results indicate that different doses of *P. anisum* and diazepam (as a positive control) are able to reduce the number of jumping in morphine-dependent mice. Also, in line with other findings, the present results showed that diazepam (as a positive control) reduced the number of jumping (20,22). Results showed that the extract reduced grooming behavior. In agreement with these results Bekar et al showed that the aqueous extract of *P. anisum* reduced the grooming behavior in open field test (23). In line with other findings that revealed the antispasmodic effects of *P. anisum*, the present results demonstrated that all doses of extract could reduce the writing behavior in morphine-dependent mice (24). Additionally, all doses of the extract reduced the behaviors of grooming, climbing, writhing, and teeth chattering. None of the used doses of the extract could reduce diarrhea significantly. In this regard, previous studies revealed the significant laxative effect of *P. anisum* when compared with placebo (17). Wet dog shakes reduced only by high dose (200 mg/kg) of the extract. Diazepam significantly suppressed other checked signs except for wet dog shakes.

Several investigations revealed that anethole is a major compound of *P. anisum* (15,25). On the other hand, Anethole is a terpenoid, found in the essential oil of anise, fennel (*Foeniculum vulgare*) and several other plants. In previous studies the antidepressant-like activity of the aqueous and ethanolic extract of *P. anisum* was attributed to anethole (19). In this regard, previous studies revealed that antidepressants might directly or indirectly decrease the abuse potential of opioids by affecting their rewarding effect or improving depressed mood resulting from opioid withdrawal, respectively (26). In line with these findings, Sahraei et al showed that essential oil of *P. anisum* might induce conditioned place aversion (CPA) in morphine-dependent mice. This may indicate that the essential oil of this plant has some aversive effects as investigated by place conditioning method. Also, they suggested that this oil has a GABAergic action. In support of this claim, pretreatment of animals with bicuculline (a GABA-A receptor antagonist) but not CGP35348 (a GABA-B receptor antagonist) inhibited the suppressive effect of the essential oil on morphine-induced conditioned place preference (CPP) (16).

Gamma-aminobutyric acid (GABA) is one of the major inhibitory neurotransmitters in the central nervous system (27). Previous studies have shown that GABAergic system is able to play a key role in the development of morphine-induced physical dependence (28,29). It has been reported that morphine causes an increase in the whole brain GABA concentration in mice. Previous studies have reported that in separate parts of the thalamus and the spinal cord of the addicted rats, GABA is increased (30,31). In support of this hypothesis, pretreatment of mice with benzodiazepines (e.g. midazolam and diazepam) suppresses morphine withdrawal signs (23,32).

Apart from anethole, *P. anisum* contains essential oil and different polyphenols including flavonoids. In line with our findings; previous studies revealed the suppressive effect of polyphenolic compounds on morphine withdrawal signs (10,33). Some flavonoids including quercetin, 3-glucuronide, rutin, and luteolin 7-glucoside were isolated from *P. anisum*. Previous studies revealed that some flavonoids decrease the morphine physical dependence (10,34). However, it may be suggested that anethole, the major component of *P. anisum*, is implicated in reducing the withdrawal syndrome in morphine-dependent mice.

Conclusion

In conclusion, the results of this study revealed that *P. anisum* L. could prevent some major signs of morphine withdrawal signs and might be beneficial in morphine dependence. Nevertheless, further studies need for determining its exact mechanism of action.

Author's contributions

SAM had a role in hypothesis making, designing the study, data analysis and preparation of the manuscript. DSH contributed to data acquisition and data collection. All authors read and approved the final manuscript.

Acknowledgments

This study was extracted from an MSc thesis (No.14750368931001) at Maragheh Branch, Islamic Azad University, Maragheh, Iran. The authors are grateful to Temad Co. for providing morphine sulfate purified powder.

Conflict of interests

The authors declare no conflict of interest.

Ethical considerations

In the present study, all experiments were carried out in accordance with guidelines of National Institutes of Health guide for the care and use of Laboratory animals (NIH Publications No. 8023, revised 1978).

Funding/Support

This project was funded by the personal finances of the authors.

References

1. Praveen KT, Law F, O'Shea J, Melichar J. Opioid dependence. Am Fam Physician. 2012;86(6):565-6.
2. Babhadiashar N, Vaseghi G, Rafieian-Kopaei M, Andalib S, Eshraghi A, Masoudian N. Neural mechanisms underlying morphine withdrawal in addicted patients: a review. Rev Clin Med. 2015;2(3):151-7.
3. Stotts AL, Dodrill CL, Kosten TR. Opioid dependence treatment: Options in pharmacotherapy. Expert Opin Pharmacother. 2009;10(11):1727-40.
4. Ahmadi Sheikh-Sarmast H, Abbasi-Maleki S. Naloxone-precipitated morphine withdrawal in male mice is attenuated by acute administration of hydroalcoholic extract of *Cymbopogon citratus* (Lemon Grass). Indian J Nat Sci. 2015;5(15):4743-9.
5. Abbasi-Maleki F, Abbasi Maleki S, Mousavi SZ. Khayatnouri MH. Effect of hydroalcoholic extract of Avena sativa L. on morphine withdrawal signs in male mice. J Sabzevar Univ Med Sci. 2014 ;20(4):408-14.
6. Abbasi-Maleki S. Effect of ethanolic extract of Safflower on naloxone-induced morphine withdrawal signs in mice. Adv Herb Med. 2015;1(4):9-15.
7. Abbasi Maleki N, Abbasi Maleki S, Bekhradi R. Suppressive effects of *Rosa damascena* essential oil on naloxone-precipitated morphine withdrawal signs in male mice. Iran J Pharmaceutic Res. 2013;12(3):357-61.
8. Hajhashemi V, Rabbani M, Asghari MR, Karami-Saravi Z. Effect of otostegia persica on naloxone-induced morphine withdrawal syndrome in mice. Iran J Pharmaceutic Res. 2004;3:171-5.
9. Hosseinzadeh H, Nourbakhsh M. Effect of *Rosmarinus officinalis* L. aerial parts extract on morphine withdrawal syndrome in mice. Phytother Res. 2003;17(8):938-41.
10. Ghannadi A, Hajhashemi V, Abrishami R. Effects of the Persian *Carum copticum* fruit extracts on morphine withdrawal syndrome in mice. Res Pharm Sci. 2012;7(3):127–31.
11. Abbasi Maleki S, Godarzi M, Mousavi SZ, Kor N. Morphine withdrawal symptoms improvement by *Ziziphora tenuior* L. ethanoic extract in male mice. Koomesh. 2016;17(4):990-5.
12. Salehi-Surmaghi MH. Medicinal plants and phytotherapy. 3rd ed. Tehran: Donyay Taghziah Press; 2010:81-3.
13. Zargari A. Medicinal Plants. 7th ed. Teharn: Tehran University Press; 2011: 532-7.
14. Heidari MR, Ayeli M. Effects of methyl alcoholic extract of *Pimpinella anisum* L. on picrotoxin induced seizure in mice and its probable mechanism. Sci J Kurdestan Univ of Med Sci. 2005; 10(3):1-8.
15. Shojai A, Abdollahi-Fard M. Review of pharmacological properties and chemical constituents of *Pimpinella anisum*. ISRN Pharm. 2012;2012:510795.
16. Sahraei H, Ghoshooni H, Hossein-Salimi S, et al. The effects of fruit essential oil of the *Pimpinella anisum* on acquisition and expression of morphine induced conditioned place preference in mice. J Ethnopharmacol. 2002;80(1):43-7.
17. Tas A, Ozbek H, Atasoy N, Altug ME, Ceylan E. Evaluation of analgesic and anti-inflammatory activity of *Pimpinella anisum* fixed oil extract. Indian Vet J. 2006;83(8):840-3.
18. Shahamat Z, Abbasi-Maleki S, Mohammadi-Motamed S. Evaluation of antidepressant-like effects of aqueous and ethanolic extracts of *Pimpinella anisum* fruit in mice. Avicenna J Phytomed. 2016;6(3):322-8.
19. Hosseinzadeh H, Parvardeh S, Masoudi A, Moghimi M, Mahboobifard F. Attenuation of morphine tolerance and dependence by thymoquinone in mice. Avicenna J Phytomed. 2016;6(1):55-66.
20. Rabbani M, Jafarian A , Sobhanian M. Comparison between acute and long-term effects of verapamil on naloxone -induced morphine withdrawal in mice. J Res Med Sci. 2004;1:26-33.
21. Broseta I, Rodríguez-Arias M, Stinus L, Miñarro J. Ethological analysis of morphine withdrawal with different dependence programs in male mice. Prog Neuropsychopharmacol Biol Psychiatry. 2002;26(2):335-347.
22. Bekara A, Hamadouche NA, Kahloula K, Harouat S, Tabbas D, Aoues AEK. Effect of Pimpinella anisum L (Aniseed) Aqueous Extract against Lead(Pb)Neurotoxicity: Neurobehavioral Study. Int J Neurosci Behav Sci. 2015;3(3): 32-40.
23. Tirapelli CR, de Andrade CR, Cassano AO, et al. Antispasmodic and relaxant effects of the hydroalcoholic extract of *Pimpinella anisum* (Apiaceae) on rat anococcygeus smooth muscle. J Ethnopharmacol. 2007;110(1):23-9.
24. EL-Hodairy FA. Neuroprotective effects of *Pimpinella anisum* on neurotoxicity induced by bisphenol an on normal and diabetic rat. Int J Pharm Pharm Sci. 2014;6(3):9-12.
25. Maldonado R. Participation of noradrenergic pathways in the expression of opiate withdrawal: biochemical and pharmacological evidence. Neurosci Biobehav Rev. 1997; 21(1):91-104.
26. Ayromlou H, Masoudian N, Ahmadi-Asl N, et al. Evaluation of chronic and acute effects of Gabapentin on

passive avoidance learning process in mice. J Chemical Health Risks. 2014;4(3):33-40.

27. Heikkilä AT, Echenko O, Uusi-Oukari M, Sinkkonen ST, Korpi ER. Morphine withdrawal increases expression of GABA(A) receptor epsilon subunit mRNA in locus coeruleus neurons. Neuroreport. 2001;12(13):2981-5.
28. Xi ZX, Stein EA. GABAergic mechanisms of opiate reinforcement. Alcohol. 2002;37(5):485-94.
29. Nakamura S, Kakinohana M, Taira Y, Iha H, Sugahara K. The effect of gamma-aminobutyric acid (GABA) receptor drugs on morphine-induced spastic paraparesis after a noninjurious interval of spinal cord ischemia in rats. Anesth Analg. 2002;95(5):1389-95.
30. Bajo M, Roberto M, Madamba SG, Siggins GR. Neuroadaptation of GABAergic transmission in the central amygdala during chronic morphine treatment. Addict Biol. 2011;16(4):551-64.
31. Cao JL, Ding HL, Zhang LC, Duan SM, Zeng YM. Pretreatment with midazolam suppresses morphine withdrawal response in mice and rats. Acta Pharmacol Sin. 2002;23(8):685-90.
32. Naidu PS, Singh A, Joshi D, Kulkarni SK. Possible mechanisms of action in quercetin reversal of morphine tolerance and dependence. Addict Biol. 2003;8(3):327-36.
33. Hanrahan JR, Chebib M, Johnston GA. Flavonoid modulation of GABA(A) receptors. Br J Pharmacol. 2011;163(2):234-45.

13

Zataria multiflora Boiss: A review study on chemical composition, anti-fungal and anti-mycotoxin activities, and ultrastructural changes

Hojjatollah Shokri[1]*, Aghil Sharifzadeh[2]

[1]Department of Pathobiology, Faculty of Veterinary Medicine, Amol University of Special Modern Technologies, Amol, Iran
[2]Mycology Research Center, Faculty of Veterinary Medicine, University of Tehran, Tehran, Iran

ARTICLE INFO

Keywords:
Zataria multiflora
Essential oil
Candida
Aspergillus
Aflatoxin

ABSTRACT

Introduction: *Zataria multiflora* is a valuable medicinal plant from Lamiaceae family with various pharmacological and therapeutic properties. In this article we reviewed the various aspects of *Z. multiflora* properties including botanical characteristics, chemical composition, anti-fungal and anti-mycotoxin activity and fungal ultrastructural changes.
Methods: Google Scholar, PubMed, EBSCO, Directory of open access journals (DOAJ), EMBASE, and Web of Science were searched using the keywords *Z. multiflora* and pathogenic and toxigenic fungi.
Results: The essential oil (EO) of *Z. multiflora* is frequently used in pharmaceutical industries. Thymol and carvacrol are the most important active components of *Z. multiflora* that are used for the treatment of a wide variety of diseases such as candidiasis and dermatophytosis. Aflatoxin production inhibitory effect of *Z. multiflora* EO was at the transcription level and this herb may cause reduction in aflatoxin biosynthesis. Ultrastructural changes showed that the main sites of action of EO were the plasma membrane and cell wall of fungi.
Conclusion: *Zataria multiflora* has the potential to be considered as a new natural drug for the treatment of some fungal infections. Morphological and structural changes may be one of the mechanisms involved in growth inhibition of the fungi and reducing aflatoxin production by *Z. multiflora* EO.

Implication for health policy/practice/research/medical education:
Zataria multiflora can be used effectively for the most clinically relevant opportunistic fungal infections. Cautious about the inhibitory effects of *Z. multiflora* against pathogenic and toxigenic fungi is very important.

Introduction

The emergence of opportunistic fungal infections, especially in immunocompromised individuals, highlights the need to elucidate new therapeutic options, especially because the fungi involved usually have remarkable morphological plasticity and express genes involved in the mechanisms of resistance to antifungal agents (1). In fact, indiscriminate use and the small number of available antifungal agents have promoted the development of resistant strains, especially in immunocompromised individuals (2). This fact justifies the development of new therapies for use in clinical practice. Among these new therapies, natural products stand out; they are considered sources of bioactive molecules with potential therapeutic applications in medicine (3).

In search of phytochemicals with potential antimicrobial activity in the past few years, attentions have been directed on *Zataria multiflora* quite reasonably. From the vegetable families, Lamiaceae is one of the biggest families, with worldwide distribution, which has 200 genuses and 2000-5000 species of aromatic bush and short shrubs producing terpenes and other types of compounds that are stored in epidermal gland of leafs, stalks and generative organs (4). *Zataria multiflora* Boiss. (Avishan-e-Shirazi in Persian and Saatar or Zaatar in the old Iranian medical books) is a thyme-like plant, which is a member of this family

***Corresponding Author:** Dr. Hojjatollah Shokri, Faculty of Veterinary Medicine, Amol University of Special Modern Technologies, Imam Khomeini Street, 24th Aftab, Amol, Iran.
Email: hshokri@ausmt.ac.ir

and is the aborigine of Iran, Afghanistan and Pakistan (5). *Zataria multiflora* can be recognized by the orbicular, densely gland-dotted, ovate leaves and the dense white, hairy, round buds on the leaf axils. It is an aromatic shrub that reaches 60-90 cm in height. Mature branches are woody and leafless whereas young branches are white with dense glandular, spreading, pilose indumentums. Leaves (5-10 × 5-10 mm^2) are orbicular ovate to orbicular. Flowering stems are usually un-branched, sometimes having short lateral branches. Flowers are white, sub-sessile, very small and often male sterile (6). *Zataria multiflora* (aerial parts) is not only a popular condimental plant but is also used in traditional folk remedies for its anti-microbial, analgesic, carminative, anthelmintic and anti-diarrheal properties (7). Modern pharmacological studies have shown that *Z. multiflora* possesses wide ranging biological properties including anti-nociceptive, anti-microbial, spasmolytic and anti-inflammatory effects (5,8-10). Currently, some pharmaceutical forms of this plant, such as syrups, oral drops, soft capsules and vaginal creams are sold as treatment remedies for various diseases. To outline the extensive uses of *Z. multiflora* in healthcare and medicine and to provide a probable scope for future research, several pharmacological and clinical studies on this plant and its active components are provided in this review article.

Methods

Google Scholar, PubMed, EBSCO, Directory of open access journals (DOAJ), EMBASE, and Web of Science were searched using the keywords *Z. multiflora* and pathogenic and toxigenic fungi.

Chemical composition of *Zataria multiflora*

Various extraction techniques like distillation, effleurage, CO_2 extraction, expression and solvent extraction are applied for essential oil (EO) extraction from various plants. But conventional methods that are usually used to extract EO oil from plants, are the distillation methods like steam-distillation, hydro-distillation and water-steam-distillation method.

Quantitatively, the most abundant components in hydrodistilled *Z. multiflora* EOs are oxygenated monoterpenes (approximately 70%), followed (in order) by monoterpene hydrocarbons, sesquiterpene hydrocarbons and oxygenated sesquiterpenes (10,11). Two studies from Pakistan identified carvacrol as the main constituent of the oil (12,13). To date, a large number of studies have focused on *Z. multiflora* EO: some reported carvacrol as the main compound, but others reported thymol, the isomer of carvacrol, as the main compound. Saei-Dehkordi et al (14) collected *Z. multiflora* from five different areas of Iran and analyzed its EOs. According to the GC–MS data, the main EO constituents remained similar between plants from different geographical regions, but their relative quantities differed among plants from different regions. Thymol was the most abundant compound among all constituents in all samples (14). In a study conducted by Shokri et al (15), *Z. multiflora* main components were carvacrol (61%) and thymol (25%). Additionally, Saleem et al (16) showed that thymol was the main constituent of the fresh plant (73.21%), while carvacrol was the primary constituent in the dried plant (62.87%). It is clear that geographical variation, cultivar differences, stage of plant growth, preparation process and other factors may influence the EO composition both quantitatively and qualitatively. According to previous studies, the EOs of *Z. multiflora* contain significant amounts of thymol and carvacrol, which are well-known anti-fungal agents (17-19). *p*-Cymene is the other main component in *Z. multiflora* EO. Zatariol, zataroside A (glycoside and non-volatile), zataroside B (glycoside and non-volatile), multiflotriol and multiflorol have been reported as new derivatives of *p*-cymene isolated from *Z. multiflora* (20,21). Linalool, caryophyllene, γ-terpinene and borneol are some of the other main components in the EOs (22).

Zataria multiflora also contains other compounds belonging to different classes of natural products, including alkanes such as n-nonacosane (C_{29}), n-hentriacontane (C_{31}), n-dotriacontane (C_{32}), n-tritriacontane (C_{33}) and n-pentatriacontane (C_{35}); fatty acids such as behenic acid (C_{22}), lignoceric acid (C_{24}), cerotic acid (C_{26}) and montanic acid (C_{28}) (23); phytosterols such as β-sitosterol and stigmasterol; triterpenes such as betulin, betulinic acid and oleanolic acid (24); and hydroxycinnamic acids such as rosmarinic acid (25). Moreover, flavonoids such as apigenin, luteolin and 6-hydroxyluteolin are also among the phytochemicals reported from *Z. multiflora* (22). This plant also contains small amounts of tannins, resins and saponins while lacking alkaloids (26).

Pharmacological and therapeutic activities of *Zataria multiflora*

1. Anti-yeast activity of *Zataria multiflora*

Various studies have shown that many species of yeasts, especially *Candida* and *Malassezia* species, have developed resistance to standard antifungal drugs. Nowadays traditional medicine and the use of herbal medicines to treat yeast infections are important because herbal medicines have fewer side effects and are less likely to develop drug resistance compared with chemical ones (27,28). Medicinal plants have been shown to eliminate the drug resistant yeasts and can be beneficial for their therapeutic effects (29). Zarei-Mahmoudabadi et al evaluated anti-*Candida* activity of three extracts of *Z. multiflora* (aqueous, ethanolic and methanolic) against 14 isolates of *Candida*. Aqueous extract of *Z. multiflora* showed no activity against *Candida* species. The ethanolic and methanolic extracts showed remarkable activities against *Candida* species. The minimum inhibitory concentration (MIC) for both extract was between 50 and 150 mg/L. The lowest MIC was for seven isolates of *C. albicans* (125 mg/L). Others MICs were respectively *C. glabrata* (126 mg/L), *C. parapsilosis* (125 mg/L) and *C. tropicalis* (131 mg/L). Totally, the MIC of ethanolic extract for 14 isolates of *Candida* was 127 mg/L. Both *C. albicans* and

C. parapsilosis were more susceptible than other species. The isolates of *C. parapsilosis* (64 mg/L) were more susceptible to methanolic extract of *Z. multiflora*, followed by *C. glabrata* (66 mg/L), *C. albicans* (76 mg/L) and *C. tropicalis* (76 mg/L). In addition, the MIC of methanolic extract for tested *Candida* was 70 mg/L. In that study methanolic extract showed more activities than ethanolic extract against 14 isolates of *Candida* (30). In Moghim et al (31) study, the obtained MIC of *Z. multiflora* extract was 0.13 mg/mL for *C. albicans*, which was lower than the effect on *C. albicans* obtained for this extract in the study of Zarei Mahmoudabadi et al (30). In another study by Fuladi et al (32), the MIC of *Z. multiflora* methanol and ethanol extracts were estimated to be 0.079 and 0.125 mg/mL, respectively. The contrasting results could be due to the different species of *Z. multiflora*, plant chemical compounds and/or methodologies. Katiraei et al (33) compared the MIC of EOs of *Z. multiflora*, *Geranium* and *Artemisia* with regard to the growth of *C. albicans* isolates resistant to azole drugs. They showed that the MIC levels of EOs of the plants were statistically significant from those of azoles. In that study, the obtained MIC of *Z. multiflora* for *C. albicans* was 0.18 mg/mL. In a study conducted by Esfandiary et al (34), a set of *C. glabrata* (29 strains), *C. krusei* (3 stains) and *C. patapsilosis* (2 strains) were studied. The results revealed that 33 isolates were resistant (MIC = 64 μg/mL), 4 isolates were susceptible (MIC ≤ 8 μg/mL) and 7 isolates had dose-dependent susceptibility (MIC = 16-32 μg/mL) to fluconazole, respectively. With regard to fluconazole, high resistance rate was observed in *C. glabrata* and *C. krusei*. However, ciclopirox olamine was found to inhibit the growth of all non-*albicans Candida* species (MIC ≤8 μg/mL). Also, favorable anti-fungal activity against *non-albicans Candida* species was obtained by *Z. multiflora* despite having a wide range of MICs (34.9-139.5 mg/mL). Mohammadi-Pourfard and Kavoosi (35) showed that EO from *Z. multiflora* significantly ($P<0.01$) inhibited the growth of *C. albicans*. MIC for *C. albicans* was 2.8 ± 0.8 mg/mL of EO. At concentration > 5 mg/mL, EO significantly ($P<0.01$) reduced the growth of *C. albicans* by 100%. However, the aqueous extract did not show any such activity at any concentration used. In addition, Zomorodian et al (36) determined the MICs and minimum fungicidal concentrations (MFCs) of the EO from *Z. multiflora* against *Candida* and *Trichosporon* species, showing strong anti-yeast activities with MIC values ranging from 0.007 to 0.5 μg/mL. This finding is similar to that of the study by Mahboubi et al (37) who reported strong anti-*Candida* activity of *Z. multiflora* EO with high thymol and carvacrol concentrations.

In a randomized clinical trial conducted by Khosravi et al (38), the application of 0.1% *Z. multiflora* cream in patients with acute vaginal candidiasis decreased vulvar pruritus in 80.9% of patients, vaginal pruritus in 65.5% of patients, vaginal burning in 73.9% of patients, urinary burning in 100% of patients, painful intercourse in 92.6% of patients, and vaginal secretion in 90% of patients. In addition, 0.1% *Z. multiflora* cream reduced erythema and satellite vulvar lesions in 100% of patients, vulvar edema in 100% of patients, vaginal edema in 83.3% of patients, vulvo-vaginal excoriation and fissures in 92% of patients, and white, sticky vaginal secretions in 86.2% of patients. After treatment with 0.1% *Z. multiflora* cream a laboratory using standard methods reported negative mycologic results on microscopic evaluation for 90% of patients; negative mycologic cultures in 86.7% of patients; and negative mycologic results on microscopy and culture combined for 93.3% of patients (38). Abou Fazeli et al (39) demonstrated the activity of the EO against *C. albicans*. They also suggested *Z. multiflora* oil-containing vaginal suppositories as a successful replacement for current drugs for the treatment of vaginitis caused by *C. albicans* (39). In a comparative study, a 7-day therapy with *Z. multiflora* as an intravaginal cream was more effective than clotrimazole vaginal cream in the treatment of Candidal vaginitis (40). An open-label, randomized and controlled study with two parallel treatment groups was conducted to evaluate the efficacy of a miconazole 2% gel compared with a *Z. multiflora* 0.1% gel applied four times daily for two weeks in the treatment of *Candida*-associated denture stomatitis. The results indicated that the *Z. multiflora* gel reduced the surface erythema of the palate more efficiently than miconazole gel but did not reduce the colony count on the denture surface as efficiently as miconazole (41). In another study, the physicochemical properties and stability of creams containing different concentrations (1%–3%) of *Z. multiflora* were evaluated and suggested as a successful replacement in the treatment of *C. albicans* induced vaginitis. In a previous study by Khosravi et al (43), intraperitoneally administration of 64 mg/kg of the EO in mice with systemic candidiasis had the highest efficacy in reducing *C. albicans* and produced 39.5, 21.8, 141.5, 174 and 501-fold reductions in mean colony forming units per 0.1 gram in *Candida* infections of the liver, spleen, lungs, brain and kidneys, respectively, as compared to itraconazole. Avaei et al (44) demonstrated that *Saccharomyces cerevisiae* (MIC = 200 μg/mL and MFC = 1600 μg/mL) was more resistant than *C. utilis* to *Z. multiflora* EO.

Naeini et al (45) showed that *Malassezia* species were susceptible to *Z. multiflora* EO ranging from 10 to > 50 mm (mean value: 28.1 mm). The highest inhibitory effect was recorded with *Malassezia obtusa*, followed by *M. furfur* and *M. globosa*. In another study conducted by Naeini et al (46), the EO from *Z. multiflora* presented anti-*Malassezia* activity against the tested yeasts. All *Malassezia* species were very susceptible to *Z. multiflora* EO, with MICs ranging from 0.015 to 0.06% (v/v), and approximately 52.4% of the strains had a MIC value of 0.015% (v/v). The mean MIC values of the EO against *M. sympodialis*, *M. furfur* and *M. pachydermatis* were 0.03, 0.024 and 0.02%, respectively. Khosravi et al (47) showed that *Z. multiflora* EO had the best anti-fungal activity against various *Malassezia* species isolated from dogs with atopic dermatitis, with MIC values ranging from 30 to 80 μg/mL. *M. nana* isolate was the most susceptible one (30 μg/mL), while *M. sloofiae* isolates showed the highest MIC value (80 μg/mL) (P<0.05).

2. Anti-dermatophyte activity of *Zataria multiflora*

Dermatophytes are the major cause of superficial mycoses, and remain a public health problem. They have the ability to invade keratinized tissues and cause dermatophytosis, the most common human contagious fungal disease (48). In recent years, the incidence of dermatophytosis has increased considerably, especially among individuals with impaired immunity, as well as in pediatric and geriatric populations (49). Some of these infections are still difficult to resolve completely, and remissions and relapses are often observed. The poor availability of antifungals and the increasing number of treatment failures have motivated current searches for therapeutic alternatives which can work effectively as potential anti-dermatophyte agents. Khosravi et al (50) showed that EO obtained from *Z. multiflora* possessed anti-fungal activity against a wide number of clinical isolates of various dermatophytes, with MIC ranging from 0.25 to 4 mg/mL. However, variation of susceptibility from one species to another was evident. The MIC values were 0.5 mg/mL for *Microsporum canis* and *M. gypseum*, 1.5 mg/mL for *Trichophyton mentagrophytes* and *Epidermophyton floccosum* and 2 mg/mL for *T. rubrum*. The MFCs recorded for plant oil tested ranged from 0.5 to 8 mg/mL. In a study conducted by Effatpanah et al (51), total (100%) fungal growth inhibition was observed from *Z. multiflora* EO at concentration of > 8 mg/mL for *T. mentagrophytes*, *T. rubrum* and *E. floccosum* (P< 0.01). In another study, the minimum inhibitory activity of *Z. multiflora* methanolic extract against various dermatophytes was found to be approximately 0.5% (w/v) (42).

3. Anti-filamentous fungi activity of *Zataria multiflora*

Literature studies indicated that there are many reports on non-dermatophytic filamentous fungi causing fungal infections in human and animals and food spoilage (18,52). Gandomi Nasr-Abadi et al (53) found that all concentrations of EO from *Z. multiflora* had a significant effect on the growth and sporulation of *Aspergillus flavus*. Also, they reported the levels of MIC and MFC 400 and 1000 ppm, respectively. In a study conducted by Mohammadi-Pourfard and Kavoosi (35), the EO from *Z. multiflora* at all tested concentrations significantly (P< 0.01) inhibited the growth of *A. niger*. MIC for *A. niger* was 2.2 ± 0.5 mg/mL of EO. At concentration > 5 mg/mL, EO significantly (P< 0.01) reduced the growth of *A. niger* by 100%. In a study by Shokri et al (18), the EO from *Z. multiflora* showed the inhibitory effects on four tested fungi including *A. flavus*, *A. parasiticus*, *A. ochraceus* and *Fusarium verticillioides* at all concentrations (500-2000 ppm). It completely inhibited four fungi at 2000 ppm. At 1000 ppm concentration, *Z. multiflora* EO significantly decreased the growth of *Aspergillus* species compared with the control, whereas it caused complete growth inhibition of *F. verticillioides* (P< 0.05). Therefore, *F. verticillioides* had a higher susceptibility than *Aspergillus* species against the EO tested. In addition, Nasseri et al (54) showed that the EO from *Z. multiflora* has anti-fungal activity; the lowest inhibition (75%) was observed in *A. niger*, while the highest inhibition (95.3%) was observed in *Alternaria solani*. The MICs for *A. solani*, *Rhizoctonia solani*, *Rhizopus stolonifer*, *A. flavus*, *A. ochraceus* and *A. niger* were 200, 200, 200, 300, 300 and 200 ppm, respectively. In addition, the MFCs for *A. solani*, *R. solani*, *R .stolonifer*, *A. niger* and *A. ochraceus* were 600, 400, 300, 900 and 700 ppm, respectively, and none of the tested concentrations were fatal for *A. flavus*. *A. solani* and *R. solani* showed a strong susceptibility to *Z. multiflora* EO at all concentrations. The fungal pathogens studied were classified according to their susceptibility to the EO in the following order: *A. solani* > *R. stolonifer* > *R. stolonifer* > *A. ochraceus* > *A. niger* > *A. flavus*. Sharif Rohani et al (55) showed that dosage of 800 ppm of *Z. multiflora* EO for *Fusarium solani* had obvious inhibitory rate. In a study by Amini et al (56), *Z. multiflora* EO was very effective on the four studied pathogenic fungi including *Pythium aphanidermatum*, *R. solani*, *Fusarium graminearum* and *Sclerotinia sclerotiorum* with growth inhibition average of 100% at 200 μL/L concentration. Nevertheless, MIC and MFC of the EO were variable depending to species of fungi. *P. aphanidermatum* and *S. sclerotiorum* were the most susceptible and most resistant to the studied EO with average growth inhibition 89.54% and 75.35%, respectively. Khosravi et al (57) determined the anti-fungal assay of EO from *Z. multiflora* against *Saprolegnia parasitica* isolated from fish eggs. The infected fish eggs were treated with EO oil at concentrations of 1, 5, 10, 25, 50, and 100 ppm daily. The MIC of *Z. multiflora* EO against *S. parasitica* was 0.9 ppm. *Z. multiflora* at concentrations of 25, 50, and 100 ppm had significant differences in comparison with negative control (P<0.05). The most hatching rates were recorded with *Z. multiflora* (11%) EO. *Z. multiflora* was effective for the treatment of *S. parasitica*-infected rainbow trout eggs in aquaculture environment (57).

4.Inhibition of mycotoxin production by *Zataria multiflora*

Fungi are significant spoilage microorganisms of foodstuffs during the storage, rendering them unfit for human consumption by retarding their nutritive value and sometimes by producing mycotoxins (58). Mycotoxins are polyketide secondary metabolites produced by the important food and feed contaminating species *Aspergillus*, *Penicillium* and *Fusarium* and are known as potent carcinogens for a wide variety of animal species, including humans (59). EOs and their phenolic compounds have been used as natural inhibitors of fungal growth and mycotoxin production to preserve foods and feeds in some countries during recent decades. Many of the spices and herbal EO which have been tested have an antagonistic effect against aflatoxigenic *Aspergillus* strains (60). Previous studies demonstrated that thymus EO, which mainly consists of thymol, has been shown to inhibit both the growth and aflatoxin production in *A.*

flavus and *A. parasiticus* (61,62). Yahyaraeyat et al (63) determined the effects of *Z. multiflora* EO on growth, aflatoxin production and transcription of aflatoxin biosynthesis pathway genes of *A. parasiticus*. The results showed that mycelial dry weight and aflatoxin production reduce in the presence of *Z. multiflora* EO (100 ppm) on day 5 of growth. It was found that the expression of *nor-1*, *ver-1*, *omt-A* and *aflR* genes was correlated with the ability of fungus to produce aflatoxins on day 5 in yeast extract sucrose medium. RT-PCR showed that in the presence of *Z. multiflora* EO (100 ppm), *nor-1*, *ver-1* and *omtA* genes expression was reduced. It was suggested that toxin production inhibitory effects of *Z. multiflora* EO on day 5 may be at the transcription level and this herb may cause reduction in aflatoxin biosynthesis pathway genes activity (63). Also, Gandomi et al (64) investigated the effect of *Z. multiflora* EO against growth, spore production and aflatoxin formation by *A. flavus* ATCC 15546. EO effectively inhibited radial growth and spore production on potato dextrose agar (PDA) in a dose-dependent manner. At 200 ppm, the radial growth and sporulation reduced by 79.4% and 92.5%, respectively. The growth was completely prevented at EO ≥400 ppm on PDA, and MFC of the oil was estimated at 1000 ppm. The EO also significantly suppressed mycelial growth and aflatoxin synthesis in broth medium at all concentrations tested ($P<0.05$). In that study, *Z. multiflora* EO had a significant inhibitory effect on aflatoxin formation, which was reduced by 31% and 99.4% at 50 and 150 ppm, respectively. In a similar study conducted by Farag et al (65), *Z. multiflora* EO was effective at concentrations ≥100 ppm in reducing aflatoxin formation by 50%. It has been suggested that the regulation of aflatoxin synthesis and conidiogenesis may be interlinked, since the loss of aflatoxigenic capabilities in the nonaflatoxigenic variant strains of *A. parasiticus* was correlated with alterations in the conidial morphology (66). Furthermore, it has been shown that lysis of the mycelia and spores of the toxigenic fungi are one of the characteristics of aflatoxin deactivation process (67).

It was shown by several investigators that chemical compounds of the EOs may cause reduction or stimulation in the toxin production and the anti-toxigenic effects of the EOs are not necessarily related to their anti-fungal activity. Values for growth inhibition were calculated as 0.79 and 0.86mM for carvacrol and thymol, while for AFB_1 and AFG_1, it was reported as 0.50 and 0.06mM for carvacrol and 0.69 and 0.55mM for thymol (68). It was also shown by Wright et al (69) that aflatoxin production by the fungus was reduced by *n*-decyl aldehyde and hexanal, but was stimulated by octanal. Their results indicated that all three volatile compounds reduced radial growth but only *n*-decyl aldehyde significantly inhibits aflatoxin biosynthesis in *A. parasiticus*. Difference in anti-fungal and aflatoxin inhibition efficacy of *Thymus* and *Zataria* EOs in different studies may be attributable to the EO compositions. Two major components of *Thyme* and *Zataria* are thymol and carvacrol. *Thyme* contains higher thymol than *Zataria* and *Zataria* contains more carvacrol. The other factors are also important for causing these differences such as differences in culture media used, culture conditions, temperature, pH and durations of culture.

There are little reports on the effect of *Z. multiflora* in inhibiting the other mycotoxins. In this regard, Vazquez et al (70) reported that phenolic compounds, i.e., thymol and eugenol, inhibited growth and citrinin production by *Penicillium citrinum* in some Galician cheeses. In another study by Noori et al (71), the EO from *Z. multiflora* significantly ($P<0.05$) suppressed citrinin formation by *P. citrinum* in mozzarella cheese at all concentrations, as citrinin accumulation was reduced by 30% and 87% at 50 and 1000 ppm, respectively.

Ultrastructural changes of fungi treated with *Zataria multiflora*

1. Scanning electron microscopy

The effect of *Z. multiflora* EO on morphology of *A. flavus* observed by Scanning electron microscopy (SEM) is illustrated in Figure 1. Hyphae grown on PDA without EO showed swollen and turgid feature with smooth and uniform surface. In presence of 50 ppm EO, hyphae lost their turgidity and uniformity to some extent and these modifications increased at higher concentrations of EO. Furthermore, 100 ppm EO induced the shrinkage of the hyphae and formation of pits along the mycelia. The severity of damage increased with 200 ppm EO and the hyphae were frequently collapsed and their destruction was often evident (72).

2. Light and transmission electron microscopy

Semi-thin sections of *A. flavus* grown in broth medium containing different concentrations of *Z. multiflora*

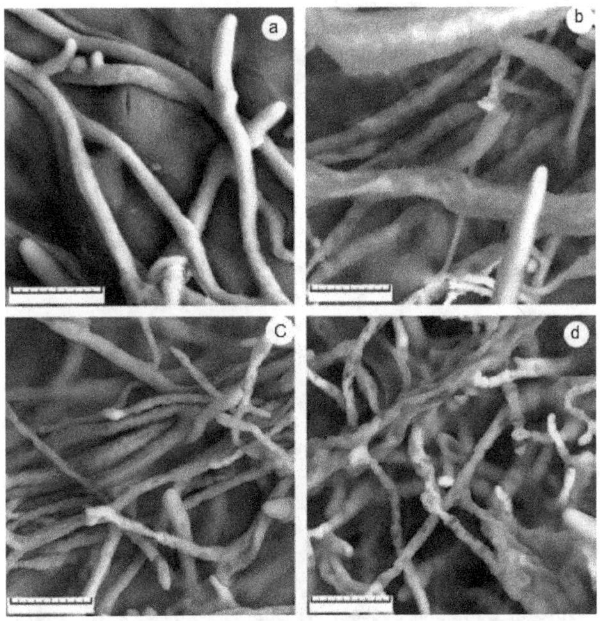

Figure 1. Scanning electron micrographs ×2000, *Aspergillus flavus* mycelia: (a) untreated; (b) treated with 50 ppm *Zataria multiflora* essential oil (EO); (c) treated with 100 ppm *Z. multiflora* EO; (d) treated with 200 ppm *Z. multiflora* EO (72).

EO are illustrated in Figure 2. Longitudinal sections of untreated culture displayed normal mycelia that had a steady arrangement with continuous and homogenous cytoplasm (Figure 2a). Vacuolization of the cytoplasm was the major effect induced in the presence of 50 ppm EO, which led to the cell swelling (Figure 2b). However, mycelia treated with 100 ppm EO revealed greater damage characterized with detachment of the cell membrane from the cell wall that was collapsed and herniated in different intervals along the longitudinal sections resulting in the deformation of mycelia (Figure 2c). In presence of 150 ppm EO, cell membrane was fully disconnected from the cell wall and mycelia obtained an electron-lucent appearance due to cytoplasm shedding from the cell (Figure 2d). Moreover, swelling and deformation of the mycelia were the other changes observed (Figure 2d). The concentration of 200 ppm EO effectively inhibited the germination of the fungal conidia and no mycelia formed at this concentration (Figure 2e). Some of the conidia had a normal shape but the others showed changes ranging from the vacuolization to cell membrane detachment and deformation (Figure 2e). With increasing EO concentration to 400 ppm, more severe damages including depletion of the cytoplasm and frequent degradation of the cell wall were observed (Figure 2f). Furthermore, deformation and destruction of conidia were often evident (Figure 2f) (72). Examination of ultrathin sections under transmission electron microscopy (TEM) resulted in more obvious findings. Untreated hypha was enclosed by the cell wall that was integrated and intact. The plasma membrane was fully attached to the cell wall along the hypha and was smooth and unwrinkled. Cytoplasm was homogeneous and dense and intercellular septum was intact and healthy. At concentration of 50 ppm of *Z. multiflora* EO, the cell wall lost its integrity and uniformity to some extent. The cell membrane in some areas was detached from the cell wall and invaginated into the cytoplasm. The loss of cytoplasm density and vacuolization were the other changes. At concentration of 100 ppm of *Z. multiflora* EO, the plasma membrane was completely separated from the cell wall and vacuolization of the cytoplasm was more evident. The presence of 150 ppm of EO increased the severity of injury characterized by the depletion of cytoplasm content, and hypha lost its normal shape and was collapsed. In addition, detachment and fragmentation of the plasma membrane and formation of the lomasome, small membrane-bound vesicles, beneath the cell wall, were seen and membrane fragments were spread over the cytoplasm. At concentration of 200 ppm EO, no evident change was observed in the cell wall, whereas cell membrane was completely destroyed and cytoplasm was released from the cell. With increase in oil concentration to 400 ppm, complete destruction of the plasma membrane and cell wall was evident and hypha was totally free of cytoplasm (73).

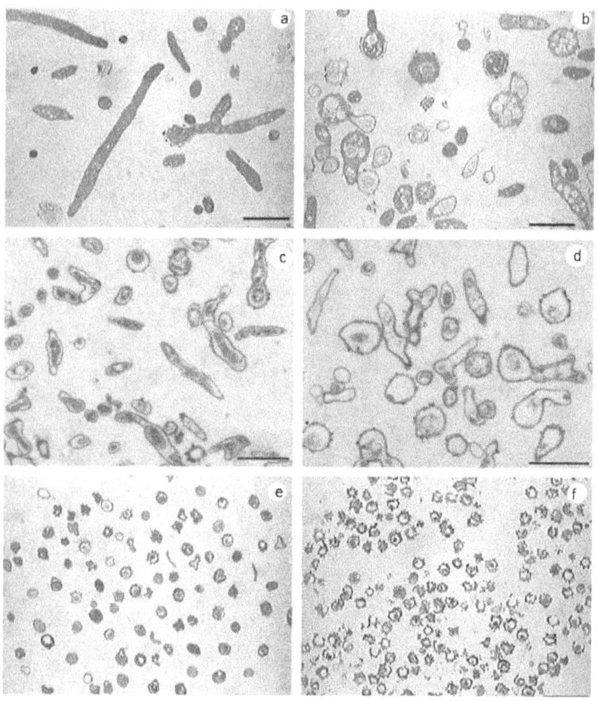

Figure 2. Semi-thin sections × 1000, *Aspergillus flavus* grown in broth medium: (a) untreated; (b) treated with 50 ppm *Zataria multiflora* essential oil (EO); (c) treated with 100 ppm *Z. multiflora* EO; (d) treated with 150 ppm *Z. multiflora* EO; (e) treated with 200 ppm *Z. multiflora* EO; (f) treated with 400 ppm *Z. multiflora* EO.

Conclusion

In summary, the microscopic examinations showed that *Z. multiflora* EO suppressed the size of the colony as well as sporulation of fungi. Mycelia treated with EO showed morphological alterations ranging from loss of turgidity and uniformity of mycelia at low concentrations of EO to evident destruction of the hyphae at higher concentration of EO. The major change at level as low as 50 ppm of EO was limited to vacuolization of cytoplasm resulting in cell swelling, while at higher concentrations, detachment of the cell membrane from the cell wall, deformation of mycelia and shedding the cytoplasm from the cell were the main alterations. These damages were well documented by TEM, which showed that the main sites of action of EO were the plasma membrane and cell wall. In conclusion, morphological and structural changes observed in this study may be one of the mechanisms involved in growth inhibition of the fungi and reducing aflatoxin production.

Authors' contributions

All authors contributed to the conception of the study, confirmed the final version of the article and approved all aspects of the study.

Conflict of interests

The authors declared no competing interests.

Ethical considerations

Ethical issues (including plagiarism, misconduct, data fabrication, falsification, double publication or submission and redundancy) were completely observed by authors.

Funding/Support

This work was supported by the Council Research of Amol University of Special Modern Technologies, Amol, Iran (Grant No. 18902).

References

1. Cornet M, Gaillardin C. pH signaling in human fungal pathogens: a new target for antifungal strategies. Eukaryot Cell. 2014;13:342-52.
2. Bondaryk M, Kurzatkowski W, Staniszewska M. Antifungal agents commonly used in the superficial and mucosal candidiasis treatment: mode of action and resistance development. Postepy Dermatol Alergol. 2013;30:293-301.
3. Newman DJ, Cragg GM. Natural products as sources of new drugs over the 30 years from 1981 to 2010. J Nat Prod. 2012;75:311-335.
4. Ettehad GH, Arab R. Evaluation of antibacterial effect of Shiraz oregano essence (*Zataria multiflora* Boiss) on *Salmonella typhi* and comparing with antibiotics. Res J Biol Sci. 2007;2:674-6.
5. Hosseinzadeh H, Ramezani M, Salmani GA. Antinociceptive, antiinflammatory and acute toxicity effects of *Zataria multiflora* Boiss extracts in mice and rats. J Ethnopharmacol. 2000;73:379-85.
6. Akhondzadeh BA, Misaghi A, Gheybi S. Effect of oregano oil on growth of *Bacillus cereus* in heart and brain broth. Herbs Quart. 2005;16:48-55.
7. Iranian Herbal Pharmacopoeia. Tehran: Ministry of Health and Medical Publications; 2002:51-6.
8. Jaffary F, Ghannadi A, Siahpoush A. Antinociceptive effects of hydroalco-holic extract and essential oil of *Zataria multiflora*. Fitoterapia. 2004;75:217-220.
9. Moosavi MH, Akhondzadeh Basti A, Misaghi A, et al. Effect of *Zataria multiflora* Boiss. Essential oil and nisin on *Salmonella typhimurium* and *Staphylococcus aureus* in a food model system and on the bacterial cell membranes. Food Res Int. 2008;41:1050-7.
10. Saei-Dehkordi SS, Razavi-Rohani SM, Tajik H, Moradi M. Antimicrobial effects of lysozyme in combination with *Zataria multiflora* Boiss. essential oil at different pH and NaCl concentrations on *E. coli* O157:H7 and *Staphylococcus aureus*. J Anim Vet Adv. 2008;7:1458-63.
11. Mohagheghzadeh A, Shams-Ardakani M, Ghannadi A. Volatile constituents of callus and flower-bearing tops of *Zataria multiflora* Boiss. (Lamiaceae). Flavour Fragr J. 2000;15:373-6.
12. Malik MS, Sattar A, Khan SA. Essential oils of the species of Labiatae Part III. Studies on the essential oil of *Zataria multiflora*. Pakistan J Sci Industr Res. 1987;30:751-753.
13. Ahmad VU, Jassbi AR, Tareen RB. Constituents of the essential oil of *Zataria multiflora* Boiss. from Pakistan. J Essent Oil Res. 1999;11:179-81.
14. Saei-Dehkordi SS, Tajik H, Moradi M, Khalighi-Sigaroodi F. Chemical composition of essential oils in *Zataria multiflora* Boiss. from different parts of Iran and their radical scavenging and antimicrobial activity. Food Chem Toxicol. 2010; 48:1562-1567.
15. Shokri H, Sharifzadeh A, Ashrafi Tamai I. Anti-*Candida zeylanoides* activity of some Iranian plants used in traditional medicine. J Mycol Med. 2012;22:211-6.
16. Saleem M, Nazli R, Afza N, Sami A, Ali MS. Biological significance of essential oil of *Zataria multiflora* Boiss. Natur Prod Res. 2004;18:493-7.
17. Baser KHC. Biological and pharmacological activities of carvacrol and carvacrol bearing essential oils. Curr Pharm Des. 2008;14:3106-20.
18. Shokri H, Khosravi AR, Mansouri M, Ziglari T. Effects of *Zataria multiflora* and *Geranium, Pelargonium* essential oils on growth-inhibiting of some toxigenic fungi. Iran J Vet Res. 2011;12:247-51.
19. Abbaszadeh S, Sharifzadeh, A, Shokri H, Khosravi AR, Abbaszadeh A. Antifungal efficacy of thymol, carvacrol, eugenol and menthol as alternative agents to control the growth of food-relevant fungi. J Mycol Med. 2014;24:e51-6.
20. Ali MS, Saleem M, Ahmad VU. Zatatriol: a new aromatic constituent from *Zataria multiflora*. J Chem Sci. 1999a;54:807-810.
21. Ali MS, Saleem M, Akhtar F, Jahangir M, Parvez M, Ahmad VU. Three p-cymene derivatives from *Zataria multiflora*. Phytochem. 1999b;52:685-8.
22. Ali MS, Saleem M, Ali Z, Ahmad VU. Chemistry of *Zataria multiflora* (Lamiaceae). Phytochem. 2000;55:933-6.
23. Gupta GS, Gupta NL. Constituents of *Zataria multiflora*. Phytochem. 1972;11:455-6.
24. Rajaei H, Khajehali M. Histochemical screening of flavonoids in secretory trichomes of *Zataria multiflora* leaves. Planta Med. 2009;75:1068-8.
25. Mohagheghzadeh A, Shams-Ardakani M, Ghannadi A, Minaeian M. Rosmarinic acid from *Zataria multiflora* tops and in vitro cultures. Fitoter. 2004;75:315-21.
26. Jaffary F, Ghannadi A, Siahpoush A. Antiinflammatory activity of *Zataria multiflora* Boiss. J Res Med Sci. 2000;5:6-9.
27. Tobudic S, Kratzer C, Presterl E. Azole-resistant *Candida* spp. - emerging pathogens? Mycoses. 2010;55:24-32.
28. Pfaller M, Neofytos D, Diekema D, Azie N, Meier-Kriesche HU, Quan SP. Epidemiology and outcomes of candidemia in 3648 patients: data from the Prospective Antifungal Therapy (PATH Alliance®) registry, 2004-2008. Diagn Microbiol Infect Dis. 2012;74:323-31.
29. Freires IA, Furletti VF, Sartoratto A, Alencar SM, Figueira GM, Murata RM. *Coriandrum sativum* L. (coriander) essential oil: antifungal activity and mode of action on *Candida* spp., and molecular targets affected in humanwhole-genome expression. PloS One. 2014;9:e99086.
30. Zarei-Mahmoudabadi A, Dabbagh MA, Fouladi Z. In-vitro anti-*Candida* activity of *Zataria multiflora* Boiss. Evid Based Complement Alternat Med. 2006;4:351-3.
31. Moghim H, Taghipoor S, Shahinfard N, Kheiri S, Panahi R. Antifungal effects of *Zataria multifora* and *Nigella sativa* extracts against *Candida albicans*. J HerbMed Pharmacol. 2015;4:138-41.
32. Fuladi Z, Afshari P, Gharibi T, Dabbagh MA. The comparison of *Zataria multiflora* boiss (Avishan Shirazi) and clotrimazol vaginal cream in the treatment of candidiasis vaginitis. Iran South Med J. 2009;12:214-24.
33. Katiraei F, Eydi S, Bahonar Ar, Zarinfar H, Khosravi A. Comparision of MICS of some Iranian herbal essences against azole resistance and azole susceptible of *Candida albicans*. J Med Plants. 2008;7:37-44.
34. Esfandiary MA, Mahmoudi S, Zaini F, et al. *In vitro* antifungal activity of *Zataria multiflora* essential oil, fluconazole and ciclopirox olamine against *non-albicans Candida* species isolated from recurrent vulvovaginal candidiasis. J Mycol Res. 2015;2:3-8.
35. Mohammadi-Pourfard A, Kavoosi G. Chemical

composition, radical scavenging, antibacterial and antifungal activities of *Zataria multiflora* Bioss essential oil and aqueous extract. J Food Safety. 2012;32:326-32.
36. Zomorodian K, Saharkhiz MJ, Rahimi MJ, et al. Chemical composition and antimicrobial activities of the essential oils from three ecotypes of *Zataria multiflora*. Pharmacog Mag. 2011;7:53-9.
37. Mahboubi M, Feizabadi MM, Safara M. Antifungal activity of essential oils from *Zataria multiflora, Rosmarinus officinalis, Lavandula stoechas, Artemisia sieberi Besser* and *Pelargonium graveolens* against clinical isolates of *Candida albicans*. Pharmacog Mag. 2008;4:15-8.
38. Khosravi AR, Eslami AR, Shokri H, Kashanian M. *Zataria multiflora* cream for the treatment of acute vaginal candidiasis. Int J Gynaecol Obstet. 2008;101:201-202.
39. Abou fazeli R, Mosadegh M, Vahidi H, Shafaati A, Nader N. Formulation, preparation and physico-chemical control of vaginal suppositories containing volatile oils of *Allium sativum* and *Zataria multiflora*. Hakim. 2000;3:231-43.
40. Eslami AR, Ansari A, Kashanian M, Bekhradi R, Akbari M, Akbari H, Darabi M. *Zataria multiflora* vaginal cream compared with clotrimazole vaginal cream in the treatment of *Candida* vaginitis. Iran J Pharm Res. 2004;3:36-7.
41. Amanlou M, Beitollahi JM, Abdollahzadeh S, Tohidast-Ekrad Z. Miconazole gel compared with *Zataria multiflora* Boiss. gel in the treatment of denture stomatitis. Phytother Res. 2006;20:966-9.
42. Aghel N, Moghimipour E, Ameri AAG. Characterization of an anti-dermatophyte cream from *Zataria multiflora* Boiss. Iran J Pharm Sci. 2007;3:77-84.
43. Khosravi AR, Shokri H, Tootian Z, Alizadeh M, Yahyaraeyat R. Comparative efficacies of Zataria multiflora essential oil and itraconazole against disseminated Candida albicans infection in BALB/c mice. Braz J Microbiol. 2009;40:439-45.
44. Avaei A, Mohamadi Sani A, Mahmoodzadeh Vaziri B. Chemical composition and antimicrobial effect of the essential oil of *Zataria multiflora* Boiss endemic in Khorasan-Iran. Asian Pac J Trop Dis. 2015;5:181-5.
45. Naeini A, Eidi S, Shokri H. Fungitoxicity of *Zataria multiflora* essential oil against various *Malassezia* species isolated from cats and dogs with *Malassezia* dermatitis. Afri J Microbiol Res. 2011;5:1057-61.
46. Naeini A, Nazeri M, Shokri H. Antifungal activity of *Zataria multiflora, Pelargonium graveolens* and *Cuminum cyminum* essential oils towards three species of *Malassezia* isolated from patients with pityriasis versicolor. J Mycol Med 2011;21:87-91.
47. Khosravi AR, Shokri H, Fahimirad S. Efficacy of medicinal essential oils against pathogenic *Malassezia* sp. isolates. J Mycol Med. 2016;26:28-34.
48. Sidat MM, Correia D, Buene TP. Tinea capitis among rural school children of the district of Magude, in Maputo province, Mozambique. Mycoses. 2006;49:480-3.
49. Jessup CJ, Warner J, Isham N. Antifungal susceptibility testing of dermatophytes: establishing a medium for inducing conidial growth and evaluation of susceptibility of clinical isolates. J Clin Microbiol. 2000;38:341-344.
50. Khosravi AR, Shokri H, Farahnejat Z, Chalangari R, Katalin M. Antimycotic efficacy of Iranian medicinal plants towards dermatophytes obtained from patients with dermatophytosis. Chinese J Natur Med. 2013;11:43-8.
51. Effatpanah H, Azar S, Kordbacheh P. Antifungal effect of *Zataria multiflora*: An in vitro evaluation. Global Vet. 2010;4:140-3.
52. Mousavi SAA, Esfandiarpour I, Salari S, Shokri H. Onychomycosis due to *Fusarium* spp. in patient with squamous cell carcinoma: A case report from Kerman, Iran. J Mycol Med. 2009;19:146-9.
53. Gandomi Nasr-Abadi H, Misaghi A, Akhoundzadeh Basti A, Khosravi AR. Effects of *Zataria multiflora* Boiss essential oil on *Aspergillus flavus*. J Med Plants. 2008;7:45-51.
54. Naseri M, Arouiee H, Golmohammadzadeh S, Jaafari MR, Neamati H. Antifungal effects of *Zataria multiflora* essential oil on the inhibitory growth of some postharvest pathogenic fungi. Not Sci Biol. 2015;7:412-6.
55. Sharif Rohani M, Dashtiannasab A, Ghaednia B, Mirbakhsh M, Yeganeh V, Vahabnezhad A. Investigation of the possibility use of *Zataria multiflora* (Avishan-e Shirazi) essence in control of fungal contamination of cultured shrimp, *Litopenaeus vannamei*. Iran J Fisheries Sci. 2013;12:454-64.
56. Amini M, Safaie N, Salmani MJ, Shams-Bakhsh M. Antifungal activity of three medicinal plant essential oils against some phytopathogenic fungi. Trakia J Sci. 2012;10:1-8.
57. Khosravi AR, Shokri H, Sharifrohani M, Ebrahimzadeh Mousavi H, Moosavi Z. Evaluation of the antifungal activity of *Zataria multiflora, Geranium herbarium*, and *Eucalyptus camaldolensis* essential oils on *Saprolegnia parasitica*-infected rainbow trout (*Oncorhynchus mykiss*) eggs. Foodborne Pathog Dis. 2012;9:674-9.
58. Kumar R, Mishra AK, Dubey NK, Tripathi YB. Evaluation of *Chenopodium ambrosioides* as a potential source of antifungal, antiaflatoxigenic and antioxidant activity. Int J Food Microbiol. 2007;115:159-64.
59. Sakuda S, Ono M, Ikeda H, et al. Blasticidin A as an inhibitor of aflatoxin production by *Aspergillus parasiticus*. J Antibiotics. 2000;68:407-12.
60. Roze LV, Koptina AV, Laivenieks M, et al. Willow volatiles influence growth, development, and secondary metabolism in Aspergillus parasiticus. Appl Microbiol Biotechnol. 2011;92:359-370.
61. Rasooli I, Razzaghi-Abyaneh M. Inhibitory effects of thyme oils on growth and aflatoxin production by *Aspergillus parasiticus*. Food Control. 2004;1:479-83.
62. Soliman KM, Badeaa RI. Effect of oil extracted from some medicinal plants on different mycotoxigenic fungi. Food Chem Toxicol. 2002;40:1669-75.
63. Yahyaraeyat R, Khosravi AR, Shahbazzadeh D, Khalaj V. The potential effects of *Zataria multiflora Boiss* essential oil on growth, aflatoxin production and transcription of aflatoxin biosynthesis pathway genes of toxigenic *Aspergillus parasiticus*. Braz J Microbiol. 2013;44:649-55.
64. Gandomi Nasrabadi H, Misaghi A, Akhondzadeh A, et al. Effect of *Zataria multiflora* Boiss. essential oil on growth and aflatoxin formation by *Aspergillus flavus* in culture media and cheese. Food Chem Toxicol. 2009;47:2397-400.
65. Farag RS, Daw ZY, Abo-Raya SH. Influence of some spice essential oil on *Aspergillus parasiticus* growth and production of aflatoxins in a synthetic medium. J Food Sci. 1989;54:74-76.
66. Kale S, Cary JW, Bhatnagar D, Bennett JW. Characterization of experimentally induced, nonaflatoxigenic variant strain of *Aspergillus parasiticus*. Appl Environ Microbiol. 1996;62:3399-404.

67. Namazi M, Allameh A, Aminshahidi M, Nohee A, Malekzadeh F. Inhibitory effect of ammonia solution on growth and aflatoxin production by *Aspergillus parasiticus* NRRL-2999. Acta Pol Toxicol. 2002;10:65-72.
68. Razzaghi Abyaneh M, Shams Ghahfarokhi M, Yoshinari T, et al. Inhibitory effects of *Satureja hortensis* L. essential oil on growth and aflatoxin production by *Aspergillus parasiticus*. Int J Food Microbiol. 2008;123:228-33.
69. Wright MS, Greene-McDowelle DM, Zeringue HJ Jr, Bhatnagar D, Cleveland TE. Effects of volatile aldehydes from *Aspergillus*-resistant varieties of corn on *Aspergillus parasiticus* growth and aflatoxin biosynthesis. Toxicon. 2000;38:1215-23.
70. Vazquez BI, Fente C, Franco CM, Vazquez MJ, Cepeda A. Inhibitory effect of eugenol and thymol on Penicillium citrinum strains in culture media and cheese. Int J Food Microbiol. 2001;67:157-63.
71. Noori N, Yahyaraeyat R, Khosravi AR, Atefi P, Akhondzadeh Basti A, Akrami F. Effect of *Zataria multiflora* Bioss. essential oil on growth and citrinin production by *Penicillium citrinum* in culture media and mozzarella cheese. J Food Safety. 2012;32:445-51.
72. Gandomi H, Misaghi A, Akhondzadeh Basti A, Hamedi H, Ramezani Shirvani Z. Effect of *Zataria multiflora* Boiss. essential oil on colony morphology and ultrastructure of *Aspergillus flavus*. Mycoses. 2010;54:e429-37.
73. Khosravi AR, Minooeianhaghighi MH, Shokri H, Emami SA, Alavi SM, Asili J. The potential inhibitory effect of *Cuminum cyminum, Ziziphora clinopodioides* and *Nigella sativa* essential oils on the growth of *Aspergillus fumigatus* and *Aspergillus flavus*. Braz J Microbiol. 2011;42:216-24.

14

Immunoadjuvant potential of *Azadirachta indica*, *Butea frondosa* and *Ficus religiosa* against Swine flu vaccine antigen

Shubham S Gaikwad[1], **Amit Gupta**[1,2*], **Bharat Shinde**[1,2]

[1]Department of Biotechnology, Vidya Pratishthan's, Arts, Science and Commerce College, Baramati, Maharashtra, India
[2]Department of Zoology, Vidya Pratishthan's, Arts, Science and Commerce College, Baramati, Maharashtra, India

ARTICLE INFO

Keywords:
Azadirachta indica
Butea frondosa
Ficus religiosa
Adjuvant
Swine flu vaccine

ABSTRACT

Introduction: In general, primary or secondary metabolites derived from medicinal plant products might be responsible for stimulating or suppressing the immune system against specific protein antigens. The objective of this study was to evaluate the adjuvant potential of aqueous leaves extract of *Azadirachta indica, Butea frondosa* and *Ficus religiosa* against Swine flu vaccine antigen.
Methods: In this study, our group evaluated the antibody (IgG) titre of Swine flu vaccine antigen (2 µg/mL) using variable doses (0.625–5 mg) of aqueous leaves extract of *A. indica, B. frondosa* and *F. religiosa*. In addition, Swiss mice were immunized subcutaneously (100 µL) on day 0 with Swine flu vaccine antigen (1:1000 dilution). Splenocytes were collected on day 7 and cultured with variable doses of aqueous leaves extract of *A. indica, B. frondosa* and *F. religiosa* pertaining to determine the total cellular content and splenocyte proliferation (Swine flu vaccine; Ovalbumin, OVA and Con A) assay. In addition, estimation of Th1 (IFN-gamma and TNF alpha) cytokines in cell culture supernatant containing swine flu vaccine antigen along with aqueous leaves extract were measured.
Results: Aqueous leaves extract of *A. indica, B. frondosa* and *F. religiosa* showed anti-Swine flu titre at higher doses. In *ex vivo* animal model studies these three medicinal plants in the form of aqueous leaves extract enhanced total cellular content at higher doses but increased in splenocyte proliferation (Swine flu vaccine, OVA and Con A) assay at lower doses. Similarly, there was enhancement in Th1 cytokines (IFN-gamma, TNF alpha) with respect to swine flu vaccine antigen containing aqueous extract at lower doses as compared to control group.
Conclusion: Aqueous leaves extract of *A. indica, B. frondosa* and *F. religiosa* showed adjuvant activity against Swine flu vaccine antigen and might be used in manufacturing active adjuvant for vaccine antigen.

Implication for health policy/practice/research/medical education:
Aqueous leaves extracts of *Azadirachta indica, Butea frondosa* and *Ficus religiosa* are capable of enhancing both antibody and cell mediated immune responses against Swine flu vaccine antigen in mice and might be used in manufacturing active adjuvant for vaccine antigen.

Introduction

Swine influenza (swine flu) is considered to be a respiratory disease of pigs caused by influenza virus (SIV, zoonotic disease). This illness was originally transmitted from pigs to humans but now easily spreads from one person to another. The symptoms of swine flu are totally similar to those of regular influenza and include fever, headaches, chills, diarrhoea, coughing and sneezing (1,2). The pandemic swine flu caused by the SIV subtype H1N1, including other subtypes H1N2, H1N3, H3N1, H3N2 and H2N3 can also cause illness. The virus was termed H1N1 because it mainly exhibited two types of antigens hemagglutinin (H) 1 and neuraminidase (N) 1 (3,4). Several vaccines are now available to prevent and/or against the disease. Generally, a healthy person may become infected by inhaling droplets expelled into the air through coughing or sneezing of an infected person or by transmission of virus-contaminated surfaces. However, the disease is not transmitted directly by eating cooked pork (1-5). The number of cases related to this virus

***Corresponding author:** Amit Gupta,
Email: amitvsbt@gmail.com; amitgupta@vsbt.res.in

shoots up during summer and monsoon season. In this regard, researchers have focused on various medicinal plants to control the burden of this disease.

Immunological exploration of these medicinal plants is totally based on phytochemical screening of primary and secondary metabolites (6). These metabolites of medicinal plants were examined for their immunopharmacological activities and approaches which lead to drug discovery and commonly referred as screening of natural products. Most of the medicinal plant products in the form of secondary metabolites i.e. flavonoids, terpenoids, saponin, etc. have shown anti-inflammatory, anti-microbial and immunosuppressive activities against specific as well as non-specific antigens (7-10). In addition, these metabolites from medicinal plant products are routinely used as raw material for extraction of active ingredients (11) that were used actually in the synthesis and manufacturing of active candidates e.g. adjuvants and vaccine antigens.

Azadirachta indica (Family *Meliaceae*; Common name, Neem) and *Butea frondosa* (Family *Fabaceae*; Common name, Palas) medicinal plants have shown many properties including anti-inflammatory, anti-hyperglycemic, antiulcer, antimalarial, antibacterial and antioxidant properties related to human health (7-13). *Ficus religiosa* (Peepal tree; family *Moraceae*) is found in tropical and subtropical regions of India. As per Ayurveda, isolation and purification of bioactive candidates from these herbal plants have shown various immunopharmacological activities so that they can be used to treat several types of diseases such as asthma, diabetes and inflammatory disorders (14). This study aimed to focus on the immunoadjuvant activities of medicinal plants namely *A. indica, B. frondosa* and *F. religiosa* against Swine flu vaccine antigen.

Materials and Methods

Plant material

Fresh leaves of *A. indica, B. frondosa* and *F. religiosa* were collected from Nakshatra Udyan of Vidya Pratishthan (Baramati, Maharashtra, India). The collected leaves were dried at room temperature and then macerated with a mortar and pestle. Powdered samples (5 g) of each plant were macerated in 50 mL of phosphate buffered saline (PBS, pH 7.2) and centrifuged at 10000 rpm. The supernatant was collected for estimation of various immunological assays. All these samples were stored at 4°C.

Qualitative analysis of secondary metabolites

The presence of secondary metabolites, i.e. terpenoids (using acetic anhydride test); flavonoids (using lead acetate test); saponins (using foam test) and phenolics (using ferric chloride test) was confirmed in aqueous leaves extracts of *A. indica, B. frondosa* and *F. religiosa.*

Swine flu vaccine

Inactivated influenza vaccines (surface antigen IP; 0.25 mL) were used in these studies. The influenza virus surface antigens (haemagglutinin and neuraminidase) were comprised of three different strains i.e. A/California/7/2009 (HIN1) pdm09-like strain (A/California/7/2009, X-181)- 7.5 µg HA; A/Hong)-Kong/4801/2014 (H3N2)-like strain (A/New Caledonia/71/2014, x-257A)- 7.5 µg HA; B/Brisbane/60/2008-like strain (B/Brisbane/60/2008, wild type)- 7.5 µg HA with a total volume of 250 µL. All strains were propagated in fertilized hens' eggs from healthy chicken flocks containing haemagglutinin as well as traces of eggs, i.e. OVA, Chicken proteins, etc.

ELISA assay

Indirect ELISA was performed using Swine flu vaccine (1:1000 dilution) as coating antigen. Variable concentrations of aqueous leaves extract of seven different medicinal plants, i.e. *Ficus religiosa, Syzygium cumini, Butea frondosa, Emblica officinalis, Terminalia arjuna, Prosopis spicigera* and *Azadirachta indica* were added and their Swine flu IgG antibody titers were determined. Horse anti-serum was used as secondary antibody and the absorbance in the form of optical density (OD) was measured at 450 nm (15).

Estimation of total cellular content

In *ex vivo* studies, Swiss mice (n = 5) were immunized subcutaneously (100 µL) on day 0 with Swine flu vaccine antigen (1:100 dilution; formulated containing three different strains in a final volume of 250 µL). On day 7, spleen cells were collected from peritoneal cavity of the mouse. Red blood cells from each spleen were then lysed with red cell lysis buffer. Finally, the cells were flushed out with PBS containing 10% FBS in order to prepare a single-cell suspension from the spleen of mouse. Splenocytes (100 µL cells containing 10^5 cells/well) were cultured in 96-well, flat-bottom tissue culture plates for 48. This incubation period was done along with variable doses of aqueous leaves extract of *A. indica, B. frondosa* and *F. religiosa* (0.312-5 mg; 50 µL) in the presence of swine flu vaccine antigen (2 µg/mL; 50 µL), OVA (50 µg/well; 50 µL) and Con A (5 µg/mL; 50 µL). Three different sets of experiments were performed simultaneously. The samples were centrifuged at 15000 rpm. The supernatant was collected in order to determine the total cellular or protein contents using NanoDrop 1000 A280 module. The Beer Lambert equation (A=E*b*c) was applied for all protein calculations to correlate absorbance with concentration.

Splenocyte proliferation assay and analysis of Th1 cytokines

Similarly, in another set of experiment performed MTT assay splenocytes were cultured and incubated at 37°C in 5% carbon dioxide incubator along with variable doses of aqueous leaves extracts in presence of swine flu vaccine antigen, OVA and Con A and determined their proliferation rate. After incubation, the medium was collected, centrifuged for the estimation of Th1 (IFN-gamma and TNF alpha) cytokines and then added fresh PBS containing 10 % FBS. MTT solution (2.5 mg/

ml; 10 µL) was added and then the plate was incubated for another 4 h at carbon dioxide incubator. Formazan crystals were appeared and settled at the bottom and then dissolved in dimethyl sulphoxide (DMSO) solution after centrifuging and discarding the supernatant. The OD was measured at 570 nm (16).

Briefly, 100 µL of diluted capture antibody (IFN-gamma and TNF alpha; 2 µg/mL) was added to each well in 96-well plates and allowed to adhere overnight at 4°C. The plates were washed properly and blocked in 1X PBS supplemented with 10% FBS for 1 hour at room temperature. After washing, serial dilutions of the standard and samples were prepared and incubated for 2 hours. The plates were then washed and the working detector solution (including detector antibody and avidin–horse radish peroxidase reagent) was added into each well. Plates were sealed and incubated at room temperature for 1 hour. After washing, 100 µL of tri-methyl benzidine (TMB) substrate was added into each well. The stop solution (2 N H2SO4) was finally added after incubation in the dark for 30 minutes at room temperature. The absorbance was read at 450 nm. The result was analyzed using softmax program and values were determined against the standard provided by the manufacturer (16).

Haemolytic activity

The haemolytic activity of human whole blood was determined using aqueous leaves extract of *A. indica, B. frondosa* and *F. religiosa*. Distilled water was used as a control. In this study, human whole blood suspension was collected from Mangal Pathology Laboratory, Baramati. Whole blood samples were prepared by diluting in PBS along with variable concentrations of aqueous leaves extracts of *A. indica, B. frondosa* and *F. religiosa*. The samples were incubated in a carbon dioxide incubator for 2 hours. After incubation, the blood samples containing aqueous leaves extract were centrifuged. The supernatants were collected and using spectrophotometer, the free hemoglobin in the supernatants was estimated. The OD was measured at 405 nm (14).

Results

ELISA assay

Determination of antibody production against Swine flu vaccine antigen was done through ELISA. As shown in Figure 1, out of seven, only three aqueous leaves extracts of *A. indica, B. frondosa* and *F. religiosa* showed enhancement in antibody production against Swine flu vaccine antigen as compared to the control group.

Total cellular content

As shown in Table 1, aqueous leaves extracts of *A. indica, B. frondosa* and *F. religiosa* showed enhancement in total cellular content with respect to Swine flu vaccine and OVA, antigen at higher doses as compared to the control group.

Proliferation assay

The effects of aqueous leaves extracts of three different medicinal plants were evaluated to determine splenocyte proliferation assay against Swine flu vaccine antigen, OVA and Con A (Figure 2). The results show that aqueous

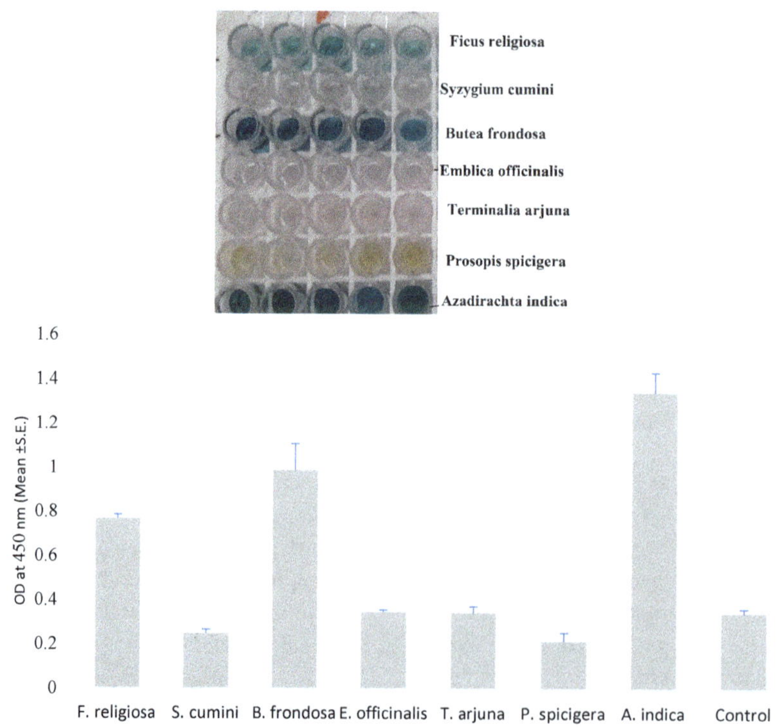

Figure 1. ELISA assay. Indirect ELISA was performed using Swine flu vaccine (1:1000 dilution) as coating antigen. Variable concentration of aqueous leaves extract of seven different medicinal plants were added and determined its Swine flu IgG antibody titre. Horse anti-serum was used as secondary antibody and absorbance in the form of optical density was measured at 450 nm.

Table 1. Effect of variable doses of aqueous leaves extract of medicinal plants on total cellular content in mouse splenocytes

Treatment		Doses (mg/mL)				
		0.156	0.312	0.625	1.25	2.5
Swine flu vaccine						
Control	0.424 ± 0.02	-	-	-	-	-
A. indica	-	0.544 ± 0.04	0.617 ± 0.02	0.982 ± 0.08	1.145 ±0.12	1.342 ± 0.22***
B. frondosa	-	0.750 ± 0.06	0.868 ± 0.14	0.912 ± 0.22	1.022 ± 0.34	1.232 ± 0.42**
F. religiosa	-	0.475 ± 0.02	0.412 ± 0.06	0.448 ± 0.04	0.568 ± 0.06	0.814 ± 0.12*
OVA						
Control	0.377 ±0.02	-	-	-	-	-
A. indica	-	0.562 ± 0.08	0.725 ± 0.06	0.986 ± 0.14	1.023 ± 0.13	1.214 ± 0.18**
B. frondosa	-	0.340 ± 0.02	0.425 ± 0.02	0.827 ± 0.08	0.924 ± 0.16	1.012 ± 0.22*
F. religiosa	-	0.319 ± 0.02	0.464 ± 0.04	0.683 ± 0.04	0.712 ± 0.06	0.784 ± 0.14

Swiss mice were immunized with swine flu vaccine on day 0. Splenocytes were collected on day 7 and cultured with variable doses of aqueous leaves extract and then further exposed with Swine flu vaccine antigen and OVA. Total cellular content was measured after high speed centrifugation and collect supernatant for estimation of total cellular content. Values are expressed as Mean ± S.E. The difference between control and variable doses of aqueous extract is controlled by one-way ANOVA test (Bonferroni multiple comparison test). *$P < 0.05$; **$P < 0.01$ and ***$P < 0.001$.

leaves extracts of *A. indica, B. frondosa* and *F. religiosa* raised splenocyte proliferation at lower doses as compared to the control group. Swine flu vaccine antigen, OVA and Con A were used as standards in this study and showed an enhancement in proliferation as compared to the control group.

Analysis of Th1 cytokines by ELISA

As shown in Figure 3, aqueous leaves extracts of *A. indica, B. frondosa and F. religiosa* raised Th1 (IFN-gamma and TNF alpha) production at lower doses as compared to the control group.

Haemolytic activity

The effects of aqueous leaves extracts of three different medicinal plants evaluated to determine their haemolytic activities in the human whole blood (Figure 4). The results showed that aqueous extracts of three medicinal plants had not any haemolytic effect at higher doses as compared to the control group. On the other hand, distilled water showed higher haemolytic activity.

Discussion

Phytochemicals are bioactive compounds that are present in medicinal plants and applied in traditional herbal medicines. Generally, these herbal medicines are used for curing various human diseases especially diabetes, cancer, HIV etc. The objective of our study was to determine qualitatively screening of phytochemicals within aqueous leaves extracts of three medicinal plants and estimating the antibody titer and proliferation rate (using specific and non-specific antigen) against Swine flu vaccine antigen. These medicinal plants were screened and evaluated in the form of aqueous leaves extracts for adjuvant activity against different vaccine antigens. These adjuvants are needed for vaccine antigen in order to enhance its immunogenicity against various infectious diseases. Searching for those active molecules derived from medicinal plants which are responsible for inducing or stimulating both humoral and cell-mediated immune responses is necessary. For the last several years, only one adjuvant has been approved for human use, i.e. alum which increases humoral response. However it poorly elicits cell-mediated immunity. In addition, emulsion-based adjuvant, i.e. MF59 provokes both humoral and cell mediated immune response. Recently, a trivalent vaccine, namely Fluad, formulated with MF59 (effective for 65 years or more; US approved) has been produced from three strains of influenza (2 subtype A and 1 type B) for prevention of seasonal influenza (17). In view of this, adjuvants are required for vaccine antigen pertaining to increase its immunogenicity, avidity and also help in decreasing the dose of antigen to decrease the toxicity. In this regard, efforts have been made in order to reduce the burden of antigen using various medicinal plants and to use as adjuvant against vaccine antigens. The most important benefit of these adjuvant-based plants is that they would remain stable for longer period of time. Generally, secondary metabolites from medicinal plants, used as adjuvant for vaccine antigen, are still under investigation, e.g. QS21 (saponin from *Quillaja saponaria*); RLJ-NE-299A (glycosides from *Picrorhiza Kurroa*) (11,18). In this study, we got similar results and these medicinal plants in the form of aqueous extract containing various phytochemicals showed enhancement in antibody production against Swine flu vaccine antigen. Further immunological *ex vivo* studies were also conducted in those splenocytes were cultured and exposed to swine flu vaccine, OVA and Con A in aqueous leaves extract and showed dose dependent changes in proliferation and total cellular content as compared to control group. In addition, specific (swine flu vaccine, OVA) and non-specific (Con A) antigens were recognized strongly by aqueous leaves extract containing primary as well as secondary metabolites and antibody-secreting cells from vaccines (11). Studying this interaction will allow us to further elucidate the effectiveness of antigen adjuvant combinations. In contrast, these medicinal plants showed no haemolytic effects as compared to distilled water.

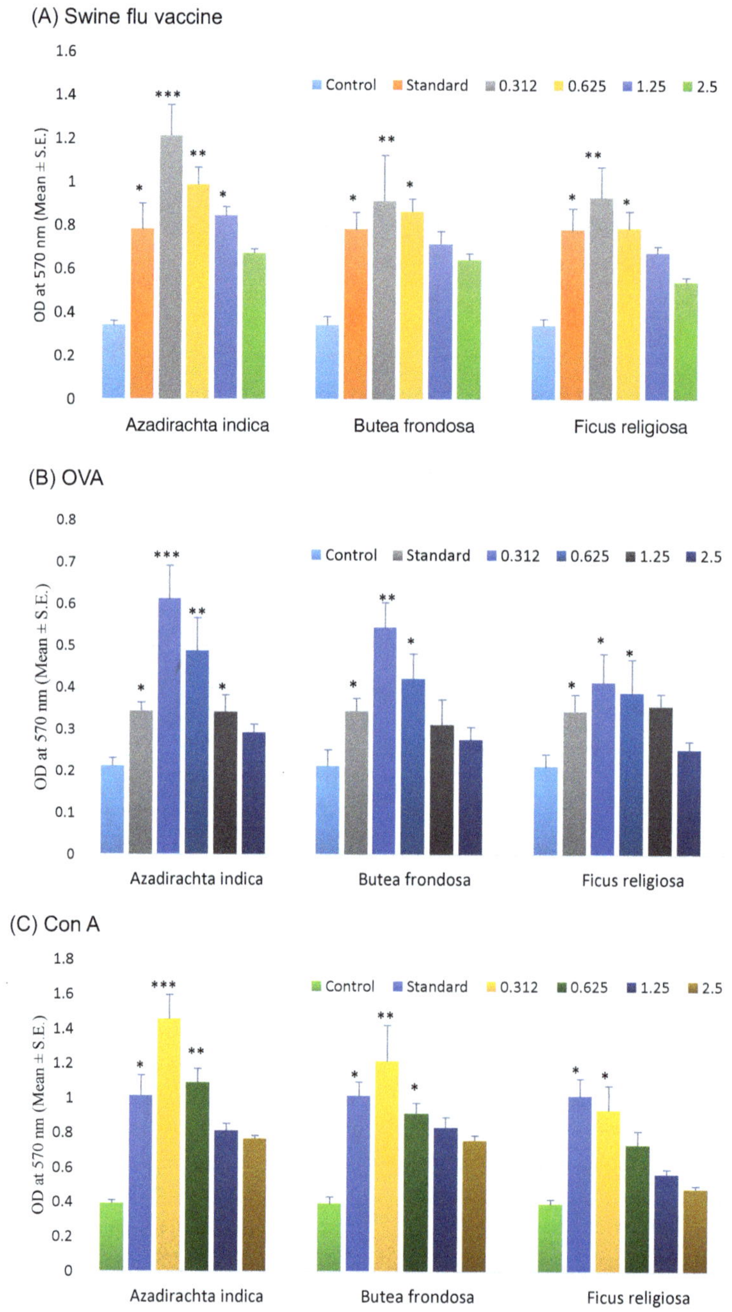

Figure 2. Splenocyte proliferation assay. Swiss mice were immunized subcutaneously on day 0 with swine flu vaccine antigen. On day 7, Splenocytes were collected and cultured with variable doses of aqueous leaves extract (0.312- 2.5 mg/mL; 50 µL) and then exposed to A) swine flu vaccine antigen (2 µg/mL; 50 µL), B) OVA (50 µg/well; 50 µL) and C) Con A (5 µg/mL; 50 µL)and determined its proliferation assay using MTT. Values are expressed as mean ± SE. The difference between control and variable doses of aqueous extract was controlled by one way ANOVA test (Bonferroni multiple comparison test). *$P < 0.05$; **$P < 0.01$ and ***$P < 0.001$.

Furthermore, aqueous leaves extract were able to induce anti-Swine flu, anti-OVA and anti-Con A T-helper cell response as shown by the strong antigen-specific/non-specific cell proliferation. Cytokine determination showed that aqueous extract adjuvanted Swine flu vaccine induced more IFN- gamma and TNF production as compared to control group. In short, we can be concluded on the basis of antibody production, proliferation and cytokines (IFN-gamma and TNF alpha) that aqueous extracts of the plants induce Th1 immune response. These observations suggest that the use of these aqueous extract as an adjuvant for swine flu vaccine antigen may provide better protection against these antigens by eliciting both humoral and cellular immune responses.

Conclusion

The results of this study indicated that aqueous leaves extracts of these plants might be considered as better vaccine adjuvant candidates in order to enhance the immunogenicity or antibody production, proliferation and Th1 cytokines against Swine flu vaccine antigen. The need for exploring alternative plant based formulation

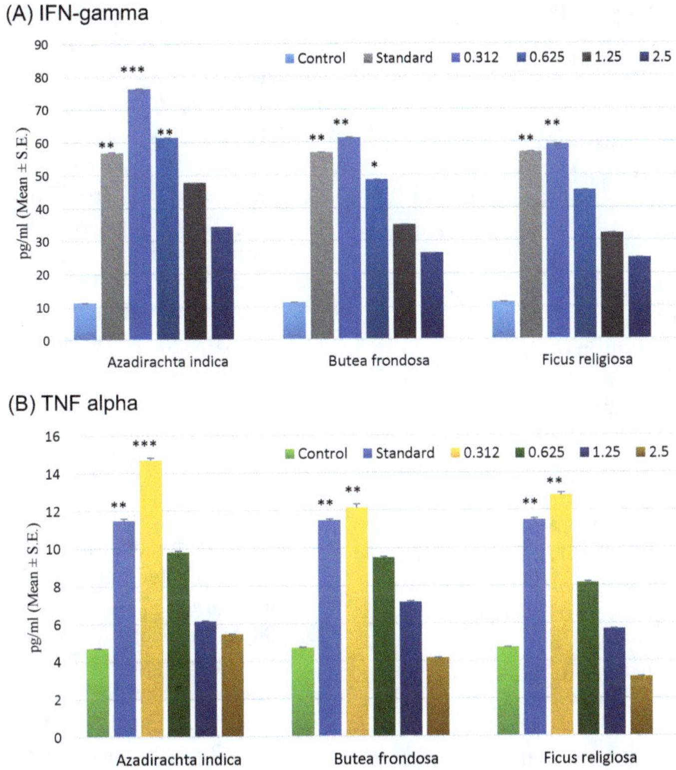

Figure 3. Th1 (IFN-gamma and TNF alpha) cytokines. Swiss mice were immunized subcutaneously on day 0 with swine flu vaccine antigen. On day 7, splenocytes were collected and cultured with variable doses of aqueous leaves extract (0.312- 2.5 mg/mL; 50 µL) and then exposed to swine flu vaccine antigen (2 µg/mL; 50 µL). Incubate the plate for another 24h. The plate was centrifuged and the supernatant was collected for the estimation of Th1 cytokines which determined by Elisa. Values are expressed as mean ± SE. The difference between control and variable doses of aqueous extract was determined by one way ANOVA test (Bonferroni multiple comparison test). $^{*}P < 0.05$; $^{**}P < 0.01$ and $^{***}P < 0.001$.

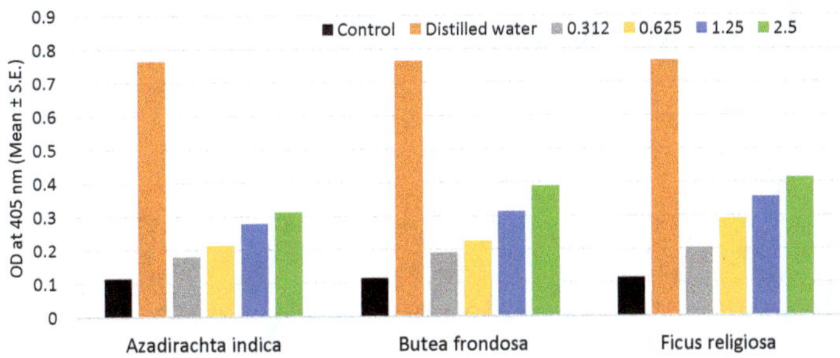

Figure 4. Haemolytic activity. Whole blood samples were diluted in PBS along with variable concentrations of aqueous leaves extracts (0.312- 2.5 mg/mL; 50 µL). The samples were incubated for 2 hours at carbon dioxide incubator. After incubation, the blood samples were centrifuged and the supernatants were collected and the free haemoglobin was estimated in the supernatants using spectrophotometer. The OD was measured at 405 nm.

for Swine flu vaccine antigen may raise the next step in this evaluation to test aqueous extract as an adjuvant with other protein antigens. Further studies with these aqueous extracts adjuvanted with Swine flu vaccine antigen are needed to establish clinically relevant proof of principles.

Authors' contribution

This work was carried out in collaboration of four authors. AG designed the study, wrote the protocol and interpreted the data where SG anchored the field study, gathered the initial data related to his M.Sc. Biotechnology dissertation work under AG guidance and performed preliminary data analysis. AG, SG and BS managed the literature searches whereas AG produced the initial draft. The final manuscript was read and approved by all authors.

Conflict of interests

The authors declared no competing interests.

Ethical considerations

This study was confirmed and conducted under ethical guidelines with registration number 1814/PO/ERE/S/15/CPCSEA.

Funding/Support

This research was financially supported by our organization

i.e. Vidya Pratishthan's School of Biotechnology, Arts, Science and Commerce College.

References

1. Simpson CR, Ritchie LD, Robertson C, Sheikh A, McMenamin J. Effectiveness of H1N1 vaccine for the prevention of pandemic influenza in Scotland, UK: A retrospective observational cohort study. Lancet Infect Dis. 2012;12(9):696-702.
2. Collignon P. H1N1 immunization: too much, too soon? Aust Prescr. 2011;33(2):30-31.
3. Murphy BR, Coelingh K. Principles underlying the development and use of live attenuated cold adapted influenza A and B virus vaccines. Viral Immunol. 2002;15(2):295-323.
4. Doroshenko A, Halperin SA. Trivalent MDCK cell culture derived influenza vaccine Optaflu (Novartis vaccines). Expert Rev Vaccines. 2009;8(6):679-688.
5. Bhakdi S, Lackner K, Doerr HW. Possible hidden hazards of mass vaccination against new influenza A/H1N1: have the cardiovascular risks been adequately weighed? Med Microbiol Immunol. 2009;198(4):205-209.
6. Gupta A, Khamkar PR, Chaphalkar SR. Applications and uses of active ingredients from medicinal plants. Indian Journal of Novel Drug Delivery. 2014;6(2):106–111.
7. Gupta A, Chaphalkar SR. Terpenoids from three medicinal plants and their potential anti-inflammatory and immunosuppressive activity on human whole blood and peripheral blood mononuclear cells. Asian Journal of Ethno Pharmacology and Medicinal Foods. 2016;4(1):13–17.
8. Gupta A, Chaphalkar SR. Cytotoxic and immunosuppressive activity of terpenoids from *Prosopis spicigera, Mimusops elengi* and *Terminalia arjuna*. International Journal of Universal Pharmacy and Biosciences. 2016;5(1):32–39.
9. Gupta A, Chaphalkar SR. Immunosuppressive activity of flavonoids isolated from *Terminalia arjuna, Prosopis spicigera* and *Mimusops elengi*. Int J Res Pharm Sci. 2015;5(4):14–17.
10. Gupta A, Chaphalkar SR. Anti-inflammatory activity of flavonoids from medicinal plants against hepatitis B vaccine antigen on human peripheral blood mononuclear cells. Asian J Pharm Clin Res. 2015;3(1):728–732.
11. Khajuria A, Gupta A, Singh S, et al. A new plant based vaccine adjuvant. Vaccine. 2007;25(14):2706–2715.
12. Gupta A, Chaphalkar SR. Analytical studies of protease extracted from *Azadirachta indica*. World J Pharm Res. 2015;4(11):1391–1398.
13. Gupta A, Chaphalkar SR. Haemolytic and immunoadjuvant effect of *Butea frondosa* on the immune response to hepatitis B vaccine containing surface antigen in mice. J Herbmed Pharmacol. 2016;5(3):103-106.
14. Gupta A, Khamkar PR, Chaphalkar SR. Immunomodulatory and anti-inflammatory activity of aqueous extract of leaf, stem and root of *Ficus religiosa* on human whole blood and peripheral blood mononuclear cells. Int J Med Pharm Res. 2014; (4):732-739.
15. Gupta A, Chaphalkar SR. Immunoadjuvant potential of *Azadirachta indica* against rabies, hepatitis and DPT vaccine antigen.Int J Med Pharm Res. 2015;5(7):1–5.
16. Khajuria A, Gupta A, Malik F, et al. A new vaccine adjuvant (BOS 2000) a potent enhancer mixed Th1/Th2 immune responses in mice immunized with HBsAg. Vaccine. 2007;25(23):4586–4594.
17. Gupta A, Chaphalkar SR. Vaccine adjuvants: Current necessity of life. Shiraz E-Medical Journal. 2015;16(7):1 -11.
18. Jacobsen NE, Fairbrother WJ, Kensil CR, Lim A, Wheeler DA, Powell MF. Structure of the saponin adjuvant QS-21 and its base-catalyzed isomerization product by 1H and natural abundance 13C NMR spectroscopy. Carbohydr Res. 1996;280:1–14.

Extraction, identification and anti-inflammatory activity of carotenoids out of *Capsicum Anuum* L.

Yurii Aleksandrovich Boiko[1*], Irina Anatolievna Kravchenko [2], Alexey Antonovich Shandra[1], Irina Anatolievna Boiko[3]

[1]Department of Physiology, Odessa National Medical University, Odessa, Ukraine
[2]Department of Pharmaceutical Chemistry, Odessa National University I.I. Mechnikova, Odessa, Ukraine
[3]Department of Pharmacognosy, Odessa National Medical University, Odessa, Ukraine

ARTICLE INFO

Keywords:
Carotenoids
Adjuvant-induced inflammation
Ukrainian bitter peppers
Acetylcholinesterase
Seromucoid

ABSTRACT

Introduction: Carotenoids extracted from dried peppers were evaluated for their anti-inflammatory activities.
Methods: Determining the concentration of carotenoids was carried out by spectrophotometry. Anti-inflammatory activity was studied on the model adjuvant-induced inflammation. In addition, the total number of white blood cells was studied by microscopic method in Gorjaev's chamber. The biochemical parameters of blood - cholinesterase activity and total number of seromucoids in blood plasma were determined by the commercial test kits for rapid analysis
Results: Peppers had a substantial carotenoid content: Ukrainian bitter 2076 ± 10 μg/g of sample in dry weight basis. The yellow fraction was 69.3%, the red fraction was 30.7%. The linear decrease of inflammatory edema in the course of therapeutic use of carotenoid extract ranged from 20% to 50%. The application of carotenoid extract reduced levels of activity acetylcholinesterase and concentration of seromucoids in serum of rats with adjuvant-induced inflammation. The use of carotenoid extract in rats with adjuvant-induced inflammation resulted in reduction of serum cholinesterase activity by 1.3 times and double decrease in the serum seromucoid concentration.
Conclusion: Ukrainian bitter pepper carotenoid extract exhibited good anti-inflammatory activity, with inhibited adjuvant-induced oedema formation and progression. The results suggest that the carotenoids in dried Ukrainian bitter peppers have significant anti-inflammatory benefits and could be useful for pain and inflammation relief. The results of this study allow to recommend carotenoid extract for further investigation as active part of anti-inflammatory drugs.

Implication for health policy/practice/research/medical education:
The results of this study show that carotenoid can be as active part of anti-inflammatory drugs

Introduction

The plant raw materials are the most important source of new biologically active substances which potentially have different types of pharmacological activities. The most high-demand compounds in the medical practice are the substances with anti-inflammatory effect. The formulations with Cayenne pepper (*Capsicum anuum* L.) have been used for a long time as anti-inflammatory drugs of plant origin (1). Therapeutic action of *Capsicum anuum* L. is primarily attributed to the presence of capsaicinoids which are the agonists of the transient receptor potential for vanilloid (TRPV-1) (2). Nevertheless the use of pepper extracts in experimental inflammation enabled to achieve effects which could not be explained solely by the action of capsaicinoids (3). The other groups of substances contained in pepper and having anti-inflammatory effects include antioxidants-carotenoids (4,5), vitamin E and vitamin C (6).

At the alteration inflammation stage the reactive oxygen intermediates (super-oxide anion radical, hydrogen peroxide, hydroxyl radical, singlet oxygen) - with high oxidation potential are accumulated and consequently may induce high damaging effect on biological membranes. Carotenoids (Figure 1) have a system of conjugated double bonds providing them with a powerful antioxidant effect, reducing the oxidative stress that accompanies the inflam-

***Corresponding author:** Boiko Yurii Aleksandrovich;
Email: yuriyalexb@gmail.com

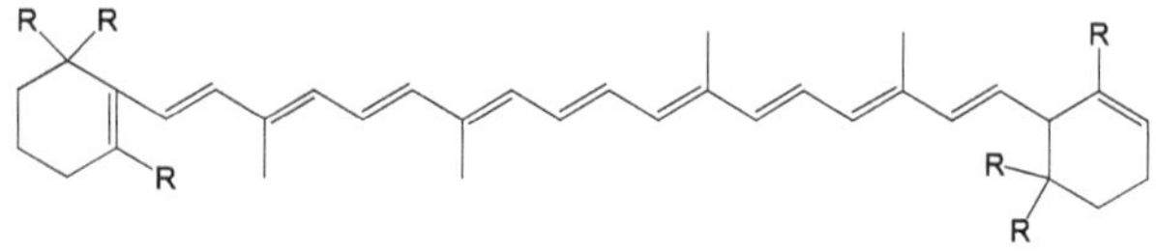

Figure 1. General formula of carotenoids, where R – various substitute.

mation processes (6).

Thus, when using the multicomponent extracts of *Capsicum anuum* L. as anti-inflammatory agents the synergistic pharmacological effect shall occur due to the effect of capsaicin and antioxidant substances on different links of the inflammation process (7).

The aim of this study was to investigate the anti-inflammatory activity of the carotenoids extract of *Capsicum anuum* L. In addition, the total content of carotenoids in generated extracts - one of the main parameters which determine the suitability of the applied plant material as a basis for the production of the pharmaceutical preparations was defined.

Materials and Methods

The plant raw materials were fresh ripe fruits of Ukrainian Cayenne pepper. For extraction of carotenoids, 25 g of finely divided plant raw material (air dried pepper pods without seeds and green part) were filled with 500 mL of acetone at 5°C for several minutes. The obtained extract was filtered under vacuum pump through paper filters No. 4. The filtrate was transferred to a separator funnel containing petroleum ether (mixture of heptane and hexane 1:1) and water. Mixing was performed without shaking, whereupon the aqueous phase was separated. The remaining mixture was washed with water several times, followed by removal of remaining water by means of anhydrous sodium sulfate. Further, the solution was stored in a tightly sealed container in a dark place at a temperature of 5°C.

In order to determine the concentrations of carotenoids of various fractions, the petroleum ether was distilled off in rotary evaporator and the resulting oily residue was dissolved in acetone. Then, the absorbance was measured at the transmitted light wavelength of 472 and 508 nm.

The concentration of carotenoids of yellow and red fractions was calculated using the following formulas:

$$C_{\text{red fraction}},\ \text{mcg/mL} = \frac{21444 \times A508 - 403,3 \times A472}{270,9}$$

$$C_{\text{yelow fraction}},\ \text{mcg/mL} = \frac{1724,3 \times A472 - 2450 \times A508}{270,9}$$

Where: A_{508} and A_{472} - absorbance of the solutions for the corresponding wavelengths.

The base for the formulation was produced by mixing 10 parts of paraffinic oil and 1 part of petrolatum. The base was supplemented with concentrated extract of the carotenoids of Cayenne pepper. The final concentration of carotenoids in the formulation was two milligrams per 1 gram of ointment.

Experiments were carried out in young male Wistar rats weighing 180-220 g, managed in standard vivarium conditions with free access to food and water. All studies conformed to the rules of the "European Convention for the Protection of Vertebrate Animals used for Experimental and Other Scientific Purposes" (8) and the principles of the Ukrainian National Congress on Bioethics (9).

Inflammatory arthritis model was reproduced by administration of Freund's complete adjuvant manufactured by FIA (the United States) underneath the plantar aponeurosis of the right limb in a volume of 0.1 mL (10).

The animals were divided into control and experimental groups by a randomized method, 10 animals per group. Treatment was carried out by applying the soft formulation with carotenoid extract to the area of limb inflammation once per day, in 24 hours after administration of phlogogen until full recovery. The control group of animals received treatment in the form of a soft base for the formulation without any carotenoid extract.

The effectiveness of the treatment was assessed by change in the morphological signs of inflammation - thickness and size of limb in the lesion area. The thickness of the limbs was measured by electronic caliper YT-7201 manufactured by YATO company, Poland, the changes in limb size were measured by means of digital Plethysmometer 37140, UgoBasile (PRC). In addition, the total number of white blood cells was studied by microscopic method in Gorjaev's chamber.

The biochemical parameters of blood - cholinesterase activity and total number of seromucoids in blood plasma were determined by the commercial test kits for rapid analysis manufactured by Research and Production Enterprise "Filicit-Diagnostika" Ltd. (Ukraine).

Results

The total content of carotenoids in the dry pods of Ukrainian Cayenne pepper was 2076 ± 10 μg/L g of plant tissue. At the same time the yellow fraction of carotenoids was 69.3%, and the red fraction 30.7%. Red fraction consisted mainly of capsanthin and yellow one of lutein (both fractions were also characterized by a high content of β-carotene).

Investigation of the effect of soft formulation, comprising carotenoid extract of Cayenne pepper fruits as active ingredient, on morphological indicators of adjuvant inflammation process development is shown in Figure 2.

Application of the studied soft formulation with carotenoid extract caused positive therapeutic dynamics reflected in decreased edema in the area of inflammation. Noticeable effect significantly different from the control was observed in 2-3 days of treatment. Linear and volumetric dimensions of the inflamed area of the limb in the experimental group were 20% to 50% lower than the corresponding indicators of the control group. On the 10th day of treatment, the size of the limb in the inflamed area in the treated group of animals was approaching the size recorded before the introduction of phlogogen. The func-

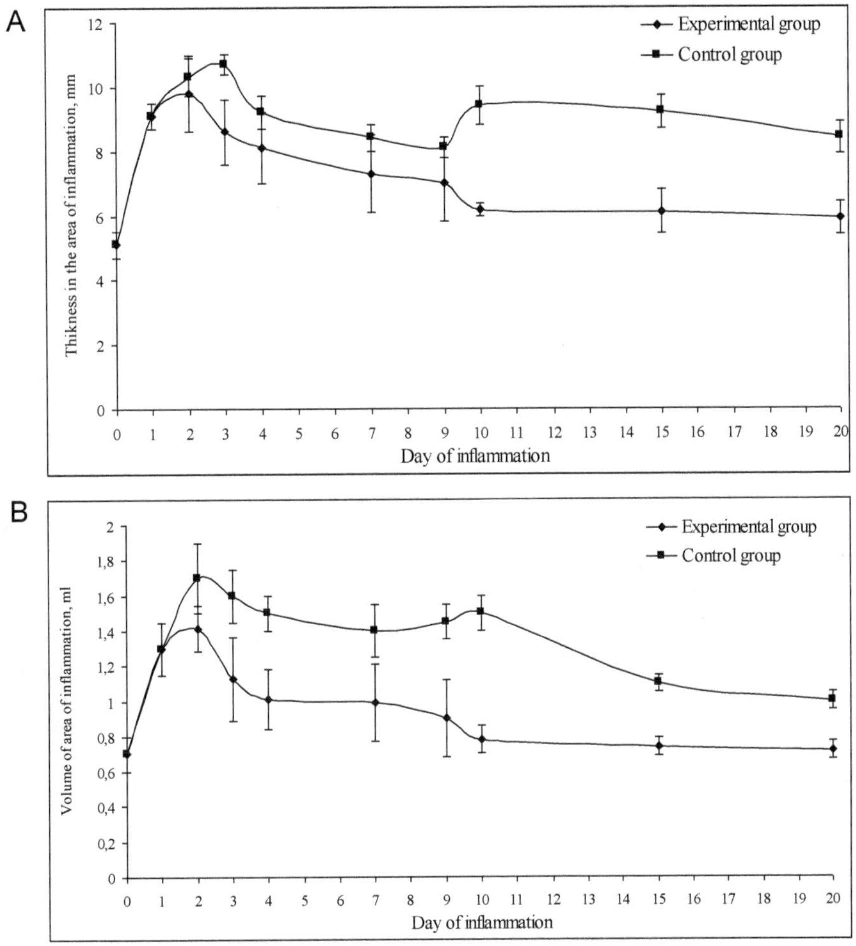

Figure 2. Effect of the formulation with soft carotenoid extract on thickness (A) and volume (B) of limb in adjuvant-induced inflammation area.

tion of the damaged limb was fully recovered. On palpation the areas of administered phlogogen were painless. In contrast, in the control group the lesion area was significantly thickened even on the 20th day after phlogogen administration. On examination, the redness and pain were detected (symptoms that completely absent in the experimental group). Thus, one can conclude that carotenoid extract of Cayenne pepper has not only antiedemic but also complex anti-inflammatory effect.

Dynamics of changes in quantitative indicators of white blood cells after inflammation induction is shown in Figure 3.

After inflammation induction the significant rise in the quantity of white blood cells was observed in the first 2 days of the experiment. The maximum content of white blood cells was observed on the second day after the phlogogen administration and reached 51 and 55 g/L for the experimental and control groups, respectively. Further, there was a decrease of white blood cells to about 30 and 40 g/L, from third to eighth days, and then the regrowth of their quantity was recorded. In the group treated with carotenoid extract ointment the quantity of white blood cells on 20th day was significantly lower than in control group. On 20th day of the inflammatory process, the number of white blood cells both in experimental and control groups exceeded the corresponding values before phlogogen administration by 2 and 2.6 times, respectively. Biochemical parameters of blood are both important markers of various pathological reactions and indicator of dynamics of the disease development. In adjuvant-induced inflammation the indicators of serum cholinesterase activity and serum seromucoid concentration are of interest (Tables 1 and 2).

Dynamics of changes in the serum seromucoid concentrations were similar to the dynamics of changes in cholinesterase activity. Maximum values of seromucoid concentrations were observed on third day for the experimental group (1.44 absorbance units) and on seventh days for the control group of animals (1.69 absorbance units). It should be noted that on 20th day of treatment the seromucoid serum concentration in the experimental group was close to intact values, while in the control group it exceeded the intact values by more than 2 times.

Discussion

Depending on the color, the quantity of carotenoids contained in the pepper fruits can vary greatly. According to data, the least quantity of carotenoids is found in green fruits, red fruits are intermediate in terms of quantity of carotenoids, and the highest concentration is observed in

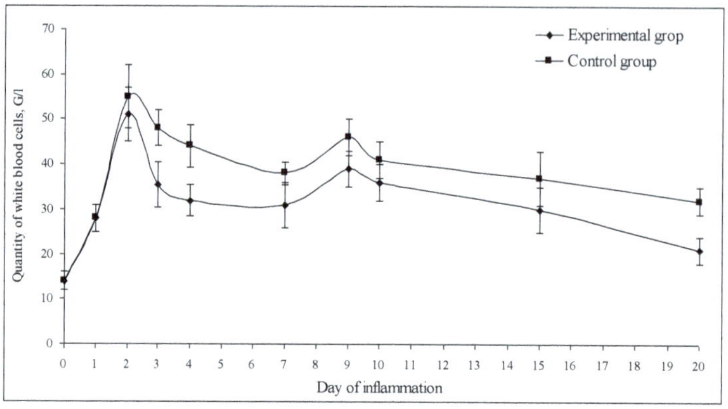

Figure 3. Dynamics of changes in the quantity of white blood cells in treatment of adjuvant-induced inflammation by carotenoid extract of *Capsicum anuum* L.

Table 1. Serum cholinesterase activity in adjuvant-induced inflammation, μmol/s*l

Day of inflammation	Control group	Treatment with soft formulation of carotenoid extract
0	28.2 ± 3.6	28.2 ± 3.6
1	83.6 ± 4.3	83.6 ± 4.3
2	129.7 ± 6.7	118.6 ± 7.1
3	138.4 ± 8.1	105.7 ± 11.2*
4	122.9 ± 6.9	92.7 ± 4.1*
7	120.5 ± 5.8	80.0 ± 9.9*
9	127.4 ± 3.1	87.4 ± 9.3*
10	130.6 ± 2.7	85.2 ± 7.6*
15	111.8 ± 7.3	70.4 ± 10.1*
20	54.9 ± 8.6	35.7 ± 8.4*

* Significant differences from control.

Table 2. The serum seromucoid concentration in treating the non-specific inflammation in rats, absorbance units

Day of inflammation	Control group	Treatment with soft formulation of carotenoid extract
0	0.47 ± 0.08	0.47 ± 0.08
1	0.91 ± 0.1	0.91 ± 0.1
2	1.24 ± 0.18	1.17 ± 0.2
3	1.52 ± 0.14	1.44 ± 0.17
4	1.57 ± 0.21	1.22 ± 0.1*
7	1.69 ± 0.16	1.08 ± 0.22*
9	1.62 ± 0.1	0.82 ± 0.18*
10	1.50 ± 0.12	0.75 ± 0.25*
15	1.33 ± 0.15	0.70 ± 0.11*
20	1.05 ± 0.1	0.62 ± 0.07*

* Significant differences from control, $P < 0.05$.

yellow fruits (11). At the same time, the color does not depend only on the total carotenoid content, but on percentage of different carotenoid fractions. In some cases related to the features of growing (low-volume hydroponics), total increase in carotenoid content can be accompanied by a fall in the quantity of yellow-orange component, which affects the final color of the fruits (12).

The quantity of carotenoids in Ukrainian Cayenne pepper is close by values to the same parameters established for chilly varieties (5). In general, we can conclude that by phytochemical composition, the fruits of Ukrainian Cayenne pepper are suitable source of bioactive compounds for the subsequent production of pharmaceutical preparations.

Pronounced anti-inflammatory effect of carotenoids of Cayenne pepper can, in part, be attributed to the effect on reactive oxygen intermediates that occur in the course of the inflammatory process. Relating to non-enzymatic antioxidant system, the carotenoids are always present in the organism providing mainly protection against the damaging effect of singlet oxygen ($^1O_2$) and peroxide radicals (ROO·). The antioxidant activity of carotenoids is directly dependent on the system of conjugated double bonds connected with different end groups. In the course of antioxidant protection provided by carotenoid the physical and chemical mechanism of utilization of $^1O_2$ is possible. At the same time the carotenoids refer to the one of the most effective natural utilizers of the singlet oxygen (13,14). Another protection feature of carotenoids is the inhibition of the Maillard reaction - glycosylation of the amino groups of proteins resulting in breach of their functional activity (15). Antinociceptive effect is associated with the α- and β-carotenes and lycopene (16,17).

Increase in the quantity of white blood cells is one of the major systemic reactions to the local inflammatory process. At this stage of primary non-specific inflammation the area of inflammation is infiltrated with neutrophils and macrophages, which is also accompanied by an increase in their quantity in the systemic circulation. In case of rheumatoid lesion due to specific autoimmune processes, there is a growing population of lymphocytes (18). Decrease in the total quantity of white blood cells in the course of the treatment demonstrates its effectiveness. Nevertheless, the absence of external local manifestations of the inflammatory response was not accompanied by the restoration of the system indicators such as the level of white blood cells. The inflammation development at the opposite limb which is sign of autoimmune lesions, typical for rheumatoid arthritis, has not been fixed. Thus, one can assume that the activation of the leukocytic cells in the focus of inflammation caused by phlogogen administration resulted in continued increase in the level of pro-inflammatory and inflammatory cytokines, which led to a stable increase in the quantity of white blood cells.

The existence of several forms of cholinesterase (acetylcholinesterase, butyrylcholinesterase, pseudocholinesterase) determines the predominant location for each type of enzyme. High concentrations of acetylcholinesterase are typical for brain, nerve fibers and erythrocytes, butyrylcholinesterase and pseudocholinesterase are found in blood serum, pancreas and liver (19). Therefore, the observed increase in cholinesterase activity may be a consequence both of direct breach of the cell integrity in the area of inflammation (particularly if skeletal muscle fibers are damaged), and activation of cellular component of the inflammatory cascade. In case of interaction of the acetylcholine with α-7H-acetylcholine receptors located on the surface of blood monocytes, the release of proinflammatory cytokines by latter is decreased, the cholinergic anti-inflammatory pathway occurs (20,21). Increase in the cholinesterase activity leads to an acceleration of acetylcholine utilization and, consequently, increase in inflammatory manifestations. In our study, the increase in cholinesterase activity correlated well with the intensity of the inflammatory response.

Subsequent decreased cholinesterase activity in animals treated with the carotenoid extract ointment in comparison with control group may be both consequence of decrease of alteration process in the inflammation area, and decreased systemic inflammatory response.

α1-Acid glycoprotein (seromucoid, orosomucoid) refers to a group of acute-phase proteins. The seromucoid level can be increased by several times in the course of inflammatory process development, which makes it an effective biomarker reflecting the development of the acute phase of inflammation (22). Seromucoid has a sufficiently long period of half-life (unlike C-reactive protein, which is 5 days). This enables it to be used as an indicator of the effectiveness of the applied treatment (23). The factors activating the seromucoid synthesis by hepatocytes are interleukin-1α (IL-1α) and interleukin-6 (IL-6). The observed decrease in serum seromucoid concentration in the experimental group can be a consequence of decreased level of IL-1α and IL-6. This assumption seems logical not only because of the direct influence of abovementioned interleukins on the products of seromucoid, but also due to the proinflammatory nature of IL-1α and IL-6. We suppose that conducted therapeutic effect has led to a decrease in the level of IL-1α and IL-6, which in turn reduced the symptoms of the acute inflammation phase and contributed to decrease in the serum seromucoid concentration.

Conclusion

The high content of carotenoids in extract of *Capsicum anuum* L. of Ukrainian Cayenne pepper makes possible its use as the base for the production of pharmaceutical anti-inflammatory products. The formulations of mixed nature containing both carotenoid extract and other antioxidants (vitamin C, E) and capsaicinoid extract are of special interest. Based on the received data on the distribution of different fractions of the carotenoids, we can recommend the use of yellow fruits due to higher carotenoid content in them.

Using of carotenoid extract as a local anti-inflammatory agent is capable of substantial decrease in all external manifestations of the inflammatory process, thus one can give findings on comprehensive anti-inflammatory effect of these drugs. The most probable mechanism of anti-inflammatory activity of carotenoids is their antioxidant effect resulting in decrease of alteration action of reactive oxygen intermediates in the area of inflammation.

Decreased serum cholinesterase activity and reduced serum seromucoid concentration in the course of inflammation process treatment by carotenoid extract may be testimony both of reduced reactions of the secondary lesion in the area of inflammation, and the general decrease in systemic inflammatory response.

Authors' contributions

BYA prepared introduction, experimental part, analysis and discussion of results, conclusion, preparation for publication. KIA and SAA analyzed the data and prepared discussion as well as conclusion of results. BIA did experimental part. All read and confirmed the article.

Conflict of interests

None of the authors has any conflict of interest to disclose.

Ethical considerations

We confirm that we have read the Journal's position on issues involved in ethical publication and affirm that this report is consistent with those guidelines.

Funding/Support

The work was performed as part of scientific programs of department of physiology (Odessa National Medical University), department of pharmaceutical chemistry (Odessa National University I.I. Mechnikova) and department of pharmacognosy (Odessa National Medical University).

References

1. Suleymanova LR, Kurkin VA. Phyto-chemical research of preparation and raw material on the basis of siliculose pepper (*Capsicum anuum* L). Proceedings of Samara Scientific Centre of Russian Academy of Sciences. 2009; 11(6):1311-1314.
2. Reyes-Escogido ML, Gonzalez-Mondragon EG, Vazquez-Tzompantzi E. Chemical and pharmacological aspects of capsaicin. Molecules. 2011;16:1253-1270.
3. Boyko Y A, Kravchenko IA, Ayat M. Pharmacotherapeutical activity of ointment based extractives *Capsicum annuum* L. at experimental inflammatory. J NAMS Ukraine. 2014;20(2):257-62.
4. Cervantes-Paz B, Yahia EM, Ornelas-Paz JJ, et al. Antioxidant activity and content of chlorophylls and carotenoids in raw and heat-processed Jalapeño peppers at intermediate stages of ripening. Food Chem. 2014;146:188-196
5. Hernández-Ortega M, Ortiz-Moreno A, Hernández-Navarro MD, Chamorro-Cevallos G, Dorantes-Alvarez L, Necoechea-Mondragón H. Antioxidant, antinociceptive,

and anti-inflammatory effects of carotenoids extracted from dried pepper (*Capsicum annuum* L.). J Biomed Biotech. 2012;2012:524019.

6. Stahl W, Sies H. Antioxidant defense: vitamins E and C and carotenoids. Diabetes. 1997;46(2):14-8.
7. Pandey V, Pandey HK, Dayal D, Joshi UC, Pant T, Ahmed Z. Studies on antioxidant constituents of some domesticated capsicums in the middle hill conditions of western Himalayas. Hort Sci. 2009;36(1):26-30.
8. European convention for the protection of vertebrate animals used for experimental and other scientific purposes. Strasbourg: Council of Europe; 1986:1-51.
9. Ethical principles of animal experiments. Endocrinology. 2003;8(1):142-5.
10. Stefanov OV. Preclinical studies of drugs. Kiev: Avicena; 2001:528.
11. Gorunova YD, Chupakhov GN. Optimization of antioxidant status of fruit bell pepper. Herald SRU. 2008;1:96-99
12. Belavkin ES, Pyshnaya ON, Mamedov MI, Golubkina NA, Dzhos EA. Environmental effect on biologically active compounds content in sweet pepper fruits. Vegetab Growing Cultivat. 2009;55:412-8
13. Sies H, Stahl W. Vitamins E and C, 3-carotene, and other carotenoids as antioxidants. Am J Clin Nutr. 1995;62:1315-21.
14. Olson JA, Krinsky NI. Introduction: the colorful fascinating world of carotenoids: important biological modulators. FASEB J. 1995;9:1547-50.
15. Khan I, Ahmad H, Ahmad B. Anti-glycation and anti-oxidation properties of Capsicum frutescens and Curcuma longa fruits: possible role in prevention of diabetic complication. Pak J Pharm Sci. 2014;27(5):1359-62.
16. Penn NW. Potentiation of morphine analgesic action in mice by β-carotene. Eur J Pharmacol. 1995;284(1-2):191–193
17. Kuhad A, Sharma S, Chopra K. Lycopene attenuates thermal hyperalgesia in a diabetic mouse model of neuropathic pain. Eur J Pain. 2008;12(5):624–32.
18. Nasonov YL, Nasonova VA, eds. Rheumatology: National Guide. Moscow: GEOTAR-Media; 2010:720.
19. Kaplay SS. Acetylcholinesterase and butyrylcholinesterase of developing human brain. Biol Neonate. 1976;28:65–73.
20. Finkin-Groner E, Moradov D, Shifrin H, Bejar C, Nudelman A, Weinstock M. Indoline-3-propionate and 3-aminopropyl carbamates reduce lung injury and pro-inflammatory cytokines induced in mice by LPS. Br J Pharmacol. 2015;172(4):1101-13.
21. Das NU. Acetylcholinesterase and butyrylcholinesterase as possible markers of low-grade systemic inflammation. Med Sci Monit. 2007;13(12):214-21.
22. Fournier T, Medjoubi-N N, Porquet D. Alpha-1-acid glycoprotein. Biochimica et Biophysica Acta. 2000;1482:157–71.
23. Minukhin VV, Kosilova OY, Tkachenko VL. Level of the proteins of the acute phase as criterions of the antibacterial therapy effectiveness in the *E. coli* associated experimental peritonitis. Zaporozhye Med J. 2013;79(4):99-101.

16

The Effects of *Glycyrrhiza glabra* L. extract use with aerobic training on inflammatory factors and cognitive state in elderly with mild cognitive impairment

Mohammad-Ali Kohanpour[1], **Maghsoud Peeri**[2*], **Mohammad-Ali Azarbayjani**[2]

[1]PhD Candidate, Department of Exercise Physiology, Islamic Azad University, Central Tehran branch, Iran
[2]Professor, Department of Exercise Physiology, Islamic Azad University, Central Tehran Branch, Iran

ARTICLE INFO

Keywords:
Aerobic training
Glycyrrhiza glabra
Cognitive state
Inflammation
Cognitive impairment

ABSTRACT

Introduction: This study was aimed to investigate the effect of a 12-week aerobic training protocol and treatment with *Glycyrrhiza glabra* extract on serum interleukin 1 beta (IL-1β) and tumor necrosis factor alpha (TNF-α) levels and cognitive state in the elderly with mild cognitive impairment (MCI).

Methods: Forty people who attained scores 21-25 on the Mini–Mental State Examination (MMSE) were selected by purposive and convenience sampling and randomly assigned to four groups of 10 each: training, *G. glabra*-treated, training+*G. glabra*-treated, and placebo. All interventions were conducted within 12 weeks. Aerobic training protocol consisted of an 8-minute running at an intensity of 75%-85% maximum heart rate in the first session. One minute was added to the duration of running per two sessions so that after 12 weeks, the duration of running in two last sessions was 26 minutes. *G. glabra* extract was orally administered in 200 mg/kg body weight capsules per day.

Results: IL-1β and TNF-α levels significantly decreased in training and *G. glabra*-treated groups but their decrease were more marked in training+*G. glabra*-treated group ($P<0.05$). Cognitive state in three intervention groups significantly improved compared to placebo group, and this improvement was more marked in training+*G. glabra*-treated group ($P<0.05$).

Conclusion: Consumption of *G. glabra* extract with aerobic training for 12 weeks can slow down or stop the progression of MCI in the elderly through improving their cognitive states probably via decreasing inflammatory factors.

Implication for health policy/practice/research/medical education:
The elderly people with mild cognitive impairment (MCI) should make attempt to improve their cognitive states to prevent intensification of this impairment through decreasing inflammatory factors via doing aerobic exercise and consuming *Glycyrrhiza glabra*.

Introduction

The population aged over 60 years in Iran will reach around 10 million in 2020 and over 26 million in 2050 that will be 23% of the total population (1). Cognitive impairment represents one of the common disorders in the elderly such that around 35% of them present with it at different severities. Alzheimer disease is the progressive stage of this disorder (2). In cognitive impairment, attention, memory, language, orientation, actions, executive performance, judgement, and problem-solving are impaired mostly due to brain memory loss (3). The normal functioning of the various brain systems is responsible for cognitive function, and cognitive impairments arise as the age increases and the elements involved in these systems develop. In

***Corresponding author**: Maghsoud Peeri, Faculty of Physical Education and Exercise Sciences, Central Tehran branch of Islamic Azad University, Iran Zamin Blvd., Shahrak-E Gharb, Tehran, Iran.
Email: m.peeri@iauctb.com

addition, different inflammatory processes and cytokines contribute fundamentally to the pathogenesis of Alzheimer disease (4). The expression of most cytokines in normal tissues is normal but in neurodegenerative diseases, their expression increases. For example, the expression of the pro-inflammatory cytokine tumor necrosis factor alpha (TNF-α) increases in neurodegenerative diseases (5,6). In this regard, it has been reported that the immunity profile of patients with mild cognitive impairment (MCI) undergoes certain variations (7).

It is essential to take into account the interventions to prevent Alzheimer disease through slowing down or even inversing the progression of MCI; and measuring inflammatory factors following such intervention can lead to better explaining the observed effects. Consumption of medicinal plants is one of such interventions that have attracted attention (8,9). Among these plants, licorice, botanically referred to as *Glycyrrhiza glabra* L., is a perennial plant from family Fabaceae which is considered important worldwide due to pharmaceutical and nutritional compounds in its root and rhizome, and therefore has attracted the attention of pharmaceutical, food, and even tobacco industries (10). *G. glabra* root has several compounds such as different sugars, flavonoids, sterols, amino acids, gum, starch, essential oils, and saponins. The most important saponin (pentacyclic triterpene) of *G. glabra* is glycyrrhizic acid or glycyrrhizin that is made up of a glucuronic acid unit and a glycerotinic acid molecule (aglycone) (10). The presence of hypolipidemic compounds and flavonoids in *G. glabra* has been reported to be associated with its potent antioxidant activity (11). In addition, this plant has been reported to exert anti-inflammatory effect (12).

However, to the best of our knowledge, no study has yet been conducted on the effects of this plant on MCI in the elderly. On the other hand, exercise training, as an inexpensive therapeutic approach, can have optimal effects on cognitive function, which can be due to decreased inflammatory factors because cross-sectional investigations have demonstrated that active people have better cognitive function compared to inactive ones (13). Training has also been reported to induce anti-inflammatory effect (14).

Because MCI is one of the common problems in the elderly and represents the onset of a course that leads to Alzheimer disease and death, and no definite treatment has yet been suggested for Alzheimer disease, it is essential to use preventive interventions that slow down, stop, or even inverse the course of MCI. Besides that, the use of medicinal plants is particularly important because they are natural and lead to comparatively fewer side effects (9). Because the roles of exercise and physical activity in improving cognitive functions (13) and inflammatory factors (14) have been confirmed, it is recommended to investigate the combined effects of training and plants on cognitive functions. However, as far as we searched, no study has yet been conducted on the combined effect of aerobic training and *G. glabra* extract on the inflammatory factors and the cognitive states in the elderly with MCI. The aim of the current study was to investigate the effect of a 12-week aerobic training protocol and treatment with *Glycyrrhiza glabra* extract on the serum IL-1β and TNF-α levels and cognitive states in the elderly with MCI.

Materials and Methods

This semi-experimental study with pretest-posttest design was conducted on four groups. Eighty-seven people aged 60-70 years volunteered to participate in the study after advertising our study among different elderly populations living in Shiraz County. Then, the Mini–Mental State Examination (MMSE) was administered to volunteers. The MMSE, developed by Folstein et al in 1975, consists of 11 subscales: Orientation to time and place, registration, attention and calculation, memory, language, executive skills, reading, writing, and doing fine works (15). The subjects that do not have any problems in these subscales are given the score 30; the scores <20 represent in-depth cognitive disabilities and the scores 20-25 represent partial cognitive damage. The reliability (Cronbach alpha) of the MMSE has been reported 0.87 with sensitivity and specificity of 90% and 84%, respectively (16). Forty volunteers who attained the MMSE scores 21-25, with the average age 68.125 ± 3.708 years, the average height 174.55 ± 6.118 cm, the average weight 78.15 ± 5.176 kg, and the average body mass index (BMI) of 25.666 ± 0.599 kg/m^2 were enrolled in the study and randomly assigned to four groups of 10 each: Training, *G. glabra*-treated, training + *G. glabra*-treated, and placebo.

Inclusion criteria were being male, being over 60 years, attending at least 90% of intervention sessions, being examined by a physician for confirming general health to do aerobic training, attaining the MMSE scores 21-25 and the scores <10 on the Geriatric Depression Scale, and not being under pharmacotherapy for cognitive impairment. Exclusion criteria were not attending over 10% of intervention sessions, being dependent to do daily routines, suffering from other physical or psychiatric illnesses, taking medicines, not providing consent to participate in the study, and being under treatment for cognitive impairment. All interventions were conducted within 12 weeks. Aerobic training protocol consisted of 8-minute running at an intensity of 75-85% maximum heart rate in the first session. One minute was added to the duration of running per two sessions so that after 12 weeks, the duration of running in two last sessions was 26 minutes. *G. glabra* extract was orally administered in 200 mg/kg body weight capsules per day.

The final 5 minutes of each session was specified to cool-down. Five milliliters of arm venous blood was taken 24 hours before and 48 hours after interventions after 12-

hour fasting. To isolate serum, blood samples were left to clot and then centrifuged at 2000 rpm for 10 minutes. The resulting samples were stored at -20°C till measurement of the variables of interest. Serum IL-1β and TNF-α levels were measured with the sensitivity of 8 and 2 pg/mL, respectively, using a kit (Dialcone, France). Cognitive states were measured using the MMSE. Data were described by average and standard deviation. Inter- and intra-subject mixed analysis of variance (ANOVA) was used to investigate inter- and intra-group changes.

In addition, independent one-way ANOVA and Tukey tests were used to compare the changes in the variables among the groups. To investigate the association between the changes in the variables, Pearson correlation coefficient was used to investigate the association between the changes in the variables. The level of significance (P) was considered ≤0.05. Data analysis was conducted in SPSS 16.

Results

Descriptive data, the results of inter- and intra-subject mixed ANOVA and Tukey test, and Pearson correlation coefficients are shown in Tables 1-4, respectively.

There were significant differences in the changes in weight, BMI, cognitive state, IL-1β and TNF-α levels among the four groups over time ($P=0.001$). Weight and BMI in training+*G. glabra*-treated group and training group significantly decreased compared to *G. glabra*-treated group and control group ($P<0.05$). There were not any significant differences in the changes in weight and BMI between training group and training+*G. glabra*-treated group ($P>0.05$) as well as between *G. glabra*-treated group and control group ($P>0.05$).

Cognitive state improved in the three intervention groups significantly compared to control group ($P<0.05$). Improvement of cognitive state was significantly more marked in training+*G. glabra*-treated group than training group and *G. glabra*-treated group ($P<0.05$), but the changes in the cognitive state in training group and *G. glabra*-treated group were not significantly different ($P>0.05$). The levels of IL-1β and TNF-α in the three intervention groups significantly decreased compared

Table 1. The mean (standard deviation) values of variables before and after interventions

Variables	Groups	Before	After
Weight (kg)	Training +*G. glabra*-treated	77.70 ± 4.547	75.30 ± 4.398
	Training	77.50 ± 3.628	75.60 ± 3.835
	G. glabra-treated	77 ± 5.537	76.90 ± 5.762
	Placebo	80.40 ± 6.619	80.40 ± 6.397
BMI (kg/m^2)	Training +*G. glabra*-treated	25.664 ± 0.432	24.877 ± 0.725
	Training	25.748 ± 0.429	25.116 ± 0.585
	G. glabra-treated	25.348 ± 0.775	25.306 ± 0.623
	Placebo	25.907 ± 0.631	25.935 ± 0.808
Cognitive State (MMSE)	Training +*G. glabra*-treated	22.20 ± 1.549	25.20 ± 1.316
	Training	22.70 ± 1.636	24.40 ± 1.429
	G. glabra-treated	22.50 ± 1.354	24.10 ± 0.994
	Placebo	24.30 ± 0.948	24.20 ± 0.632
TNF-α (pg/ mL)	Training +*G. glabra*-treated	8.516 ± 1.204	5.926 ± 0.691
	Training	7.863 ± 1.341	6.723 ± 0.930
	G. glabra-treated	9.224 ± 1.285	8.114 ± 1.268
	Placebo	7.572 ± 1.612	7.897 ± 1.466
IL-1β (pg/mL)	Training +*G. glabra*-treated	3.561 ± 0.453	2.270 ± 0.295
	Training	3.344 ± 0.770	2.778 ± 0.432
	G. glabra-treated	3.598 ± 0.712	3.023 ± 0.620
	Placebo	3.345 ± 0.721	3.514 ± 0.635

Table 2. The results of inter- and intra-subject mixed ANOVA regarding the comparison of variables among 4 groups

Variables	*F* value	*P* value	Effect size
Weight	8.76	0.001 *	0.42
BMI	8.59	0.001 *	0.41
Cognitive State	21.24	0.001 *	0.64
TNF-α	11.33	0.001 *	0.49
IL-1β	10.96	0.001 *	0.48

*Significant at 0.05.

Table 3. The results of Tukey test regarding the points of significant difference

Pair wise comparison	Weight	BMI	Cognitive State	TNF-α	IL-1β
Training+*G. glabra*-treated/training	0.83	0.86	0.010 *	0.031 *	0.035 *
Training+*G. glabra*-treated/*G. glabra*-treated	0.002 *	0.003 *	0.005 *	0.027 *	0.038 *
Training+*G. glabra*-treated/placebo	0.001 *	0.001 *	0.001 *	0.001 *	0.001 *
Training/*G. glabra*-treated	0.021 *	0.026 *	0.99	1	1
Training/placebo	0.013 *	0.011 *	0.001 *	0.029 *	0.032 *
G. glabra-treated/placebo	0.99	0.98	0.001 *	0.033 *	0.029 *

*Significant at 0.05.

Table 4. Pearson correlation coefficients to examine the association between the changes in variables

Variables	Weight	BMI	Cognitive state	TNF-α	IL-1β
Weight	-	r = 0.99, *P* = 0.001 *	r = - 0.44, *P* = 0.004 *	r = 0.43, *P* = 0.005 *	r = 0.30, *P* = 0.054
BMI	r = 0.99, p = 0.001 *	-	r = - 0.44, *P* = 0.004 *	r = 0.44, *P* = 0.004 *	r = 0.31, *P* = 0.051
Cognitive state	r = - 0.44, p = 0.004 *	r = - 0.44, *P* = 0.004 *	-	r = - 0.66, *P* = 0.001 *	r = - 0.56, *P* = 0.001 *
TNF-α	r = 0.43, p = 0.005 *	r = 0.44, *P* = 0.004 *	r = - 0.66, *P* = 0.001 *	-	r = 0.52, *P* = 0.001 *
IL-1β	r = 0.30, p = 0.054	r = 0.31, *P* = 0.051	r = - 0.56, *P* = 0.001 *	r = 0.52, *P* = 0.001 *	-

*Significant at 0.05.

to control group ($P<0.05$). These levels in training+*G. glabra*-treated group significantly decreased compared to training group and *G. glabra*-treated group ($P<0.05$), but the changes in IL-1β and TNF-α levels in training group and *G. glabra*-treated group were not significantly different ($P>0.05$).

Results indicated that the changes in weight and BMI were significantly and inversely correlated with changes in cognitive state ($P<0.05$), and were significantly and directly correlated with changes in TNF-α levels ($P<0.05$). The changes in weight and BMI were not significantly associated with the changes in serum IL-1β levels ($P>0.05$). In addition, the cognitive state of the elderly improved significantly with decreasing their serum TNF-α levels ($r=-0.66$, $P=0.001$) and IL-1β serum levels ($r=-0.56$, $P=0.001$)

Discussion

After the interventions, cognitive state improved significantly and inflammatory factors (IL-1β and TNF-α) decreased significantly in training group and *G. glabra*-treated group, but the corresponding changes in training+*G. glabra*-treated group were more marked. Besides that, results indicated that in the elderly with MCI, cognitive state improved and TNF-α levels decreased with decreasing weight and BMI. The current study also demonstrated that cognitive state in these elderly improved with decreasing IL-1β and TNF-α, and this association was more marked for TNF-α. Accordingly, although such associations cannot be considered causal relationships, the significant association between the changes in cognitive state and the variations in inflammatory factors may be explained by the role that decreased inflammatory factors, following doing aerobic training and using *G. glabra* extract, play in improving the cognitive states of the elderly with MCI. Indeed, doing aerobic training and using *G. glabra* extract prevent MCI from progressing toward more advanced cognitive impairments and Alzheimer disease through preventing its progression. However, this argument should be further investigated

The effect of *G. glabra* on inflammatory factors has already been studied. Jung et al studied the effect of this plant on alcohol-induced fatty liver due to inflammation and oxidative stress in mouse model. To achieve this purpose, they treated mice with an alcohol-containing diet with and without *G. glabra* extract. Consumption of alcohol led to increase in TNF-α levels and fat accumulation, but consumption of *G. glabra* led to decrease in the levels of triglyceride and TNF-α. Taken together, the study of Jung et al that consumption of *G. glabra* resulted in improvement of kidney damage due to decreased inflammation (17). Nakamura et al studied the effect of glycyrrhizin on the inflammatory factors macrophage inflammatory protein, TNF-α, interleukin 6 (IL-6), and interferon gamma due to fungal infection, and glycyrrhizin caused decrease in inflammation in fungal infection (18). Studying the anti-inflammatory effects of *G. glabra*, Yu et al measured IL-6, IL-1β, and TNF-α, and observed that *G. glabra* and its three bioactive compounds could be used for treating inflammation-associated disorders such as hepatic oxidative stress and hepatic inflammation (19). Li et al also reported that *G. glabra* caused decrease in the levels of IL-6, IL-1β, and TNF-α (20). The study of Yu et al showed that *G. glabra* extract caused decrease in the levels of the inflammatory factors cyclooxygenase-2 (COX-2), interleukin 1 (IL-1), IL-6, IL-1β, and TNF-α in inflammation-induced kidney damage while the expression of IL-6, IL-1β, and TNF-α decreased (19). In addition, Yang et al reported that the consumption of *G. glabra* root led to down-regulation of the gene expression of COX-2, IL-6, and IL-1β (21).

Overall, studies have demonstrated that *G. glabra* exerts anti-inflammatory effect (22-25). It has even been reported that this plant can be used for treating inflammation-associated disorders including kidney damage (19,26). Farag et al argued that *G. glabra* is a popular plant-based supplement for treating chronic inflammatory diseases that plays role in decreasing inflammation due to different active compounds including glycyrrhizin (27). Consistently, Bernela et al investigated the pharmaceutical properties of glycyrrhizic acid, a *G. glabra*-derived saponin, and demonstrated that it has anti-inflammatory properties (28). Wang et al also reported the anti-inflammatory effects of this compound (29). The antioxidant and anti-inflammatory effects of *G. glabra*-derived glycyrrhizic acid have been confirmed (29). In this regard, the anti-inflammatory effects of *G. glabra*-derived have been studied in vivo.

Results showed that this compound caused decrease in the inflammatory factors IL-6, IL-1β, and TNF-α (30). Maurya et al argued that glycerrhizic acid is the main factor for anti-inflammatory properties of *G. glabra* (31). In agreement with available evidence, Chakravarthi and Avadhani studied the effects of *G. glabra* root on memory and learning in 1-month and adult male rats. Aqueous *G. glabra* root extract was administered at 75, 150, 225, and 300 mg/kg of body weight (BW) concentrations for 6 weeks. Results showed that the treatment with this extract led to a significant improvement of memory, and in 150 and 225 mg/kg BW, significant improvement of memory and learning. Chakravarthi and Avadhani concluded that these findings are probably due to the anti-inflammatory effects of *G. glabra* (32).

Consistent with our study, Farinha et al studied the levels of TNF-α, IL-1β, and IL-23 in the women without training before and after 12-week treadmill training and without any change in diet, and observed that the aerobic training course caused significant decrease in serum TNF-α and IL-1β levels (33). However, Isanejad et al reported that 8-week endurance training led to significant increase in IL-1β and significant decrease in TNF-α (34). Knudsen and Pedersen studied the effect of training on the inflammatory factors in type 2 diabetes patients, and found that training caused significant increase in IL-6 that led to anti-inflammatory effects through inhibiting TNF-α, stimulating IL-1 receptor antagonist, and therefore restricting IL-1β signaling (14). In our study, aerobic training led to both decrease in the inflammatory factors and improvement of cognitive state. Consistently, Miller et al reported that cognitive state and physical activity were significantly and directly correlated (35), which can be due to decreased oxidative stress and inflammation, increased angiogenesis, secretion of neurotrophins and catecholamines, and neurogenesis especially in the hippocampus (36).

To date, no study has yet been conducted on the combined effects of *G. glabra* and training on inflammatory factors and cognitive state especially in the elderly with MCI, and therefore it is difficult to interpret our evidence with reference to previous findings. Altogether, according to the findings of our study, the consumption of *G. glabra* alongside aerobic training, can help decrease inflammatory factors and improve cognitive state in the elderly with MCI. However, the current study was first to investigate this issue and additional studies are needed.

Conclusion

Probably, both aerobic training and consumption of *G. glabra* extract can slow down and even stop the progression of MCI in the elderly through improving cognitive state via decreasing inflammatory factors. It seems that combining these two interventions leads to more efficient prevention of MCI progression. It is likely that decreased inflammation plays a significant role in this regard, but other mediators should be investigated in additional studies.

Acknowledgements

This article was derived from the Ph.D thesis of Mohammad-Ali Kohanpour approved at the Islamic Azad University, Central Tehran Branch, Tehran, Iran. Hereby, we gratefully appreciate the spiritual assistance of the Research Deputy of this university and are also grateful to the participants of this study.

Authors' contributions

MAK contributed to data collection and manuscript drafting, MP revised and copyedited the manuscript, and MAA made necessary corrections to the methodology especially data analysis. All read and confirmed the final version of the manuscript for publication.

Conflict of interests

The authors declared no competing interests.

Ethical considerations

The study was confirmed by the Ethical Committee of the university and the ethical issues (including plagiarism, misconduct, data fabrication, falsification, double publication or submission, redundancy) have been completely observed by the authors.

Funding/Support

This research was financially supported by Islamic Azad University, Central Tehran Branch, Iran.

References

1. Sharif-Zadeh QR, Moudi M, Akhbari H. Health situation of

elderly supported by Imam Khomeini charity. Iran Elderly Mag. 2010; 5(17):52-60.
2. Sohrabi MB, Zolfaghari P, Mahdizade F, Aghayan SM, Ghasemian-Aghmashhadi M, Shariat Z, et al. Evaluation and comparison of cognitive state and depression in elderly admitted in sanitarium with elderly sited in personal home. Knowledge and Health. 2008;3(2):27.
3. Torpy JM, Lynm C, Glass RM. JAMA patient page. Dementia. JAMA. 2010;304(17):972.
4. Greig NH, Mattson MP, Perry T, Chan SL, Giordano T, Sambamurti K, et al. New therapeutic strategies and drug candidates for neurodegenerative diseases: p53 and TNF-α inhibitors, and GLP-1 receptor agonists. Ann N Y Acad Sci. 2004;1035:290-315.
5. Jiang H, Hampel H, Prvulovic D, Wallin A, Blennow K, Li R, et al. Elevated CSF levels of TACE activity and soluble TNF receptors in subjects with mild cognitive impairment and patients with Alzheimer's disease. Mol Neurodegener. 2011;6:69.
6. Swardfager W, Lanctôt K, Rothenburg L, Wong A, Cappell J, Herrmann N. A meta-analysis of cytokines in Alzheimer's disease. Biol Psychiatry. 2010;68:930-41.
7. Ha I. Mild cognitive impairment (MCI): pathogenesis and treatments. Clin Psychopharmacol Neurosci. 2009;7(1): 3-8.
8. Karamian R, Mohammadian A, Hassanimoghadam E, et al. Identification and comparison of the yield and composition of essential oil constituents of four Eucalyptus species adapted to the climatic conditions of Khorramabad. J Herbmed Pharmacol. 2015;4(1):25-8.
9. Kohanpour MA, Peeri M, Azarbayjani MA, lizadeh L, Abdali N, Keshvari M, et al. The effects of aerobic exercise with lavender essence use on cognitive state and serum brain-derived neurotrophic factor levels in elderly with mild cognitive impairment. J Herbmed Pharmacol. 2017;6(2):80-4.
10. Amani M, Sotudeh-Gharebagh R, Mostaoufi N. Optimal exteraction of Glycyrrhetinic acid from Licorice root. J Technol. 2005;3(4):376-580.
11. Saleem M, Mohammad A, Al-Tameemi JA, et al. Biological study of the effect of licorice roots extract on serum lipid profile, liver enzymes and kidney function tests in albino mice. African J Biotech. 2011;10(59):12702-6 .
12. Chang CZ, Wu SC, Kwan AL. Glycyrrhizin attenuates proinflammatory cytokines through a peroxisome proliferator-activated receptor-γ-dependent mechanism and experimental vasospasm in a rat model. J Vasc Res. 2015;52(1):12-21.
13. Hillman CH, Motl RW, Pontifex MB, Posthuma D, Stubbe JH, Boomsma DI, et al. Physical activity and cognitive function in a cross-section of younger and older community-dwelling individuals. Health Psychol. 2006;25:678-87.
14. Knudsen SH, Pedersen BK. Targeting inflammation through a physical active lifestyle and pharmaceuticals for the treatment of type 2 diabetes. Curr Diab Rep. 2015;15(10):82.
15. Nillson J, Parker MG, Kabir ZN. Assessing health – related quality of life among older people in rural Bangladesh. J Trans Cult Nurs. 2004;15(4):298-307.
16. Frooghian M, Jafari Z, Shirinbaiani P. Standardization of brief examination of cognitive status of elderly in Tehran. Advanced Cognitive Science Journal. 2008;10(2):29-37.
17. Jung JC, Lee YH, Kim SH, Kim KJ, Kim KM, Oh S, et al. Hepatoprotective effect of licorice, the root of *Glycyrrhiza uralensis* Fischer, in alcohol-induced fatty liver disease. BMC Complement Altern Med. 2016;16:19.
18. Nakamura T, Nishibu A, Yoshida N, Yasoshima M, Anzawa K, Watanabe Y, et al. Glycyrrhetinic acid inhibits contact hypersensitivity induced by trichophytin via dectin-1. Exp Dermatol. 2016; 25(4):299-304.
19. Yu JY, Ha JY, Kim KM, Jung YS, Jung JC, Oh S. Anti-inflammatory activities of licorice extract and its active compounds, glycyrrhizic acid, liquiritin and liquiritigenin, in BV2 cells and mice liver. Molecules. 2015;20(7):13041-54.
20. Li C, Eom T, Jeong Y. *Glycyrrhiza glabra* L. extract inhibits LPS-induced inflammation in RAW macrophages. J Nutr Sci Vitaminol. 2015;61(5):375-81.
21. Yang XL, Liu D, Bian K,Zhang DD. Study on in vitro anti-inflammatory activity of total flavonoids from Glycyrrhizae Radix et Rhizoma and its ingredients. Zhongguo Zhong Yao Za Zhi. 2013;38(1):99-104.
22. Man S, Wang J, Gao W, Guo S, Li Y, Zhang L, Xiao P. Chemical analysis and anti-inflammatory comparison of the cell culture of Glycyrrhiza with its field cultivated variety. Food Chem. 2013;136(2):513-7.
23. Zhang J, Gao W, Yan S, Zhao Y. Effects of space flight on the chemical constituents and anti-inflammatory activity of licorice (*Glycyrrhiza uralensis* Fisch). Iran J Pharm Res. 2012;11(2):601-9.
24. Siracusa L, Saija A, Cristani M, Cimino F, D'Arrigo M, Trombetta D, et al. Phytocomplexes from liquorice (*Glycyrrhiza glabra* L.) leaves--chemical characterization and evaluation of their antioxidant, anti-genotoxic and anti-inflammatory activity. Fitoterapia. 2011;82(4):546-56.
25. Wu TY, Khor TO, Saw CL, Loh SC, Chen AI, Lim SS, et al. Anti-inflammatory/Anti-oxidative stress activities and differential regulation of Nrf2-mediated genes by non-polar fractions of tea *Chrysanthemum zawadskii* and licorice *Glycyrrhiza uralensis*. AAPS J. 2011;13(1):1-13.
26. Dunlap TL, Wang S, Simmler C, Chen SN, Pauli GF, Dietz BM, et al. Differential effects of *Glycyrrhiza* species on genotoxic estrogen metabolism: licochalcone a downregulates P450 1B1, whereas Isoliquiritigenin stimulates it. Chem Res Toxicol. 2015;28(8):1584-94.
27. Farag MA, Porzel A, Wessjohann LA. Unequivocal glycyrrhizin isomer determination and comparative in vitro bioactivities of root extracts in four *Glycyrrhiza* species. J Adv Res. 2015;6(1):99-104.
28. Bernela M, Ahuja M, Thakur R. Enhancement of anti-inflammatory activity of glycyrrhizic acid by encapsulation in chitosan-katira gum nanoparticles. Eur J Pharm Biopharm. 2016;105:141-7
29. Wang J, Li J, Wu X, Liu S, Li H, Gao W. Assessment of genetic fidelity and composition, mixed elicitors enhance triterpenoids and flavonoids biosynthesis of *Glycyrrhiza uralensis* Fisch. tissue cultures. Biotechnol Appl Biochem. 2017;64(2):211-217.
30. Wang CY, Kao TC, Lo WH, Yen GC. Glycyrrhizic acid and 18β-glycyrrhetinic acid modulate lipopolysaccharide-

induced inflammatory response by suppression of NF-κB through PI3K p110δ and p110γ inhibitions. J Agric Food Chem. 2011;59(14):7726-33.

31. Maurya SK, Raj K, Srivastava AK. Antidyslipidaemic activity of *Glycyrrhiza glabra* in high fructose diet induced dsyslipidaemic Syrian golden hamsters. Indian J Clin Biochem. 2009;24(4):404-9.
32. Chakravarthi KK, Avadhani R. Beneficial effect of aqueous root extract of *Glycyrrhiza glabra* on learning and memory using different behavioral models: An experimental study. J Nat Sci Biol Med. 2013;4(2):420-5.
33. Farinha JB, Steckling FM, Stefanello ST, Cardoso MS, Nunes LS, Barcelos RP, et al. Response of oxidative stress and inflammatory biomarkers to a 12-week aerobic exercise training in women with metabolic syndrome. Sports Med Open. 2015;1(1):19.
34. Isanejad A, Saraf ZH, Mahdavi M, Gharakhanlou R, Shamsi MM, Paulsen G. The effect of endurance training and downhill running on the expression of IL-1β, IL-6, and TNF-α and HSP72 in rat skeletal muscle. Cytokine. 2015;73(2):302-8.
35. Miller DI, Taler V, Davidson PS, Messier C. Measuring the impact of exercise on cognitive aging: methodological issues. Neurobiol Aging. 2012;33:622-629.
36. Adlard PA, Perreau VM, Pop V, Cotman CW. Voluntary exercise decreases amyloid load in a transgenic model of Alzheimer's disease. J Neurosci. 2005;25:4217-21.

17

Chemical composition and antioxidant activities of different parts of *Ficus sur*

Kossivi Issa Saloufou[1*], Pakoupati Boyode[1], Oudjaniyobi Simalou[1], Kodjo Eloh[2], Kokou Idoh[3], Mamatchi Melila[4], Outéndé Toundou[1], Kafui Kpegba[1], Amegnona Agbonon[3]

[1]Laboratoire de chimie organique et des substances naturelles (Lab COSNat), Département de Chimie, Faculté Des Sciences, Université de Lomé, 01 BP 1515 Lomé 01, Lomé, TOGO
[2]Department of Life and Environmental Sciences, Unversity of Cagliari, Via Ospedale 72, 09124, Cagliari, Italy
[3]Laboratoire de Physiologie, Pharmacologie et Toxicologie, Faculté des Sciences, Université de Lomé, 01 BP 1515 Lomé 01, Lomé,TOGO
[4]Département de Biochimie, Université de Lomé, 01 BP 1515 Lomé 01, Lomé, TOGO

ARTICLE INFO

Keywords:
Ficus sur
Antioxidant
Phenolic compounds
Flavonoids
HPLC-QTOF-HRMS

ABSTRACT

Introduction: *Ficus sur* is a plant widely used in traditional pharmacopoeia in Togo. So, this study aimed the assessment of antioxidant properties and identification of some compounds from the ethanolic extracts of different parts of the plant (leaves, fruits, roots, and barks).
Methods: The phenolic and flavonoid contents of the ethanolic extracts of different organs of *Ficus sur* were assessed using conventional known methods. The DPPH radical scavenging and the ferric-reducing antioxidant power (FRAP) assays were used to highlight the antioxidant activities. The different extract samples were also analysed by liquid chromatography coupled to a quadrupole-time of flight mass detector (ESI-QTOF).
Results: Total phenolic contents (TPCs) for 1 mg of dry extract ranged from 489.40 ± 7.48 µg GAE (gallic acid equivalents) for the bark to 62.34 ± 2.66 µg GAE for unripe fruits. The bark exhibited the highest flavonoid content, which was closed to 90.20 ± 3.72 µg QE (quercetin equivalents)/mg of dry extract. The radical scavenging activities of the bark and unripe fruits were 56.50 ± 0.29 and 7.3 ± 0.30 µg QE/mg of dry extract, respectively. In the same order, the FRAP values of the two organs were 104.57 ± 4.75 and 19.61 ± 0.22 µmol $FeSO_4$ Eq/mg of dry extract. Many compounds including notoginsenoside R10; 4',5,7-trihydroxyflavan-3-ol; catechin; and boviquinone 4 were identified.
Conclusion: The various organs of *Ficus sur* are a source of bioactive compounds especially phenolic compounds and flavonoids with antioxidant activity.

Implication for health policy/practice/research/medical education:
Well established as source of bioactive compounds, medicinal plants have long been used in treatment of human ailments. The validation of traditional use of medicinal plants can be achieved by screening a collection of extracts for bioactivity using *in vitro, in cellulo* and even *in vivo* assays. The results of this work are consistent with the traditional use of the various parts of *Ficus sur* to cure hepatic pain, cardiovascular and neurodegenerative diseases, cancer, and diabetes. Although the bark extract is more active than the extracts of the other organs, it would be better to use the leaves to preserve the plant, as these contain all the metabolites present in the bark and much more.

Introduction

In recent years, there has been growing interest in alternative therapies by the use of natural products. So, during the last decade, focus has been made on the investigation of phytochemistry of plants for pharmaceutical and nutritional purposes. In Togo, plants are widely used in traditional medicine, especially in the rural areas. Among the plants used in Togolese pharmacopoeia, there is *Ficus sur* (Moraceae) commonly called "Petit sycamore" in French and "Wild fig" in English. This plant is usually found in tropical and subtropical areas along the rivers. The plant can grow up to 30-35 m of height while trunk diameter can reach 150 cm (1). The fruits and leaves of *Ficus sur* are used as food in the northern Togo. In addition, several medicinal properties have been attributed to various parts of the plant since

***Corresponding author**: Kossivi Issa Saloufou,
Email: salkos@hotmail.fr

its roots, barks, leaves, and fruits are used to treat, relieve and heal several pathologies. Indeed, the roots are braised and crushed with grilled corn cobs, then the sieved are used against female infertility. The crushed and macerated fruits in water are used for the care of women during childbirth and after delivery (promotion of lactation) (1). The beverage obtained by decoction after mixing roots and leafy twigs is used to treat eczema (1). Decocted trunk bark is used against amenorrhea, dysentery, hepatic, and cardiovascular pain (2-4).

It is known that oxidative stress is involved in many inflammatory processes related to chronic diseases such as cardiac dysfunction, neurodegenerative diseases or diabetes (5). Indeed, a large number of phenolic compounds such as flavonoids, isoflavones, and phenolic acids have shown antioxidant activity (6-9). Moreover, the benefits of phenolic antioxidant compounds from plants in prevention of chronic diseases have been reported (10,11).

In our preliminary work on this plant, two bioactive phytosterols were identified in the cyclohexanic extract of the leaves (12). The aim of the current work was to assess the antioxidant properties, the total phenolic and flavonoid contents, and then identify some more compounds from various organs of this medicinal plant.

Materials and Methods

Plant material

The leaves, roots, bark, ripe and unripe fruits of *Ficus sur* were harvested at north latitude 11°05'31" and east longitude 00°19'38" in the northern region of Togo (Dapaong). Samples were dried at room temperature inside the laboratory and then reduced to a fine powder using a mill (Thomas Scientific Laboratory Mill Model 4, USA) with a sieve of 1 mm porosity. The extracts were obtained by macerating in ethanol (95°) for 72 hours. After filtration, the solvent was evaporated under reduced pressure at 30°C.

Antioxidant activity

The antioxidant activities of the extracts were evaluated by the DPPH radical-scavenging activity and the ferric-reducing antioxidant power (FRAP).

Determination of DPPH radical-scavenging activity

The method, inspired by the works of Molyneux (13) and Constantin et al (14), is based on the reduction of the violet DPPH• radical by an H atom donor (AH) leading to the formation of the colorless 2,2-diphenyl-1-picrylhydrazine (DPPH-H) and the radical (A•) according to the following equation: DPPH• + AH ⟶ DPPH-H + A•

One hundred microliters (100 μL) of each extract or standard methanolic solutions was mixed and vortexed with a 2 mL methanolic solution of DPPH (10^{-4} M). Only methanol was used as extract solution in the control sample. The fading of the purple free radical DPPH solution by effect of the extracts was measured at 517 nm using a Genesys 10S UV-Vis spectrophotometer (USA), after incubating samples at room temperature in the dark for 30 minutes. A quercetin calibration curve was established for concentrations ranging from 0 to 30 μg/mL. Results were expressed in mg of quercetin equivalents/g of dry extract (mg QE/g).

Determination of ferric-reducing antioxidant power

The FRAP assay consists in reducing the intense blue tripyridyltriazine-ferric complex (Fe^{3+}-TPTZ). At pH 3.5, the Fe^{3+}-TPTZ complex is added to the sample whose antioxidant compounds have effect to reduce this complex into its reduced form Fe^{2+}-TPTZ. The test was carried out according to the method described by Nair et al (15). In tubes containing 300 μL of freshly prepared FRAP solution (25 mL of acetate buffer, 2.5 mL of 10 mM Fe^{3+}-TPTZ in 40 mM HCl and 2.5 mL of 20 mM $FeCl_3$,$6H_2O$), 30 μL of distilled water and 10 μL of sample were added. The change in absorbance from the red to blue was followed at 593 nm after a process of 10 minutes of incubation. A calibration curve was established from a concentration range of 0 to 2000 μM of iron sulphate ($FeSO_4$,$7H_2O$) solution dissolved in methanol (blank). The obtained results were expressed in μmol of $FeSO_4$ equivalents/mg of dry extract.

Phytochemical profiles of the different organs of *Ficus sur*

An initial rapid screening of molecular families present in the different organ extracts was done using specific reagents and procedures described in the literature (16-18).

Determination of total phenolic content

The colorimetric method developed by Singleton et al (19) and slightly modified by Al-Farsi et al (20) was used. An aliquot of 100 μL of each extract at 1 mg/mL was mixed with 750 μL of Folin-Ciocalteu reagent diluted up to 1/10. After 5 minutes of incubation at 25°C, 750 μL of Na_2CO_3 aqueous solution (20%) was added. The obtained mixture was incubated for 90 minutes in the dark and the change in absorbance was followed at λ = 765 nm. The extract was substituted by distilled water for blank. Gallic acid at different concentrations (0-500 μg/mL) was used as standard and the results were expressed in μg of gallic acid equivalents per milligram of dry extract (μg of GAE/mg of dry extract) by extrapolating the calibration line ($y = 0.005018x + 0.055190$, $R^2 = 0.9925$) obtained from the different concentrations of gallic acid. The Genesys 10S UV-Vis Spectrophotometer, USA was used.

Determination of flavonoid content

The total flavonoid contents (TFCs) of the extracts were estimated via the colorimetric aluminum trichloride

($AlCl_3$) method described by Kim et al (21). One hundred microliters (100 µL) of ethanolic extracts solution was added to 400 µL of distilled water. Thirty microliters (30 µL) of a 5% sodium nitrite ($NaNO_2$) solution was added to the former mixture. After 5 minutes of incubation at room temperature, 20 µL of a 10% aqueous solution of $AlCl_3$ was added. Finally, 200 µL of a Na_2CO_3 aqueous solution (1M) and 5 minutes later, 250 µL of distilled water (blank) were added, successively. The whole mixture was vortexed and the absorbance was measured directly with UV-Vis spectrophotometer (Genesys 10S UV-Vis Spectrophotometer, USA) at λ = 510 nm. The concentration of total flavonoids was deduced from the calibration curve established with quercetin (0-500 µg/mL) and the results were expressed in µg quercetin equivalents/mg of dry extract (µg EQ/mg of extract).

Statistical analysis

Results were analyzed statistically using the OriginPro 9.0 software. Data were expressed as means ± standard deviation (SD) of experiments performed in triplicate. One-way analysis of variance (ANOVA), principal component analysis (PCA) and Pearson correlation coefficient (ρ) were used to evaluate and correlate the results with each other. Differences with *P* values less than 0.05 were considered significant.

HPLC-ESI+-QTOF-HRMS analysis

A methanolic solution (1000 µg/mL) was prepared from the ethanolic extracts of different organs. The chromatographic analysis for the separation of the compounds was carried out in reverse phase on an Agilent series 1200 HPLC system equipped with a C18 column from Microchip Technology (Agilent, Zorbax 300 SB-C18, 5 µm, 43 mm, 75 µm). An Agilent 6530 quadrupole - time of flight (QTOF) mass detector (Agilent Technologies, Santa Clara, Calif., USA) coupled to an electrospray ionizer (ESI) was used. Chromatographic conditions were as follows: flow rate: 0.4 $\mu L.min^{-1}$; solvent A: 0.1% formic acid in water; solvent B: 0.1% formic acid in methanol. The solvent gradient (v/v) was generated starting from 20% B and reaching 100% B in 10 minutes and maintaining at 100% B for 10 minutes for a total run of 20 min. Two microliters of the samples were analyzed by ESI in positive mode. Mass spectral data were acquired in the range m/z 100–1500, with an acquisition rate of 1.35 $spectra.s^{-1}$, averaging 10 000 transients. The source parameters were adjusted as follows: drying gas temperature 250°C, drying gas flow rate 5 $L.min^{-1}$, nebuliser pressure 45 psi and fragmentor voltage 150 V. Data acquisition and processing were done by Agilent MassHunter Workstation Acquisition software v. B.02.00. The METLIN database (https://metlin.scripps.edu/index.php) was used to predict plausible structures of detected metabolites.

Results

Evaluation of antioxidant activity

To investigate the antioxidant activity of the various organs of *Ficus sur*, two *in vitro* assays were used, the DPPH radical scavenging and the FRAP assays. Results are resumed in Figure 1. The bark extract had the best DPPH radical scavenging activity closed to 56.50 ± 0.29 µg QE/mg of dry extract; the ripe fruit extract being the least active with an activity of 7.3 ± 0.30 µg QE/mg of dry extract. The evaluation of the ferric ion reduction power yielded FRAP values ranging from 104.57 ± 4.75 µmol $FeSO_4$ Eq/mg dry extract for the bark to 19.61 ± 0.22 µmol $FeSO_4$ Eq/mg of dry extract for ripe fruits.

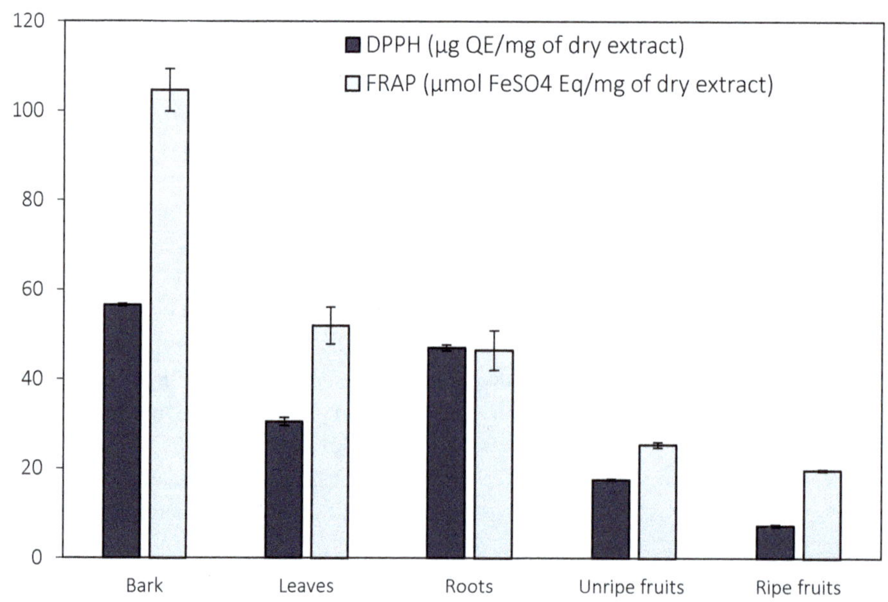

Figure 1. Antioxidant abilities in µg QE (quercetin equivalents)/mg of dry extract (for the DPPH radical scavenging assay) and in µmol $FeSO_4$ Eq/mg of dry extract (for the FRAP assay). Values are expressed as mean ± SEM; n = 3.

Table 1. Phytochemical analysis of the various organs of *Ficus sur*

Phyto-chemicals	Ripe fruits	Unripe fruits	Leaves	Bark	Root
Alkaloids	+	+	+	+	+
Flavonoids	+	+	+	+	+
Saponosides	+	+	+	+	+
Quinones	-	-	-	-	-
Glycosides	+	+	+	+	+
Tannins	+	+	+	+	+
Sterols and terpenoid	+	+	+	+	+
Anthocyanins	+	+	+	+	+

(+) = present ; (-) = absent.

Phytochemical screening

The phytochemical screening revealed the presence of alkaloids, flavonoids, saponosides, glycosides, anthocyanins, tannins, sterols, and terpenoid in the various organs of *Ficus sur* (Table 1).

Total phenolic content

Figure 2 reports the different values of total phenolic contents (TPCs) of the various organs of *Ficus sur*. For 1 mg of the dry extracts, the TPC ranged from 489.40 ± 7.48 µg GAE for the bark to 62.34 ± 2, 66 µg GAE for unripe fruits. For the other organs, the values are as follows: 177.79 ± 3.29 µg GAE for the roots, 84.86 ± 15.06 µg GAE for the ripe fruits and 66.06 ± 7.44 µg GAE for leaves.

Total flavonoid content

The TFCs of the various organs of *Ficus sur* are reported in Figure 2. The bark had the highest flavonoids content, 90.20 ± 3.72 µg QE/mg of dry extract. This was followed by ripe fruit (78.07 ± 10.23 µg QE/mg of dry extract), roots (48.55 ± 3.19 µg QE/mg of dry extract), unripe fruits (31.57 ± 5.72 µg QE/mg dry extract) and leaves (27.06 ± 5.19 µg QE/mg of dry extract).

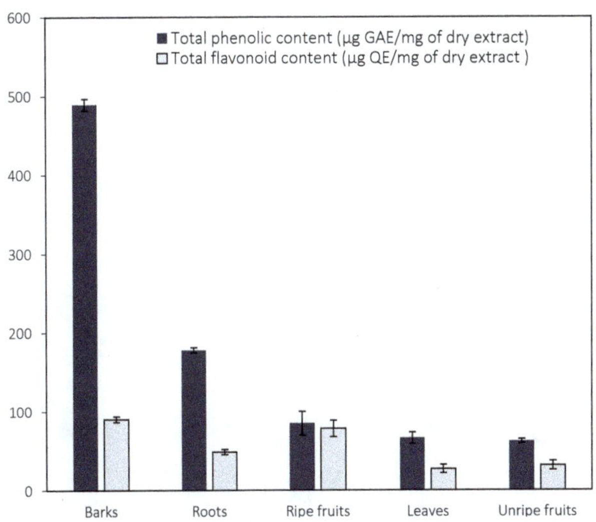

Figure 2. Total phenolic and flavonoid content of extracts from different organs of *Ficus sur*. Values are expressed as mean ± SEM; n = 3.

Results of the descriptive statistical analyses

Figure 3 shows the principal component analysis (PCA) carried out taking into account the different parameters (TFC, TPC, FRAP and DPPH). The Pearson correlation coefficients (ρ) determined in order to quantify correlation between those parameters are resumed in Table 2.

Identification of the main compounds of the various extracts

The HPLC analysis of each tested extract yielded the chromatograms which are shown in Figure 4. The comparative chromatographic profile of roots, barks, leaves, and ripe fruit shows (Figure 4), on the one hand, common peaks to all the four extracts (peaks 1-23) and on the other hands, some peaks that discriminate different organs (peaks a-q). This comparison shows that the root extract has the simplest chromatographic profile, followed by barks, leaves, and finally by fruits which exhibit complex profile.

The ESI$^+$-QTOF-HRMS analysis offered the possibility to determine the exact masses of the different compounds detected. Many characteristics of the different compounds identified are summarized in Tables 3 and 4.

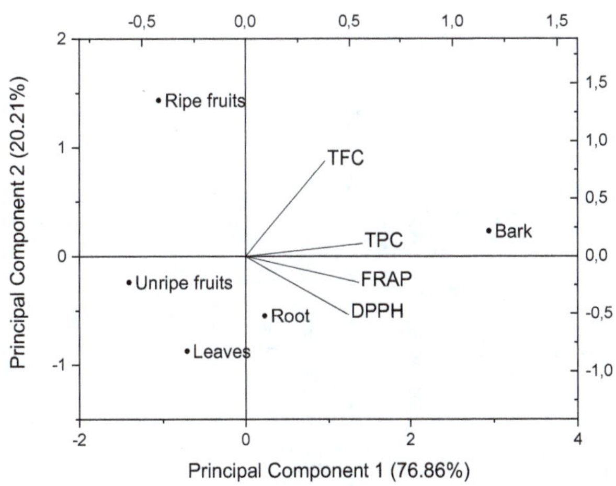

Figure 3. Comparison of the different organs by principal component analysis.

Table 2. Correlation matrix between DPPH, FRAP, TFC and TPC

	DPPH	TPC	TFC	FRAP
DPPH	1	0.79994	0.25466	0.8747
TPC	0.79994	1	0.72076	0.92075
TFC	0.25466	0.72076	1	0.46917
FRAP	0.8747	0.92075	0.46917	1

Discussion

All extracts from the various organs of *Ficus sur* showed antioxidant activities considering the two assays: DPPH and FRAP. Indeed, the different extracts exhibited positive effect to the total phenolics and flavonoids contents. The PCA allowed a better understanding of the relative behavior of the different parameters studied. In fact, the determination of the Pearson correlation coefficient between FRAP and DPPH ($\rho = 0.8747$) indicated that the two methods of assessing the antioxidant activity progress together and could be complementary. Moreover, the TPC is strongly correlated with the FRAP values ($\rho = 0.92075$) and DPPH values ($\rho = 0.79994$). The similar observations were made by Michel et al (22). Flavonoids are a subclass of phenolic compounds recognized as an important source of antioxidants (23). In this work, although the TFCs are well correlated with those of the total phenolic compounds ($\rho = 0.72076$), the antioxidant activity is very weakly related to the TFCs; the coefficients being 0.25466 between the TFC and the DPPH values and 0.46917 with those of the FRAP. This weak correlation could be explained by the non-specificity of the flavonoid assay method. Indeed, as illustrated by Cornard and Merlin (24), quercetin is able to form stable compounds in the presence of aluminum chloride since three different complexation sites (3-hydroxy-4-keto, 5-hydroxy-4-keto, 3′,4′-o-diphenolic) exist in its structure. The extracts showing positive responses to this assay might contain derivatives of quercetin and more generally flavonoids. However, it should be noted that some terpene compounds with adjacent hydroxyl, acidic or coumaryl groups that favour the complexation of aluminum may also respond

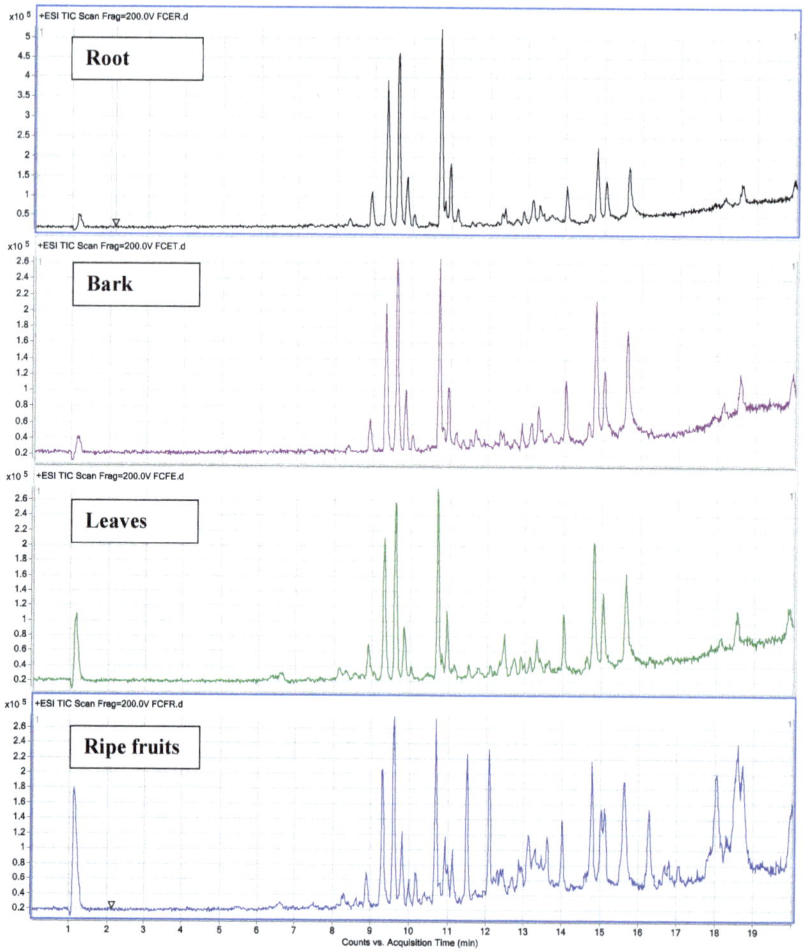

Figure 4. Chromatographic profiles of the extracts from various organs.

Table 3. Characteristics of the common compounds of the extracts of the various organs of *Ficus sur*

Peak	RT (min)	$[M + H]^+$ m/z	Proposed molecular formula	Proposed compound identification	Class
1	8.31	453.3470	$C_{20}H_{36}O_{11}$	2-Cyclohexyl-1-ethyl-β-D-maltoside	Glycoside
2	8.89	567.4323	N.I.	-	-
3	9.28	555.3575	$C_{30}H_{50}O_9$	Notoginsenoside R10	Glycoside
4	9.60	396.8035	N.I.	-	-
5	9.81	453.8481	N.I.	-	-
6	9.99	509.8878	N.I.	-	-
7	10.69	275.2768	$C_{15}H_{14}O_5$	4′,5,7-trihydroxyflavan-3-ol	Flavonoid
8	10.93	291.2711	$C_{15}H_{14}O_6$	Catechin or isomer	Flavonoid
9	11.13	304.3010	$C_{21}H_{37}N$	3,5-dipentyl-2-hexyl-pyridine	Alkaloid
10	12.35	579.2985	N.I.	-	-
11	12.69	277.2176	$C_{18}H_{28}O_2$	α-Parinaric acid	Fatty acid
12	12.86	425.2159	$C_{22}H_{32}O_8$	Dihydrovaltrate	Fatty acid
13	13.10	502.3760	N.I.	-	-
14	13.28	470.2553	N.I.	-	-
	13.29	491.1869	N.I.	-	-
15	13.60	637.3068	N.I.	-	-
16	13.98	257.2486	$C_{16}H_{32}O_2$	Palmitic acid	Fatty acid
	13.99	353.2673	$C_{21}H_{36}O_4$	Ceriporic acid C	Fatty acid
17	14.66	522.5984	N.I.	-	-
18	14.78	285.2799	$C_{18}H_{36}O_2$	Stearic acid or isomer	Fatty acid
	14.78	381.2989	$C_{23}H_{40}O_4$	Persine or isomer	Fatty acid
19	15.02	413.2679	$C_{26}H_{36}O_4$	Boviquinone 4	terpenoid
20	15.42	437.2887	$C_{25}H_{40}O_6$	Salvisyriacolide	terpenoid
21	18.16	520.4382	N.I.	-	-
22	18.59	685.4381	N.I.	-	-
23	19.9	569.4346	$C_{40}H_{56}O_2$	Lutein	Carotenoid

N.I. = Not Identified.

Table 4. Characteristics of compounds discriminating extracts of the various organs of *Ficus sur*

Peak	RT (min)	$[M + H]^+$ m /z	Proposed molecular formula	Proposed compound identification	Class	Organ
a	6.35	377.0863	$C_{18}H_{16}O_9$	5,7,3',6'-Tetrahydroxy-6,8,2'-trimethoxyflavone	Flavonoid	Le
b	6.63	235.0612	$C_{12}H_{10}O_5$	Armillarisin A or isomer	Coumarin	Le, Fr
c	8.18	608.3866	N.I.	-	-	Le
d	8.66	393.1897	N.I.	-	-	Le, Fr
e	8.76	481.1690	N.I.	-	-	Le
f	10.16	293.0432	N.I.	-	-	Fr
g	11.25	479.1722	N.I.	-	-	Ba
h	11.49	415.2132	$C_{24}H_{30}O_6$	Armillarine	Sesquiterpene aryl ester	Ba, Le, Fr
i	11.76	288.2570	N.I.	-	-	Ba, Le, Fr
j	12.07	452.3259	$C_{28}H_{41}N_3O_2$	Teleocidin B1 or isomer	Alkaloid	Le, Fr
k	13.37	468.3925	$C_{30}H_{49}N_3O$	Lucidine B	Alkaloid	Fr
ℓ	16.25	484.3889	N.I.	-	-	Fr
m	16.47	469.3321	$C_{30}H_{44}O_4$	Uralenolide	Terpenoid	Fr
n	16.77	429.3746	$C_{29}H_{48}O_2$	Saringosterol	Sterol	Fr
o	17.11	427.3940	$C_{30}H_{50}O$	alpha-amyrin or isomer	terpenoid	Fr
p	18.16	520.4382	N.I.	-	-	Fr
q	18.62	703.4176	N.I.	-	-	Fr

positively to this assay (25).

Figure 3 provides an excellent comparison of the various organs studied. In that figure one may notice the eccentricity of two organs: on the one hand, the bark which seems more antioxidant and richer in phenolic compounds and on the other hand the ripe fruits with less antioxidant activity and less rich in phenolic compounds. Unripe fruits, leaves and roots have more or less similar behaviour in relation to the parameters studied. This trend is confirmed by the one-way ANOVA. In fact, with the DPPH radical scavenging assay, the bark extract is significantly more antiradical ($P<0.0001$) than the extracts of the other organs. All antiradical activities are significantly different from each other and decrease in the following order: bark, roots, leaves, unripe fruits, ripe fruits. This order is almost confirmed by the FRAP test, except that the leaves are significantly more active than the root. Similarly, for phenolic compound contents, the bark is significantly richer in those metabolites ($P<0.0001$). The HPLC-ESI$^+$-QTOF-HRMS analysis provided important information on the nature of the metabolites contained in the various extracts. Positive ionization yielded proton molecular ions $[M + H]^+$ and the approximate value of the mass of each $[M + H]^+$ ion was given with the corresponding molecular structure in the METLIN database. Mass analysis showed more than one compound for some peaks (peaks 14 and 18), demonstrating that the problem of coelution of some compounds in HPLC can be solved by mass spectrometry. Based on the $[M + H]^+$ quasi-molecular ions provided by the high-resolution mass spectra, some common compounds from the various extracts might be notoginsenoside R10 (peak 3) and 4',5,7-trihydroxyflavan-3-ol (peak 7). According to previous studies, the latter compound (a flavonoid), has been identified in *Ficus sur* (26). In the present work, other major compounds such as catechin, palmitic acid, saringosterol and α-amyrin have been identified. The presence of some of these compounds in *Ficus sur* extracts has been previously reported (27,28).

Conclusion

This study shows that the different organs of *Ficus sur* constitute an important source of phenolic compounds and flavonoids. The immature fruit extract which is poor in phenolic compounds contains 62.34 ± 2.66 µg GAE for 1 mg of dry extract while the extract of the bark (the most active) contains 489.40 ± 7.48 µg GAE/mg dry extract. The correlation assessment shows that about 72% of the phenolic compounds found in the *Ficus sur* would be flavonoids. Moreover, the FRAP technique and the inhibition of the DPPH radical confirmed that the various organs of *Ficus sur* contain metabolites with potential antioxidant activity. Above all, statistical analyses such as PCA and ANOVA showed that the bark is the organ that contains both the most important phenolic content and presents the best antioxidant activity. The bark of *Ficus sur* would therefore be a natural source for the search for active ingredients against cardiovascular diseases, neurodegenerative diseases, cancer, and diabetes.

Acknowledgement

The authors thank Professor Pierluigi Caboni for his help concerning the use of the HPLC-ESI-HRMS device.

Authors' contributions

KIS, PB, OS and MM conceived and designed the experiments; KIS, KE, KI, performed the experiments; KIS, OS, KE, KI and OT analysed the data; PB, OS, KK and AA supervised the experiments; all authors contributed to the writing of the manuscript and confirmed publication of the final version.

Conflict of interests

The authors have no conflicts of interest.

Ethical considerations

Ethical consideration has been completely observed by the authors.

Funding/Support

This research was financially supported by Université de Lomé (Togo) and Agence Universitaire de la Francophonie/ Bureau Afrique de l'Ouest.

References

1. Malgras D. Arbres et arbustes guérisseurs des savanes maliennes. Paris: Karthala & ACCT; 1992.
2. Nadel H, Frank JH, Knight RJ. Escapees and Accomplices: The Naturalization of Exotic Ficus and Their Associated Faunas in Florida. Fla Entomol. 1992;75(1):29-38. doi: 10.2307/3495478.
3. Kapoor M, Jasani N, Acharya N, Acharya S, Kumar V. Phytopharmacological evaluation and anti-asthmatic activity of Ficus religiosa leaves. Asian Pac J Trop Med. 2011;4(8):642-4. doi: 10.1016/s1995-7645(11)60163-6.
4. Amandeep K, Rana AC, Vineeta T, Ramica S, Sunil K. Review on ethanomedicinal and pharmacological properties of *Ficus religiosa*. J Appl Pharm Sci. 2011;1(8):6-11.
5. Kazemi S, Shirzad H, Rafieian-Kopaei M. Recent findings in molecular basis of inflammation and anti-inflammatory plants. Curr Pharm Des. 2018. doi: 10.2174/1381612824666180403122003.
6. Fattouch S, Caboni P, Coroneo V, Tuberoso CI, Angioni A, Dessi S, et al. Antimicrobial activity of Tunisian quince (Cydonia oblonga Miller) pulp and peel polyphenolic extracts. J Agric Food Chem. 2007;55(3):963-9. doi: 10.1021/jf062614e.
7. Cai Y, Luo Q, Sun M, Corke H. Antioxidant activity and phenolic compounds of 112 traditional Chinese medicinal plants associated with anticancer. Life Sci. 2004;74(17):2157-84. doi: 10.1016/j.lfs.2003.09.047.
8. Balasundram N, Sundram K, Samman S. Phenolic

compounds in plants and agri-industrial by-products: Antioxidant activity, occurrence, and potential uses. Food Chem. 2006;99(1):191-203. doi: 10.1016/j.foodchem.2005.07.042.

9. Zheng W, Wang SY. Antioxidant activity and phenolic compounds in selected herbs. J Agric Food Chem. 2001;49(11):5165-70. doi: 10.1021/jf010697n.
10. Sies H, Hollman PC, Grune T, Stahl W, Biesalski HK, Williamson G. Protection by flavanol-rich foods against vascular dysfunction and oxidative damage: 27th Hohenheim Consensus Conference. Adv Nutr. 2012;3(2):217-21. doi: 10.3945/an.111.001578.
11. Watson RR, Preedy VR, Zibadi S. Polyphenols in human health and disease. London: Academic Press; 2013.
12. Saloufou KI, Boyode PB, Simalou O, Eloh K, Melila M, Kpegba K, et al. Identification de deux phytosterols biologiquement actifs de l'extrait cyclohexanique des feuilles de *Ficus sur* (Moraceae). Int J Biol Chem Sci. 2017;11(5):2510-20. doi: 10.4314/ijbcs.v11i5.44.
13. Molyneux P. The use of the stable free radical diphenylpicrylhydrazyl (DPPH) for estimating antioxidant activity. Songklanakarin J Sci Technol. 2004;26(2):211-9.
14. Dabire C, Nebie RHC, Belanger A, Nacro M, Sib FS. Effet du séchage de la matière végétale sur la composition chimique de l'huile essentielle et l'activité antioxydante d'extraits de *Ocimum basilicum* L. Int J Biol Chem Sci. 2011;5(3):1082-95. doi: 10.4314/ijbcs.v5i3.72218.
15. Nair VD, Dairam A, Agbonon A, Arnason JT, Foster BC, Kanfer I. Investigation of the Antioxidant Activity of African Potato (Hypoxis hemerocallidea). J Agric Food Chem. 2007;55(5):1707-11. doi: 10.1021/jf0619838.
16. Evans WC. Trease and Evans' Pharmacognosy. London: Saunders Elsevier; 2009.
17. Dohou N, Yamni K, Tahrouch S, Idrisi Hassani LM, Badoc A, Gmira N. Screening phytochimique d'une endémique ibero-marocaine, *Thymelaea lythroides*. Bull Soc Pharm Bord. 2003;142:61-78.
18. N'Guessan K, Kadja B, Zirihi G, Traore D, Ake-Assi L. Screening phytochimique de quelques plantes médicinales ivoiriennes utilisées en pays Krobou (Agboville, Côte-d'Ivoire). Sci Nat. 2009;6(1):1-15. doi: 10.4314/scinat.v6i1.48575.
19. Singleton VL, Orthofer R, Lamuela-Raventos RM. Analysis of total phenols and other oxidation substractes and antioxidants by means of Folin Ciocaleu Reagent. Methods Enzymol. 1999;299:152-78. doi: 10.1016/S0076-6879(99)99017-1.
20. Al-Farsi M, Alasalvar C, Morris A, Baron M, Shahidi F. Comparison of antioxidant activity, anthocyanins, carotenoids, and phenolics of three native fresh and sun-dried date (*Phoenix dactylifera* L.) varieties grown in Oman. J Agric Food Chem. 2005;53(19):7592-9. doi: 10.1021/jf050579q.
21. Kim DO, Jeong SW, Lee CY. Antioxidant capacity of phenolic phytochemicals from various cultivars of plums. Food Chem. 2003;81(3):321-6. doi: 10.1016/S0308-8146(02)00423-5.
22. Michel T, Destandau E, Le Floch G, Lucchesi ME, Elfakir C. Antimicrobial, antioxidant and phytochemical investigations of sea buckthorn (*Hippophaë rhamnoides* L.) leaf, stem, root and seed. Food Chem. 2012;131(3):754-60. doi: 10.1016/j.foodchem.2011.09.029.
23. Bors W, Michel C, Stettmaier K. Antioxidant effects of flavonoids. Biofactors. 1997;6(4):399-402. doi: 10.1002/biof.5520060405.
24. Cornard JP, Merlin JC. Complexes of aluminium(III) with isoquercitrin: spectroscopic characterization and quantum chemical calculations. Polyhedron. 2002;21(27-28):2801-10. doi: 10.1016/S0277-5387(02)01288-3.
25. Grigoras CG, Destandau E, Fougere L, Elfakir C. Evaluation of apple pomace extracts as a source of bioactive compounds. Ind Crops Prod. 2013;49:794-804. doi: 10.1016/j.indcrop.2013.06.026.
26. Dafalla HAA. Studies on the constituents of *Ficus capensis* (Thunb). Pak J Soc Sci. 2005;3(5):751-4.
27. Feleke S, Brehane A. Triterpene compounds from the latex of *Ficus sur* I. Bull Chem Soc Ethiop. 2005;19(2):307-10. doi: 10.4314/bcse.v19i2.21137.
28. Muanda NF, Dicko A, Soulimani R. Chemical composition and biological activities of *Ficus capensis* leaves extracts. J Nat Prod. 2010;3(1):147-60.

18

The effect of hydro-alcoholic *Ferulago angulata* extract on locomotor activity and anxiety caused by hypoperfusion ischemia in adult male rats

Shahrbanoo Alami-Rostami[1*], Maryam Rafieirad[2]

[1]Department of Biology, Islamic Azad University, Gomishan Center, Gorgan Branch, Gorgan, Iran
[2]Department of Biology, Faculty of Sciences, Izeh Branch, Islamic Azad University, Izeh, Iran

ARTICLE INFO

Keywords:
Ferulago angulata
Ischemia
Locomotor activity
Anxiety
Rat

ABSTRACT

Introduction: Ischemia in rat brain causes severe neuronal damage and causes anxiety disorders. *Ferulago angulata* extracts contain phenolic compounds with powerful antioxidant activity. Therefore, the aim of this study was to evaluate the protective effect of *F. angulata* (Chevilan) extract on locomotor activity and anxiety in ischemia model in rats.
Methods: In this experimental study, 50 male Wistar rats weighing 200 to 250 g were randomly divided into 5 groups including intact (control), ischemic hypoperfusion without extract and three groups of ischemic hypo-perfusion, for 14 days, received 100, 200 and 400 mg/kg Chevilan extracts by gavage method daily. For ischemia common bilateral carotid arteries were isolated, blocked in two parts and cut from the middle section. Locomotor activity and anxiety were evaluated during an open field testing.
Results: The ischemic group showed a significant increase in anxiety and decrease in motor activity in the open field test. Administration of 100, 200 or 400 mg/kg doses of the extract significantly reduced the number of raising hands, especially at the dose of 200 ($P<0.05$), and all three doses reduced the number of defecations ($P<0.001$). Consumption of 400 mg/kg dose of the *F. angulata* extracts showed a significant increase in the number of movements in the central house in the open field and between houses margins ($P<0.05$).
Conclusion: *Ferulago angulata* extract reduces anxiety in animal models of ischemia, which is probably due to some phenolic compounds and its antioxidant activity.

Implication for health policy/practice/research/medical education:
Ferulago angulata extract reduces anxiety in animal models of ischemia, which is probably due to some phenolic compounds and its antioxidant activity and might be beneficial in these patients.

Introduction

Stress is a factor that by affecting living organisms, leads to reactions causing compliance and adjustment in the body's internal environment (1). However, when stress is prolonged or repetitive, it can be very harmful (2). The most common cause of ischemic stroke is the lack of adequate blood flow to the brain tissue and cut off blood flow to any part of the brain can lead to irreversible nerve damage (3). Hypoxia in the ischemic areas of the brain causes difficulties in mitochondrial function and also causes free radical damage (4), decreasing the activity and capacity of antioxidant enzymes. Increased free radicals lead to a serious damage to cellular components such as lipids, proteins and nucleic acids and eventually causes cell death (2). As time passes, the ischemia causes various complications such as learning and memory disorders, some types of pain, anxiety, fear, reproductive disorders and depression (2). Reducing the ischemia complications using herbal anti-ischemia and anti-oxidant active ingredients is of great clinical importance (5). *Ferulago angulata* with the name of Chevilan in Persian belongs to the family of Apiaceae (Umbelliferae) that is an extended

***Corresponding author**: Shahrbanoo Alami-Rostami,
Email: sh_alemi_r@yahoo.com

family consisted of 300 genera and 3000 aromatic plants species (6). The Ferulago angulata extract has phenolic compounds and antioxidant properties and is known as an important medicinal plant of Iran (6-8). Due to their antioxidant activities, phenolic compounds are able to control free radicals. For this reason, they can be effective in preventing many diseases such as cancer, cardiovascular disease and neurological diseases and play an important role in human health (8). Therefore, in this study, the effect of *F. angulata* extract has been evaluated in the animal model of cerebral hypo-perfusion ischemia through investigating its effect on anxiety and movement activities.

Materials and Methods

Animals

The present study was carried out using adult male Wistar rats purchased from the proliferation and maintenance center of animals' house in Ahvaz Medical Science University with a weight range of 200 to 250 g. Animals were kept in standard conditions of 20 ± 2°C and 12-hour photoperiodic cycle (light started from 7 am) and adequate access to intensive food from Tehran Pars Animal Companies and Chavdaneh of Shahreza in Isfahan and purified piped water in Izeh in the animal care center of Islamic Azad University of Izeh, inside standard cages in groups of four. To facilitate the process and for more compatibility with the environment and experimenter, animals were trained daily for a few minutes before the experiment (Ethical No. 1739608130014)

In this study, 50 male Wistar rats weighing 200 to 250 g were divided randomly into 5 equal groups as follows:

1. The control group without inducing ischemia and without receiving medication (control)
2. Ischemic hypo-perfusion group without receiving medication (ischemia)
3. Ischemic hypo-perfusion group, receiving a daily dose of 100 mg/kg of *F. angulata* extract for 14 days through gavage method (ischemia + F.A E100 mg/kg)
4. Ischemic hypo-perfusion group, receiving a daily dose of 200 mg/kg of *F. angulata* extract for 14 days through gavage method (ischemia + F.A E 200 mg/kg)
5. Ischemic hypoperfusion group, receiving a daily dose of 400 mg/ kg of *F. angulata* extract for 14 days through gavage method (ischemia + F.A E 400 mg/ kg) (10).
6.

Preparing the hydroalcoholic extract of Ferulago angulata

In early May, *F. angulata* were collected from the Zagros mountain range in Khozestan province. The plant twigs were kept in a dark and dry environment for 2 weeks to dry them. After being dried and ground, they were placed in 72% ethanol and after three days of storage at room temperature we spread them out on a flat surface to dry out. After that, doses of 100, 200 and 400 of *F. angulata* extract were administered by normal saline and based on the prepared weight and through gavage for 14 days, every day at a certain hour (7-8 AM) (9).

Hypo-perfusion ischemia surgery procedure

In this study, Schty method was used with slight modifications (10). In a way that after anesthetizing rats with ketamine/xylazine (90/10 mg/kg), and neck midline incision, carotid artery appeared and then was slowly separated from the vagus nerve and carotid artery was blocked within a week of each other.

Open field test

The open field test is used to evaluate stress and movement activities. The test was done by using a 72 × 72 cm wooden field that was evenly divided into 16 homes (18 × 18 cm) and had walls with a height of 36 cm that were white (11). A central house of 18 × 18 cm was drawn in the middle of the open field. The rats were individually placed in the central square. In these circumstances, animals were passing from the central and outer lines and between the tests the considered environment was cleaned with cotton dipped in alcohol. For measuring the movement system time, the time duration of animals' mobility and immobility was recorded by the stopwatch during a specific time limit. The environmental conditions were the same for all groups and the test time was about 10 minutes and also in this test, the number of raised hands and the number of defecations were used to assess anxiety (11).

Statistical methods

Data were presented in the form of mean standard error of mean (mean + SEM) and one-way analysis of variance (ANOVA) was used followed by Tukey test. After obtaining information from different experimental groups, the results of the above groups were analyzed and $P<0.05$ was proposed as the indicator of significance. SPSS software was used for data analysis.

Results

Animal movement activity was evaluated by open field devices. The number of motor units in the open field test was significantly declined in ischemia group animals compared with the control group. Motor activity scores (number of passes in the marginal squares/number of passes in the central square) and the number of stools were recorded. In the assessment of anxiety, there was a significant difference between the control and ischemia group, reducing movement in the central square ($P<0.01$), reduction in raising hands or rearing ($P<0.05$), reducing movements in margin squares ($P<0.001$) and increase in the number of defecation ($P<0.001$), in ischemia group which shows that anxiety has increased in ischemia group compared to the control group. Administration of 100, 200 and 400 mg/kg of *F. angulata* extract caused a reduction in raising hands/rearing especially in the dose of 200 mg/kg ($P < 0.05$) (Figure 1). Only the dose of 400 mg/kg of extract in ischemia rat was able to show a significant increase in the number of movements between the central houses in the open field (Figure 2) and the number of movements between the margin houses ($P < 0.05$) (Figure 3). Also a significant reduction was observed in the number of defecations in all 3 doses of 100 ($P < 0.01$), 200 and 400 mg/kg ($P < 0.001$) (Figure 4).

Discussion

According to the survey results, 14 days of oral prescription of *F. angulata* extract to the ischemic rats, improved anxiety and depression. Cerebral ischemia leads to neurological disorders such as mental and cognitive

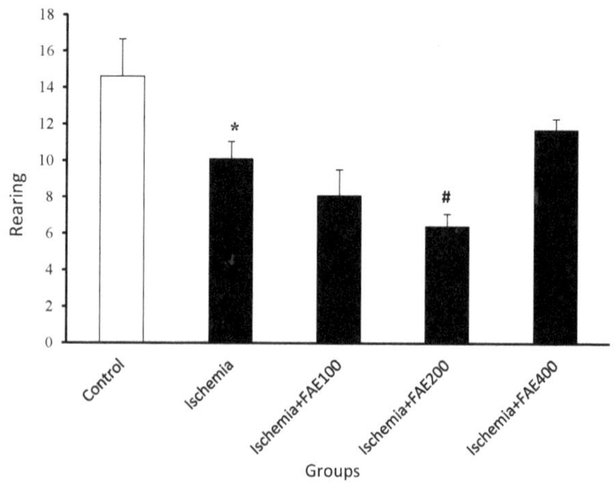

Figure 1. Comparison of the average anxiety (the number of raising hands/ Rearing) among the groups receiving different doses of *Ferulago angulata* extracts with ischemia and control group. The graph is plotted according to (mean ± SD). As can be seen, *F. angulata* extract caused a significant decrease in anxiety only at the dose of 200 mg/kg. The sign of (*) indicates a significant difference with the control group and the sign of (#) indicates a significant difference with the ischemia group (#$P < 0.05$, *$P < 0.05$, n=10, one-way ANOVA and Tukey test).

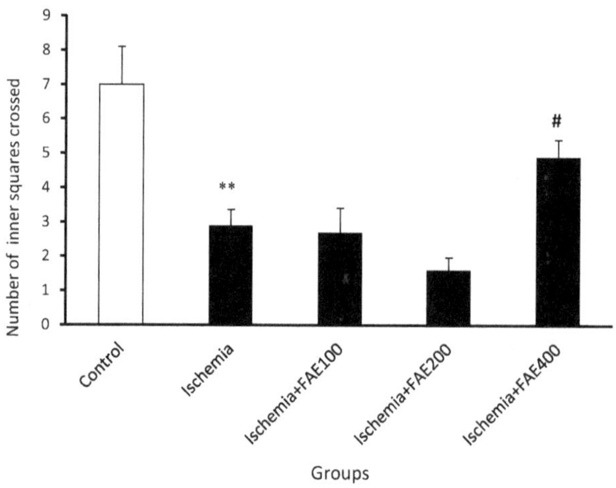

Figure 2. Comparison of the average movement activity (number of inner squares crossed in the open field) among the groups receiving different doses of the extract with ischemia and control group, the graph is plotted according to (mean ± SD), in this figure, *Ferulago angulata* extract at the dose of 400 mg/kg has led to a significant increase in the movement activities. The sign of (**) indicates a significant difference with the control group and the sign of (#) indicates a significant difference with the ischemia group (#$P < 0.05$, **$P < 0.05$, n=10, one-way ANOVA and Tukey test).

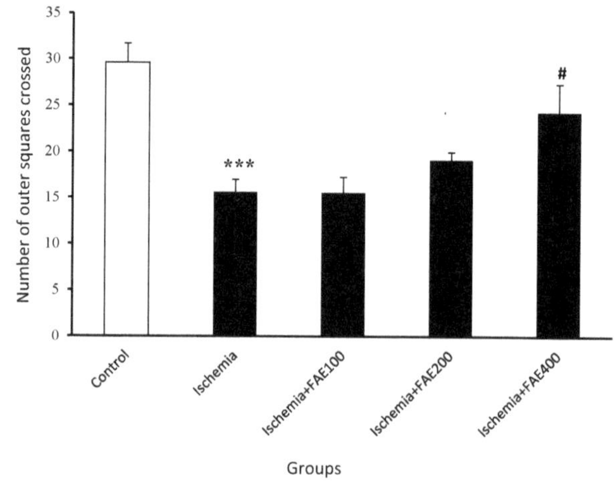

Figure 3. Comparison of the average movement activity (number of outer squares crossed in the open field) among the groups receiving different doses of the extract with ischemia and control group, the graph is plotted according to (mean ± SD), in this figure, Ferulago angulata extract at the dose of 400 mg/kg has led to a significant increase in the movement activities. The sign of (*) indicates a significant difference with the control group and the sign of (#) indicates a significant difference with the ischemia group (#$P < 0.05$, *$P < 0.05$, n=10, one-way ANOVA and Tukey test).

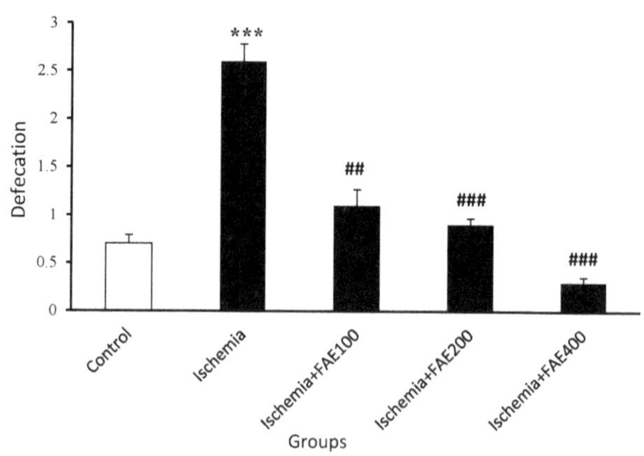

Figure 4. Comparison of the average number of defecation (anxiety) in the open field test among the groups receiving different doses of *Ferulago angulata* extract with ischemia and control group, the graph is plotted according to (mean ± SD), as can be seen, *F. angulata* resulted in a significant decrease in the number of defecation at all three doses. The sign of (*) indicates a significant difference with the control group and the sign of (#) indicates a significant difference with the ischemia group (###$P < 0.001$, ##$P < 0.01$, ***$P < 0.001$, n=10, one-way ANOVA and Tukey test).

disorders, behavioral disorders including anxiety, mania and bipolar disorders (12). Oxidative stress, as a major cause of cerebral ischemic complication, leads to disorder in oxidant-antioxidant balance and potential damages (3). It has also a pivotal role in the pathogenesis of neurodegenerative and neurological diseases such as, Alzheimer's and Parkinson's diseases, as well as trauma and brain stroke (13). Several studies have shown that the production of free radicals will increase considerably after ischemia and Sesjo in 1984 suggested that there are many routes where free radicals are produced during ischemia such as proxy nitrite (13). Scientific evidence shows that free radicals have an undeniable role in the formation and extension of secondary brain lesions after brain stroke (14). Oxidative stress will arise due to the lack of balance among the formation of reactive oxygen species (ROS) and cellular antioxidant defense system and brain is very sensitive to oxidative stress. The expression of the genes of antioxidant enzymes (such as superoxide dismutase, glutathione peroxidase and glutathione reductase) are usually increased in the natural environment in response to the uncontrolled production of ROS (15). High levels of anxiety have been reported in rats with significant production of ROS in blood lymphocytes granulocytes and monocytes. These results confirm that there is a relationship between the levels of intracellular ROS in blood cells and anxiety-related behavior in rats. In addition, Yasunari et al presented a significant relationship between anxiety and ROS formation in individuals' monocytes (16). In recent researches, a close relationship has been observed between oxidative stress and anxiety both in human beings who suffer from anxiety disorders (intellectual-practical obsession disorder and panic disorder) and also in animals and humans that have shown high levels of anxiety (17). Phenolic compounds act as the electron donor and may neutralize unwanted reactions created by free radicals in the body (18). They also have various biological properties including antioxidant, anti-radical, anti-microbial and anti-inflammatory activities (19). For this reason, they are effective in stopping the process of nervous system destruction, prevention and treatment of many diseases including ischemia by inhibiting free radicals and protecting cells against oxidative reactions (20,21). Therefore, considering the high prevalence of chronic and erosive diseases, plants should be used to provide antioxidants needed by the body especially plants that have high phenol and flavonoid compounds (19). According to many studies, it can be said that *F. angulata* extract with phenolic and antioxidant properties, it has the potential to be used as a natural antioxidant in the food and pharmaceutical industries (22,23). It can be said that the extraction of *F. angulata*, having phenolic compounds and antioxidant properties, has the potential to be used in food and pharmaceutical industries as a natural antioxidant (6). In our previous studies, *F. angulata* was able to decline the oxidative stress factors in a quite significant way in both ischemia (24) and Parkinson (25) models.

Conclusion

Ferulago angulata extract reduces anxiety in animal models of ischemia, which is probably due to some phenolic compounds and its antioxidant activity. Probably, phenolic compounds of Ferulago angulata extract, through sweeping the free radicals produced by the procedure of brain ischemia, will lead to behavioral disorders recovery including the anxiety after ischemia.

Acknowledgments

The authors would like to thank the Research Deputy of Islamic Azad University, Izeh Branch, Gomishan Branch, Gorgan Center, who supported this research.

Authors' contributions

MRR: Design of the study and laboratory methods, preparation of PGSE and laboratory methods. ShAR: Preparation of the paper draft, statistical analysis and help in laboratory methods. Both authors read the final version of the article and confirmed its publication.

Conflict of interests

The authors declared no competing interests.

Ethical considerations

The experiments were confirmed by Ethical Committee in Vice Chancellor of Research of Islamic Azad University. (Ethical No: 1739608130014) Ethical issues (including plagiarism, misconduct, data fabrication, falsification, double publication or submission, redundancy) have been completely observed by the authors.

Funding/Support

Financial costs for this research was provided of an approved project at the Islamic Azad University Gomishan Branch, Gorgan Center (Grant No: 1739608130014).

References

1. Tsigos C, Chrousos GP. Hypothalamic-pituitary-adrenal axis, neuroendocrine factors and stress. J Psychosom Res. 2002;53(4):865-71.
2. Chan PH. Reactive oxygen radicals in signaling and damage in the ischemic brain. J Cereb Blood Flow Metab. 2001;21(1):2-14. doi: 10.1097/00004647-200101000-00002.
3. Tarawneh R, Galvin JE. Potential future neuroprotective therapies for neurodegenerative disorders and stroke. Clin Geriatr Med. 2010;26(1):125-47. doi: 10.1016/j.cger.2009.12.003.
4. Sabban EL, Kvetnansky R. Stress-triggered activation of gene expression in catecholaminergic systems: dynamics of transcriptional events. Trends Neurosci. 2001;24(2):91-8.
5. Sarkaki A, Farbood Y, Hashemi S, Rafiei Rad M. Pomegranate seed hydroalcoholic extract improves memory deficits in ovariectomized rats with permanent

cerebral hypoperfusion /ischemia. Avicenna J Phytomed. 2015;5(1):43-55.

6. Hosseini N, Akbari M, Ghafarzadegan R, Shahmohammadi R, Changizi-Ashtiyani S. Total phenol, antioxidant and antibacterial activity of the essential oil and extracts of *Ferulago angulata* ssp. Angulate. J Med Plants. 2012;11(43):80-9.
7. Demetzos C, Perdetzoglou D, Gazouli M, Tan K, Economakis C. Chemical analysis and antimicrobial studies on three species of *Ferulago* from Greece. Planta Med. 2000;66(6):560-3. doi: 10.1055/s-2000-8652.
8. Taran M, Ghasempour HR, Shirinpour E. Antimicrobial activity of essential oils of *Ferulago angulata* subsp. Jundishapur J Microbiol. 2010;3(2):10-4.
9. Mirzapour S, Rafieirad M, Rouhi L. Hydroalcoholic extract of *Ferulago angulata* Improves memory and pain in brain hypoperfusion ischemia in rats. Jundishapur J Nat Pharm Prod. 2015;10(1):e17451.
10. Sarkaki A, Rafieirad M, Farbood Y, Mansouri SFM. Cognitive deficiency induced by cerebral hypoperfusion/ ischemia improves by exercise and grape seed extract. Health Med J. 2012;6(4):1097-105.
11. Rafieirad M, Zangeneh Nezhad Z, Allahbakhshi E. Neuroprotective effects of oral ellagic acid on locomotor activity and anxiety-induced by ischemia/hypoperfusion in rat. Adv Environ Biol. 2014;8(1):83-8.
12. Acikgoz O, Gonenc S, Kayatekin BM, Uysal N, Pekcetin C, Semin I, et al. Methamphetamine causes lipid peroxidation and an increase in superoxide dismutase activity in the rat striatum. Brain Res. 1998;813(1):200-2.
13. Siesjo BK. Cell damage in the brain: a speculative synthesis. Acta Psychiatr Scand Suppl. 1984;313:57-91.
14. Heo JH, Han SW, Lee SK. Free radicals as triggers of brain edema formation after stroke. Free Radic Biol Med. 2005;39(1):51-70. doi: 10.1016/j.freeradbiomed.2005.03.035.
15. Hovatta I, Tennant RS, Helton R, Marr RA, Singer O, Redwine JM, et al. Glyoxalase 1 and glutathione reductase 1 regulate anxiety in mice. Nature. 2005;438(7068):662-6. doi: 10.1038/nature04250.
16. Yasunari K, Watanabe T, Nakamura M. Reactive oxygen species formation by polymorphonuclear cells and mononuclear cells as a risk factor of cardiovascular diseases. Curr Pharm Biotechnol. 2006;7(2):73-80.
17. Bouayed J, Rammal H, Soulimani R. Oxidative stress and anxiety: relationship and cellular pathways. Oxid Med Cell Longev. 2009;2(2):63-7.
18. Manian R, Anusuya N, Siddhuraju P, Manian S. The antioxidant activity and free radical scavenging potential of two different solvent extracts of *Camellia sinensis* (L.) O. Kuntz, *Ficus bengalensis* L. and Ficus racemosa L. Food Chem. 2008;107(3):1000-7. doi: 1016/j.foodchem.2007.09.008.
19. Jamshidi M, Ahmadi Ashtiani HR, Rezazadeh SH, Fathi Azad F, Mazandarani M, Khaki A. Study on phenolicd and anioxidant activity of some selected plant of Mazandaran province. J Med Plants. 2010;9(34):177-83.
20. Gupta R, Singh M, Sharma A. Neuroprotective effect of antioxidants on ischaemia and reperfusion-induced cerebral injury. Pharmacol Res. 2003;48(2):209-15.
21. Helbecque N, Cottel D, Codron V, Berr C, Amouyel P. Paraoxonase 1 gene polymorphisms and dementia in humans. Neurosci Lett. 2004;358(1):41-4. doi: 10.1016/j.neulet.2003.12.100.
22. Khanahmadi M, Janfeshan K. Study on antioxidation property of *Ferulago angulata* plant. Asian J Plant Sci. 2006;5(3):521-6.
23. Ghasempour H, Shirinpour E, Heidari H. The Constituents of essential oils of *Ferulago angulata* (SCHLECHT) boiss at two different habitate, nevakoh and shahoo, zagross mountain, western IRAN. Iran J Sci Technology, Transaction. 2007;31:814-7.
24. Baser KH, Demirci B, Demirci F, Hashimoto T, Asakawa Y, Noma Y. Ferulagone: a new monoterpene ester from *Ferulago thirkeana* essential oil. Planta Med. 2002;68(6):564-7. doi: 10.1055/s-2002-32557.
25. Sharifi F, Rafieirad M, Sazegar H. Effects of *Ferulago angulata* extract against oxidative stress induced by 6-hydroxydopamine in rats. J Med Plants. 2015;1(53):34-44.

Antispasmodic activity of apigenin and luteolin, two components of *Dracocephalum kotschyi* extract, on rat ileum contractions

Hassan Sadraei[1*], Mostafa Ghanadian[2], Gholamreza Asghari[2], Nastaran Sekhavati[1,2]

[1]Department of Pharmacology and Toxicology, School of Pharmacy and Pharmaceutical Sciences, Isfahan University of Medical Sciences, Isfahan, Iran
[2] Isfahan Pharmaceutical Sciences Research Center, School of Pharmacy and Pharmaceutical Sciences, Isfahan University of Medical Sciences, Isfahan, Iran

ARTICLE INFO

Keywords:
Apigenin
Luteolin
Dracocephalum kotschyi
Medicinal plants
Ileum
Antispasmodic activity

ABSTRACT

Introduction: Aerial parts of *Dracocephalum kotschyi* have been used as antispasmodic agents in Iranian traditional medicine. Recent pharmacological studies confirmed antispasmodic activity of *D. kotschyi* extract. The objective of this research was to investigate antispasmodic activities of apigenin and luteolin to find out if they are responsible for the spasmolytic activity of hydroalcoholic extract of *D. kotschyi.*
Methods: Aerial parts of *D. kotschyi* were extracted with ethanol. Antispasmodic effect of hydroalcoholic extract of *D. kotschyi*, apigenin and luteolin were examined on KCl and/or acetylcholine (ACh)-induced contractions in rat isolated ileum.
Results: Hydroalcoholic extract of *D. kotschyi* concentrations-dependently inhibited KCl and ACh induced contractions with IC_{50} values of 41 ± 10 μg/mL and 133 ± 19 μg/mL, respectively. Apigenin concentrations-dependently inhibited KCl and ACh induced contractions with IC_{50} values of 57 ± 12 μM and 80 ± 18 μM, respectively. Luteolin concentrations-dependently inhibited KCl induced contractions with IC_{50} values of 68 ± 14 μM. Loperamide reduced both KCl and ACh induced contraction with IC_{50} values of 189 ± 44 nM and 82 ± 20 μM, respectively.
Conclusion: In this study apigenin and luteolin were identified as two active ingredients responsible for antispasmodic activities of *D. kotschyi* extract.

Implication for health policy/practice/research/medical education:
Apigenin and luteolin, two active ingredients of *Dracocephalum kotschyi* extract, are responsible for its antispasmodic activity and might be used for this purpose in patients having abdominal spasm.

Introduction

Dracocephalum kotschyi (Labiatae family) is an endemic herbaceous plant of Iran (1-3). *Dracocephalum* genus plants are used in traditional medicine as carminative and tonic and treatment of ailment such as congestion, headache, stomachache and liver diseases (1-4). Recent pharmacological studies have confirmed some medicinal properties of *D. kotschyi* including antihyperlipidemic (5), immunomodulatory (6), anti-inflammatory (7) and anticancer (8) effects.

In traditional herbal books there are substantial reports about use of *D. Kotschyi* as antispasmodic herbal medicine (9). Recent pharmacological studies have supported the antispasmodic effects of *D. Kotschyi* extract in both isolated ileum and rat uterus smooth muscles (10,11). The *D. kotschyi* extract inhibited the response to KCl, acetylcholine and electrical field stimulations in rat isolated ileum (10). In addition, it has been reported that hydroalcoholic extract of *D. kotschyi* possesses relaxant effect on uterus responses to KCl, acetylcholine and electrical nerve stimulation as well as oxytocin-induced contractions (11). Above findings confirms that *D.*

*Corresponding author: Dr. Hassan Sadraei,
Email: sadraei@pharm.mui.ac.ir

kotschyi extract possesses components with antispasmodic activities on smooth muscle of ileum and uterus. Furthermore, hydroalcoholic and hexane extracts of *D. kotschyi* attenuated the intestinal charcoal meal transit, confirming the antispasmodic action *in vivo* (12). The hydroalcoholic and hexane extracts of *D. kotschyi* also significantly inhibited the castor oil and $MgSO_4$-induced diarrhea in mice which could be related to its antispasmodic activity (12). In a separate experiment, the anti-inflammatory effect of hydroalcoholic extract of *D. kotschyi* was examined on acetic acid-induced colitis in rats and it was found to be very effective (13). From these experiments, it can be concluded that *D. kotschyi* extract possesses potent antispasmodic activities both *in vitro* and *in vivo* and could be used as a remedy for the treatment of gastrointestinal disorders especially those associated with intestinal spasm. Therefore, identification of the activity of plants constituents is necessary for drug development. *Dracocephalum kotschyi* is an aromatic medicinal plant enrich in essential oils (5,14), valuable flavonoids (15), monoterpene glycosides and trypanocidal terpenoids (16). Some of the constituents of the *D. kotschyi* extract have already been published (15). These include calycopterin, xanthomicrol, isokaempferide, luteolin, apigenin, luteolin 7-O-beta-D-glucopyranoside, lutcolin 3'-O-beta-D-glucuronide, apigenin 4'-O-beta-D-glucopyranoside, acacetin 7-O-beta-D-glucopyranoside and rosmarinic acid (15). However, so far there is no report about the antispasmodic activity of these components. Therefore, in this research we have investigated antispasmodic effects of apigenin and luteolin and compared with antispasmodic action of hydroalcoholic extract of *D. kotschyi* and loperamide.

Materials and Methods

Plant materials

Aerial parts of *D. kotschyi* Boiss. (Labiatae family) were collected in June 2015 from Chadegan (in Isfahan province-Iran) and identified at the Botany Department of the Faculty of Sciences, University of Isfahan. A voucher specimen of the plant (No. 1519) deposited in the herbarium of the Faculty of Pharmacy and Pharmaceutical Sciences, Isfahan University of Medical Sciences. The plant materials were dried in shadow and grained to powder using electrical miller (Moulinex, France). The dried plant material was used for extraction by maceration (17). Powdered plant material was thoroughly mixed with 70% ethanol and left for two hours. Wetted plant materials were packed into percolator and soaked in 70% ethanol for three days, with occasional shaking. Plant extract was evacuated from bottom tap passing through cotton cloth placed on the bottom of the percolator. This procedure was repeated three times and the combined filtrate was evaporated using rotary evaporator (Buchi Rotavapor RE) at 50°C to get the final hydroalcoholic extract of *D. kotschyi*. After evaporating the ethanol, amount of dried crude extract was determined (w/w).

Antispasmodic assessment

Experiments were conducted on adult male Wistar rats (180-220 g) bred in School of Pharmacy, animal house. All animals were handled in compliance with the principles of the guide for care and use of laboratory animal care approved by the university committee (18). On the day of experiment, a rat was killed by a blow on the head, followed by exsanguinations. A portion of ileum was removed and placed in oxygenated Tyrode's solution at room temperature. A section of ileum (2-3 cm) was mounted for isotonic contraction under 1 g tension in 20 mL organ bath (Harvard, England) containing Tyrode's solution and continuously gassed with O_2 at 37°C. Ileum contraction was measured using a Harvard isotonic transducer and recorded on a Harvard Universal Oscillograph (England) pen recorder device. Initially the oscillograph was calibrating, and 3 successive washes were given and the tissue was allowed to relax to a stable baseline. When the tissue baseline was established, KCl (80 mM) was added in to the organ bath in order to induce a sustained tonic contraction. The inhibitory effect of *D. kotschyi* extract or drugs were examined on isolated rat ileum contraction induced by KCl. Fifteen minutes after addition of KCl, extract or drugs were added to the bath at 5 minutes intervals in a cumulative manner using two-fold increments in concentration, until maximum inhibition was obtained. In the case of acetylcholine (ACh), non-cumulative manner was used. ACh was added into the tissue bath to give the final bath concentration of 5 µg/mL. ACh was allowed to act for 30 seconds before it was washed with fresh Tyrode's solution. The time-matched control tissues were treated with an equivalent volume of the vehicle.

Drugs and solutions

Solidified extract was weighted and prepared as 20 mg/mL stock solution in dimethyl sulfoxide (DMSO). Further dilutions were made in distilled water. Apigenin and luteolin (Sigma, China) were made up in DMSO as 10mM stock solutions. Loperamide was dissolved in DMSO as 20 mM stock solution. KCl was prepared as 2M stock solution. Acetylcholine (Sigma) was prepared in distilled water as 1mM stock solution. Tyrode's solution (NaCl, 136.9; KCl, 2.68; $CaCl_2$, 1.8; $MgCl_2$, 1.05; $NaHCO_3$, 11.9; NaH_2PO_4, 0.42 and glucose 5.55 mM) was prepared in distilled water. Unless stated, all the chemicals were purchased from Merck (Germany).

Data analysis

The tissue contractile responses were measured as maximum amplitude from pretreatment baseline and expressed as the percentage of the initial contraction induced by KCl or ACh. All values were quoted as mean ± standard error of the mean (SEM). The IC_{50} value (Drug concentration causing 50% of maximum inhibitory response) was calculated for each tissue and mean and SEM was determined for each group of results. SigmaPlot computer program was used for statistical analysis and plotting the graphs. The IC_{50} values were used as an index for comparison of antispasmodic activities.

Results

Dried hydroalcoholic extract of *D. kotschyi* had dark greenish color. A sample of concentrated extract was thoroughly dried on a hot pate and the yield of dried extract was calculated to be 23% (w/w).

Antispasmodic studies

Rat isolated ileum suspended in Tyrode's solution gradually relaxed to a stable baseline over 15-30 min. KCl (80 mM) caused a tonic contraction which maintained for the duration of the study. Acetylcholine (ACh, 5 μM) caused a rapid phasic contraction in rat ileum during 30 seconds of contact time. KCl and ACh concentrations were chosen to produce maximum contractile responses in the tissue.

Antispasmodic activities of apigenin and luteolin were examined on isolated ileum contraction for comparison with the total extract of hydroalcoholic extract of *D. kotschyi* by constructing full concentration-response curve. Loperamide, an opioid agent with antimotility action, was used as a positive standard drug in this research. As expected, loperamide concentration-dependently inhibited rat ileum contractile responses induced by both KCl and ACh with IC_{50} values of 189±44 nM and 82±20 μM respectively (Figure 1).

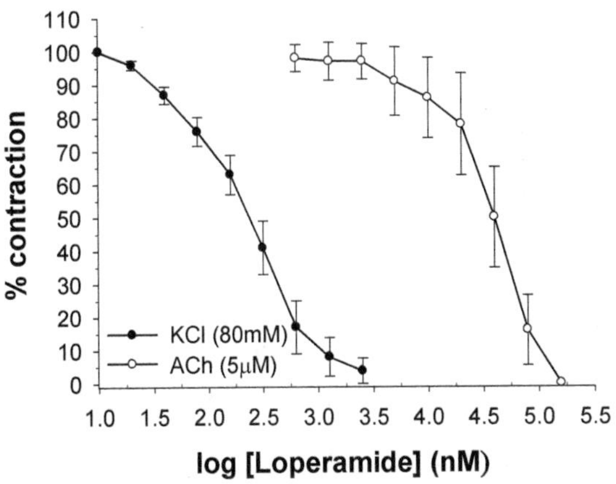

Figure 1. Inhibitory concentration-responses curves for loperamide on contractions induced by KCl and acetylcholine (ACh) in rat isolated ileum.
Ordinate scales: spasm remaining as a % of the contraction prior to drugs addition. Abscissa scales: log_{10} concentration of loperamide. Each point is mean of six experiments and the vertical lines show the SEM (n=6).

Hydroalcoholic extract of *D. kotschyi,* concentration-dependently inhibited both KCl and ACh induced contraction in the rat ileum. The inhibitory effect on KCl response was seen with bath concentration of 8 μg/mL and complete inhibition was achieved with extract concentration of 256 μg/ml (Figure 2). Inhibitory effect of *D. kotschyi* extract on ACh response started with bath concentration of 64 μg/mL and total inhibition was

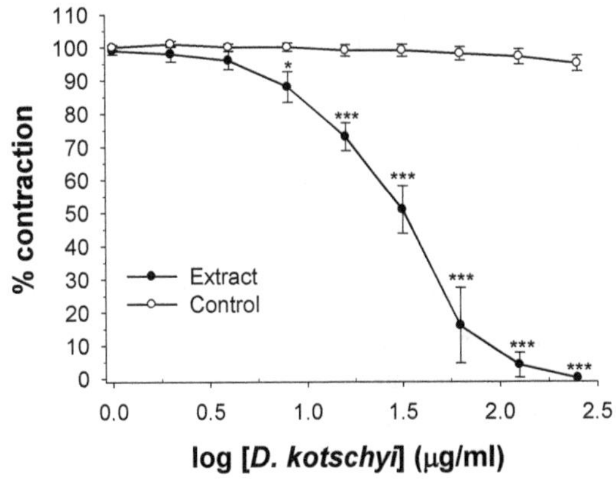

Figure 2. Inhibitory concentration response curves for hydroalcoholic extract obtained from *D. kotschyi* on tonic contractions induced in rat isolated ileum by KCl (80mM).
Ordinate scales: spasm remaining as a % of the contraction prior to drugs addition. Abscissa scales: log10 concentration of extract. Each point is mean of six experiments and the vertical lines show the SEM (n=6). The control groups were treated with equivolume amount of vehicle (DMSO). The stars show the statistically significant difference with corresponding point in the time-matched control groups. **P*< 0.05, ****P*< 0.001 (Student's t-test).

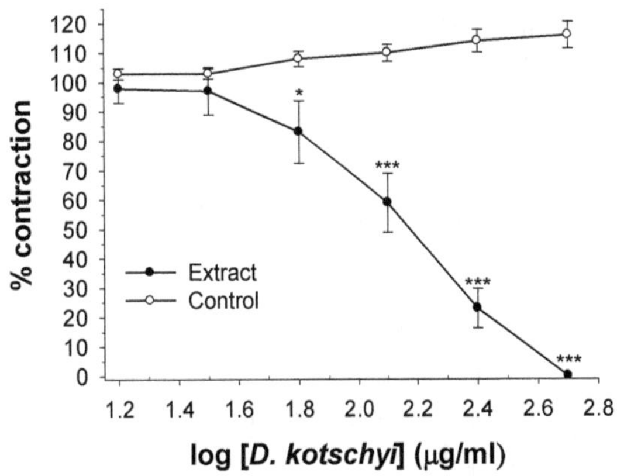

Figure 3. Inhibitory concentration responses curve for hydroalcoholic extract of *D. Kotschyi* on phasic contractions induced in rat isolated ileum by acetylcholine (5 μM). Ordinate scales: spasm remaining as a % of the contraction prior to addition of extract. Abscissa scales: log_{10} concentration of extract. Each point is mean of six experiments and the vertical lines show the SEM (n=6). The control groups were treated with equivolume amount of vehicle (DMSO). Gradual increase in tissue responses in the control group is statistically significant (ANOVA, *P*< 0.05). The stars show the statistically significant difference with corresponding point in the time-matched control groups. **P*< 0.05, ****P*< 0.001 (Student's *t* test).

seen with 512 μg/mL extract in the bath (Figure 3). The inhibitory concentrations causing 50% of maximum response (IC_{50} value) were 41 ± 10 μg/mL and 133 ± 19 μg/mL for KCl and ACh respectively.

Apigenin, a known component of *D. kotschyi*, also in a concentration-dependent manner inhibited KCl, as well as ACh induced contractions with IC_{50} values of 57 ± 12 μM and 80 ± 18 μM respectively. First sign of attenuation of KCl response was seen with 8 μM apigenin in the bath and at bath concentration of 480 μM, apigenin totally removed the KCl response in the rat ileum (Figure 4). Inhibitory effect of apigenin on ACh response was seen with similar concentration ranges (Figure 5). Luteolin, another component of *D. kotschyi* extract, in a concentration-dependent manner inhibited KCl induced contraction in rat ileum with IC_{50} value of 80 ± 18 μM (Figure 5). Initial reduction was observed with bath concentration of 14 μM and at bath concentration of 450 μg/mL, luteolin wiped out the tonic contraction induce by KCl (Figure 6). Potencies of apigenin, luteolin and loperamide are compared in Table 1. In the vehicle treated control groups, equivalent volume of DMSO not only did not reduce ACh response but also was observed a gradual increase in contractile response (Figures 3 and 5). Low concentration of DMSO had no effect on KCl response (Figure 2).

Discussion

Dracocephalum kotschyi hydroalcoholic extract is a relaxant of ileum and uterus smooth muscles and possessed antispasmodic and antidiarrheal activities (10-12). However, *D. kotschyi* extract contains a mixture of several active substances with various pharmacological properties including, anti-inflammatory, anti-cancer, anti-dyslipidimea, etc (5-8). Therefore, it is essential to identify the active substances which could be responsible for antispasmodic activities on smooth muscle. Preparation of standard drug form purified compound is more convenient and administrations of unwanted substances are avoided. Although several constituents of *D. kotschyi* extract are known (15), however, the main problem is that we had no idea which chemical components were

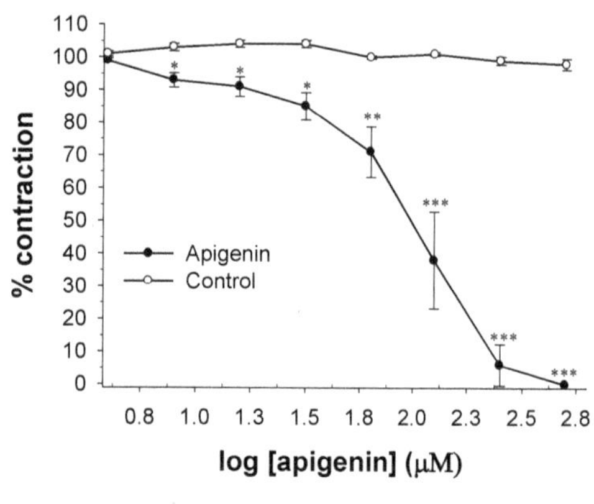

Figure 4. Inhibitory concentration-responses curve of apigenin on the tonic contraction induced by KCl in rat isolated ileum.
Ordinate scales: spasm remaining as a % of the contraction prior to apigenin addition. Abscissa scales: $\log_{10}$ concentration of apigenin. Each point is mean of six experiments and the vertical lines show the SEM (n=6). The control groups were treated with equivolume amount of vehicle (DMSO). There are not statistically significant changes in the fluctuation seen in the vehicle treated control group (ANOVA). The stars show the statistically significant differences of the test tissues with the corresponding points in the time-matched control groups. *$P < 0.05$, **$P < 0.01$, ***$P < 0.001$ (Student's *t* test).

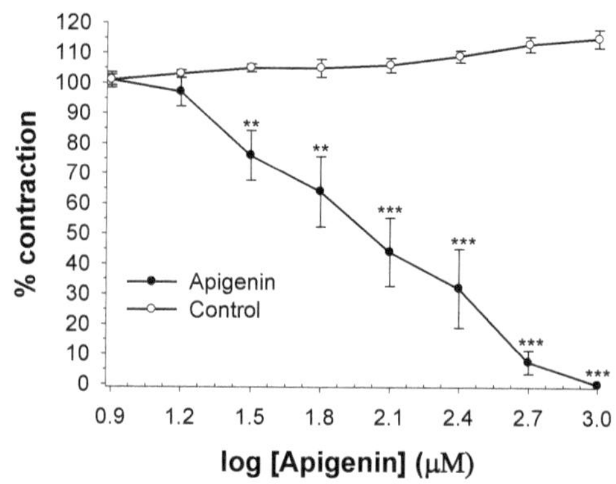

Figure 5. Inhibitory concentration responses curve for apigenin on phasic contraction induced in rat isolated ileum by acetylcholine (5 μM).
Ordinate scales: spasm remaining as a % of the contraction prior to apigenin addition. Abscissa scales: $\log_{10}$ concentration of apigenin. Each point is mean of six experiments and the vertical lines show the SEM (n=6). The control groups were treated with equivolume amount of vehicle (DMSO). Gradual increase in tissue response in the control group is statistically significant (ANOVA, $P < 0.05$). The stars show the statistically significant difference with corresponding point in the time-matched control groups. **$P < 0.01$, ***$P < 0.001$ (Student's *t* test).

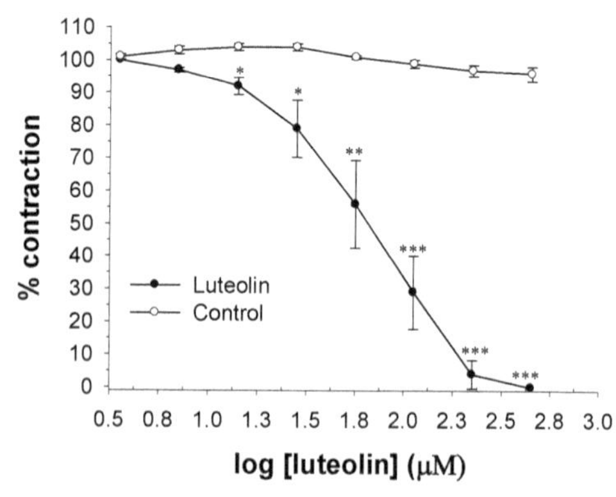

Figure 6. Inhibitory concentration responses curve of luteolin in rat isolated ileum for the tonic contraction induced by KCl (80 mM).
Ordinate scales: spasm remaining as a % of the contraction prior to luteolin addition. Abscissa scales: $\log_{10}$ concentration of luteolin. Each point is mean of six experiments and the vertical lines show the SEM (n=6). The control groups were treated with equivolume amount of vehicle (DMSO). Observed fluctuation in the vehicle treated control group response was not statistically significant (ANOVA). The stars show the statistically significant differences of the test tissues with the corresponding points in the time-matched control groups. *$P < 0.05$, **$P < 0.01$, ***$P < 0.001$ (Students *t* test).

Table 1. Comparison of potency of loperamide, apigenin and luteolin for inhibiting KCl (80 mM) and acetylcholine (ACh, 5 μM) responses in rat isolated ileum

	pD_2 values		
	Loperamide	Apigenin	Luteolin
KCl	6.72	4.24	4.10
ACh	4.09	4.10	-

Potency has expressed as pD_2 value (log_{10} potency in molar concentration).

responsible for the antispasmodic activities. Apigenin and luteolin are two flavonoids that have been identified in the hydroalcoholic extract *D. kotschyi* (15). Therefore, antispasmodic activities of apigenin and luteolin were examined on isolated ileum contractions.

In this study loperamide was used as a standard drug and as expected it reduced ileum contraction in a concentration-dependent manner. Loperamide is an opioid agent with antimotility action which inhibits peristalsis and slows gastrointestinal motility by the effect on circular and longitudinal muscle of the intestine (19,20). Loperamide act by several different mechanisms, mediated by various opioid receptors on the enteric nerves and smooth muscles (19,20).

This study revealed that apigenin and luteolin as well as hydroalcoholic extract of *D. kotschyi* have direct relaxant effects on rat ileum smooth contractions by KCl and ACh. ACh is cholinergic neurotransmitter which acts on muscarinic M_3-receptors on smooth muscle of ileum. Muscarinic receptors are G-protein couple receptors (GPCR) and cause the release of Ca^{2+} ions from intracellular stores via increasing phospholipase-C activities and generation of inositol triphosphate (21,22). Addition of high potassium concentration (80 mM KCl) into extracellular solution results in cell membrane depolarization and activation of voltage-gated calcium channels (23). Increase in intracellular Ca^{2+} ion concentrations results in smooth muscle contraction (23). However, other studies have shown that membrane depolarization induced by high concentrations of extracellular KCl can also cause Ca^{2+} sensitization in many smooth muscles (23). In the case of KCl induced tonic contraction it has been proposed that tonic force maintenance in the smooth muscle is dependent on rhoA kinase activity (23). However, some isotype of protein kinase C (PKC) may also play a role in causing KCl-induced sensitization (24). Flavonoids such an apigenin and luteolin are reported to inhibit PKC activities (25-27). Inhibition of PKC by apigenin and luteolin indicates that both apigenin and luteolin are acting intracellulary and this is consistent with inhibition of both ACh and KCl induced contractions. In addition, luteolin is a non-selective competitive inhibitor of phosphodiesterases (28) which could also play a role in its antispasmodic activity. Therefore, apigenin and luteolin are two active ingredients of *D. kotschyi* extract with potent antispasmodic activities.

Comparison of inhibitory concentration at molar concentration showed that potencies of apigenin and luteolin were close to that of loperamide especially for inhibiting acetylcholine response (Table 1). However, *D. kotschyi* extract is a mixture of several substances and comparison of potency in molar concentration was not feasible. Nevertheless, as luteolin and apigenin are found to be relatively potent antispasmodic agents, it can be concluded that they are responsible for antispasmodic activity of *D. kotschyi* extract, although, contribution of other components could not be excluded.

Drugs that reduce spasm in the gut are of great value in gastrointestinal disorders including irritable bowel syndrome and diverticular disease (29). It has been shown that apigenin as well as *D. kotschyi* extract reduce the intestinal transit and has anti-diarrheal activity in mice (12). Therefore, apigenin has been shown to have antispasmodic activities both *in vitro* and *in vivo*. Furthermore, apigenin has anti-inflammatory activities in acetic acid-induced colitis (13). These findings confirm that apigenin is a suitable candidate for the treatment of irritable bowel syndrome in which intestinal spasms and diarrhea are part of the clinical signs.

Conclusion

In this research relaxant effects of apigenin and luteolin were examined on rat ileum and it was found to have direct relaxation actions on gastrointestinal smooth muscle. Apigenin and luteolin not only inhibited contraction induced by ACh but they also were as much potent as loperamide. Therefore, it can be concluded that apigenin and luteolin are two components responsible for antispasmodic activity of *D. kotschyi* extract. However, *D. kotschyi* extract is enriched in bioactive substances. Therefore, further pharmacological researches for identification of other active components with antispasmodic activities are recommended.

Acknowledgments

This project was part of Pharm. D thesis of Nastaran Sekhavati as Pharm. D student at Isfahan University of Medical Sciences.

Authors' contributions

MG and GA were responsible for preparation of extract while HS supervised the pharmacological studies. NS was responsible for performing the laboratories work. All contributed to the preparation of the article and confirmed final edition for publication.

Ethical considerations

Ethical issues have been observed by the authors.

Funding/Support

This research project financially was supported by

Research Department of Isfahan University of Medical Sciences (Grant No. 395862).

References

1. Mozaffarian V. A Dictionary of Iranian Plant Names. Tehran: Farhng Moaser; 2012:292-3. [Persian].
2. Zargari A. Medicinal plants. 4th ed. Tehran: Tehran University Publication; 1990:42-5. [Persian].
3. Rechinger KH. Labiatae. In: Rechinger KH, Hedge IC, eds. Flora Iranica, Akademische Druck Verlagsantalt. Vol 150, Graz, Austria; 1986:218-31.
4. Mirheydar H. Maaref Giahi. Vol 2. Tehran: Daftare Nasher Farhange Eslami;1995:170-76. [Persian].
5. Ebrahim Sajjadi S, Movahedian Atar AM, Yektaian A. Antihyperlipidemic effect of hydroalcoholic extract, and polyphenolic fraction from *Dracocephalum kotschyi* Boiss. Pharm Acta Helv. 1998;73(3):167-70.
6. Amirghofran Z, Azadbakht M, Karimi MH. Evaluation of the immunomodulatory effects of five herbal plants. J Ethnopharmacol. 2000;72(1-2):167-72.
7. Golshani S, Karamkhani F, Monsef-Esfehani HR, Abdollahi M. Antinociceptive effects of the essential oil of *Dracocephalum kotschyi* in the mouse writhing test. J Pharm Pharm Sci. 2004;7(1):76-9.
8. Jahaniani F, Ebrahimi SA, Rahbar-Roshandel N, Mahmoudian M. Xanthomicrol is the main cytotoxic component of *Dracocephalum kotschyi* and a potential anti-cancer agent. Phytochemistry. 2005;66(13):1581-92. doi: 10.1016/j.phytochem.2005.04.035.
9. Naghibi F, Mosaddegh M, Mohammadi Motamed M, Ghorbani A. Labiatae family in folk medicine in Iran: from ethnobotany to pharmacology. Iran J Pharm Res. 2005;4(2):63-79.
10. Sadraei H, Asghari G, Kasiri F. Antispasmodic effect of *Dracocephalum kotschyi* hydroalcoholic extract on rat ileum contraction. Res Pharm Sci. 2015;10(5):446-52.
11. Sadraei H, Asghari G, Alinejad M. Comparison of antispasmodic effect of hydroalcoholic extract of *Dracocephalum kotschyi* Boiss. in rat uterus and ileum. Res Pharm Sci. 2016;11(4):284-92. doi: 10.4103/1735-5362.189295.
12. Sadraei H, Asghari G, Shahverdi F. Antidiarrhoeal assessment of hydroalcoholic and hexane extracts of *Dracocephalum kotschyi* Boiss. and apigenin in mice. Res Pharm Sci. 2016;11(3):200-9.
13. Sadraei H, Asghari G, Khanabadi M, Minaiyan M. Anti-inflammatory effect of apigenin and hydroalcoholic extract of *Dracocephalum kotschyi* on acetic acid-induced colitis in rats. Res Pharm Sci. 2017;12(4):322-9. doi: 10.4103/1735-5362.212050.
14. Sadraei H, Asghari G, Kasiri F. Comparison of antispasmodic effects of *Dracocephalum kotschyi* essential oil, limonene and alpha-terpineol. Res Pharm Sci. 2015;10(2):109-16.
15. Gohari AR, Saeidnia S, Matsuo K, Uchiyama N, Yagura T, Kiuchi F, et al. Flavonoid constituents of *Dracocephalum kotschyi* growing in Iran and their trypanocidal activity. Natural Medicines. 2003;57(6):250-2.
16. Saeidnia S, Gohari AR, Uchiyama N, Ito M, Honda G, Kiuchi F. Two new monoterpene glycosides and trypanocidal terpenoids from *Dracocephalum kotschyi*. Chem Pharm Bull (Tokyo). 2004;52(10):1249-50.
17. Samuelsson G. Drugs of natural origin. Stockholm: Swedish Pharmaceutical Press; 1999:48-9.
18. Committee for the update of the guide for the care and use of laboratory animals National Research Council. Guide for the Care and Use of Laboratory Animals. Washington DC: The National Academies Press; 2010:11-37.
19. Ooms LA, Degryse AD, Janssen PA. Mechanisms of action of loperamide. Scand J Gastroenterol Suppl. 1984;96:145-55.
20. Reynolds IJ, Gould RJ, Snyder SH. Loperamide: blockade of calcium channels as a mechanism for antidiarrheal effects. J Pharmacol Exp Ther. 1984;231(3):628-32.
21. Eglen RM, Hegde SS, Watson N. Muscarinic receptor subtypes and smooth muscle function. Pharmacol Rev. 1996;48(4):531-65.
22. Unno T, Matsuyama H, Sakamoto T, Uchiyama M, Izumi Y, Okamoto H, et al. M(2) and M(3) muscarinic receptor-mediated contractions in longitudinal smooth muscle of the ileum studied with receptor knockout mice. Br J Pharmacol. 2005;146(1):98-108. doi: 10.1038/sj.bjp.0706300.
23. Ratz PH, Berg KM, Urban NH, Miner AS. Regulation of smooth muscle calcium sensitivity: KCl as a calcium-sensitizing stimulus. Am J Physiol Cell Physiol. 2005;288(4):C769-83. doi: 10.1152/ajpcell.00529.2004.
24. Ratz PH, Miner AS. Role of protein kinase Czeta and calcium entry in KCl-induced vascular smooth muscle calcium sensitization and feedback control of cellular calcium levels. J Pharmacol Exp Ther. 2009;328(2):399-408. doi: 10.1124/jpet.108.142422.
25. Ferriola PC, Cody V, Middleton E, Jr. Protein kinase C inhibition by plant flavonoids. Kinetic mechanisms and structure-activity relationships. Biochem Pharmacol. 1989;38(10):1617-24.
26. Lin JK, Chen YC, Huang YT, Lin-Shiau SY. Suppression of protein kinase C and nuclear oncogene expression as possible molecular mechanisms of cancer chemoprevention by apigenin and curcumin. J Cell Biochem Suppl. 1997;28-29:39-48.
27. Agullo G, Gamet-Payrastre L, Manenti S, Viala C, Remesy C, Chap H, et al. Relationship between flavonoid structure and inhibition of phosphatidylinositol 3-kinase: a comparison with tyrosine kinase and protein kinase C inhibition. Biochem Pharmacol. 1997;53(11):1649-57.
28. Yu MC, Chen JH, Lai CY, Han CY, Ko WC. Luteolin, a non-selective competitive inhibitor of phosphodiesterases 1-5, displaced [3H]-rolipram from high-affinity rolipram binding sites and reversed xylazine/ketamine-induced anesthesia. Eur J Pharmacol. 2010;627(1-3):269-75. doi: 10.1016/j.ejphar.2009.10.031.
29. Rang HP, Dale MM, Ritter JM, Flower RJ. Rang and Dale's Pharmacology. 6th ed. London: Churchill Livingstone; 2007;385-96.

Hypoglycemic and hypolipidemic effects of *Nelumbo nucifera* flower in Long-Evans rats

Dipa Islam[1*], Amdadul Huque[1], Sheuly[2], Liton Chandra Mohanta[1], Sadhan Kumar Das[1], Abida Sultana[3], Evena Parvin Lipy[1], U. K. Prodhan[4]

[1]Biomedical and Toxicological Research Institute (BTRI), Institute of Food Science and Technology, Bangladesh Council of Scientific and Industrial Research (BCSIR), Dhaka, Bangladesh
[2]Science, Secondary Education Quality and Access Enhancement Project (SEQAEP), Ministry of Education, Dhaka, Bangladesh
[3]Department of Food Technology, Kishoreganj Polytechnic Institute, Kishoreganj, Bangladesh
[4]Department of Food Technology and Nutritional Science, Mawlana Bhashani Science and Technology University, Bangladesh

ARTICLE INFO

Keywords:
Alloxan monohydrate
Diabetes
Hypoglycemia
Hypolipidemia
Medicinal plant

ABSTRACT

Introduction: The study was conducted to assess the hypolipidemic and hypoglycemic effects of *Nelumbo nucifera* flowers powder in Long-Evans rats.
Methods: Experimental rats were made hyperlipidemic and diabetic (type 2) by feeding high fat diet (Lab diet, Dalda and Coconut oil = 4: 3: 1) and injecting alloxan respectively. *N. nucifera* flowers powder in different percentages was mixed with the regular Lab Diet for 21 days feeding. Serum total cholesterol, triglyceride, low-density lipoprotein (LDL), high-density lipoprotein (HDL) and blood glucose levels were evaluated in various groups.
Results: Feeding with *N. nucifera* flowers powder at different percentages to hyperlipidemic groups showed diverse but a significant ($P < 0.05$) decrease in serum total cholesterol, triglyceride and LDL-cholesterol levels when compared to control group while HDL-cholesterol level was increased significantly ($P < 0.05$). Routine feeding with *N. nucifera* flowers powder for 21 days resulted in significant decrease in the blood glucose levels of alloxan-induced diabetic rats. Both 20% and 10% of *N. nucifera* flower powders with Lab Diet significantly ($P < 0.05$) decreased blood glucose level up to 48% and 34%, respectively in comparison to the drug control group treated with glibenclamide which was found with the decreasing capability up to 66% where the higher percentage of *N. nucifera* flower powder was found to exert more prominent effect in lowering blood glucose level. During comparison to the control group, the above mentioned percentages of *N. nucifera* flowers powder was found to reduce the blood glucose level around 32.05% and 47.92% respectively. Although not prominent, but the data revealed that the sample was endowed with the body weight declining capability.
Conclusion: Results of the experiments affirm that the flower of *N. nucifera* has potent hypoglycemic and hypolipidemic properties and might be useful in these patients.

Implication for health policy/practice/research/medical education:
Flowers of *N. nucifera* may be utilized for both diabetic and hyperlipidemic patients. Thus, further studies on it may reveal new active compounds having anti-diabetic and lipid lowering properties.

Introduction

Lipid abnormalities are generally connected with diabetes which ultimately is considered as one of the most contributory factors for cardiovascular morbidity and mortality in patients suffering from diabetes. Type II diabetes is the most common one which accounts for about 90% of the diabetic population affecting minimum 15 million people. It is directly connected with other difficulties including hypertension, atherosclerosis and microcirculatory disorders. Among all the endocrine disorders, diabetes mellitus (type 2) is highly reported and is projected that almost three hundred million will be affected by the disease by 2025 and greater portion of diabetic population will be from India, China and

***Corresponding author**: Dipa Islam,
Email: btrl5071@gmail.com

United States (1-6). According to recent epidemiological studies, in Bangladesh more than 11% diabetic patients are suffered from type II diabetes and the presence of atypical fasting glucose, which triggers the initiation of diabetes, goes beyond 6% in Dhaka city (7). Therefore, it is now inevitable to search for novel oral drugs that will be therapeutically effective both as hypoglycemic and hypolipidemic agents at affordable cost particularly both for the developing and under-developed countries. In the experiments of hypoglycemic effects evaluation, animals are made diabetic usually by injecting alloxan or streptozotocin (STZ) intraperitoneally (IP) or intravenously (IV). For the studies of hypolipidemic activity, the subjected animals are generally fed with high fat diet to produce hyperlipidemia in those animals.

Nelumbo nucifera is an aquatic perennial which belongs to the family of Nelumbonaceae and is familiar by many local names (e.g. Indian lotus, Chinese water lily, and Sacred lotus). Lotus flowers powder is utilized in traditional medicine to treat high blood pressure, diarrhea, fever, weakness, infection, skin inflammation, and body heat imbalance (8). It is also an effective treatment against abnormal bleeding such as hematemesis, epistaxis, hemoptysis, hematuria, and metrorrhagia (9). Lotus flowers extracts are found to possess a powerful antioxidant and radical scavenging ability along with inhibitory activity of diabetic complications (10-13). Lotus flower extract has been reported to treat obesity, too (14-16). Furthermore, lotus flowers extracts were observed to modulate lipolysis-activity and decrease adipogenesis in human pre-adipocytes (17) as well as to increase cholesterol profile in mice and reduce levels of phospholipids and triglycerides (18). It is notable to mention that anti-HIV principles have also been constructed using the ethanolic extract of the lotus flowers (19). This study was conducted to assess the hypolipidemic and hypoglycemic effects of *N. nucifera* flowers powder in Long-Evans rats.

Materials and Methods

Experimental design

This experiment was conducted according to Figure 1.

The study was carried out in Biomedical and Toxicological Research Institute (BTRI), Bangladesh Council for Scientific and Industrial Research (BCSIR), Dhaka, Bangladesh. Flowers of *N. nucifera* were brought from National Botanical Garden, Mirpur, Dhaka, Bangladesh and identified by the Bangladesh National Herbarium, Dhaka. At first, the flowers of *N. nucifera* were washed vigorously using water and then dried at room temperature. The flowers were then air dried and subsequently oven dried at 37°C temperature. Later on, the dried flowers were grinded to powder form which then screened to find out the fine powder. Powder size of <0.5 mm after passing through a 35-mesh sieve was considered for the experiment.

Healthy male rats (Long-Evans) of local strain, having around 150-200 g and 200-250 g weights were taken for the hypolipidemic and hypoglycemic effects studies, respectively. The proper environmental condition for the experimental rats was confirmed, kept under firm supervision for a week and maintained at a constant room temperature of 25°C ± 5°C with humidity of 40% to 70%

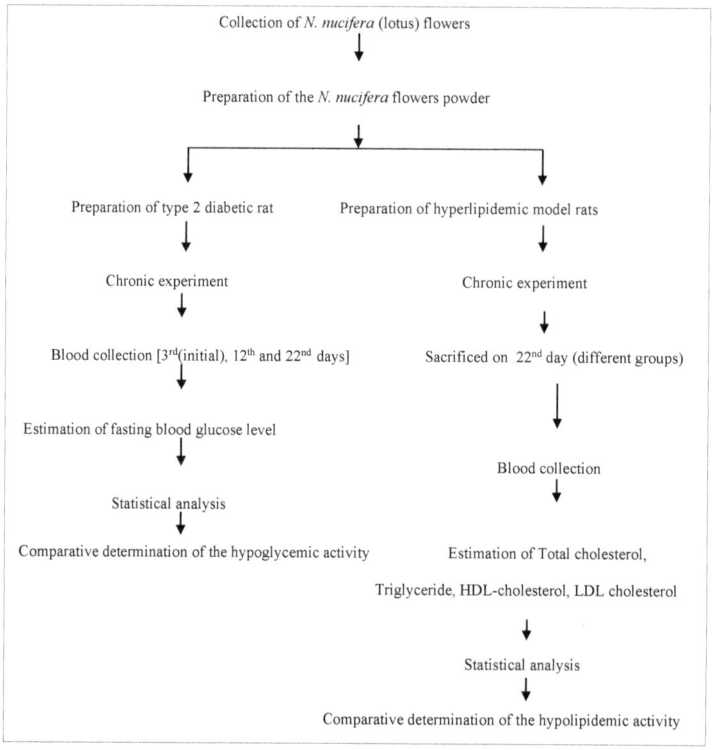

Figure 1. Experimental design.

with natural day-night cycle.

For the hypolipidemic effect studies, the rats were segregated into a total of eight groups consisting of six in each maintaining the congruity of body weight. These included:

Group-A (feeding with lab diet).

Group-B1 (feeding with 10% powder of *N. nucifera* flower and 90% lab diet).

Group-B2 (feeding with 20% powder of *N. nucifera* flower and 80% lab diet).

Group-B3 (feeding with 30% powder of *N. nucifera* flower and 70% lab diet).

Group-C (feeding with high fat diet after inducing hyperlipidemia).

Group-D1 (feeding with 10% powder of *N. nucifera* flower and 90% high fat diet after inducing hyperlipidemia).

Group-D2 (feeding with 20% powder of *N. nucifera* flower and 80% high fat diet after inducing hyperlipidemia).

Group-D3 (feeding with 30% powder of *N. nucifera* flower and 70% high fat diet after inducing hyperlipidemia).

For evaluation of hypoglycemic activity of *N. nucifera* flower, the rats were segregated into five groups comprising of six in each with the congruence of body weight. These included:

1) Group-A (Normal Control, rats fed with 100% lab diet)

2) Group-B (Alloxan induced diabetic rats fed with 100% lab diet, diabetic control).

3) Group-C (Alloxan induced diabetic rats fed with Lab Diet plus glibenclamide, given at a dose of 5 mg/10 mL (9.9 mL H_2O + 0.1 mL Twin 20)/kg body weight, drug control (23).

4) Group-D (Alloxan induced diabetic rats fed with 10% powder of *N. nucifera* flower plus 90% lab diet).

5) Group-E (Alloxan induced diabetic rats fed with 20% powder of *N. nucifera* flower plus 80% lab diet).

Before starting the experiment, the weights of the rats were taken precisely and the rats were marked on the tail, right front, right back, left front, left back and kept unmark which was subsequently applied as identification purpose for a particular rat, so that the reaction of a specific rat before and after the drug administration could be observed individually.

Preparation of hyperlipidemic rats and estimation of the lipid profile

The rats were made hyperlipidemic by feeding high fat diet for 10 days containing Lab Diet, Dalda and Coconut oil in 4:3:1 ratio.

For evaluation of hypolipidemic activity, the powder of the *N. nucifera* flower was administered orally with high fat diet and lab diet at doses of daily 10%, 20% and 30% of the regular diet for 21 days.

Blood samples were collected on the 22nd day by sacrificing the rats after making anesthesia using ketamine hydrochloride. After sacrificing about 2 mL of blood was taken cautiously. The blood samples were then centrifuged after 20 minutes at 4000 rpm for 10 minutes and re-centrifuged at 2000 rpm for 5 minutes. After that the serums samples were separated and taken into Eppendorf tubes. Then the serum triglyceride, total cholesterol, high-density lipoprotein cholesterol (HDL-C) and low-density lipoprotein cholesterol (LDL-C) were measured. One milliliter of serum was aliquoted and kept frozen at -20°C until analysis of serum for lipid profile.

Serum total cholesterol was measured by enzymatic colorimetric (Cholesterol Oxidase /Peroxidase, CHOD-PAP) method (Randox Laboratories Ltd., UK) using autoanalyzer, AutoLab. Serum HDL-cholesterol was estimated by enzymatic colorimetric (Cholesterol CHOD-PAP) method (Randox Laboratories Ltd., UK) using micro-plate reader (Bio-Tec, ELISA) and Serum triglyceride (TG) was examined by enzymatic colorimetric (GPO-PAP) method (Randox Laboratories Ltd., UK) using auto analyzer, Auto Lab. Then, serum LDL cholesterol was calculated manually. The calculated formula was:

$$LDL - C = TC - (\frac{TG}{5} + HDL - C)$$

All the groups of rats were remained under similar environmental conditions and provided with the measured food and water throughout the experiment. The body weight of each rat was measured and compared with the controls.

Preparation of diabetic rats and measurement of blood glucose level

Alloxan monohydrate ($C_4H_2N_2O_4.H_2O$) was available in colored bottles containing 25 g powder. The solution was prepared by dissolving 10 g in 100 mL of distilled water (10%).

The rats were made diabetic (diabetes mellitus) by injecting alloxan monohydrate 150-mg/kg-body weight intravenously (20). Three days after injection of the alloxan monohydrate, blood glucose of all the surviving rats was determined by the Diagnostics EliTech method. The rats with blood glucose levels above 6 mmol/L were considered as diabetic and considered for further study.

For the assessment of hypoglycemic effect, *N. nucifera* flowers powder was fed orally with Lab Diet at doses of daily 10% and 20% of regular diet for 21 days. The drug, glibenclamide was administrated orally as a drug control, at a dose of 5 mg/10 mL (9.9 mL H_2O + 0.1 ml Twin 20)/kg body weight to the respective grouped rats.

Fasting blood glucose level was measured using glucometer on the 3rd (initial), 12th and 22nd days by collecting blood samples nicking the lateral tail vein using a sterile scalpel blade under ketamine hydrochloride anesthesia. Just before cutting, the tail was immersed into warm water (40°C) for around 25 seconds for vasodilatation.

Data analysis

The data analysis was performed using SPSS. 11.5

windows program. $P<0.05$ was considered significant. For charts and graphical representation Microsoft Word and Microsoft Excel were used.

Results

During the entire study period laboratory protocols described in Materials and Methods section were followed strictly. The findings based on experimental data are depicted below:

Chronic effect of *Nelumbo nucifera* flower powder on body weight of rats

Chronic effect of N. nucifera flower powder on body weight of normal control rats fed with lab diet and rats fed with lab diet plus sample

The impacts of *N. nucifera* flowers powder on body weight of the rats during 21 days of feeding with Lab Diet plus sample in different percentages are shown in Table 1. Body weight of each rat was measured at every 11-day intervals and compared with that of the normal control group fed with 100% Lab Diet.

Chronic effect of Nelumbo nucifera flower powder on body weight of hyperlipidemic model rats fed with high fat diet plus sample in comparison to hyperlipidemic model rats fed with only high fat diet

The impacts of *N. nucifera* flower powder on body weight of hyperlipidemic rats administered with 100% high fat diet and the grouped rats fed with high fat diet plus sample at various percentages during 21 days of feeding are delineated in Table 2. Body weight of each rat was measured at every 11-day intervals.

Chronic effects of *Nelumbo nucifera* flower powder on lipid status (total cholesterol & triglyceride) of rats

Chronic effects of Nelumbo nucifera flower powder on lipidemic status (total cholesterol & triglyceride) of rats fed with Lab Diet plus sample in comparison to normal control rats fed with lab diet

The mean serum total cholesterol and triglyceride levels of normal control rats administered with lab diet and model rats, administered with Lab Diet plus *N. nucifera* flowers powder for 21 days followed by blood collection on 22nd day are presented in Table 3. To find out whether there was a statistically significant difference in hypolipidemia obtained by the powder sample on the 22nd day.

Chronic effect of Nelumbo nucifera flowers powder on lipidemic status (total cholesterol & triglyceride) of hyperlipidemic rats fed with high fat diet Plus Sample in comparison to hyperlipidemic model rats fed with only high fat diet

The mean serum total cholesterol and triglyceride levels of high fat diet treated hyperlipidemic rats administered with only high fat diet (treated as control) and model rats administered with high fat diet plus powder of *N. nucifera* flower for 21 days followed by blood collection on 22nd day are presented in Table 4.

Chronic effect of *Nelumbo nucifera* flower powder on lipidemic status (HDL-C and LDL-C) of rats

Chronic effect of Nelumbo nucifera flower powder on lipidemic status (HDL-C and LDL-V) of rats fed with lab diet plus sample in comparison to normal control rats fed with lab diet

The effect of *N. nucifera* flower powder on atherogenic

Table 1. Chronic effect of *Nelumbo nucifera* flower powder on body weight (BW) of rats fed with lab diet plus sample in comparison to normal control rats fed with lab diet

Group		BW, Initial day (g)	BW, 12th day (g)	BW, 22nd day (g)
Group A (100% high diet) (n=6)		174.17±8.04 (100%)	178.17±7.78 (102.30%)	183.17±7.31 (105.18%)
Group B (lab diet + sample)	B1 (90% lab diet + 10% sample) (n=6)	172±7.04 (100%)	173.83±7.68 [a] (101.06%)	176±7.82 [a] (102.33%)
	B2 (80% lab diet + 20% sample) (n=6)	171.17±6.43 (100%)	172.83±6.11 [a] (100.97%) [a]	174.83±6.11 [a] (102.12%)
	B3 (70% lab diet + 30% sample) (n=6)	172.67±6.19 (100%)	174.50±6.09 [a] (101.06%)	174.83±5.67 [a] (101.25%)

Data are presented as Mean ± SD and compared using one-way ANOVA (Duncan post hoc test), n = number of rats.
[a] Statistically significant in comparison to the control group ($P<0.05$).

Table 2. Chronic effect of *Nelumbo nucifera* flower powder on body weight (BW) of hyperlipidemic rats fed with high fat diet plus sample in comparison to hyperlipidemic rats fed with only high fat diet

Group		BW, Initial day (g)	BW, 12th day (g)	BW, 22nd day (g)
Group C (100% high fat diet (n=6)		172.33±10.46	176.83±10.52	180.33±9.63
Group D (high fat diet + sample)	B1 (90% lab diet + 10% sample) (n=6)	171.67±11.00	172.20±11.62 [a]	172.14±12.58 [a]
	B2 (80% lab diet + 20% sample) (n=6)	171.50±8.17	172.58±7.06 [a]	172.59±7.17 [a]
	B3 (70% lab diet + 30% sample) (n=6)	174±5.93	174.88±5.47 [a]	174.79±5.92 [a]

Data are presented as Mean ± SD and compared using one-way ANOVA (Duncan post hoc test), n = number of rats.
[a] Statistically significant in comparison to the control group ($P<0.05$).

Table 3. Chronic effects of *Nelumbo nucifera* flower powder on lipidemic status (total cholesterol & triglyceride) of rats fed with lab diet plus sample in comparison to normal control rats fed with lab diet

Group		BW, Initial day (g)	BW, 12th day (g)	BW, 22nd day (g)
Group C (100% high fat diet) (n=6)		172.33±10.46 (100%)	176.83±10.52 (102.61%)	180.33±9.63 (104.64%)
Group D (high fat diet + sample)	D1 (90% high fat diet + 10% sample) (n=6)	171.67±11.00 (100%)	172.20±11.62 [a] (100.31%)	172.14±12.58 [a] (100.27%)
	D2 (80% high fat diet + 20% sample) (n=6)	171.50±8.17 (100%)	172.58±7.06 [a] (100.58%)	172.59±7.17 [a] (100.64%)
	D3 (70% high fat diet + 30% sample (n=6)	174±5.93 (100%)	174.88±5.47 [a] (100.51%)	174.79±5.92 [a] (100.45%)

Data are presented as Mean ± SD and compared using one-way ANOVA (Duncan post hoc test), n = number of rats.
[a] Statistically significant in comparison to the control group ($P < 0.05$).

Table 4. Chronic effect of *Nelumbo nucifera* flowers powder on lipidemic status (total cholesterol & triglyceride) of hyperlipidemic rats fed with high fat diet plus sample in comparison to hyperlipidemic model rats fed with only high fat diet

Group		TC, 22nd day (mg/dL)	TG, 22nd day (mg/dL)
Group C (100% high fat diet) (n=6)		119.33±11.13	100.83±18.49
Group D (high fat diet + sample)	D1 (90% high fat diet + 10% sample) (n=6)	85.17±9.26 [a]	89.83±16.39 [a]
	D2 (80% high fat diet + 20% sample) (n=6)	72.67±8.14 [a]	83±15.28 [a]
	D3 (70% high fat diet + 30% sample)(n=6)	60.17±8.18 [a]	77.83±14.16 [a]

Data are presented as mean ± SD and compared using one-way ANOVA (Duncan post hoc test), n = number of rats.
[a] Statistically significant in comparison to the control group ($P < 0.05$).

lipids (HDL-C and LDL-V) of rats fed with lab diet plus sample and normal control rats fed with lab diet is shown in Table 5.

Chronic effect of Nelumbo nucifera flowers powder on lipidemic status (HDL-C and LDL-V) of high fat diet induced hyperlipidemic rats fed with high fat diet plus sample in comparison to hyperlipidemic rats fed with only high fat diet

The effect of *N. nucifera* flower powder on atherogenic lipids (HDL-C and LDL-V) is presented in Table 6.

Chronic effect of *Nelumbo nucifera* flowers powder on fasting blood glucose concentration of alloxan induced type 2 diabetic model rats

The effects of *N. nucifera* flower powder 10% with 90% Lab Diet and 20% with 80% Lab Diet, expressed as change in blood glucose level, are depicted in Table 7. Fasting blood glucose level of each rat was taken at every 11-day intervals.

Discussion

It is obvious that there was a tendency to decline the body weight in all sample fed rat groups whereas normal control rats displayed increase in body weights at the end of study period (Table 1). Mathematically around a maximum 0.90% body weight reduction was observed in comparison to the body weights measured at first day considered as 100%.

It is noticed from the data presented in Table 2 that there was a raise in body weight in each group. But the sample administered groups displayed slower enhancement in body weight than high fat diet fed groups. Data also suggest that after feeding of only high fat diet for 21 days, body weight augmentation was almost maximum of 10% if the initial body weight was considered as 100%. But, when along with the high fat diet, the sample at different percentages was given, the body weight increase was only a maximum of 0.20% considering the initial body weight as 100%.

According to data presented in Table 3, a significant diminution ($P < 0.05$) of TC and TG values in group B1 (90% lab diet + 10% sample), group B2 (80% lab diet + 20% sample) and group B3 (70% lab diet + 30% sample) compared to group A (100% Lab Diet) was observed and this diminution was more significant in higher percent of

Table 5. Chronic effect of *Nelumbo nucifera* flower powder on lipidemic status (HDL-C and LDL-C) of rats fed with lab diet plus sample in comparison to normal control rats fed with lab diet

Group		HDL-C, 22nd day	LDL-C, 22nd day
Group A (100% lab diet) (n=6)		55.50±4.42	16.85±2.44
Group B (lab diet + sample)	B1 (90% lab diet + 10% sample) (n=6)	69.83±7.91 [a]	9.00±1.21 [a]
	B2 (80% lab diet + 20% sample) (n=6)	76±9.78 [a]	8.33±1.08 [a]
	B3 (70% Lab diet + 30% sample) (n=6)	80.83±9.70 [a]	7.28±1.01 [a]

Data are presented as mean ± SD and compared using one-way ANOVA (Duncan post hoc test), n = number of rats.
[a] Statistically significant in comparison to the control group ($P < 0.05$).

Table 6. Chronic effect of *Nelumbo nucifera* flower powder on lipidemic status (HDL-C and LDL-C) of high fat diet induced hyperlipidemic model rats fed with high fat diet plus sample in comparison to hyperlipidemic model rats fed with only high fat diet

Group		HDLC, 22nd day	LDLC, 22nd day
Group C (100% high fat diet) (n=6)		50.67±2.42	21.20±4.53
Group D (high fat diet + sample)	D1 (90% high fat diet + 10% sample) (n=6)	75±7.46 [a]	14.03±2.54 [a]
	D2 (80% high fat diet + 20% sample) (n=6)	79±6.90 [a]	12±1.92 [a]
	D3 (70% high fat diet + 30% sample) (n=6)	89.17±5.42 [a]	9.60±1.16 [a]

Data are presented as mean ± SD and compared using one-way ANOVA (Duncan post hoc test), n = number of rats.
[a] Statistically significant in comparison to the control group ($P < 0.05$).

Table 7. Chronic effect of *Nelumbo nucifera* flower powder on fasting blood glucose (FBG) concentration of alloxan induced type 2 diabetic model rats

Group	FBG, initial day (mmol/L)	FBG, 12th day (mmol/L)	FBG, 22nd day (mmol/L)
Group-A (normal control)	4.80 ± 0.51 (100%)	4.76 ± 0.43 (99.17%)	4.74 ± 0.39 (98.75%)
Group-B (diabetic control)	15.42 ± 0.23 (100%)	15.38 ± 0.18 (99.74%)	15.64 ± 0.25 (101.43%)
Group-C (drug control)	15.50 ± 0.28 (100%)	9.41 ± 0.38 [a] (60.71%)	5.32 ± 0.16 [a] (34.32%)
Group-D (sample 10% + lab diet 90%)	15.07 ± 0.47 (100%)	11.49 ± 0.87 [a] (76.24%)	10.24 ± 0.96 [a] (67.95%)
Group-E (sample 20% + lab diet 80%)	15.13 ± 0.58 (100%)	9.76 ± 0.57 [a] (64.51%)	7.88 ± 0.33 [a] (52.08%)

Data are presented as mean ± SD and compared using one-way ANOVA (Duncan post hoc test), n = number of rats.
[a] Statistically significant in comparison to the control group ($P < 0.05$).

Sample treated groups. Data reveal that the TC and TG values of the highest percentage sample treated group, group B3 in comparison to the group A after 21 days of feeding, were found to be lowered by around 43% and 44%, respectively.

Data shown in Table 4, confirm that samples have the characteristics of TC and TG diminishing abilities at a significant level in comparison to that of control one.

In Table 5, significant variations were observed in the HDL-C and LDL-C levels among all the test groups after 21 days of sample treatment. In case of group B3 (70% lab diet + 30% sample) HDL-cholesterol was mostly augmented compared to the group A (100% lab diet). In Groups B1 (90% lab diet + 10% sample) and B2 (80% lab diet + 20% sample) the HDL-C levels were also found to be augmented in a significant level although lower than group B3. Furthermore, LDL-C level was observed to be reduced significantly in all the studies groups. Among all the groups, group B3 (70% lab diet + 30% sample) was found with the lowest level of LDL-C. In group B3, the HDL-C level was observed to be augmented by almost 49% and the LDL-C level was found to be reduced to 60% in comparison to that of group A after 21 days of sample treatment.

It was found according to data presented in Table 6 that, overall, HDL-C level increased significantly while that of LDL-C decreased which was also significant among all the studied groups after 21 days of chronic trial. The lipidemic profile was checked on 22nd day of the study. In case of group D3 (70% lab diet + 30% sample) HDL-C level was found to be increased maximum compared to the group C (100% lab diet). It is worth mentioning that in case of group D1 (90% lab diet + 10% sample) and group D2 (80% lab diet + 20% sample) the HDL-C level was also observed to be augmented significantly while LDL-C level in all experimental groups was found to be decreased significantly. More specifically, in case of group D3 where the maximum of around 48% of HDL-C level was observed to be increased and the highest of 62% of LDL-C level seen to be reduced in comparison to that of group C.

It is worth mentioning from Table 5 and Table 6 that the increase of HDL cholesterol level was prominently higher in sample diet fed groups compared to that of normal control groups (both group A and group C). Significantly increment tendency of HDL cholesterol level was observed with the higher percentage of sample diet. It is also clear from Table 5 and Table 6 that the reduction of LDL cholesterol level was higher with the higher percentage of sample diet which surely implies to the hypolipidemic activities of the sample, *N. nucifera* flowers powder.

In Table 7, blood glucose levels were depicted and more significant ($P < 0.05$) anti-diabetic activity was observed on 22nd day in alloxan induced type 2 diabetic model rats. In a study it has been suggested that a 25% reduction in blood glucose level is considered a significant hypoglycemic effect. The results of the study were satisfactory and revealed that the 10% & 20% *N. nucifera* flowers powder exhibited significant ($P < 0.05$) hypoglycemic activity. In case of 10% sample induced group, the reduction of blood glucose level was 33%. The reduction of blood glucose level in alloxan induced rat was found highest, 44% with the *N. nucifera* of 20%.

Conclusion

According to the experimental results, it can be affirmed that *N. nucifera* flowers powder is endowed with strong hypoglycemic and hypolipidemic properties. Therefore, powder of *N. nucifera* flower may be utilized for the management of diabetes mellitus and other related complications directly linked to the lipid disorders. On the whole, *N. nucifera* is a very promising herbal plant having enormous medicinal values. The plant should be examined vigorously to find out for its active ingredients for which hypoglycemic and hypolipidemic activities are being exerted and mode of actions behind the observed effects.

Acknowledgements

We are expressing our heartfelt gratitude to the Biomedical and Toxicological Research Institute (BTRI), IFST, BCSIR, Dhaka, Bangladesh, for protruding the required hands during the study in all respects including financial and logistic supports.

Authors' contribution

DI generated the idea. AH, S, LCM, SKD, AS and EPL executed the studies in accordance with the designed procedure working in the laboratories and capturing data. DI, AH and UKP performed data analysis. S and AS prepared the initial draft. AH revised the draft and produced the final manuscript with the consent of DI. All are well concerned about the latest version and agreed for publication.

Conflict of interests

The authors of the manuscript affirm that they have no conflict of interest.

Ethical considerations

The research protocol and all the tests performed in this study were approved by the Animal Care Committee of BCSIR (No. 39.307.099.00.00.166.2010-455). All the associated ethical matters were considered to the best by the authors.

Funding/Support

Financial and logistic supports were provided by Biomedical and Toxicological Research Institute (BTRI), (BTRI), IFST, BCSIR, Dhaka, Bangladesh, Tel: +880 2 58610717.

References

1. Ramachandran A, Snehalatha C, Ma RC. Diabetes in South-East Asia: an update. Diabetes Res Clin Pract. 2014;103(2):231-7.
2. Kesari AN, Kesari S, Singh SK, Gupta RK, Watal G. Studies on the glycemic and lipidemic effect of Murraya koenigii in experimental animals. J Ethnopharmacol. 2007;112:305-11.
3. Edem DO. Hypoglycemic effects of ethanolic extracts of alligator pear seed (*Persea americana* Mill) in rats. Eur J Sci Res. 2009;33:669-678.
4. Bastaki S. Review diabetes mellitus and Its treatment. Int J Diab Met. 2005;13:111-34.
5. King H, Auburt RE, Herman WH. Global burden of diabetes 1995-2025: prevalence, numerical estimates and projections. Diab Care. 1998;21:1414-1431. doi: 10.2337/diacare.21.9.1414.
6. Ramachandran A, Snehalatha C, Kapur A, Vijay V, Mohan V, Das AK, et al. High prevalence of diabetes and impaired glucose tolerance in India: National Urban Diabetes Survey.. Diabetologia. 2001;44:1094-100. Doi: 10.1007/s001250100627.
7. Sayeed MA, Rumi MAK, Ali L. Effect of socioeconomic risk factors on the difference in prevalence of diabetes between rural and urban populations in Bangladesh. Biol Med Res Council. 2007;33:1-12.
8. Sridhar KR, Rajeev B. Lotus—a potential nutraceutical source. J Agr Technol. 2007;3:143-155.
9. Moro CF, Yonekura M, Agrawal GK. Lotus—a source of food and medicine: current status and future perspectives in context of the seed proteomics. Int J Life Sci. 2013;7:1-5. Doi: 10.3126/ijls.v7i1.6394.
10. Wu MJ, Wang L, Weng CY, Yen JH. Antioxidant activity of methanol extract of the lotus leaf. Am J Chin Med. 2003;31:687-698. doi: 10.1142/S0192415X03001429.
11. Saengkhae C, Arunnopparat W, Sungkhajorn P. Antioxidative activity of the leaf of *Nelumbo nucifera* Gaertn. on oxidative stress-induced erythrocyte hemolysis in hypertensive and normotensive rats. Thai J Physiol Sci. 2008;20:70-78.
12. Jung HA, Jung YJ, Yoon NY, Jeong DM, Bae HJ, Kim DW, et al. Inhibitory effects of *Nelumbo nucifera* leaves on rat lens aldose reductase, advanced glycation endproducts formation, and oxidative stress. Food Chem Toxicol. 2008;46:3818-26. Doi: 10.1016/j.fct.2008.10.004.
13. Huang B, He J, Ban X, Zeng H, Yao X , Wang Y. Antioxidant activity of bovine and porcine meat treated with extracts from edible lotus (*Nelumbo nucifera*) rhizome knot and leaf meat Science. 2001;87:46-53. doi: 10.1016/j.meatsci.2010.09.001.
14. Cour B, Molgaard P, Yi Z. Traditional Chinese medicine in treatment of hyperlipidaemia. J Ethnopharmacol. 1995;46:125-9. doi: 10.1016/0378-8741(95)01234-5.
15. Onishi E, Yamada K, Yamada T, Kaji K, Inoue H, Seyama Y, et al. Comparative effects of crude drugs on serum lipids. Chem Pharmaceut Bull. 1984;32:646-650. doi: 10.1248/cpb.32.646.
16. Ono Y, Hattori E, Fukaya Y, Imai S, Ohizumi Y. Anti-obesity effect of *Nelumbo nucifera* leaves extract in mice and rats. J Ethnopharmacol. 2006;106:L238-244. doi: 10.1016/j.jep.2005.12.036.
17. Siegner R, Heuser S, Holtzmann U, Söhle J, Schepky A, Raschke T, et al. Lotus leaf extract and l-carnitine influence different processes during the adipocyte life cycle. Nutr Metab. 2010;7:66. doi: 10.1186/1743-7075-7-66.
18. Kashiwada Y, Aoshima A, Ikeshiro Y, Chen YP, Furukawa H, Itoigawa M, et al. Anti-hiv-benzylisoquinoline alkaloids and flavonoids from the leaves of *Nelumbo nucifera*, and structure-activity correlations with related alkaloids. Bioorgan Med Chem. 2005;13:1443-1448. doi: 10.1016/j.bmc.2004.10.020.
19. Ali L, Khan AK, Mamun MI, Mosihuzzaman M, Nahar N, Nur-e-Alam M, R, et al. Studies on hypoglycemic effects fruit pulp, seed and whole plant of Momordica charantia on normal and diabetic model rats. Planta Med. 1993;59:408-412. doi: 10.1055/s-2006-959720.
20. Akhtar MS, Athar MA, Yaqub M. Effect of Momordica charantia on blood glucose levels of normal and alloxan diabetic rabbits. Planta Med. 1981;42:205-212. doi: 10.1055/s-2007-971629.

21

Medicinal plants: Past history and future perspective

Fatemeh Jamshidi-Kia[1], Zahra Lorigooini[1*], Hossein Amini-Khoei[1]

[1]Medical Plants Research Center, Basic Health Sciences Institute, Shahrekord University of Medical Sciences, Shahrekord, Iran

ARTICLEINFO

Keywords:
Medicinal herbs
Medicinal plant history
Medicinal plant perspective

ABSTRACT

Human societies have been in close contact with their environments since the beginning of their formation and used the ingredients of the environment to obtain food and medicine. Awareness and application of plants to prepare food and medicine have been realized through trial and error, and gradually human became able to meet his needs from his surroundings. Information about medicinal plants has long been transmitted gradually and from generation to generation, a human knowledge has gradually become complete with the formation of civilizations and the provision of more facilities. Medicinal plants are used as a medical resource in almost all cultures. Ensuring the safety, quality and effectiveness of medicinal plants and herbal drugs very recently became a key issue in industrialized and developing countries. By standardizing and evaluating the health of active plant-derived compounds, herbal drugs can help the emergence of a new era of the healthcare system to treat human diseases in the future. Awareness of traditional knowledge and medicinal plants can play a key role in the exploitation and discovery of natural plant resources. In order to maintain this knowledge, comprehensive approach and collaboration are needed to maintain historical records on medicinal plants and use these resources in favour of human beings, before they are destroyed forever. Therefore, this review was conducted to investigate and describe the process of using medicinal plants throughout history. This review focuses on the recent various important challenges in quality evaluation of medicinal plants in the authenticity, efficacy, toxicity and consistency.

Implication for health policy/practice/research/medical education:
Medicinal plants play a golden role not only as traditional medicine but also as trade commodities, meeting the demand of distant markets for the development of new drugs. In fact, to realize the effective integration of plants into a medical system, researchers and practitioners should be trained in both modern and traditional medicine in the use of plant compounds. In addition, to build credibility for the use of plants in conventional medicine, the empirical arguments should be converted into evidence-based arguments.

Introduction

Nature is always a golden sign to show the prominent phenomena of coexistence. Natural products from plants, animals and minerals are the basis for treating human diseases (1). Medicinal plants are presently in demand and their acceptance is increasing progressively. Undoubtedly, plants play an important role by providing essential services in ecosystems. Without plants, humans and other living organisms cannot live in a way living should be. Anyway, herbals especially medicinal herbs have constantly acted as an overall indicator of ecosystem health (2). Medicinal plants have undoubtedly been considered by human beings since ancient times. It can be said that before the history and since the early humans recognized and exploited the plants around them for use as fuel, clothing, shelter and food, they became aware of their properties more or less. Medicinal plants have been transformed into one of the oldest sciences in countries such as China, Greece, Egypt and India. In ancient Persia, plants were commonly used as a drug and disinfectant

*Corresponding author: PhD of Pharmacognosy, Assistant professor of Medical Plants Research Center, Basic Health Sciences Institute, Shahrekord University of Medical Sciences, Shahrekord, Iran.
Email: zahralorigooini@gmail.com

and aromatic agent (3). In fact, the use of medicinal plants for the treatment of diseases dates back to the history of human life, that is, since human beings have sought a tool in their environment to recover from a disease, the use of plants was their only choice of treatment (4). More than a tenth of the plant species (over 50 000 species) are used in pharmaceutical and cosmetic products. However, the distribution of medicinal plants across the world is not uniform (5,6), and medicinal herbs are mainly collected from the wildlife population. Indeed, the demand for wildlife sources has increased by 8%-15% per year in Europe, North America and Asia in recent decades (7).

The term *medicinal plant* refers to a variety of plants that have medicinal properties. These plants are a rich source of compounds that can be used to develop drug synthesis (8). The parts of medicinal plants that may be used are different types of seeds, root, leaf, fruit, skin, flowers or even the whole plant. The active compounds in most parts of the medicinal plants have direct or indirect therapeutic effects and are used as medicinal agents. In the body of these plants, certain materials are produced and stored that are referred to as active compounds (substances), which have physiological effects on the living organisms (9). Human is mainly dependent on raw plant materials in order to meet medical needs to maintain health and cure diseases (10). Medicinal plants are used for treatment because they have certain properties, including synergistic actions. The constituents of the plant may interact with each other, and this interaction can be beneficial for both or adverse to either of them or eliminate the harmful effects of both. Plant-derived compounds can dramatically improve hard-to-treat illnesses, such as cancer. Plant components are also characterized by their ability to prevent the development of certain diseases. The toxicity and adverse effects of conventional and allopathic medicines have also been important factors in the sudden increase in population demands and increase in the number of herbal drug manufactures as well as a reduction in the use of chemical drugs (8).

Knowing the history of any science is effective in understanding and using that science. Hence, the historical significance of the past and present and future to medicinal herbs will continue to be addressed. In this perspective review, we have highlighted and discussed the history, current challenges, development and future outlook of using medicinal plants and their active compounds.

History of the use of medicinal herbs

Determining the exact time of using plants as drug is very difficult. Evidence indicates that plants have been cultivated as drugs approximately 60 000 years ago (11). Scripts about medicinal plants date back to almost 5000 years ago in India, China and Egypt, and at least 2500 years in Greece and Central Asia (12). Since ancient times, people have sought to cure their own illness using nature. As the use of animals was initially instinctive, such instinctive use was also applied to plants (13).

Given the fact that at that time there was insufficient information about the causes of the disease, useful plants for treating them, and the ways of using them for such purpose, everything was empirical. Over time, the reasons for the use of certain medicinal plants for treatment of certain diseases were discovered; consequently, the use of medicinal plants gradually rejected the empirical framework and was limited to the facts. The earliest written evidence of the use of medicinal plants for preparation of drugs has been found on a Sumerian clay slab from Nagpur dating back to nearly 5000 years ago (14). According to some inscriptions, Egyptians and Chinese who used plants as medicine since more than 27 centuries BC were among the earliest human beings who did so (15). Ancient Greek people were also familiar with the medicinal properties of some medicinal plants, and Hippocrates, the founder of Greek medicine and Aristotle, pupil of Hippocrates, used medicinal plants for the treatment of diseases. After that, Theophrastus, a Greek scientist, founded the *School of Medicinal Plants*. Then, Pedanius Dioscorides (He lived in the first century A.D), a physician and surgeon in the years 75-45 BC, wrote an encyclopedia, called *De Materia Medica*, to describe 600 therapeutic medicinal plants in the form of a series of scientific studies on medicinal plants (16-18).

History of medicinal plants in Iran

The results of Iranian historical studies have shown that the history of the use of medicinal herbs in Iran dates back to the time of Aryan civilization from about 6500 to 7000 BC when Zarathustra referred to the properties of medicinal plants in his writings. In Zoroastrianism in Iran, a plant called *Haoma* or Ephedra (Ephedra major host) was considered a sacred plant (Figure 1) (17). In Iran, the traditional science of medicine and pharmacy is the result of the integration of nation's prehistorical beliefs and traditions of the early inhabitants of Mesopotamia and then the Babylonians, Assyrians, Elamites and other ancient civilizations (19,20). Iranians have long enjoyed advanced knowledge about medicinal plants and their properties. The most prominent example of this argument is *Avesta*, the sacred book of Zoroastrianism. Many sections of *Dorandiyud*, one of the 5 books of the *Avesta*,

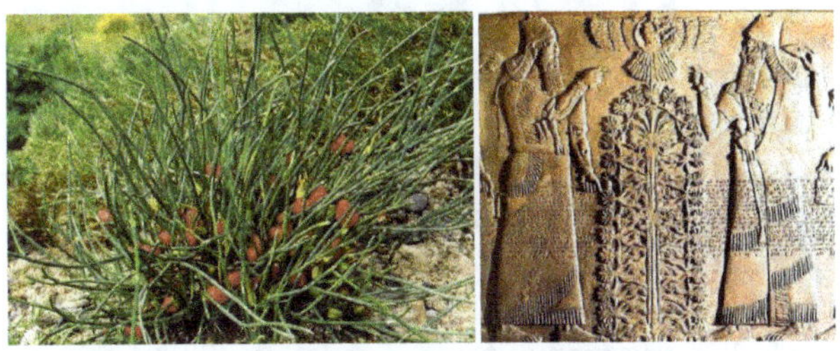

Figure 1. The holy plant called *Haoma* or Ephedra (Ephedra major host) in Zoroastrianism.

addresses phytotherapy, medicinal plants and their use (21). But unfortunately, in the Alexander Macedonian campaign, the famous library of Alexandria was deliberately destroyed in a fire. Thus, the botanical history of Iran lacked any long-standing evidence. Later, due to the destruction of the Castles of Ismailis and the burning of their libraries by Hulagu Khan, a Mongol ruler, the rest of the books of medicinal plants that had been collected by this sect were also destroyed. Then, in the eighth and ninth centuries, Iranian physicians, including Avicenna and Razi, made great progress in Persian medicine, evidenced by great works such as Avicenna's *Canon* and Razi's *al-Hawi.* In the 13th century, Ibn al-Baitar described the properties of over 1400 plants, which he personally knew, in his book (22).

Medicinal herbs and traditional medicine

The World Health Organization (WHO) defines traditional medicinal plants as natural plant materials which are used at least or in the absence industrial processing for the treatment of diseases at a local or regional scale (23). Traditional herbal medicine has been used in developing and developed countries for thousands of years because it is natural and causes comparatively fewer complications (24). Early medical history is consistent with the history of herbal medicine. The first books written about medicine were the first books written about plants, including the texts of the *Ebers Papyrus*, written 1500 BC, in which the names of many plants have been appeared (25). Different types of traditional drugs are widely used in Asia, Africa and Latin America to meet basic health needs. This use is growing rapidly in industrialized countries, which is often referred to as *complementary* or *alternative* medicine.

In the United States, the National Institutes of Health (NIH) uses the complementary and alternative medicine (CAM) to cover health systems, practices, and products are not presently considered to be part of conventional medicine. Across the world, among all the various traditional medical systems, traditional Chinese medicine (TCM) is currently the most popular, followed by Indian medicine. In Western countries, *Oriental Medicine* refers to Chinese, Japanese, and Korean medicines selected by immigrants from Korea, while "Asian medicine" often includes TCM, India (Ayurveda) and Tibetan medicine. Among all treatments in traditional medicine systems, medicinal plants are most frequently used (26).

Medicinal plants and conventional medicine

Today, according to the WHO, more than 80% of the world's population rely more often on traditional drugs, mainly plants, serving as the main source of health care (27). This figure includes not only a large population of China, India and all the developing countries of the world but also many advanced countries (28). Although diseases are currently being treated more often through medicines of synthetic origin and specifically developed in laboratories, and their definite effects in the treatment of diseases have contributed to the development of their use, the use of some medications leads to certain damages to the body. Therefore, the importance of medicinal plants and their products is increasingly recognized and the public confidence in their use is constantly strengthened (18).

Currently, the clinical, pharmaceutical and chemical studies of these traditional drugs, which are mainly derived from plants, are the basis of many early drugs such as Aspirin (from willow bark), Digoxin (from Foxglove), Morphine (from Opium poppy), Quinine (from Cinchona skin) and Pilocarpine (from Maranham Jaborandi). Currently, it is estimated that over 50% of the available drugs are somehow derived from medicinal plants (30,31). Phytotherapy is widely being used across the world on a constantly growing basis. Therefore, the global trend of synthetic compounds has turned to herbal drugs, which we can refer to it as a return to nature to prevent diseases and pains. Nature has been served as the source of medicinal herbs (32).

Drug discovery of natural compounds

Traditional processes

In traditional methods, plant materials are tested for pharmaceutical purposes. If any evidence of activity is observed, the extract is fractioned, and the active compound is isolated and identified. Each step of decomposition and isolation is usually guided by biological tests, which is referred to as bioassay-guided fractionation. Figure 2 illustrates a summary of a bioassay-guided drug discovery process. Sometimes, a direct product isolation method, regardless of bioactivity, is also used, which leads to the isolation of a number of natural compounds suitable for measuring any biological activity. However, this process can be slow and inefficient, and also does not guarantee isolation of lead compounds from screening would be in chemically successful or even recordable (33).

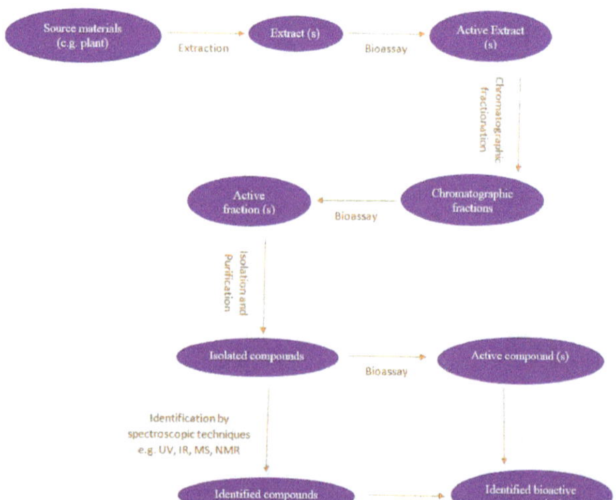

Figure 2. The traditional process of discovering natural drugs.

Modern processes of discovering natural drugs

The methods of discovering natural drugs by using modern processes including high-throughput screening (HTS) in which, using full and robotic automation, hundreds of molecules can be screened in several tests quickly and with small amounts of compounds. In order to integrate natural products into modern HTS programs, a library of natural compounds should be founded.

While in the past, the foundation of such a library was complex, time-consuming and challenging, the conditions have improved significantly with the advent of new and advanced technologies for the isolation and identification of natural products. The best result can be obtained from a library of fully naturally identified products that enables scientists to quickly isolate lead compound for faster progression of novel drug formulation, such as full or partial synthesis, *in vivo* experiments and clinical trials (Figure 3) (33).

Medicinal herbs in the future

Medicinal herbs have a hopeful future since there are about half a million plants around the world, most of them have not yet been studied in medical practice, and current and future studies on medical activities can be effective in treating diseases (34). The use of medicinal plants has a long history; however, the use of the whole plant or raw materials for treatment or experimentation has many drawbacks, including changes in the plant's compounds in different climates, simultaneous development of synergistic compounds that lead to adverse effects of antagonists, or other unexpected changes in bioactivity, and changes or loss of bioactivity due to the variability and accumulation, storage and preparation of raw materials; therefore, advancing towards the isolation of compounds and the use of pure substances with bioactivity, instead of the plant benefits, has certain benefits including convenient examination of therapeutic effects and determination of toxic doses to control the quality of the therapeutic formulation (35). The beginning of the development of herbal medicines was concurrent with the development of chemistry and isolation, purification, and determination of plant compounds (36).

In the past, the drug discovery of the biological compounds from plant materials and the process of identifying the structures of active compounds from the extracts were problematic depending on the complexity of the compounds and might take weeks, months or even years. Nowadays, the rate of bioassay-guided fractionation has been significantly enhanced by the development of precision instruments such as high-performance liquid chromatography (HPLC/MS), liquid chromatography-mass spectrometry (LC/MS), magnetic field and nuclear magnetic resonance (NMR) is a recent major breakthrough for the categorization (NMR) is a recent major breakthrough for the categorization of compounds that are extremely limited in quantity in their organisms of origin (37). Despite the success of research to produce medicinal plants over the past few decades, future efforts face many challenges. The quality of the herbal product has been studied. Standardization of raw materials is an important issue for the plant industry (38).

Herbaceous plants can be easily infected during growth, processing and collection. Contamination and pollution with heavy metals are two main problems with herbal drugs. It is therefore necessary to improve the quality and quantity of bioactive compounds for the production of herbal drugs while making effort to discover more new herbal drugs (39). Due to expanding the use of natural substances around the world, the quality and safety of plant-derived medicines should be comprehensively and accurately studied issues and the traditional and the millennial beliefs about these issues cannot be surely

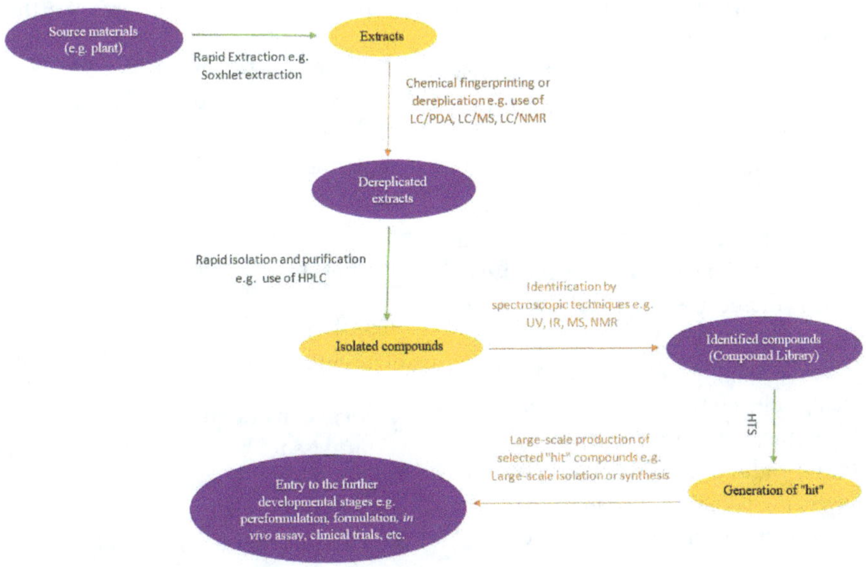

Figure 3. The modern process of discovering natural drugs.

trusted; therefore, scientific and enlightening studies are essential to obtain reliable information for the use of medicinal plants in health care (40).

On the other hand, one of the challenges facing medicinal plants is the loss of medicinal plant species due to the non-principled use of these resources. According to the International Union for Conservation of Nature, there are between 50 000 and 80 000 flowering plant species that are used for pharmaceutical purposes around the world. Among these numbers, about 15 000 species are exposed to a risk of extinction due to high harvesting and destruction of habitats (41) and 20% of their wildlife resources are decreasing due to growing human populations and excessive consumption of plants (42). Therefore, the environmental code of ethics that preserves biodiversity in the processes of exploiting natural resources to discover natural drugs should be considered (43). Good agricultural practice (GAP) for medicinal plants are planned to regulate production and ensure quality and facilitate the standardization of herbal drugs (44). GAP is an approach that uses high-quality, safe and non-contaminated (raw drugs) herbal medicines to help solve various problems (45). GAP includes comprehensive items such as environmental ecology, production locations, germplasm, cultivation, collection and quality aspects of pesticide detection, macroscopic or microscopic validation, chemical identification of active compounds, and checking of metal elements (46). Many countries seriously implement and promote the GAP. For example, in China, GAP has promoted the growth of conventional medicinal plants in areas where these plants are traditionally cultivated (47).

Although many people nowadays use herbal medicines as a constituent of primary health care, there are still many concerns about the safety and efficacy of using plants. While herbal medicines can potentially contribute to the advancement of healthcare, many major challenges need to be addressed before effective adherence of herbal medicines to traditional medicine. The lack of accurate translation and interpretation of the texts and research findings on plants by scientists around the world is one of the main challenges in this field. In fact, to realize the effective integration of plants into a medical system, researchers and practitioners should be trained in both modern and traditional medicine in the use of plant compounds. In addition, to build credibility for the use of plants in conventional medicine, the empirical arguments should be converted into evidence-based arguments. Finally, several questions about safety, accurate dose, duration of treatment, side effects, acute and chronic toxicities as well as the standardization of herbal medicines and natural products should be answered. If these issues are resolved, medicinal plants can be used as a safe, effective, and affordable form of health care.

Conclusion and future outlook

Undoubtedly, the demand for plant-derived products has increased across the world. In the Middle East, Latin America, Africa and Asia more than 85 percent of the populations predominantly rely on traditional medicine, especially on herbal medicines, for their health care needs. About 100 million people in the European Union and in some countries as high as 90% of the population, still use traditional, complementary or herbal medicines. The herbal medicine has an increasing big market. In 2012, the whole sales of Chinese herbal medicines reached more than US$83 billion which was 20% more than the market in 2011. It has been suggested that the whole market for all herbal supplements will reach more than US$115 billion by 2020, which in Asia-Pacific is the fastest and in Europe is the largest growing markets. These demands are predominantly driven by women subjects by growing emphasis on concerns on the adverse effects of synthetic drugs. Therefore, investing in human resource training can be the main source of research development in order to move from production to the production of crops. The importance of research in the field of medicinal plants is felt more than ever. Some medicinal plants are the sources of adjuvant therapy in the health systems worldwide, not only to treat diseases but also to prevent them and maintain health. Despite the extensive experiences in use of medicinal plants in traditional medicine, scientific study and identification of active plant compounds and their effects can lead to the discovery of new therapeutic benefits and the production of nature-based products in the future. To achieve this purpose, extensive research is fundamentally important to control the quality of raw drugs and the formulation to justify their use in the modern medicine system; subsequently, animal studies and clinical trials are required to use the benefits of these plants. In addition, in the development of medicine from medicinal plants, among other things, a practical plan should be developed to preserve these resources.

Authors' contributions

ZL contributed to design of the study, supervised the research and manuscript editing, HA helped the preparation of the manuscript. FJ performed the searching, data collection and prepare manuscript drafting. All authors read and confirmed the final version of the manuscript for publication.

Conflict of interests

The authors declare no conflict of interest.

Ethical considerations

Ethical issues have been observed by the authors.

Funding/Support

This research was financially supported by Shahrekord

University of Medical Sciences, Shahrekord, Iran (Grant No. 1874). Authors are so thankful to research council of Shahrekord University of Medical Sciences.

References

1. Firenzuoli F, Gori L. Herbal medicine today: clinical and research issues. Evid Based Complement Alternat Med. 2007;4(Suppl 1):37-40. doi: 10.1093/ecam/nem096.
2. Singh JS. The biodiversity crisis: A multifaceted review. Curr Sci. 2002;82(6):638-47.
3. Hamilton AC. Medicinal plants, conservation and livelihoods. Biodivers Conserv. 2004;13(8):1477-517. doi: 10.1023/b:bioc.0000021333.23413.42.
4. Halberstein RA. Medicinal plants: historical and cross-cultural usage patterns. Ann Epidemiol. 2005;15(9):686-99. doi: 10.1016/j.annepidem.2005.02.004.
5. Huang H. Plant diversity and conservation in China: planning a strategic bioresource for a sustainable future. Bot J Linn Soc. 2011;166(3):282-300.
6. Rafieian-Kopaei M. Medicinal plants and the human needs. J HerbMed Pharmacol. 2012;1(1):1-2.
7. Verma S, Singh SP. Current and future status of herbal medicines. Vet World. 2008;1(11):347-50. doi: 10.5455/vetworld.2008.347-350.
8. Rasool Hassan BA. Medicinal plants (importance and uses). Pharmaceut Anal Acta. 2012;3:e139. doi: 10.4172/2153-2435.1000e139.
9. Phillipson JD. Phytochemistry and medicinal plants. Phytochemistry. 2001;56(3):237-43.
10. Jack DB. One hundred years of aspirin. Lancet. 1997;350(9075):437-9. doi: 10.1016/s0140-6736(97)07087-6.
11. Solecki R, Shanidar IV. a Neanderthal flower burial in Northern Iraq. Science. 1975; 190(4217):880-1. doi: 10.1126/science.190.4217.880.
12. Ang-Lee MK, Moss J, Yuan CS. Herbal medicines and perioperative care. JAMA. 2001;286(2):208-16.
13. Stojanoski N. Development of health culture in Veles and its region from the past to the end of the 20th century. Veles: Society of science and art. 1999:13-34.
14. Qiu J. Traditional medicine: a culture in the balance. Nature. 2007;448(7150):126-8.doi:10.1038/448126a.
15. Schippmann UW, Leaman D, Cunningham AB. A comparison of cultivation and wild collection of medicinal and aromatic plants under sustainability aspects. Frontis. 2006;17:75-95.
16. Lindberg Madsen H, Bertelsen G. Spices as antioxidants. Trends Food Sci Technol. 1995;6(8):271-7. doi: 10.1016/S0924-2244(00)89112-8.
17. Rios JL, Recio MC. Medicinal plants and antimicrobial activity. J Ethnopharmacol. 2005;100(1-2):80-4. doi: 10.1016/j.jep.2005.04.025.
18. Zargari A. Medicinal Plants. Tehran University Press; 1992: 889.
19. Elgood C. A medical history of Persia and the Eastern Caliphate: From the earliest times until the year AD 1932. Cambridge University Press; 2010.
20. Levey M. Early Arabic Pharmacology: An Introduction Based on Ancient and Medieval Sources. Brill Archive; 1973.
21. Malandra WW. An introduction to ancient Iranian religion: Readings from the Avesta and Achaemenid inscriptions. U of Minnesota Press; 1983.
22. Gurib-Fakim A. Medicinal plants: traditions of yesterday and drugs of tomorrow. Mol Aspects Med. 2006;27(1):1-93. doi: 10.1016/j.mam.2005.07.008.
23. Tilburt JC, Kaptchuk TJ. Herbal medicine research and global health: an ethical analysis. Bull World Health Organ. 2008;86(8):594-9.
24. Wichtl M. Herbal drugs and phytopharmaceuticals: a handbook for practice on a scientific basis. Boca Raton: CRC press; 2004.
25. Ackerknecht EH. Therapeautics, from the primitives to the 20th century. New York: Hafner Press; 1973.
26. Liu WJH. Traditional Herbal Medicine Research Methods: Identification, Analysis, Bioassay, and Pharmaceutical and Clinical Studies. John Wiley Sons Inc; 2011. 477.
27. Farnsworth NR, Akerele O, Bingel AS, Soejarto DD, Guo Z. Medicinal plants in therapy. Bull World Health Organ. 1985;63(6):965-81.
28. Ganesan A. The impact of natural products upon modern drug discovery. Curr Opin Chem Biol. 2008;12(3):306-17. doi: 10.1016/j.cbpa.2008.03.016.
29. Butler MS. The role of natural product chemistry in drug discovery. J Nat Prod. 2004;67(12):2141-53. doi: 10.1021/np040106y.
30. Yarnell E, Abascal K. Dilemmas of traditional botanical research. Herbal Gram. 2002;55:46-54.
31. Harvey AL. Natural products in drug discovery. Drug Discov Today. 2008;13(19-20):894-901. doi: 10.1016/j.drudis.2008.07.004.
32. Fabricant DS, Farnsworth NR. The value of plants used in traditional medicine for drug discovery. Environ Health Perspect. 2001;109 Suppl 1:69-75.
33. Sarker SD, Nahar L. Chemistry for Pharmacy Students: General, Organic, and Natural Product Chemistry. John Wiley Sons Inc; 2013:1-383.
34. Singh R. Medicinal plants: A review. J Plant Sci. 2015;3(1-1):50-5. doi: 10.11648/j.jps.s.2015030101.18.
35. Zhang H. Bioactive Natural Products: Detection, Isolation, and Structural Determination. Phytomedicine. 2011;18(10):902-3.
36. Shakya AK, Sharma N, Saxena M, Shrivastava S, Shukla S. Evaluation of the antioxidant and hepatoprotective effect of Majoon-e-Dabeed-ul-ward against carbon tetrachloride induced liver injury. Exp Toxicol Pathol. 2012;64(7-8):767-73. doi: 10.1016/j.etp.2011.01.014.
37. Schroeder FC, Gronquist M. Extending the scope of NMR spectroscopy with microcoil probes. Angew Chem Int Ed Engl. 2006;45(43):7122-31. doi: 10.1002/anie.200601789.
38. Yadav M, Chatterji S, Gupta SK, Watal G. Preliminary phytochemical screening of six medicinal plants used in traditional medicine. Int J Pharm Pharm Sci. 2014;6(5):539-42.
39. Clark AM. Natural Products as a Resource for New Drugs. Pharmaceutical Research. 1996;13(8):1133-41. doi: 10.1023/a:1016091631721.
40. Firenzuoli F, Gori L. Herbal medicine today: clinical and research issues. Evid Based Complement Alternat Med. 2007;4(Suppl 1):37-40. doi: 10.1093/ecam/nem096.
41. Bentley RE. Medicinal Plants. London: Domville-Fife Press;

2010:23-46.
42. Ross IA. Constituents, Medicinal Plants of the World (volume 3): Chemical Traditional and Modern Medicinal Uses. Humana, New Jersey: Humana Press; 2005;110-30.
43. Pan SY, Zhou SF, Gao SH, Yu ZL, Zhang SF, Tang MK, et al. New Perspectives on How to Discover Drugs from Herbal Medicines: CAM's Outstanding Contribution to Modern Therapeutics. Evid Based Complement Alternat Med. 2013;2013:627375. doi: 10.1155/2013/627375.
44. Chan K, Shaw D, Simmonds MS, Leon CJ, Xu Q, Lu A, et al. Good practice in reviewing and publishing studies on herbal medicine, with special emphasis on traditional Chinese medicine and Chinese materia medica. J Ethnopharmacol. 2012;140(3):469-75. doi: 10.1016/j.jep.2012.01.038.
45. Muchugi A, Muluvi GM, Kindt R, Kadu CA, Simons AJ, Jamnadass RH. Genetic structuring of important medicinal species of genus Warburgia as revealed by AFLP analysis. Tree Genetics Genomes. 2008;4(4):787-95. doi: 10.1007/s11295-008-0151-3.
46. Makunga NP, Philander LE, Smith M. Current perspectives on an emerging formal natural products sector in South Africa. J Ethnopharmacol. 2008;119(3):365-75. doi: 10.1016/j.jep.2008.07.020.
47. Ma J, Rong K, Cheng K. Research and practice on biodiversity in situ conservation in China: progress and prospect. Biodiversity Science. 2012;20(5):551-8. doi: 10.3724/sp.j.1003.2012.08118.

Therapeutic effect of *Melissa officinalis* in an amyloid-β rat model of Alzheimer's disease

Siamak Beheshti*, Bahareh Shahmoradi

Department of Biology, Faculty of Sciences, University of Isfahan, Isfahan, Iran

ARTICLE INFO

Keywords:
Alzheimer's disease
Memory
Melissa officinalis
Amyloid-β
Passive avoidance task

ABSTRACT

Introduction: Medicinal herbs have several components with different pharmacological effects. It has been described that *Melissa officinalis* is able to improve memory in different models of learning. Nevertheless, its influence has not been studied in animal models of AD. Here, we studied the potential therapeutic effect of *M. officinalis* in intracerebroventricular (i.c.v) amyloid-β (Aβ) model of Alzheimer's disease (AD).
Methods: Male Wistar rats weighing 260-330 g received the hydro-alcoholic extract of *M. officinalis* (50, 100, 200, 400 mg/kg; P.O), chronically for 30 consecutive days. The control group received solvent of the drug. Memory retrieval was assessed, using the passive avoidance task. Three groups of the rats received Aβ (1-42; 10 μg/rat bilaterally; i.c.v). One group received DMSO 1% (2 μL/rat; i.c.v). Twenty days later memory retrieval was assessed. The Aβ-treated rats, received *M. officinalis* (50, 100 mg/kg; P.O) or saline (1 mL/kg; P.O), chronically for 30 consecutive days. The DMSO 1%-treated rats received saline (1 mL/kg; P.O).
Results: The hydro-alcoholic extract of *M. officinalis* (50, 100, 200, 400 mg/kg; P.O) did not have a significant effect on step-through latency (STL). Aβ impaired memory retrieval by decreasing STL and increasing the time spent in the dark compartment (TDC). *M. officinalis* (50, 100 mg/kg; P.O) improved memory retrieval in AD rats by increasing STL and decreasing TDC, significantly.
Conclusion: The outcomes of the study show that *M. officinalis* has a therapeutic effect in the Aβ model of AD. It seems that the extracts of *M. officinalis* can be suggested as a powerful therapeutic herb for AD patients.

Implication for health policy/practice/research/medical education:
Melissa officinalis has the potential to improve memory deficiency and might be advantageous in patients with Alzheimer's disease.

Introduction

Alzheimer's disease (AD) is an enduring, progressive and irreversible neurodegenerative syndrome and is the central cause of dementia in later life. Two neuropathological features of AD are neuritic plaques and neurofibrillary tangles which are respectively related to the buildup of the amyloid-beta peptide (Aβ) in the brain, and to cytoskeletal alterations that appear due to the hyper-phosphorylation of tau protein in neurons. Aβ-peptide has a crucial impact to the pathogenesis of AD (1). Based on the amyloid theory, accretion of Aβ in the brain is the major impact driving AD pathogenesis. Other aspect of the disease progression, including creation of neurofibrillary tangles comprising tau protein, is suggested to result from an inequality between Aβ production and Aβ clearance. Aβ deposit leads to oxidative stress, mitochondrial abnormalities and depletion of cellular ATP, elevated intracellular calcium and excitotoxicity and induction of inflammatory responses. All these mechanisms result in synaptic dysfunction and cause neuronal loss through activation of apoptotic and necrotic cell death pathways (2). Intracerebroventricular (i.c.v) injection of Aβ molecules leads to the buildup of Aβ plaques in the brain tissue, oxidative stress and neurotoxicity, which results in impairment of memory characteristic of the AD (3). It has been commonly used as an animal model of AD (4-6). The step-through passive

***Corresponding author**: Siamak Beheshti,
Email: s.beheshti@sci.ui.ac.ir

avoidance paradigm is a learning task that has been widely utilized to assess the involvement of various treatments in learning and memory (7).

Treatment of AD is a great clinical challenge. Despite all the advances in this field, there is not a complete curative strategy for patients with AD. Due to the multifaceted pathology of AD, novel therapeutic strategies aim to stop disease progress through different pathways (8). Medicinal herbs have numerous constituents with diverse pharmacological properties and may be effective in complex diseases like AD. Hence, several studies have been considered to evaluated therapeutic effects of herbal medicines in AD therapy (9). *Melissa officinalis* is a medicinal herb from Lamiaceae family. It has been consumed as a medicinal plant for more than 2000 years (10). It has putative anti-inflammatory, antioxidant, neuro-protective, binding capacity to cholinergic receptors and anti-cholinesterase activity. It is suggested to be effective in the hindrance of various neurological diseases accompanied with oxidative stress (11) and has the potential to provide a natural treatment for AD (12). Acute injection of *M. officinalis* modulated mood and memory performance in healthy young individuals. Meanwhile, no side effects or toxicities have been described with its use (13).

Melissa officinalis is traditionally used to improve memory, however, there are not any reports assessing its effect in animal models of AD. Due to the central role of Aβ in AD pathogenesis, here we investigated the potential therapeutic activity of chronic injections of the hydro-alcoholic extract of *M. officinalis* in the Aβ rat model of AD.

Materials and Methods

Chemicals

Ketamine and xylazine were purchased from Alfasan (the Netherland). Aβ (1-42) was purchased from Sigma (USA) and dissolved in DMSO 1%. Dried leaves of *M. officinalis* were a gift from Iraninoosh Company which gathered it from Kamfiruz, Fars province, Iran in 2014.

Animals

Adult male Wistar rats (260–330 g) were obtained from the breeding colony of Department of Biology, University of Isfahan. Rats were kept four per cage in a temperature (24±1°C) well-ordered room that was upheld on a 12:12 light cycle (light on at 07:00 AM). The rats had unrestricted access to food and water. After the surgery for cannula embedding, the rats were housed alone in standard cages. All experiments were performed in agreement with the guide for the care and use of laboratory animals (USA National Institute of Health publication No. 80-23, revised 1996) and were approved by the graduate studies committee of the Department of Biology, University of Isfahan.

Preparation of the hydro-alcoholic extract of *Melissa officinalis*

One hundred grams of dried leaves of *M. officinalis* were pulverized, using a mixing instrument (Molineux, France), then were soaked in 400 mL of 96% ethanol, while mixing in a stirrer. The solution was filtered and put in a dark glass after 24 hours. The remaining crude was again soaked in 400 mL of 70% ethanol for 24 hours. The solution was again filtered and mixed with the previous solution. The extract was then concentrated in a rotary evaporator and dried in an oven in 40°C for 72 hours. The resulting extract was dissolved in saline to a final concentration of 100 mg/mL. The animals received the extract through gavage.

Surgical procedures

Rats were anesthetized with a combination of ketamine (100 mg/kg, i.p) and xylazine (10 mg/kg, i.p) and were bilaterally embedded with guide cannula (22-gauge) targeted at site 1 mm dorsal to the lateral ventricles (anterior-posterior: −0.9 mm from bregma, midline: ±1.4 mm from midline, and dorsal-ventral: −2.5 mm from dura) based on the atlas of Paxinos and Watson (14). A screw was implanted into the skull and cannulas were fixed to it with dental cement. The cannulas were locked with stainless steel stylets smeared with mineral oil to avoid clogging with blood.

Microinjection procedure

Intracerebroventricular injections were done via guide cannula with needles (27-gauge) that were joined by polyethylene tubing (PE20, Stoelting) to a 2 μL Hamilton micro syringe. The injections (2 μL total volume) were conveyed over 4 minutes bilaterally (1 μL each side), and the injection needles (extending 1mm from the end of the guide cannula) were left in place an extra minute, then they were slowly withdrawn.

Passive avoidance task

The step-through passive avoidance task was executed to evaluate memory performance, as formerly described (15). Briefly, each rat was positioned in the white compartment of the PAT apparatus facing the sliding door. After 5 seconds the door was elevated. When the animal walked into the dark compartment with all four paws, the door was closed and the rat stayed there for 20 seconds. Then the animal was removed to be sited in a temporary cage. 30 minutes later, the rat was again positioned in the white compartment for 5 seconds, then the door was elevated to let the animal enter the dark compartment and after entrance, the door was shut, but this time a controlled electrical shock of 0.3 mA lasting for 1 second was delivered. After 20 seconds, the rat was sited into the temporary cage. Two minutes later, the same testing process was reiterated. When the rat stayed in the white compartment for a 2-minute times period, the training was ended. On the second day, a retrieval test was done to assess long-term memory. Each animal was positioned in the white start compartment for 20 seconds, then the door was elevated and the step-through latency (STL) and the time spent in the dark compartment (TDC), were recorded, up to 600 seconds.

Experiment 1

Eight rats were used in each experimental group. In this experiment, the effect of chronic injection of different doses of the hydro-alcoholic extract of *M. officinalis* was assessed on memory performance. Five groups of animals received the hydro-alcoholic extract of *M. officinalis* (50, 100, 200 and 400 mg/kg; P.O) or Saline (1 mL/kg; P.O) for 30 consecutive days. Memory retrieval was assessed using a passive avoidance paradigm.

Experiment 2

In this experiment, the effect of i.c.v administration of Aβ was assessed on memory performance in rats. One group of animals received Aβ (10 μg/rat), bilaterally. The dose of Aβ was selected according to previous reports (16). The control group received DMSO 1%. Twenty days following the injection, memory retrieval was evaluated.

Experiment 3

In this experiment, the effect of the hydro-alcoholic extract of *M. officinalis* was assessed on memory performance in Aβ-treated rats. The animals were allocated into four groups. Group 1 received DMSO 1% (2 μL/rat; i.c.v). Groups 2, 3 and 4 received Aβ (10 μg/rat; i.c.v), bilaterally. Twenty days later, memory performance was assessed. Afterwards, groups 1 and 2 received saline (1 mL/kg; P.O) for 30 consecutive days. Groups 3 and 4 received the hydro-alcoholic extract of *M. officinalis* (50 or 100 mg/kg; P.O), respectively for 30 consecutive days. Memory performance was assessed again after completion of the treatment regimen (Figure 1).

Statistical analysis

One-way analysis of variance (ANOVA) followed by Tukey-Kramer multiple comparison post-hoc test, unpaired or paired *t* tests were performed using GraphPad Prism version 5.04 for Windows. In all experiments, differences were considered statistically significant at the level of $P < 0.05$. The data are presented as mean ± standard error of the mean (SEM).

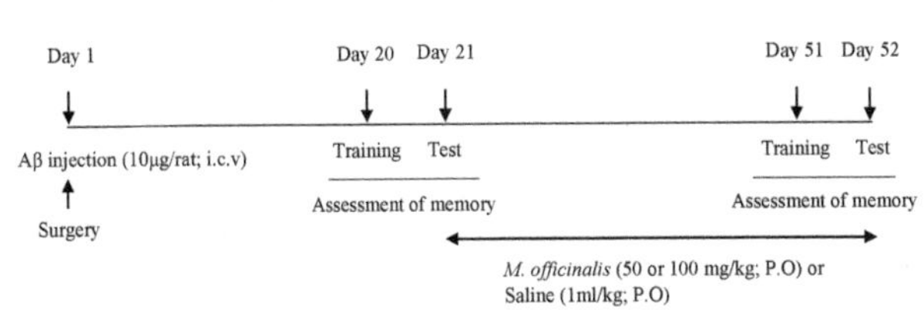

Figure 1. Diagram illustrating experimental design.

Results

Verification of cannulas placements

At the end of the experiments, each animal was euthanized with an overdose of chloroform. The brain was removed and fixed in a 10% formalin solution and sectioned 5 days later. Sections were inspected to determine the site of the cannulas targeted for the lateral ventricles. The cannula placements were confirmed using the atlas of Paxinos and Watson (14). Data from the animals with the injection sites placed outside the lateral ventricles were not used for the analysis.

The effect of the hydro-alcoholic extract of *Melissa officinalis* on memory retrieval

In the passive avoidance task, the decrease in STL and the increase in TDC indicate loss of fear memory. One-way ANOVA showed that the hydro-alcoholic extract of *M. officinalis* (50, 100, 200 and 400 mg/kg) did not have a significant effect on STL ($P > 0.05$; Figure 2).

The effect of Aβ on memory retrieval

Intracerebroventricular injection of Aβ impaired memory retrieval by decreasing STL and increasing TDC, significantly compared with the control group (Figure 3; $P < 0.05$).

The effect of the hydro-alcoholic extract of *Melissa officinalis* on memory retrieval in rats treated with Aβ

One-way ANOVA indicated a significant main effect of STL following chronic i.c.v injections of the hydro-alcoholic extract of *M. officinalis* in the Aβ-treated rats ($F[3, 31] = 5.21$; $P = 0.005$). Post hoc comparison showed that *M. officinalis* (50 and 100 mg/kg; P.O) significantly increased STL as compared to the group received Aβ-saline (Table 1; $P < 0.05$). Data analysis of this experiment

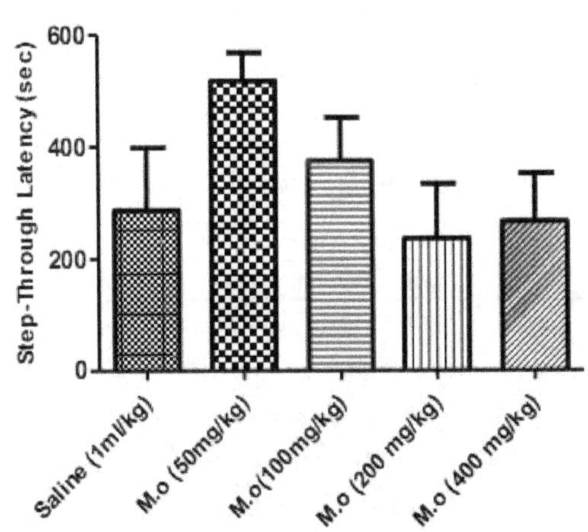

Figure 2. The effect of the hydro-alcoholic extract of *Melissa officinalis* on step-through latency (STL). Data are shown as means ±SEM and were analyzed by ANOVA.

also revealed main effect of TDC ($F [3, 31] = 4.30$; $P = 0.01$). Post hoc comparisons showed that *M. officinalis* (50 mg/kg; P.O), significantly decreased TDC in the Aβ-treated rats as compared to the group received Aβ-saline (Table 2; $P < 0.05$). Post-hoc comparisons also revealed that *M. officinalis* (100 mg/kg; P.O), significantly reduced TDC in the Aβ-treated rats as compared to the group received Aβ-saline (Table 2; $P < 0.01$).

Discussion

The main finding of the current study was that chronic consumption of the hydro-alcoholic extract of *M. officinalis* has a therapeutic effect in rats with AD induced by i.c.v injections of Aβ. In AD there is a gradual loss of cholinergic neurons in basal forebrain which has been suggested to cause the cognitive deficits observed in patients with AD (17). Drugs used for AD treatment are acetylcholinesterase inhibitors, which can improve cognitive impairment but cannot prevent disease progression (18). *M. officinalis* has a variety of components, of which the most important are phenolic compounds, rosmarinic acid, caffeic acid, cholinergic acid, metrilic acid; flavonoids such as luteolin, apigenin and monoterpene derivatives; the sesquiterpenes including beta-caryophyllene and germacrene; triterpenes such as oleanolic and ursolic acid; volatile oil, and tannins (19). Some of these compounds have binding capacity to nicotinic and muscarinic acetylcholine receptors and also inhibit the effects of acetylcholinesterase enzyme (20-22). Thus, by regulating the cholinergic system it might be helpful in Alzheimer's treatment and adjusting mood and cognitive processes. In *M. officinalis* extract the affinity for acetylcholine nicotinic receptor is more than muscarinic receptor (23). It was reported that nicotinic receptor stimulation, may be able to protect neurons from degeneration induced by Aβ and may have effects that stand the progress of AD.

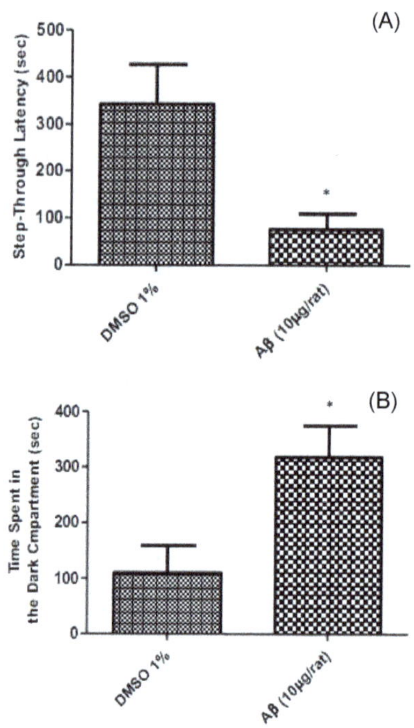

Figure 3. The effect of bilateral injection of Aβ (10 µg/rat; i.c.v) on (A) step-through latency (STL) and (B) TDC (the time spent in the dark compartment). Data are shown as means ± SEM and were analyzed by un-paired *t* test. $*P < 0.05$.

Oxidative stress is the mechanism that was assumed for Aβ toxicity and Alzheimer's etiology (24). Aβ is accumulated and creates more free radicals in the presence of free radicals. In this regard, *M. officinalis* total extract could attenuate the Aβ-induced toxicity and oxidative stress (22). Direct free radical scavenging activity has been reported for *M. officinalis*. The total extract could defend PC12 cells against hydrogen peroxide-induced cell death and oxidative stress (25). Antioxidants can ameliorate disease progression (26), so it is supposed that antioxidant activity of *M. officinalis* may have contributed to neuro-protective effect against Aβ toxicity.

Different biological activities have been designated for the major polyphenol component of *M. officinalis*, rosmarinic acid, including anti-oxidative and anti-inflammatory activities (27). Rosmarinic acid could protect against Aβ-induced memory impairment in mice, due to the direct

Table 1. The effect of *Melissa officinalis* on step-through latency (STL) in Aβ-treated rats

	21 days after surgery	52 days after surgery
	Aβ treatment of rats (single injection)	***M. officinalis* treatment of rats (30 days) treated with Aβ**
Group 1	DMSO 1% (2 µL/rat; i.c.v)	Saline (1 mL/kg; P.O)
	274±79.00	400±97.00
Group 2	Aβ (10 µg/rat; i.c.v)	Saline (1 mL/kg; P.O)
	51.28±15.00	66.50±20
Group 3	Aβ (10 µg/rat; i.c.v)	*M. officinalis* (50 mg/kg; P.O)
	76.33±29.41	365.70±93.23*
Group 4	Aβ (10 µg/rat; i.c.v)	*M. officinalis* (100 mg/kg; P.O)
	60.63±20.29	309.00±63.97*

Data are shown as means ± SEM and were analyzed by paired *t* test. $* P<0.05$.

Table 2. The effect of *Melissa officinalis* on TDC (the time spent in the dark compartment) in Aβ-treated rats

	21 days after surgery	52 days after surgery
	Aβ treatment of rats (single injection)	***M. officinalis* treatment of rats (30 days) treated with Aβ**
Group 1	DMSO 1% (2 μL/rat; i.c.v)	Saline (1 mL/kg; P.O)
	86.43±25.10	95±15.00
Group 2	Aβ (10 μg/rat; i.c.v)	Saline (1 mL/kg; P.O)
	231.10±40.00	250±49.00
Group 3	Aβ (10 μg/rat; i.c.v)	*M. officinalis* (50 mg/kg; P.O)
	228.40±38.16	79.56±40.90*
Group 4	Aβ (10 μg/rat; i.c.v)	*M. officinalis* (100 mg/kg; P.O)
	291.70±59.91	8.71± 2.63**

Data are shown as means ± SEM and were analyzed by paired *t* test. * $P<0.05$.

peroxynitrite scavenging activity (28). Rosmarinic acid protected mice against impairment of memory induced by i.c.v injection of Aβ (28). It could also lower Aβ depositions in ovariectomized rats and improve short-term spatial memory (29).

The caffeic acid and the ursolic acid found in *M. officinalis* were reported to have neuro-protective effects. Ursolic acid is a triterpenoid with hydroxyl radical scavenging activity and it augmented the activities of antioxidant enzymes like superoxide dismutase, catalase and glutathione peroxidase (30). Caffeic acid improved Aβ-induced cognitive damage through inhibition of lipid peroxidation and NO production (31). Caffeic acid also exerted neuro-protective and anti-dementia effects by preventing the loss of neural cells and synapses in mice ischemic brain injury (32).

Another active component of *M. officinalis*, luteolin could improve Aβ-induced memory deficiency and increased the activity of choline acetyl transferase, superoxide dismutase and glutathione peroxidase in hippocampal tissue. Luteolin also inverted the augmented activity of acetylcholine esterase. In hippocampi homogenate, the amount of acetylcholine augmented, but malondialdehyde reduced. Moreover, luteolin could raise Bcl-2/Bax ratio. Luteolin could protect AD rats against Aβ-induced memory deficiency through regulating the cholinergic system and inhibiting oxidative damages (33). Luteolin also improved learning and memory in Aβ-induced cognition damage in rats by activating the anti-oxidation system (34). Luteolin reduced the impairment of passive avoidance memory induced by scopolamine by increasing the activities of the brain muscarinic and nicotinic receptors (35).

Apigenin, another component of *M. officinalis*, attenuated cognitive deterioration in diabetic rats via suppressing oxidative stress, nitric oxide and apoptotic cascades synthase pathway (36). Oral administration of apigenin for three month rescued learning deficits and improved memory retention in APP/PS1 double transgenic AD mice. Apigenin also affected APP processing and prevented Aβ load, the relief of Aβ deposition, and the decrease of insoluble Aβ levels. Moreover, apigenin showed superoxide anion scavenging effects and enhanced antioxidative enzyme activity of superoxide dismutase and glutathione peroxidase (37).

Oral administration of β-Caryophyllene, another compound found in *M. officinalis* prohibited cognitive deficiency in APP/PS1 mice, and this positive cognitive effect was concomitant with reduced β-amyloid load in the hippocampus and the cerebral cortex. Moreover, β-caryophyllene reduced astrogliosis and microglial activation and the levels of cyclooxygenase-2 protein and the mRNA levels of the tumor necrosis factor-α and interleukin-1β in the cerebral cortex (38).

Due to the above mentioned beneficial effects of the components of *M. officinalis* on improvement of memory, oxidative stress, inflammatory conditions, neuro-protection, anti-cholinesterase activities and Aβ clearance, it seems that *M. officinalis* can be suggested as a powerful therapeutic herb for AD patients.

In accordance with our results, *M. officinalis* enhanced spatial memory in the Morris water maze in streptozotocin-induced memory impairment in rats and reduced amyloid plaques (39). Also, in a clinical trial it could improve disease signs in patients with mild to moderate AD (40). Based on the outcomes of the current study and these studies, it appears that *M. officinalis* have components with a great potential to treat AD.

Conclusion

As a conclusion, the outcomes of the current study indicated potential therapeutic effects of the hydro-alcoholic extract of *M. officinalis* in the i.c.v Aβ model of AD. The anti-inflammatory, anti-oxidant, neuro-protective and anti-cholinesterase activities of the extract are proposed to be involved in the observed results. Further studies are requisite to clarify the mechanisms of this activity and identify the responsible components of the extract.

Acknowledgments

The authors would like to thank Iraninoosh Company, for donating *M. officinalis* dried leaves.

Authors' contributions

SB contributed to the conception and design of the work, drafting and revising the draft, approval of the final version of the manuscript, and agreed for all aspects of the work. BS contributed to conducting the study.

Conflict of interests

Authors declare no conflict of interests.

Ethical considerations

Ethical issues (including plagiarism, misconduct, data fabrication, falsification, double publication or submission, redundancy) have been completely observed by the authors.

Funding/Support

Supports from the Vice-chancellorships for Research and Technology, University of Isfahan (grant No: 13525/93) are acknowledged.

References

1. Walsh DM, Selkoe DJ. A beta oligomers - a decade of discovery. J Neurochem. 2007;101(5):1172-84. doi: 10.1111/j.1471-4159.2006.04426.x.
2. Hardy J, Selkoe DJ. The amyloid hypothesis of Alzheimer's disease: progress and problems on the road to therapeutics. Science. 2002;297(5580):353-6. doi: 10.1126/science.1072994.
3. Butterfield DA. Amyloid beta-peptide (1-42)-induced oxidative stress and neurotoxicity: implications for neurodegeneration in Alzheimer's disease brain. A review. Free Radic Res. 2002;36(12):1307-13.
4. Caughlin S, Hepburn JD, Park DH, Jurcic K, Yeung KK, Cechetto DF, et al. Increased Expression of Simple Ganglioside Species GM2 and GM3 Detected by MALDI Imaging mass spectrometry in a combined rat model of abeta toxicity and stroke. PLoS One. 2015;10(6):e0130364. doi: 10.1371/journal.pone.0130364.
5. Sachdeva AK, Chopra K. Lycopene abrogates Abeta(1-42)-mediated neuroinflammatory cascade in an experimental model of Alzheimer's disease. J Nutr Biochem. 2015;26(7):736-44. doi: 10.1016/j.jnutbio.2015.01.012.
6. Dao AT, Zagaar MA, Levine AT, Salim S, Eriksen JL, Alkadhi KA. Treadmill exercise prevents learning and memory impairment in Alzheimer's disease-like pathology. Curr Alzheimer Res. 2013;10(5):507-15.
7. Beheshti S, Shahrokhi S. Blocking the ghrelin receptor type 1a in the rat brain impairs memory encoding. Neuropeptides. 2015;52:97-102.doi:10.1016/j.npep.2015.05.003.
8. Carreiras MC, Marco JL. Recent approaches to novel anti-Alzheimer therapy. Curr Pharm Des. 2004;10(25):3167-75.
9. Anekonda TS, Reddy PH. Can herbs provide a new generation of drugs for treating Alzheimer's disease? Brain Res Brain Res Rev. 2005;50(2):361-76. doi: 10.1016/j.brainresrev.2005.09.001.
10. Sun ZK, Yang HQ, Chen SD. Traditional Chinese medicine: a promising candidate for the treatment of Alzheimer's disease. Transl Neurodegener. 2013;2(1):6. doi: 10.1186/2047-9158-2-6.
11. Pereira RP, Fachinetto R, de Souza Prestes A, Puntel RL, Santos da Silva GN, Heinzmann BM, et al. Antioxidant effects of different extracts from *Melissa officinalis, Matricaria recutita* and *Cymbopogon citratus*. Neurochem Res. 2009;34(5):973-83. doi: 10.1007/s11064-008-9861-z.
12. Perry EK, Pickering AT, Wang WW, Houghton P, Perry NS. Medicinal plants and Alzheimer's disease: Integrating ethnobotanical and contemporary scientific evidence. J Altern Complement Med. 1998;4(4):419-28. doi: 10.1089/acm.1998.4.419.
13. Kennedy DO, Scholey AB, Tildesley NT, Perry EK, Wesnes KA. Modulation of mood and cognitive performance following acute administration of *Melissa officinalis* (lemon balm). Pharmacol Biochem Behav. 2002;72(4):953-64.
14. Paxinos G, Watson C. The Rat Brain in Stereotaxic Coordinates. New York: Academic Press; 2007.
15. Beheshti S, Hosseini SA, Noorbakhshnia M, Eivani M. Role of hippocampal CA1 area gap junction channels on morphine state-dependent learning. Eur J Pharmacol. 2014;745:196-200. doi: 10.1016/j.ejphar.2014.10.040.
16. Doost Mohammadpour J, Hosseinmardi N, Janahmadi M, Fathollahi Y, Motamedi F, Rohampour K. Non-selective NSAIDs improve the amyloid-beta-mediated suppression of memory and synaptic plasticity. Pharmacol Biochem Behav. 2015;132:33-41. doi: 10.1016/j.pbb.2015.02.012.
17. Schliebs R. Basal forebrain cholinergic dysfunction in Alzheimer's disease--interrelationship with beta-amyloid, inflammation and neurotrophin signaling. Neurochem Res. 2005;30(6-7):895-908. doi: 10.1007/s11064-005-6962-9.
18. Lane RM, Kivipelto M, Greig NH. Acetylcholinesterase and its inhibition in Alzheimer disease. Clin Neuropharmacol. 2004;27(3):141-9.
19. Rasmussen P. Lemon balm--*Melissa officinalis*; also known as lemon balm, bee balm, garden balm, Melissa, melissengeist. J Prim Health Care. 2011;3(2):165-6.
20. Perry EK, Pickering AT, Wang WW, Houghton PJ, Perry NS. Medicinal plants and Alzheimer's disease: from ethnobotany to phytotherapy. J Pharm Pharmacol. 1999;51(5):527-34.
21. Dastmalchi K, Ollilainen V, Lackman P, Boije af Gennas G, Dorman HJ, Jarvinen PP, et al. Acetylcholinesterase inhibitory guided fractionation of *Melissa officinalis* L. Bioorg Med Chem. 2009;17(2):867-71. doi: 10.1016/j.bmc.2008.11.034.
22. Sepand MR, Soodi M, Hajimehdipoor H, Soleimani M, Sahraei E. Comparison of neuroprotective effects of *Melissa officinalis* total extract and its acidic and non-acidic fractions against a beta-induced toxicity. Iran J Pharm Res. 2013;12(2):415-23.
23. Wake G, Court J, Pickering A, Lewis R, Wilkins R, Perry E. CNS acetylcholine receptor activity in European medicinal plants traditionally used to improve failing memory. J Ethnopharmacol. 2000;69(2):105-14.
24. Christen Y. Oxidative stress and Alzheimer disease. Am J Clin Nutr. 2000;71(2):621s-9s. doi: 10.1093/ajcn/71.2.621s.

25. Lopez V, Martin S, Gomez-Serranillos MP, Carretero ME, Jager AK, Calvo MI. Neuroprotective and neurological properties of *Melissa officinalis*. Neurochem Res. 2009;34(11):1955-61. doi: 10.1007/s11064-009-9981-0.
26. Aliev G, Obrenovich ME, Reddy VP, Shenk JC, Moreira PI, Nunomura A, et al. Antioxidant therapy in Alzheimer's disease: theory and practice. Mini Rev Med Chem. 2008;8(13):1395-406.
27. Petersen M, Simmonds MS. Rosmarinic acid. Phytochemistry. 2003;62(2):121-5.
28. Alkam T, Nitta A, Mizoguchi H, Itoh A, Nabeshima T. A natural scavenger of peroxynitrites, rosmarinic acid, protects against impairment of memory induced by Abeta(25-35). Behav Brain Res. 2007;180(2):139-45. doi: 10.1016/j.bbr.2007.03.001.
29. Kantar Gok D, Ozturk N, Er H, Aslan M, Demir N, Derin N, et al. Effects of rosmarinic acid on cognitive and biochemical alterations in ovariectomized rats treated with D-galactose. Folia Histochem Cytobiol. 2015;53(4):283-93. doi: 10.5603/fhc.a2015.0034.
30. Liu J. Pharmacology of oleanolic acid and ursolic acid. J Ethnopharmacol. 1995;49(2):57-68.
31. Kim JH, Wang Q, Choi JM, Lee S, Cho EJ. Protective role of caffeic acid in an Abeta25-35-induced Alzheimer's disease model. Nutr Res Pract. 2015;9(5):480-8. doi: 10.4162/nrp.2015.9.5.480.
32. Pinheiro Fernandes FD, Fontenele Menezes AP, de Sousa Neves JC, Fonteles AA, da Silva AT, de Araujo Rodrigues P, et al. Caffeic acid protects mice from memory deficits induced by focal cerebral ischemia. Behav Pharmacol. 2014;25(7):637-47. doi: 10.1097/fbp.0000000000000076.
33. Yu TX, Zhang P, Guan Y, Wang M, Zhen MQ. Protective effects of luteolin against cognitive impairment induced by infusion of Abeta peptide in rats. Int J Clin Exp Pathol. 2015;8(6):6740-7.
34. Tsai FS, Cheng HY, Hsieh MT, Wu CR, Lin YC, Peng WH. The ameliorating effects of luteolin on beta-amyloid-induced impairment of water maze performance and passive avoidance in rats. Am J Chin Med. 2010;38(2):279-91. doi: 10.1142/s0192415x10007841.
35. Tsai FS, Peng WH, Wang WH, Wu CR, Hsieh CC, Lin YT, et al. Effects of luteolin on learning acquisition in rats: involvement of the central cholinergic system. Life Sci. 2007;80(18):1692-8. doi: 10.1016/j.lfs.2007.01.055.
36. Mao XY, Yu J, Liu ZQ, Zhou HH. Apigenin attenuates diabetes-associated cognitive decline in rats via suppressing oxidative stress and nitric oxide synthase pathway. Int J Clin Exp Med. 2015;8(9):15506-13.
37. Zhao L, Wang JL, Liu R, Li XX, Li JF, Zhang L. Neuroprotective, anti-amyloidogenic and neurotrophic effects of apigenin in an Alzheimer's disease mouse model. Molecules. 2013;18(8):9949-65. doi: 10.3390/molecules18089949.
38. Cheng Y, Dong Z, Liu S. beta-Caryophyllene ameliorates the Alzheimer-like phenotype in APP/PS1 Mice through CB2 receptor activation and the PPARgamma pathway. Pharmacology. 2014;94(1-2):1-12. doi: 10.1159/000362689.
39. Sabbaghziarani F, Rasapour S, Mortezaee K, Oryan S, Sharifzadeh M, Khanavi M, et al. Could *Melissa officinalis* extract restore streptozotocin-induced spatial memory impairment in rats? Anatomical Sciences Journal. 2014;11(1):25-32.
40. Akhondzadeh S, Noroozian M, Mohammadi M, Ohadinia S, Jamshidi A, Khani M. *Melissa officinalis* L. extract in the treatment of patients with mild to moderate Alzheimer's disease: a double blind, randomized and placebo-controlled trial. Journal of Medicinal Plants. 2002;4(4):47-57.

23

Toxicology of solvent extract and fractions of *Alstonia boonei* (DC.) wild stem bark in rats

Oludele John Olanlokun[*], Olufunso Olabode Olorunsogo

Laboratories for Biomembrane Research and Biotechnology, Department of Biochemistry, Faculty of Basic Medical Sciences, College of Medicine, University of Ibadan

ARTICLE INFO

Keywords:
Hematological parameters
Marker enzymes
Hepatotoxicity
Nephrotoxicity
Recovery

ABSTRACT

Introduction: Toxic effects arising from the use of medicinal herbs have been frequently overshadowed by the therapeutic efficacy of phytomedicines. This study was carried out to assess the safety of extract and fractions of *Alstonia boonei* (de wild) stem bark, popularly used in the treatment of malaria especially in Africa.
Methods: Rats were orally exposed to different doses (200 and 400 mg/kg body weight) of methanol extract (ME), *n*-hexane (HF), chloroform (CF), ethylacetate (EF) and aqueous fractions (AF) of *A. boonei* for 7 days. Furthermore, 10 mg/ kg body weight (bw) of chloroquine (CQN) was administered as standard drug for 7 days while, 5% tween 80 (TT) and distilled water (TW) were administered as control for 7 days. Group I (treatment group) was sacrificed after 7 days while group II (recovery group) was left for 21 days to recover and thereafter sacrificed. The effects of treatment and recovery were analyzed using serum biomarkers, hematological parameters and tissue histopathological evaluation.
Results: There was reduction in hematological parameters after 7 days but recovered after 21 days. There was also increase in serum alanine aminotransferase (ALT), aspartate aminotransferase (AST) and alkaline phosphatase (ALP), after 7 days. Compared to TW and TT treated groups, histopathological scores of liver and kidney were critical for all groups at 400 mg/kg bw after 21 days.
Conclusion: The animals did not fully recover after 21 days, suggesting that 400 mg/kg bw of extract and fractions of *A. boonei* were both hepatotoxic and nephrotoxic. Hence this plant should be used with caution.

Implication for health policy/practice/research/medical education:
The extract and fractions of *A. boonei* are not only toxic, but also recovery from the toxic effects is also not within a short-term limit. Hence, in general the safety of herbs must be considered when using them for therapeutic and prophylactic purposes.

Introduction

Plants are cheap sources of medicinal intervention both for curative and preventive measures. In African and Asian continents, a greater percentage of the entire population relies solely on phytomedicine because of their folkloric and high efficiency. Herbs are prepared as infusion of a mixture of plants, a whole plant or plant parts containing phytochemical components some of which may not be necessary for the reasons why the decoction was prepared. *Alstonia boonei* (de wild), a deciduous plant of the *Apocynaceae* family is well known for its antimalarial activity and other therapeutic efficacies. The folkloric use of this plant for therapeutic and prophylactic antimalarial purposes has been justified with scientific research (1,2). A herbal medicine may be taken in a toxic dose because of self-treatment (3), management and preparation of the phytomedicine by unqualified practitioners (4), substandard phytomedical products and the presence of heavy metals and toxins in the herbal decoctions (5) and/or improper intake (6). Herbal drugs may be nephrotoxic (7), hepatotoxic (8), cardiotoxic (9) or neurotoxic (10). It has been reported that Africans that are vulnerable to kidney diseases are mostly those that rely on traditional medicines and that herbal medicines account for about

*Corresponding author: Oludele John Olanlokun,
Email: jodel72000@yahoo.com, iyanuife@gmail.com

30%-35% of acute kidney diseases in Africa (11). Because of its central role in metabolizing herbs and herbal products ingested, the liver is one of the internal organs affected directly by herbs or indirectly by their metabolites (12). While some common plants used as herbal medicines have shown clinical signs of cardiotoxicity due to their adverse effects on some cardiac events such as blood pressure and inflammation of myocardium, some have neurotoxic effects (10,13). Few researches have been done to assess the toxicity of *A. boonei*. The ethanol extract of *A. boonei* stem bark might be toxic when co-administered with DDVP (2, 2-dichlorovinyl dimethyl phosphate) (14). However, there is paucity of information on the duration of recovery from the toxic effects of administration of various solvent fractions of the stem bark extract or if a permanent damage is to be established as a result of the toxicity of this plant. Besides, the doses of extract and fractions of *A. boonei* used in this work and duration have been used in antimalarial works (1,2) and so it is a representative of expected toxicity of such experimental design. It is against this background that we assessed the toxic effects of oral administration of extracts and fractions of *A. boonei* and levels of recovery after 21 days of drug withdrawal.

Materials and Methods

Chemicals

Methanol, *n*-hexane, chloroform and ethylacetate were obtained from Sigma-Aldrich chemicals, St. Louis MO, USA; chloroquine phosphate was obtained from Jopan Pharmaceuticals Nig. Ltd, Ajao Estate, Lagos Nigeria; Alnine and aspartate aminotransferases assay kits were obtained from Randox laboratories ltd. (Antrim, UK). All other chemicals used were of analytical grade and were obtained from British Drug Houses (Poole, Dorset, UK).

Plant material

Stem bark peels of *A. boonei* were obtained from Ekiti State University, Nigeria and were identified by Mr. Omotayo, F.O. of the University Herbarium, Ekiti State University and a voucher number (UHAE013) was assigned to the sample. The peels were washed and air-dried in the laboratory for 3 weeks after which they were pulverized, and soaked in methanol for 3 days. The filtrate was concentrated using rotary evaporator (Stuart, UK) to yield a dark brown methanol extract (ME).

Partitioning of the methanol extract

Methanol extract (50 g) was mixed with 250 mL of distilled water and partitioned successively between *n*-hexane, chloroform and ethylacetate to yield hexane (HF), chloroform (CF), ethylacetate (EF) and aqueous fractions (AF) using a separating funnel. These were concentrated using rotary evaporator and were further concentrated in water bath at 40°C until constant weights were obtained. In this way, the solvents were removed and the dry fractions were stored in the refrigerator until used.

Animals

Seventy male rats (100-120 g) were obtained from the Central Animal House, College of Medicine, University of Ibadan, Nigeria and were broadly divided into two groups of thirty-five animals each for the acute and recovery experiments. Each fraction, extract, chloroquine and untreated control group had five animals each. Similar animal groupings were used for the recovery experiment. The animals were housed in clean cages and had access to clean water and standard rat pellets (Ladokun Feeds, Nigeria) a*d libitum*.

Animal treatment and sample collection

The animals were exposed to 200 and 400 mg/kg bw doses of ME, HF, CF, EF AF and 10 mg/kg bw of chloroquine (CQN) orally, once daily for 7 days. The untreated control group received the vehicle -- water (TW) and 5% v/v tween 80 (TT) for those days. After 7 days, the acute treated groups were sacrificed via cervical dislocation, opened up and blood was collected from the heart into plain sample bottles, spun at 3000 rpm for 5 minutes and the serum was collected into another plain bottle. The recovery groups were left for 21 days without treatment and sacrificed after an overnight fast. Liver and kidney sections used for histopathology were excised and fixed in ten percent formalin until used.

Biochemical assays

Serum alanine, aspartate aminotransferases (ALT and AST) and alkaline phosphatase (ALP) were analyzed using Randox kits.

Hematological parameters

Packed cell volume (PCV), hemoglobin (Hb), total white blood cell count (TWBC), neutrophils (N), and lymphocytes (L) were estimated according to a previously defined method (15).

Tissue histopathology

The fixed liver and kidney tissues were dehydrated by ascending grades of isopropyl alcohol for an hour. The dehydrated organs were cleared in xylene and transferred into two changes of liquid paraffin wax. The tissue sections were stained in Ehrlich's hematoxylin for 8 minutes, washed in water and dipped in acid alcohol to remove excess stain. These were counter stained in 10% aqueous eosin, incubated and mounted for photomicrography.

Statistical analysis

All values were expressed as mean ± standard deviation (SD). Data were analyzed using Duncan's multiple range test and level of significance was set at $P < 0.05$.

Results

Tables 1 and 2 respectively show the effects of oral administration of 200 mg/kg bw of the extract and

Table 1. Hematological effects of 200 mg/kg bw of extract and fractions of *Alstonia boonei* in rats after 7 days

Drugs	PCV (%)	TWBC (cumm^{-1})	Hb (g/dL)	N (%)	L (%)
ME	38.50^{a}±4.93	5975.00^{a}±1078.19	12.65^{a}±1.70	14.75^{ab}±6.07	85.00^{a}±6.37
HF	36.00^{a}±4.24	5350.00^{a}±1799.07	11.97^{a}±1.39	26.00^{ab}±9.34	73.50^{a}±9.03
CF	34.25^{a}±4.34	4500.00^{a}±1000.00	11.35^{a}±1.39	30.75^{b}±14.17	71.25^{a}±12.09
EF	35.50^{a}±4.04	6750.00^{b}±613.73	11.80^{a}±1.33	23.25^{ab}±9.21	76.00^{a}±9.20
AF	37.00^{a}±4.08	5600.00^{a}±1564.18	12.05^{a}±1.02	12.75^{ab}±2.42	87.25^{a}±12.41
TW	40.00^{b}±8.49	6500.00^{b}±282.84	13.30^{a}±1.61	14.50^{ab}±6.36	89.50^{a}±15.90
CQN	34.25^{a}±8.96	4600.00^{a}±743.86	12.03^{a}±1.61	11.50^{a}±3.79	88.50^{a}±4.03
TT	37.50^{a}±2.65	4725.00^{a}±1791.42	12.42^{a}±0.89	20.25^{ab}±5.35	78.75^{a}±6.36

Methanol extract (ME); n-Hexane fraction (HF); Chloroform fraction (CF); Ethylacetate fraction (EF); Aqueous fraction (AF); Treated with water only (TW); Chloroquine (CQN); Tween 80 (5% v/v) only (TT); Packed cell volume (PCV); Total white blood cell (TWBC); Hemoglobin (Hb); Neutrophil (N); Lymphocyte (L). Values are mean of five determinations ± standard deviation. Values with different superscripts within the column are significantly different at $P < 0.05$.

Table 2. Hematological effects of 200 mg/kg bw of extract and fractions of *Alstonia boonei* in rats after 21 days

Drugs	PCV (%)	TWBC (cumm^{-1})	Hb (g/dL)	N (%)	L (%)
ME	41.25^{b}±2.63	6675.00^{a}±665.21	13.73^{b}±0.8	5.50^{b}±2.38	90.25^{a}±2.62
HF	33.50^{a}±7.3	7675.00^{b}±607.59	11.13^{b}±2.41	13.25^{a}±11.35	86.00^{a}±12.11
CF	38.00^{b}±0.81	6775.00^{ab}±2085.47	12.63^{b}±0.29	8.50^{b}±8.06	91.50^{a}±8.06
EF	41.75^{b}±0.96	8075.00^{b}±991.21	13.88^{b}±0.34	12.50^{a}±3.87	87.50^{a}±3.87
AF	34.00^{a}±6.38	6650.00^{ab}±2389.56	11.30^{b}±0.34	15.75^{a}±4.92	84.00^{a}±5.23
TW	46.00^{b}±0.00	6700.00^{ab}±0.00	15.60^{a}±0.00	7.00^{b}±0.00	93.50^{a}±0.00
CQN	40.00^{b}±4.32	4675.00^{a}±1379.31	13.30^{b}±1.44	6.25^{a}±5.18	93.00^{a}±5.68
TT	37.00^{b}±6.27	7400.00^{b}±1557.78	12.30^{b}±2.12	10.00^{a}±5.29	91.00^{a}±6.06

Methanol extract (ME); n-Hexane fraction (HF); Chloroform fraction (CF); Ethylacetate fraction (EF); Aqueous fraction (AF); Treated with water only (TW); Chloroquine (CQN); Tween 80 (5% v/v) only (TT); Packed cell volume (PCV); Total white blood cell (TWBC); Hemoglobin (Hb); Neutrophil (N); Lymphocyte (L). Values are mean of five determinations ± standard deviation. Values with different superscripts within the column are significantly different at $P < 0.05$.

fractions of the methanol stem bark extract of *A. boonei* on blood parameters. The PCV, TWBC, Hb and L values increased albeit insignificantly after a recovery period of 21 days among groups administered with ME, HF, CF, EF and CQN while there was no significant difference when values of the hematological parameters were compared among the extract and fractions. In all these parameters, animals treated with water (TW) had the highest values both after 7 days treatment and 21 days recovery except in TWBC.

Tables 3 and 4 respectively show the effects of the extract and fractions of the methanol stem bark extract of *A. boonei* on some hematological parameters at 400 mg/kg bw dose after 7 days treatment and 21 days recovery period. The results obtained showed a similar trend with 200 mg/kg bw dose but with severe and critical effects. Biochemical studies on AST, ALT and ALP activities (Tables 5, 6, 7 and 8) at 200 and 400 mg/kg bw dose of *A. boonei* extract and fractions showed that the enzyme activities increased dose dependently with maximal effect noticed in the CF group. There was no significant decrease in the activities of these enzymes after 21 days.

Histopathological studies (Figure 1) revealed the lesions both in the liver and kidney of animals treated with 400

Table 3. Hematological effects of 400 mg/kg bw of extract and fractions of *Alstonia boonei* in rats after 7 days

Drugs	PCV (%)	TWBC (cumm^{-1})	Hb (g/dL)	N (%)	L (%)
ME	39.00^{a}±2.82	5325.00^{a}±1650	12.95^{a}±0.96	24.73^{a}±3.40	74.25^{a}±3.30
HF	38.50^{a}±4.12	6200.00^{a}±983.19	12.82^{a}±1.36	17.50^{a}±1.63	74.75^{a}±4.73
CF	32.25^{a}±4.03	5900.00^{a}±2824.89	10.72^{a}±1.33	13.50^{a}±1.18	85.75^{a}±5.11
EF	31.50^{a}±5.80	5925.00^{a}±1740.45	10.42^{a}±1.99	26.25^{ab}±1.90	72.75^{a}±10.53
AF	34.00^{a}±1.41	4950.00^{a}±1791.42	11.32^{a}±0.47	27.75^{a}±1.08	71.50^{a}±9.77
TW	40.00^{b}±8.49	6500.00^{b}±282.84	13.30^{a}±1.61	14.50^{ab}±6.36	89.50^{a}±15.90
CQN	34.25^{a}±8.96	4600.00^{a}±743.86	12.03^{a}±1.61	11.50^{a}±3.79	88.50^{a}±4.03
TT	37.50^{a}±2.65	4725.00^{a}±1791.42	12.42^{a}±0.89	20.25^{ab}±5.35	78.75^{a}±6.36

Methanol extract (ME); n-Hexane fraction (HF); Chloroform fraction (CF); Ethylacetate fraction (EF); Aqueous fraction (AF); Treated with water only (TW); Chloroquine (CQN); Tween 80 (5% v/v) only (TT); Packed cell volume (PCV); Total white blood cell (TWBC); Hemoglobin (Hb); Neutrophil (N); Lymphocyte (L). Values are mean of five determinations ± standard deviation. Values with different superscripts within the column are significantly different at $P < 0.05$.

Table 4. Hematological effects of 400 mg/kg bw of extract and fractions of *Alstonia boonei* in rats after 21 days

Drugs	PCV (%)	TWBC (cumm^{-1})	Hb (g/dL)	N (%)	L (%)
ME	42.333^{a}±1.52	5633.33^{a}±981.49	14.06^{b}±0.50	10.67^{a}±2.08	88.69^{a}±3.21
HF	39.25^{b}±2.22	7625.00^{ab}±1102.65	13.05^{b}±0.71	8.75^{a}±6.80	91.00^{a}±7.25
CF	41.00^{a}±1.41	9200.00^{b}±1414.21	13.65^{b}±0.49	19.00^{a}±2.21	80.50^{a}±21.92
EF	39.00^{b}±1.83	5900.00^{a}±2426.25	12.95^{b}±0.34	17.25^{a}±14.89	82.50^{a}±14.02
AF	37.33^{b}±2.31	6666.67^{ab}±1553.49	12.43^{b}±0.75	11.00^{a}±2.00	89.00^{a}±2.02
TW	46.00^{b}±0.00	6700.00^{ab}±0.00	15.60^{a}±0.00	7.00^{b}±0.00	93.50^{a}±0.00
CQN	40.00^{b}±4.32	4675.00^{a}±1379.31	13.30^{b}±1.44	6.25^{a}±5.18	93.00^{a}±5.68
TT	37.00^{b}±6.27	7400.00^{b}±1557.78	12.30^{b}±2.12	10.00^{a}±5.29	91.00^{a}±6.06

Methanol extract (ME); n-Hexane fraction (HF); Chloroform fraction (CF); Ethylacetate fraction (EF); Aqueous fraction (AF); Treated with water only (TW); Chloroquine (CQN); Tween 80 (5% v/v) only (TT); Packed cell volume (PCV); Total white blood cell (TWBC); Hemoglobin (Hb); Neutrophil (N); Lymphocyte (L). Values are mean of five determinations ± standard deviation. Values with different superscripts within the column are significantly different at $P < 0.05$.

mg/kg bw of the drug candidates after 21 days. The results obtained showed that there was portal congestion (ME), diffuse vacuolar degeneration (HF, EF CQN and AF), and severe diffuse hepatic vacuolation with central venous congestion (CF) after 21 days. The kidney showed few tubules with protein cast (ME and HF), and moderate renal cortical congestion (EF and AF). The kidney section of the CF showed marked renal cortical congestion and hemorrhage.

Table 5. Effects of 200 mg/kg bw of extract and fractions of *Alstonia booneion* AST, ALT and ALP after 7 days

Drugs	ALT (U/L)	AST (U/L)	ALP (U/L)
ME	120.70^{ab}±10.14	57.20^{bcd}±2.47	220.81^{a}±28.61
HF	83.03^{a}±8.25	33.72^{a}±2.09	227.03^{ab}±20.49
CF	126.83^{b}±8.34	61.16^{cd}±9.82	243.57^{ab}±20.49
EF	115.20±6.25	53.44^{abcd}±8.92	200.19^{a}±44.46
AF	110.78^{ab}±3.90	48.20^{abc}±3.25	222.18^{a}±6.11
TW	46.25^{c}±3.18	48.24^{abcd}±3.62	75.90^{a}±0.74
CQN	98.55^{ab}±2.73	40.68^{abc}±3.98	517.50^{ab}±13.21
TT	40.95^{c}±7.33	37.24^{ab}±8.82	51.75^{a}±6.83

Methanol extract (ME); n-Hexane fraction (HF); Chloroform fraction (CF); Ethylacetate fraction (EF); Aqueous fraction (AF); Treated with water only (TW); Chloroquine (CQN); Tween 80 (5% v/v) only (TT); Aspartate aminotransferase (AST); Alanine aminotransferase (ATL); alkaline phosphatase (ALP). Values are mean of five determinations ± standard deviation. Values are mean of five determinations ± standard deviation. Values with different superscripts within the column are significantly different at $P < 0.05$.

Discussion

Malaria is a fatal parasitic infection especially in the tropical African and Asian continent and it is believed that it kills more than AIDS and the most vulnerable are children under the age of 5 years (16). Herbal remedy, which in most cases, is a combination of two or more plants is usually taken *ad libitum* for the treatment or prevention of malaria in Africa. This good intention but with fatal consequences has its deleterious effects in terms of toxicities. The results obtained showed that PCV, Hb, and TWBC decreased after 7 days but slightly increased after 21 days. The significant decrease in PCV observed in the HF and AF groups showed that these fractions might contain phytochemicals capable of causing hemolytic anemia possibly via the destabilization of the erythrocyte membrane (17,18). The observed significant decrease in

Table 6. Effects of 200 mg/kg bw of extract and fractions of *Alstonia booneion* AST, ALT and ALP after 21 days

Drugs	ALT (U/L)	AST (U/L)	ALP (U/L)
ME	117.90^{ab}±7.14	52.11^{ab}±22.00	200.01^{a}±5.86
HF	80.13^{a}±3.24	33.00^{a}±6.90	218.04^{a}±10.73
CF	120.88^{c}±0.07	60.42^{c}±7.90	220.12^{b}±3.14
EF	110.20^{c}±3.14	49.09^{abc}±2.41	190.14^{d}±0.00
AF	106.90^{bc}±3.14	47.00^{ab}±2.91	215.11^{b}±3.20
TW	44.21^{c}±0.00	45.00^{ab}±0.00	78.04^{a}±0.00
CQN	96.41^{ab}±7.71	32.01^{a}±7.81	476.50^{c}±5.99
TT	46.21^{c}±9.36	36.11^{ab}±14.82	53.44^{a}±2.93

Methanol extract (ME); n-Hexane fraction (HF); Chloroform fraction (CF); Ethylacetate fraction (EF); Aqueous fraction (AF); Treated with water only (TW); Chloroquine (CQN); Tween 80 (5% v/v) only (TT); Aspartate aminotransferase (AST); Alanine aminotransferase (ATL); alkaline phosphatase (ALP). Values are mean of five determinations ± standard deviation. Values are mean of five determinations ± standard deviation. Values with different superscripts within the column are significantly different at $P < 0.05$.

Table 7. Effects of 400 mg/kg bw of extract and fractions of *Alstonia booneion* AST, ALT and ALP after 7 days

Drugs	ALT (U/L)	AST (U/L)	ALP (U/L)
ME	127.95^{ab}±16.85	58.84^{abc}±5.69	302.82^{a}±9.73
HF	121.35^{ab}±29.3	52.92^{b}±13.06	448.64^{abc}±4.39
CF	130.13^{b}±9.36	81.68^{abc}±10.41	536.65^{bc}±1.99
EF	123.23±6.07	58.92^{b}±14.02	250.65^{abc}±1.99
AF	121.73^{abc}±4.28	49.12^{ab}±7.16	445.91^{a}±11.28
TW	46.25^{c}±3.18	48.24^{abcd}±3.62	75.90^{a}±0.74
CQN	98.55^{ab}±2.73	40.68^{abc}±3.98	517.50^{ab}±13.21
TT	40.95^{c}±7.33	37.24^{ab}±8.82	51.75^{a}±6.83

Methanol extract (ME); n-Hexane fraction (HF); Chloroform fraction (CF); Ethylacetate fraction (EF); Aqueous fraction (AF); Treated with water only (TW); Chloroquine (CQN); Tween 80 (5% v/v) only (TT); Aspartate aminotransferase (AST); Alanine aminotransferase (ATL); alkaline phosphatase (ALP). Values are mean of five determinations ± standard deviation. Values are mean of five determinations ± standard deviation. Values with different superscripts within the column are significantly different at $P < 0.05$.

Table 8. Effects of 400 mg/kg bw of extract and fractions of *Alstonia booneion* AST, ALT and ALP after 21 days

Drugs	ALT (U/L)	AST (U/L)	ALP (U/L)
ME	$120.01^{abc}\pm11.34$	$50.10^{c}\pm15.61$	$200.49^{d}\pm10.03$
HF	$100.01^{bc}\pm38.12$	$39.40^{bc}\pm21.27$	$341.42^{bc}\pm4.98$
CF	$126.40^{ab}\pm30.33$	$70.62^{c}\pm4.29$	$490.04^{ab}\pm4.87$
EF	$119.00^{c}\pm19.34$	$47.48^{ab}\pm9.92$	$200.41^{c}\pm9.75$
AF	$115.90^{a}\pm43.05$	$40.44^{ab}\pm21.48$	$296.11^{b}\pm8.78$
TW	$44.21^{c}\pm0.00$	$45.00^{ab}\pm0.00$	$78.04^{a}\pm0.00$
CQN	$96.41^{ab}\pm7.71$	$32.01^{a}\pm7.81$	$476.50^{c}\pm5.99$
TT	$46.21^{c}\pm9.36$	$36.11^{ab}\pm14.82$	$53.44^{a}\pm2.93$

Methanol extract (ME); n-Hexane fraction (HF); Chloroform fraction (CF); Ethylacetate fraction (EF); Aqueous fraction (AF); Treated with water only (TW); Chloroquine (CQN); Tween 80 (5% v/v) only (TT); Aspartate aminotransferase (AST); Alanine aminotransferase (ATL); alkaline phosphatase (ALP). Values are mean of five determinations ± standard deviation. Values are mean of five determinations ± standard deviation. Values with different superscripts within the column are significantly different at $P < 0.05$.

Hb of the test groups compared with the animals treated with water (TW) showed that the extract and fractions interfered with oxygen carrying capacity of blood cells or that the administration of the drug candidates impaired erythropoiesis (19). The significant increase in TWBC levels after 21 days compared with its levels after 7 days could be as a result of phytochemicals eliciting immune response to chemicals or as a result of secondary infections (20).

The reduction in the levels of neutrophils after the withdrawal of the drug candidates indicated that the extract and fractions repressed neutrophil production or enhanced its destruction maybe to minimize cellular injury because in addition to their immune response, neutrophils are implicated in tissue damage (21). An increase in the lymphocyte values showed that the extract and fractions enhanced the proliferation. This showed that the extract and fractions of *A. boonei* had immunosuppressive effects on neutrophils and immunostimulatory on lymphocyte proliferation. Some herbal preparations have immunomodulatory effects like this (22). The hematological parameters did not fall below a threshold which could pose danger to the animals, however, an increase in these hematological parameters following the withdrawal of the drug candidates showed that oral administration of the extract and fractions had reducing effects on them. A basal level of AST and ALT is found in the plasma which may increase when there is damage to tissues such as liver, kidney and heart. Increase in the serum level of ALP indicates liver injury or hepatitis (23). The reference values for AST (0 to 40 U/L) and ALT (0 to 45 IU/L) in human (24) showed that all values obtained for these enzymes from all the drug candidates at both doses and at 7 and 21 days were significantly higher than normal and it was evidently clear that damage was done to the liver. The increase in the activities of these enzymes after 7 days is indicative of the toxic effects of the extract and fractions of the stem bark extract of *A. boonei.* Subsequent decrease in the serum activities of these enzymes after 21 days did not reveal complete recovery. Microscopic examination of the liver and kidney sections after the recovery period of 21 days showed various lesions such as vacuolar degeneration, portal cellular infiltration by mononuclear cells and severe, diffuse hepatic vacuolation with central venous congestion, diffuse hepatic vacuolation and severe portal congestion with cellular infiltration by mononuclear cells and mild

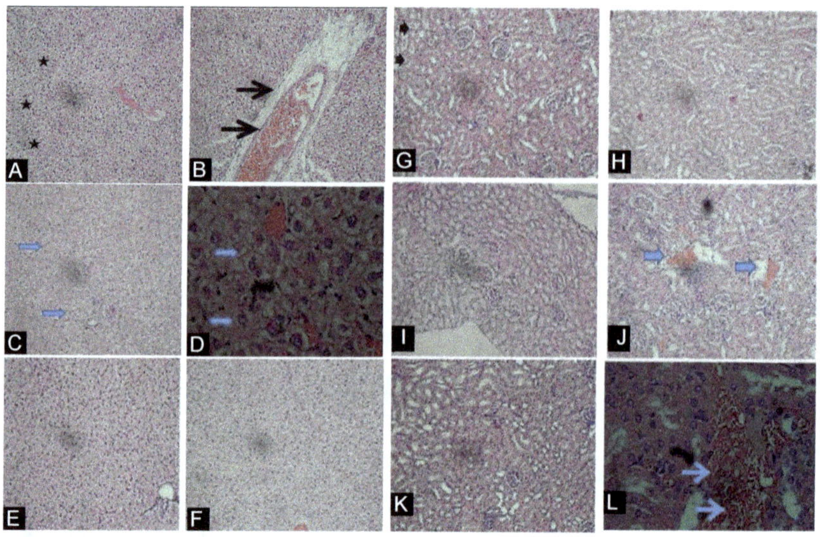

Figure 1. Histopathology of liver and kidney tissue sections of rats exposed to 400mg/kg of ME (A), HF (B), EF (C), AF (D), CQN (E) and CF (F) after 21 days of recovery. The result showed hepatic vacuolation (black stars in A), severe portal congestion with cellular infiltration by mononuclear cells and mild fibroplasias (blue arrows in C and D). The kidney sections of the same treated groups (G-L respectively) showed renal cortical congestion and tubules with protein casts (black arrows in G) and hemorrhage (blue arrows in J and L). ME= Methanol Extract, CQN= Chloroquine, HF, CF, EF and AF are *n*-hexane, chloroform, ethylacetate and aqueous fractions respectively.

fibroplasias, renal cortical congestion and hemorrhage. The congestion observed in the liver is evidence that the liver is involved in the biotransformation of xenobiotics. The kidney is an organ for excretion; therefore, it is exposed to both metabolized and un-metabolized toxicant for their removal from the body; the heavy task for the removal of toxicant from the body may cause much damage for the kidney. Again, some herbs may contain compounds such as oxalate which may chelate calcium and thus cause kidney stone. This means that high dose of extract and fractions of the methanol stem bark extract of *A. boonei* is both hepatotoxic and nephrotoxic and 21 days after the withdrawal of the drug did not give complete recovery. However, treatment of the negative control groups with water (TW) and 5% v/v (TT) did not show any noticeable effects on the hematological parameters, marker enzymes and histological evaluation.

Conclusion

Taking together, the results obtained from this research work suggested a moderate intake of herbal formulation for the treatment of diseases because of the possible side effects. The extract and fractions of *A. boonei* are not only toxic, but also recovery from the toxic effects is not within a short-term limit. Although, administration of herbal medicines may be useful in the treatment of diseases, the secondary adverse effects must not be overlooked because in some cases, these side effects are more deleterious than the diseases these phytochemicals are originally used to treat. In conclusion, the safety of the administration of herbs must be considered when using them for therapeutic and prophylactic purposes.

Authors' contribution

OJO carried out the experiments and wrote the draft manuscript, OOO designed the experiment, supplied reagents and equipments and proofread the manuscript. All authors read and approved the manuscript.

Conflict of interests

The authors declared no conflict of interest.

Ethical considerations

All experimental procedures conform to the guiding principles for research as recommended by the Declaration of Helsinki and National Institute of Health.

Funding/Support

The authors were the financiers of this research project.

Acknowledgements

We acknowledge the priceless and invaluable efforts of Mr. Omotayo, F.O. of the University Herbarium, Ekiti State University, Nigeria who authenticated the samples used in this study. We also appreciate the efforts of Mr. Ogunsakin, E.R., PhD student at Kwazulu Natal University, South Africa, for the statistical analysis.

References

1. Olanlokun JO, Bolaji OM, Agbedahunsi JM, Olorunsogo OO. Therapeutic effects of various solvent fractions of *Alstonia boonei* (apocynaceae) stem bark on Plasmodium berghei-induced malaria. Afr J Med Med Sci. 2012;41 Suppl:27-33.
2. Olanlokun JO, Bolaji OM, Agbedahunsi JM, Olorunsogo OO. Prophylactic potentials of extract of *Alstonia boonei* stem bark on chloroquine-sensitive *P. berghei*-induced malaria in mice. Arch Basic App Med. 2013;1:49-53.
3. Barrueto F, Tarabar A. Medscape. Herb Poisoning. http://emedicine.medscape.com/article/817427-overview. Accessed December 2016.
4. Jennifer K. Medicine Management in Nursing Times, Toxicity and Adverse Effects of Herbal Complementary Therapy. https://www.nursingtimes.net/clinical-archive/medicine-management/toxicity-and-adverse-effects-of-herbal-complementary-therapy/197707.article. 1 May 2002.
5. Barrett B, Kiefer D, Rabago D. Assessing the risks and benefits of herbal medicine: an overview of scientific evidence. Altern Ther Health Med. 1999;5(4):40-9.
6. Asif M. A brief study of toxic effects of some medicinal herbs on kidney. Adv Biomed Res. 2012;1:44. doi: 10.4103/2277-9175.100144.
7. Allard T, Wenner T, Greten HJ, Efferth T. Mechanisms of herb-induced nephrotoxicity. Curr Med Chem. 2013;20(22):2812-9.
8. Bunchorntavakul C, Reddy KR. Review article: herbal and dietary supplement hepatotoxicity. Aliment Pharmacol Ther. 2013;37(1):3-17. doi: 10.1111/apt.12109.
9. Andrade RJ, Robles M, Fernandez-Castaner A, Lopez-Ortega S, Lopez-Vega MC, Lucena MI. Assessment of drug-induced hepatotoxicity in clinical practice: a challenge for gastroenterologists. World J Gastroenterol. 2007;13(3):329-40.
10. Nielsen E, Brant J. Chemotherapy-induced neurotoxicity: assessment and interventions for patients at risk. Am J Nurs. 2002;102 Suppl 4:16-9; quiz 49-52.
11. Brown AC. Kidney toxicity related to herbs and dietary supplements: Online table of case reports. Part 3 of 5 series. Food Chem Toxicol. 2017;107(Pt A):502-19. doi: 10.1016/j.fct.2016.07.024.
12. Au JS, Navarro VJ, Rossi S. Review article: Drug-induced liver injury--its pathophysiology and evolving diagnostic tools. Aliment Pharmacol Ther. 2011;34(1):11-20. doi: 10.1111/j.1365-2036.2011.04674.x.
13. Pai VB, Nahata MC. Cardiotoxicity of chemotherapeutic agents: incidence, treatment and prevention. Drug Saf. 2000;22(4):263-302.
14. Ojo OA, Ajiboye B, Oyinloye BE, Akintayo CO. Prophylactic Effects of Ethanolic Extract of *Alstonia boonei* Stem Bark Against DDVP-induced Toxicity in Albino Rats. J Pharm Biomed Sci. 2014; 4(7): 650-657.
15. Jain NC. Schalm's Veterinary Hematology. 4th ed. Philadelphia, USA: Lea and Febiger; 1986.

16. World Health Organization. World Malaria Report. Geneva: WHO; 2014.
17. Ileke KD, Odeyemi OO, Ashamo MO. Phytochemical Screening and Effectiveness of Alstonia boonei De Wild oils as an Entomocides in the Management of *Cowpea bruchid, Callosobruchus maculatus* (Fab.) [Coleoptera: Chrysomelidae]. International Journal of Horticulture. 2014;4(6):24-31.
18. Opoku F, Akoto O. Antimicrobial and phytochemical properties of *Alstonia boonei* extracts. Organic Chemistry: Current Research. 2015;4(1):137. doi: 10.4172/2161-0401.1000137.
19. Chattopadhyay RR. Possible mechanism of hepatoprotective activity of *Azadirachta indica* leaf extract: part II. J Ethnopharmacol. 2003;89(2-3):217-9.
20. Adebayo AH, Abolaji AO, Opata TK, Adegbenro IK. Effects of ethanolic leaf extract of *Chrysophyllum albidum* G. on biochemical and haematological parameters of albino Wistar rats. Afr J Biotechnol. 2010;9(14):2145-50.
21. Kruger P, Saffarzadeh M, Weber AN, Rieber N, Radsak M, von Bernuth H, et al. Neutrophils: Between host defence, immune modulation, and tissue injury. PLoS Pathog. 2015;11(3):e1004651. doi: 10.1371/journal.ppat.1004651.
22. Adebiyi OE, Abatan MO. Phytochemical and acute toxicity of ethanolic extract of *Enantia chlorantha* (oliv) stem bark in albino rats. Interdiscip Toxicol. 2013;6(3):145-51. doi: 10.2478/intox-2013-0023.
23. Gowda S, Desai PB, Hull VV, Math AA, Vernekar SN, Kulkarni SS. A review on laboratory liver function tests. Pan Afr Med J. 2009;3:17.
24. Melissa P. Guide of hepatitis and liver disease. Am J Biochem. 2004;13:234-6.

Anticancer potential of *Tinospora cordifolia* and arabinogalactan against benzo(a)pyrene induced pulmonary tumorigenesis

Vandana Mohan, **Ashwani Koul***

Department of Biophysics, Basic Medical Science Block II, South campus, Panjab University, Chandigarh, India

ARTICLE INFO

Keywords:
Arabinogalactan
Benzo(a)pyrene
Lactate dehydrogenase
Medicinal plant
Tinospora cordifolia

ABSTRACT

Introduction: Aqueous *Tinospora cordifolia* stem extract (Aq.Tc) and arabinogalactan (AG), its bioactive polysaccharide, which are antioxidant remedies were evaluated on pulmonary cancer and associated tumor markers.

Methods: Mice were randomly segregated into 6 groups. Group I: animals served as control. Group II: animals which were administered Aq.Tc extract (200 mg/kg, orally), thrice a week. Group III: animals which received AG (7.5 mg/kg, orally) thrice a week. Group IV: animals which were instilled with benzo(a)pyrene (B(a)P) (50 mg/kg, orally) twice within an interval of 2 weeks. Group V: animals which received Aq.Tc extract as in group II, along with B(a)P after 2 weeks of Aq.Tc administration. Group VI: animals which received AG as in group III along with B(a)P after 2 weeks of AG administration.

Results: As expected, B(a)P treated mice exhibited high tumor incidence and multiplicity with concomitant increase in serum/plasma markers like carcinoembryonic antigen (CEA), circulating tumor DNA (ctDNA), lactate dehydrogenase (LDH) and tumor necrosis factor. However, Aq.Tc and AG supplementation to B(a)P abused animals significantly attenuated these parameters at different stages of cancer, depicting their anti-cancer effects in lung carcinogenesis. Also, treatment of Aq.Tc and AG to tumor bearing mice reduced the degree of histopathological alterations as compared to B(a)P installed mice. The apoptotic index in case of Aq.Tc and AG fed mice treated with B(a)P was higher as compared to only B(a)P treated mice. Further it was observed that Aq.Tc could induce higher degree of apoptosis when compared to AG group, suggesting Aq.Tc as a more effective modulator of tumorigenesis.

Conclusion: Overall, these findings substantiate the chemopreventive potential of Aq.Tc and AG against lung tumorigenesis. Aq.Tc was found to be more effective than AG in modulating the process of lung carcinogenesis as reflected by various observations.

Implication for health policy/practice/research/medical education:
Tinospora cordifolia plant and its various bioactive components have wide range of pharmacological properties. Aqueous extract of Tinospora cordifolia stem and arabinogalactan (AG), its bioactive polysaccharide, act as anti-cancer agents and have the potential for preparation of new drugs against lung cancer.

Introduction

Lung cancer is the prime cause of cancer mortality and is a growing economic burden worldwide (1). Primary factors that lead to induction of lung cancer include use of tobacco, automobile exhausts, occupational exposure and indoor air pollution (2). Polycyclic aromatic hydrocarbons (PAHs) are the major constituents of these pollutants (3). One of the most potent PAH, Benzo(a)pyrene {B(a)P} is known to induce lung cancer in humans as well as experimental animals (4).

In spite of various advancements in lung cancer diagnosis and treatment, survival rates remain low (5). Generally, tumor size and its extent of invasion detected histopathologically (biopsy) is considered to be the gold

***Corresponding author**: Prof. Ashwani Koul,
Email: drashwanikoul@yahoo.co.in, ashwanik@pu.ac.in

standard for evaluating the disease (6). Since the procedure of biopsy is invasive and could add to the agony of the patient, different serological markers of tumor could be taken into account for specific diagnosis and evaluation of progress of cancer (7). Sensitive and specific diagnostic markers of lung cancer could facilitate the early detection of the cancer lowering the associated mortality rates (8). Various serum markers include circulating tumor DNA (ctDNA), carcinoembryonic antigen (CEA), neuron specific enolase (NSE), carbohydrate antigen 125 (CA125) and squamous cell carcinoma antigen (SCC) (9). These markers when combined with other diagnostic tools could classify tumor into different molecular subtypes and monitor disease relapse and treatment response (10).

Since, there is no magic bullet to combat cancer, lung cancer is no exception to it, never the less, the risk could be reduced by eliminating contact or exposure to putative carcinogens. But this may not be feasible always, considering the quality of air, soil and water in the present scenario. Therefore, it presses the need for adopting other practical measures to control the dreadful disease. The complexity of this hyperproliferative disease necessitates the adoption of secondary prevention as a rational way to control it (11). The use of botanicals in the form of vegetables, fruits and other dietary supplements as chemopreventive agents seem to be relevant (12). Chemoprevention is a reasonable and cost-effective approach to decrease cancer mortality by inhibiting the pre-cancerous events and/or delaying its progression (13). Most of the drugs that are available to combat cancer have shown severe side effects. Synthetic chemopreventive drugs are cytotoxic, immune suppressants and may cause a variety of ill effects in various organs of the body (14). Various drugs that are currently being used are based on folk remedies and subsequent ethnopharmacological studies. There are more than 100 drugs of known structure that are extracted from medicinal plants. As modern medicine came up, people started looking for active components from the crude extract but due to their higher/acute side effects they are not much being used (15). Various medicinal plants have been identified for their anticancer properties and in varied number of ailments (16,17). *Tinospora cordifolia* is a known medicinal plant having a wide spectrum of pharmacological activity. It is commonly known as 'Guduchi' or 'Amrita' and is considered as an important drug of Indian Systems of Medicine (18). Different parts of this plant including leaves, roots and stem have been widely used for their variety of medicinal properties (19). However, use of stem has been widely reported, so far (20). *T. cordifolia* is known to exhibit anti-inflammatory and anti-cancer properties in various experimental models (21). There are several experimental reports which document the anticancer potential of aqueous, methanolic as well as ethanolic extracts of *T. cordifolia* in various cancer models (22,23). One of the active constituents in its polysaccharide fraction is arabinogalactan (AG) (24). Its potent biological activity and immune-enhancing properties have received increased attention as a clinically useful nutraceutical agent (25). AG has several properties which make it an ideal adjunct supplement to be considered in cancer protocols (26).

Aqueous extract of *T. cordifolia* is enriched in the polysaccharide fraction containing AG when compared with other types of extract (27). Many biological activities of *T. cordifolia* have been attributed to its polysaccharide fraction (28). The above mentioned observations warrant further investigations with respect to preparations rich in AG or its use as such active principle.

The polysaccharide fraction of *T. cordifolia* in lung has shown profound anti-metastatic activity against lung cancer cell lines (29). However, not much has been explored about its effect in *in vivo* lung cancer models and the underlying mechanism involved. Considering this, the present study was designed to assess the effects of aqueous *T. cordifolia* extract and its bioactive polysaccharide AG in *in vivo* benzo(a)pyrene induced pulmonary carcinogenesis model.

Material and Methods

Chemicals and kits

1,1-diphenyl 2-picrylhydrazyl (DPPH), 2,2'-azino-bis(3-ethylbenzothiazoline-6-sulphonic acid) (ABTS), Benzo(a) pyrene (B(a)P) and AG (99% pure) were obtained from Sigma-Aldrich Co. (St. Louis, MO, USA). Rest of the chemicals used were of analytical grade. Terminal deoxynucleotidyl transferase dUTP nick end labelling (TUNEL) assay kit was procured from Trevigen Inc. (Gaithersburg, Maryland, USA). FitAmp™ Circulating DNA Quantification kit was procured from Epigenetek (Farmingdale, New York, USA).

Preparation of aqueous Tinospora cordifolia stem extract

Tinospora cordifolia stems were collected from the Panjab University Botanical Garden after identification by a qualified Botanist. Aqueous powder of *T. cordifolia* was prepared according to method described by Tiwari et al, with minor modifications (30,31). Dried Aq. Tc powder (500 mg) was reconstituted in 10 mL of distilled water and was subjected to preliminary screening for the presence of phytoconstituents by standard protocol (32).

Free radical scavenging activity assays

Free radical scavenging activity of Aq.Tc as well as AG was analysed using DPPH (1,1-diphenyl 2-picrylhydrazyl) radical scavenging assay (33) and ABTS radical cation ($ABTS^{\cdot+}$) assay (34).

Animals and experimental conditions

Male Balb/c mice (25–30 g) were procured from the Central

Animal House, Panjab University, Chandigarh (Approval no PU/IAEC/S/15/61 Panjab University, Chandigarh). Mice were housed in polypropylene cages bedded with sterilized rice husk and were provided with standard pellet diet (Ashirwad Industries Ltd., Ropar, Punjab, India) and water *ad libitum* with standard conditions of relative humidity (50%–60%) and temperature (24±2°C). Mice were acclimatized to the experimental conditions for one week after which various treatments were given.

Experimental design

Mice were randomly segregated into 6 groups (n=6-8). Group I animals served as control and received no special treatment. Group II animals were administered aqueous *T. cordifolia* extract (Aq.Tc) (200 mg/kg, orally) on the alternate days (thrice a week). Group III animals were administered AG (7.5 mg/kg, orally) on alternate days (thrice a week). Group IV animals were instilled with B(a)P (50 mg/kg, i.p.) twice, within an interval of two weeks. Group V animals received Aq.Tc extract as in group II, along with B(a)P was installed after 2 weeks of Aq.Tc administration following the same protocol as for group IV. Group VI animals received AG as in group III along with B(a)P was instilled after 2 weeks of AG administration following the same protocol as in group IV. Changes in body weight, diet and water intake were observed every week in all the groups throughout the treatment period. Dose of Aq.Tc in the present study was standardized according to the available literature (200 mg/kg) (35). Dose of AG was deduced considering the amount of AG (active polysaccharide) present in 200 mg of Aq.Tc which amounted to 7.5 mg/kg (Figure 1A).

Tumor assessment studies

Tumor statistics

At the end of the treatment period (22 weeks), the lung tissue/lung tumors were excised and analyzed for (*a*) tumor incidence (*b*) tumor size (*c*) tumor multiplicity following the protocol of Gupta et al (36).

Histopathological evaluation

Lung tissue/tumors were excised at the end of 10th and 22nd weeks, fixed in 10% formaldehyde in phosphate buffer saline (pH 7.4) for Haematoxylin and eosin (H&E) staining as per the conventional laboratory procedures (37). H&E stained slides were evaluated under light

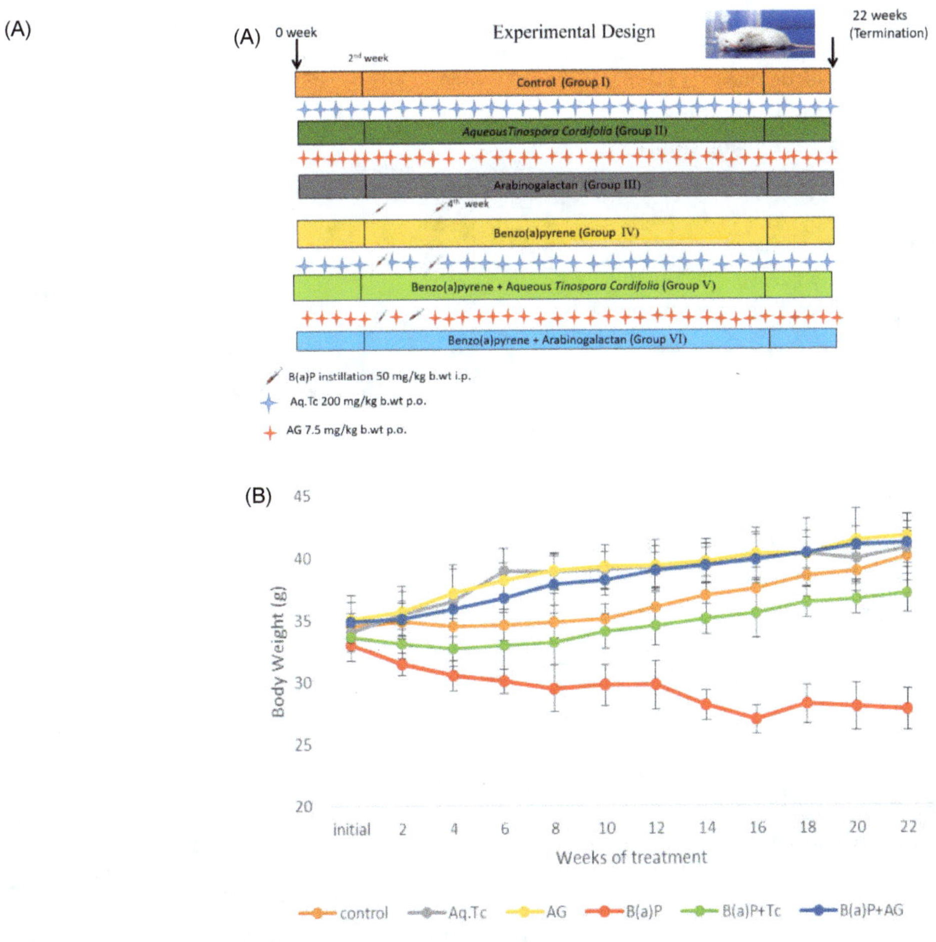

Figure 1. (A) Animal treatment schedule to study the effect of Aq.Tc and AG in B(a)P induced pulmonary carcinogenesis. (B) Alterations in average body weight of the animals during the treatment period. Data were represented as Mean ± S.D. (n=6-10)

microscope (LEICA DM 3000).

Tumor markers

Various tumor markers were estimated in the plasma/serum of mice from different treatment groups. Blood samples from the mice of various treatment groups were collected by retro-orbital puncture. Prior to retro-orbital puncture, a drop of 0.5% pro-paracaine hydrochloride ophthalmic solution (Sunways Pvt. Ltd. India) was applied to anesthetize the eyes so that pain was reduced.

Carcinoembryonic antigen

Quantification of tumor marker CEA was estimated in blood serum using the Qayee-Bio Mouse carcinoembryonic antigen ELISA kit. The detection range of the kit lies between 78 pg/mL to 5000 pg/mL.

Circulating tumor DNA

Circulating tumor DNA was quantified using the FitAmp™ Circulating DNA Quantification kit for mouse. The linear detection range of the kit lies between 0.1 ng to 100 ng (1-1000 ng/mL) in 96-well plate assay. DNA was fluorescently quantified at Ex 480-500 and Em 520-550 nm using a fluorescence microplate reader (Biotek Synergy H1 microplate reader).

Lactate dehydrogenase

The specific activity of Lactate dehydrogenase (LDH) in blood serum was estimated according to the method described by Bergmeyer and Bernt (38) using molar extinction coefficient 6.22 $mM^{-1}cm^{-1}$.

Quantification of tumor necrosis factor-alpha

Quantitative estimation of tumor necrosis factor-α (TNF-α) in blood serum samples of various treatment groups was carried out by using *in vitro* enzyme linked immunosorbent assay (ELISA) (Ray Biotech). The minimum detectable dose of mouse TNF-α is 30 pg/ml.

TUNEL assay

The TUNEL assay was performed on deparaffinised and rehydrated lung sections with the TACS-XL DAB *in situ* apoptosis detection kit according to the manufacturer's specifications. Apoptotic index was calculated as the percentage of TUNEL (+ve) cells were quantified over the total number of cells in the selected lung tissue section.

Statistical analysis

The data were represented as mean ± standard deviation (SD). and analysed by one-way ANOWA followed by LSD post hoc test using the SPSS software package (version 16) for windows (SPSS Inc., Chicago, IL).

Results

Phytochemical screening

In the present study, preliminary phytochemical analysis of Aq.Tc stem extract showed the presence of alkaloids, phenols, flavonoids, carbohydrates, and proteins. However, steroids were found to be absent in the extract.

Free radical scavenging activity

In DPPH and ABTS free radical scavenging assay Aq.Tc extract exhibited free radical scavenging activity in a concentration dependent manner when compared with other strong antioxidants like BHT and tannic acid (Figure 2A and 2B). It showed a higher antiradical activity with IC_{50} of 432 μg and 49.8 μg in DPPH and ABTS assays, respectively. However, AG showed a greater antiradical activity at higher concentrations when compared with Aq.Tc, BHT and tannic acid. The IC_{50} of AG was found to be 648 μg and 384.17 μg in DPPH and ABTS assay, respectively (Table 1).

Body status, diet and water intake

Mice in all the experimental groups did not show any significant change in the diet and water consumption throughout the treatment period. A considerable decrease in the body weight of animals in B(a)P group was observed when compared with their control counterparts. There was no significant difference in the body growth patterns in animals treated with Aq.Tc and AG i.e., Aq.Tc, AG, B(a)P + Aq.Tc and B(a)P + AG group when compared with control group (Figure 1B).

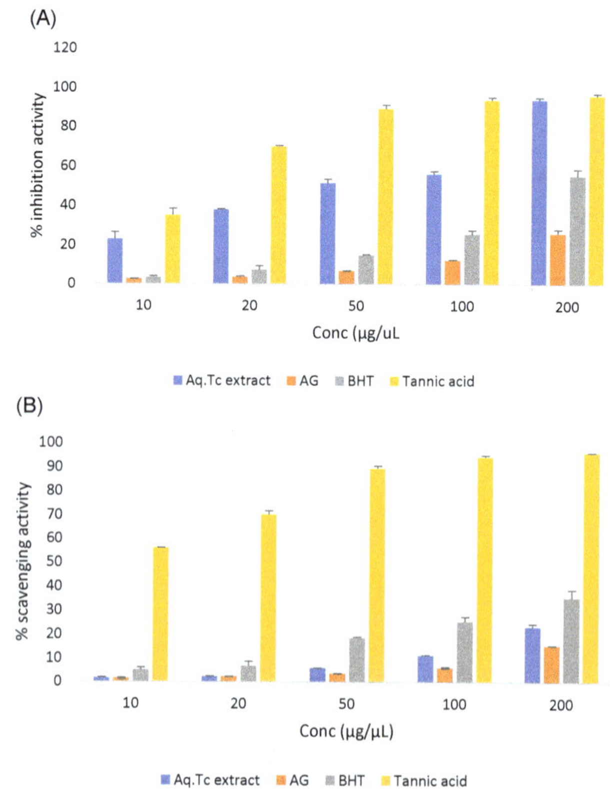

Figure 2. (A) Radical scavenging effects of Aq.Tc. Extract and AG on ABTS radicals. (B) Radical scavenging effects of Aq.Tc. extract and AG on DPPH radicals. Data were represented as mean ± SD (n = 3).

Table 1. IC_{50} values of Aq.Tc. extract, AG, BHT and tannic acid using ABTS and DPPH scavenging activity

Extract/ Compound	IC_{50} value (μg/μL) ABTS assay	IC_{50} values (μg/μL) DPPH assay
Tannic acid	14.24	103.21
BHT	49.80	282.40
Aq.Tc	180.66	432.52
AG	384.17	648.50

Morphological changes in lung/lung tumors

Normal architecture was observed in Aq.Tc and AG treated lung when compared with control animals (Figure 3A). However, in B(a)P challenged mice lung, large number of superficial lesions and hematomas were observed. Prominent tumor nodules around different lobes of lung were also present (Figure 3B). Mice bearing tumors co-administered with Aq.Tc and AG showed a significant reduction in tumor nodules and tumor mass (Figure 3C, D, E and F, respectively).

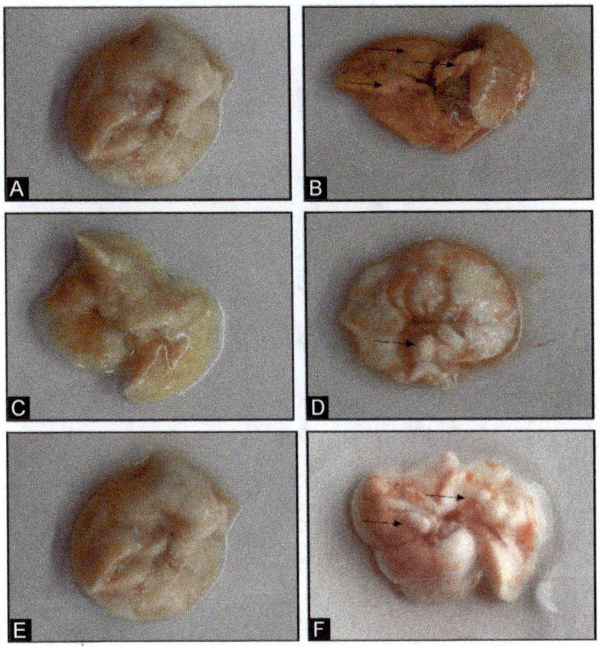

Figure 3. Gross morphology of lungs in mice of different treatment groups.
(A) Control, **(B)** Pulmonary lesions in B(a)P treated mice, **(C),** Aq.Tc, **(D)** B(a)P treated mice co-administered with Aq.Tc. extract, **(E)** AG, **(F)** B(a)P treated mice co-administered with AG. (arrow indicates tumor).

Tumor statistics

After 22 weeks of the B(a)P treatment, the mice from B(a)P, B(a)P +Aq.Tc and B(a)P + AG group developed lung tumors, whereas no tumor/lesion was observed in control, Aq.Tc and AG group.

The total number of tumors/lesions formed in various experimental groups and the associated parameters are summarised in Table 2.

Histopathology

Tenth week of B(a)P treatment showed loss of normal pulmonary architecture and higher number of hyper chromatic nuclei with air space enlargement (Figure 4B). However, in animals from B(a)P +Aq.Tc and B(a)P+AG groups showed decreased number of hyperchromatic irregular cells in the alveolar wall at 10th week of treatment (Figure 4D-F). Histopathological changes in the pulmonary tissue at 22nd week post instillation of B(a)P revealed extensive proliferation of alveolar epithelium, large number of eosinophilic macrophages infiltrating the pulmonary parenchyma with more number of hyper chromatic nuclei in the alveolar wall (Figure 5B). Number of hyperproliferative cells in B(a)P + Aq.Tc and B(a)P + AG group decreased when compared to B(a)P group at 22nd week of treatment (Figure 5D-F).

Tumor markers

Carcinoembryonic antigen

Instillation of B(a)P showed a significant ($P \leq 0.001$) increase in the CEA levels in a time dependent manner when compared with the rest of the groups (158±1.36 to 288± 21.0 pg/mL). However, in B(a)P+AG group the increase was less intense (162±6.20 to 228±2.12 pg/mL). Interestingly, the levels of CEA in B(a)P +Aq.Tc group dropped from 165±6.20 to 143±16.4 pg/mL (Table 3).

Circulating tumor DNA

A significant increase in ctDNA levels was observed in B(a)P group at different time intervals when compared with other respective groups (1.15±0.012 to 3.28±0.140 ng/mL). However, Aq.Tc administration to the cancer bearing animals, significantly ($P \leq 0.001$) lowered the

Table 2. Effect of Aq.Tc and AG on B(a)P induced lung tumorigenesis at end of the treatment period where (n=6-10)

Parameters/Groups	Control	Aq.Tc	AG	B(a)P	B(a)P+Aq.Tc	B(a)P+AG
Tumor incidence (%)	-	-	-	100%	66.6%	83.3%
Tumor multiplicity	-	-	-	2.45±0.365	1.22±0.057 *	1.52±0.125 **
Total no of tumors	-	-	-	96	53	71
Big tumors (>2 mm)	-	-	-	83	44	63
Small tumors (<2 mm)	-	-	-	13	9	8

Data is expressed as Mean±SD and are analysed by Student's *t* test.
* $P \leq 0.01$, ** $P < 0.05$ with regard to B(a)P.

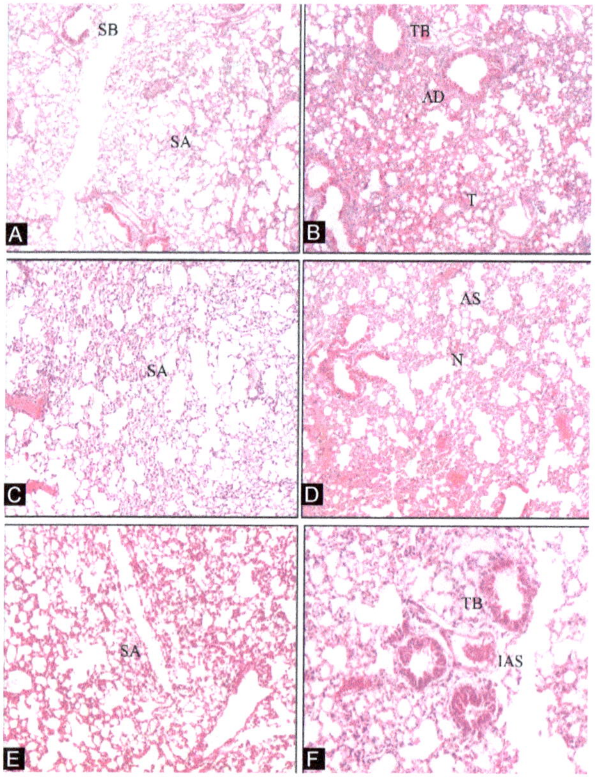

Figure 4. Hematoxylin and eosin stained lung tissue at 10th week of treatment at 200 X.
(A). Control mice showing normal histoarchitecture, (**B**) B(a)P treated mice, (**C**) Aq.Tc treated mice, (**D**) B(a)P installed mice co-treated with Aq.Tc, (**E**) AG treated mice, **(F)** B(a)P installed mice co-treated with AG. **SB**; small bronchiole, **SA**; single squamous epithelium, **AW**; alveolar wall, **AS**; alveolar space, **AD**; Widespread alveolar destruction, **N**; thinning of alveolar walls, **T**; thickening of alveolar wall, **IAS**; increased alveolar sac, **TB**; thickened bronchiolar epithelium.

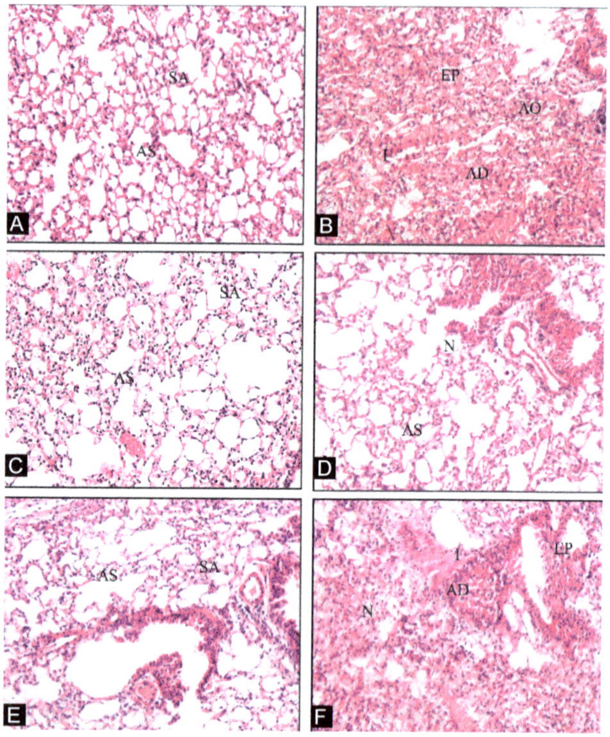

Figure 5. Haematoxylin and Eosin stained lung tissue/lung tumors at 200X.
(A) Control mice showing normal histoarchitecture, **(B)** B(a)P treated mice, **(C)** Aq.Tc treated mice, **(D)** B(a)P induced tumor co-treated with Aq.Tc, **(E)** AG treated mice, **(F)** B(a)P induced tumor co-treated with AG. (**EP:** extensive proliferation of alveolar epithelium and presence of hyperchromatic nuclei in the alveolar wall; **SB**; small bronchiole, **SA**; single squamous epithelium, **AW**; alveolar wall, **AS**; alveolar space, **AD**; Widespread alveolar destruction, **N**; thinning of alveolar walls, **T**; thickening of alveolar wall, **IAS**; increased alveolar sac, **TB**; thickened bronchiolar epithelium, **I**; Inflammatory cellular infiltrations.

levels of ctDNA to their near normal values. Also, the levels of ctDNA were found to significantly ($P \leq 0.001$) decreased in B(a)P + AG animals when compared to the B(a)P group (Table 3).

Lactate dehydrogenase

A significant increase in LDH activity in B(a)P group was observed when compared to various treatment groups (259 ± 54.1 to 628 ± 16.5 IU/L). However, treatment of Aq.Tc to the cancer bearing animals significantly ($P \leq 0.001$) restored the levels of LDH to their near normal values. Also, the levels of LDH were found to significantly ($P \leq 0.001$) reduced in B(a)P+AG animals when compared to the B(a)P group (Table 3).

Quantification of TNF-alpha

TNF-alpha levels were significantly increased in B(a)P group when compared to control, Tc and AG groups at different time intervals. Whereas, Aq.Tc treatment to cancer bearing animals significantly ($P \leq 0.001$) restored the level of TNF-alpha to their near normal values. Also, the levels of TNF-alpha significantly decreased ($P \leq 0.001$) in B(a)P+AG animals when compared to the B(a)P group (Table 3).

TUNEL assay

A significant increase in the apoptotic index in B(a)P + Aq.Tc group was observed when compared with rest of the four groups i.e., control, AG, B(a)P and Aq.Tc. There was a significant increase in extent of apoptosis in B(a)P + AG group but much less than the B(a)P + Aq.Tc group (Figure 6A,B).

Discussion

Lung and the associated respiratory system is the prime target of the inhaled contaminated air which include pollutants and carcinogens like B(a)P that have been established as important etiological agents in causation of lung cancers (39). Majority of lung cancers are diagnosed at late stages when the options for treatment are mostly palliative (40). Management of lung cancer requires monitoring of the tumor burden to determine the response to treatment and therefore, improved biomarkers are

Table 3. Effect of Aq.Tc and AG on various blood tumor markers at different time intervals during B(a)P induced lung tumorigenesis

Parameters/Groups	Weeks	Control	Aq.Tc	AG	B(a)P	B(a)P+Aq.Tc	B(a)P+AG
CEA (pg/ml)	0	160.5± 1.56	160.3±9.30	164.5±6.82	159.5±1.36	162.2±10.7	162.9±6.20
	10	164.8± 4.54	146.8±12.9	168.1±11.73	251.1±8.64 $a_1b_1c_1$	165.5±11.6 d_1	205.3±11.0 c_3e_3
	22	164.2±5.49	176.0±15.4	174±6.57	288.3±21.0 $a_3b_1c_1$	143.1±16.4 d_1	228.7±2.12 b_2d_2
ctDNA (ng/ml)	0	1.28±0.012	1.11±0.013	1.21±0.010	1.15±0.012	1.17±0.010	1.19±0.020
	10	1.29±0.015	1.27±0.062	1.34±0.219	2.95±0.060 $a_1b_1c_1$	1.65±0.189 $a_1b_1c_1d_1$	2.37±0.210 $a_1b_1c_1d_2$
	22	1.41±0.010	1.30±0.010	1.31±0.005	3.28±0.140 $a_1b_1c_1$	2.33±0.100 d_1	2.52±0.136 $a_1b_1c_1d_2e_2$
LDH(IU/L)	0	249.5±58.8	304.0±33.9	278.1±45.6	259.1±54.1	259.9±53.0	252.1±51.9
	10	233.9±63.8	311.8±46.7	278.1±50.7	688.7±50.7 $a_1b_1c_1$	465.2±62.5 $a_2b_2c_2d_2$	491.2±56.2 $a_2b_2c_2d_2$
	22	246.9±67.2	218.3±48.6	155.4±41.2	628.9±16.5 $a_2b_2c_1$	293.7±16.2 d_3	343.3±27.0 d_3
TNF-α (pg/ml)	0	44.6±0.01	46.1±0.01	48.2±2.99	45.4±2.30	44.0±1.70	46.4±2.83
	10	46.0±2.35	46.3±2.71	43.6±2.02	59.6±2.91 $a_1b_1c_1$	49.6±2.04 c_1d_1	49.4±1.55 c_2d_1
	22	44.6±2.64	46.2±2.71	48.2±2.11	66.9±4.16 $a_1b_1c_1$	49.8±0.20 d_1	51.2±1.44 a_3d_1

Data is expressed as Mean ± SD (n = 6-8). Data is analysed using one-way ANOVA followed by post-hoc test. a_1 $P \leq 0.001$, a_2 $P \leq 0.01$, a_3 $P \leq 0.05$ significant with respect to control group; b_1 $P \leq 0.001$, b_2 $P \leq 0.01$ significant with respect to Tc group; c_1 $P \leq 0.001$, c_2 $P \leq 0.01$, c_3 $P \leq 0.05$ significant with respect to Arb group; d_1 $P \leq 0.001$, d_2 $P \leq 0.01$, significant with respect to B(a)P group; e_2 $P \leq 0.01$, e_3 $P \leq 0.05$ significant with respect to B(a)P+ Tc group.

needed (41). The present study was aimed to evaluate the efficacy of Aq.Tc extract and its active component, AG, in B(a)P induced lung tumorigenesis and to demonstrate the effect on various plasma/serum markers at different stages of pulmonary carcinogenesis.

To assess the chemopreventive efficacy of Aq.Tc/AG in *in vivo* system various parameters were studied in Balb/c mice pulmonary tumor model. The considerable weight loss observed in tumor bearing mice could be related to cancer cachexia, anorexia or malabsorption, which resulted in wasting of skeletal muscle and adipose tissue (42). Several studies have shown similar observations of decrease in body weight of animals following administration of B(a) P (43). However, Aq.Tc and AG seem to prevent this alteration in body weight of lung tumor bearing mice.

Chemopreventive response of Aq.Tc and AG administered animals challenged with B(a)P induced carcinogenesis was monitored on the basis of tumor incidence, multiplicity, size and gross morphology. All these parameters serve as a valuable reference to study the development of carcinogenesis in *in vivo* studies. Aq.Tc was successful in reducing the extent of carcinogenesis as depicted by different parameters like tumor morphology, multiplicity and incidence when compared to B(a)P group. Mean number of large and small tumors was also observed to be significantly altered in Aq.Tc treated animals. However, in B(a)P+AG mice less reduction in mean number of small tumors was observed but the number of large tumors varied, significantly. Earlier studies also supported our observation depicting that various plant extracts were successful in reducing lung adenoma incidence and multiplicity induced by B(a)P in mice. To the best of our knowledge no reports are available of chemopreventive effects of Aq.Tc extract and AG in in vivo lung tumor model.

Mode of cell death can be a useful parameter to assess the severity of the cancer (44). Dysregulation of apoptosis is pivotal to tumorigenesis and the development of most cancers (45). Aq.Tc treated animals bearing tumors revealed enhanced apoptosis in comparison to the B(a) P treated mice bearing pulmonary tumors. Increase in apoptotic index may also be responsible for the decrease in the size of the tumors in the B(a)P+Aq.Tc group. The induction of apoptosis by Aq.Tc extract has already been documented in the literature as a potential candidate in therapy to glioblastomas (46). Pure active component AG of *T. cordifolia* was found to be less effective in inducing apoptosis in lung tumor bearing mice. Our lab also reported the induction of apoptosis by using different plant extracts in cancer models (47).

Pro-inflammatory cytokines such as TNF-α are the major molecular players involved in inflammation to cancer axis. As a representative inflammatory cytokine with pleiotropic functions, TNF-α plays a dual role in carcinogenesis (48). In the present study, the gradual increased levels of TNF-α at 10th and 22nd week of treatment in lung cancer bearing animals may be due to pronounced inflammatory response and increased cell

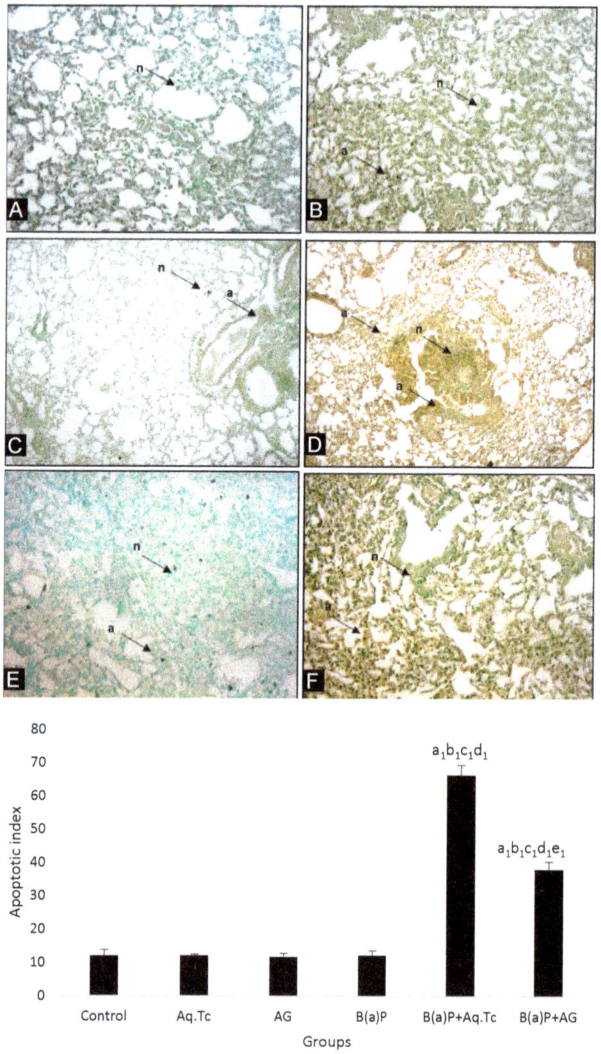

Figure 6. (**A**) TUNEL assay performed in paraffin embedded lung/tumor tissue sections at 200X.
a. Control, **b**. Benzo(a)pyrene, **c**. *Tinospora cordifolia* extract, **d**. Benzo(a)pyrene+ *Tinospora cordifolia* extract group, **e**. AG treated, **f**. Benzo(a)pyrene+ AG treated group.
Green stained cells represent non-apoptotic cells (**n**), brown stained cells represent apoptotic cells (**a**). (**B**) Attenuation in apoptotic index of B(a)P induced lung tumors and its chemoprevention by Aq.Tc and AG.
Data is represented as mean ± SD (n= 5) and analysed by one-way ANOVA followed by the post hoc test. Statistical significance and symbols: a_1 $P \leq 0.001$ w.rt control group; b_1 $P \leq 0.001$ w.rt B(a)P group; c_1 $P \leq 0.001$ w.rt Aq.Tc group.

death by B(a)P administration. Also, there is increasing evidence that TNF-α is mainly produced by cancers and act as an endogenous tumor promoter (49). Studies have shown that B(a)P administration promotes the increase of TNF-α levels in pulmonary tumor bearing mice (50). At 10th week of Aq.Tc and AG treatment to cancer bearing animals significantly downregulated the levels of TNF-α to near normal values. The results of the present study are in collaboration with several other reports which suggested that *T. cordifolia* administration to cancer bearing mice downregulated the levels of TNF-α suggesting the immunomodulating activity of *T. cordifolia* extract (51). Surprisingly, there was no change in TNF-α levels after 10th week of the treatment protocol in B(a)P +Aq.Tc and B(a)P +AG treated groups which could be because of higher apoptotic index found in both these groups.

LDH is a sensitive marker for solid tumors and enhanced activity of this enzyme has been reported in serum of various lung tumor patients (52). Serum LDH was observed to be increased at the promotion stage (10th week) followed by progression stage (22nd week) of tumorigenesis in B(a)P treated mice which could be due to the increased glycolysis in cancerous conditions or the cellular leakage of these enzymes in circulation. Our results are in agreement with earlier findings which depicted that B(a)P administration increased the levels of LDH in cancer bearing animals (53). A subsequent decrease in LDH activity on treatment with Aq.Tc aids in the protection against abnormal cell growth by changing the permeability of membrane or by affecting the cellular growth of the tumor. Our lab also reported, reduction of pulmonary and serum levels of LDH upon administration of *Aloe vera* gel extract to cigarette smoke exposed mice (54). In the present study, AG administration was less efficient in normalising the LDH activity when compared to the Aq.Tc extract. AG was found to be less effective in protecting the membrane permeability and cellular proliferation of cells damaged by B(a)P insult.

CEA is one of the extensively studied tumor markers which has also shown prognostic value and has been found to overexpress on the cell surface of malignant epithelial-type (55). It is considered as a sensitive tumor marker for diagnosis, prognosis, and therapy monitoring of lung cancer (56). Gradual increase in serum CEA levels (10th and 22nd week) in B(a)P installed animals was observed which could be associated with increase in tumor growth and cellular proliferation rate. Available literature also suggests that CEA levels increase concomitantly in lung tumor bearing mice (53). Reduction in levels of CEA in Aq.tc and AG treated animals could be due to decrease in tumor growth that reveal the anti-tumor effects of these compounds. Reduction in levels of CEA was more pronounced in B(a)P+Aq.Tc than B(a)P+AG group which shows Aq.Tc extract has more potent anticancer activity. An earlier finding suggested that thymoquinone, which is the main active constituent of black seed and essential oil, reduced the serum CEA levels in benzo(a) pyrene induced lung cancer (57).

Evaluation of plasma ctDNA is a promising diagnostic and prognostic marker which circumvents the complications associated with use of invasive techniques used for biological sampling (58). In the present study, a spike in ctDNA concentration was prominent at 10th week of the treatment with B(a)P administration which could be because of the increase in necrosis of tumor cells, or release of the intact cells into the bloodstream and their lysis. Further increase in ctDNA in lung tumor bearing animals at 22nd week of the treatment could be because of the severe progression of the tumor cells or the increase of micro metastatic cells in the blood, which can also shed their DNA into the blood circulation (59). A significant drop in ctDNA level was visible in Aq.Tc treated animals which almost reached the level observed in normal healthy animals. Also, in animals treated with AG, the drop in ctDNA level was not as striking as compared to Aq.Tc treated animals bearing pulmonary tumors. This decrease in DNA level is either because plasma DNA is released at lower rates or is due to rapid degrade. ctDNA release in blood stream could be also correlated to the mode of cell death as its concentration depends whether the cell is undergoing apoptotic cell death or necrotic cell death (60). Histopathological findings were also in concordance with altered levels of CEA, LDH, ctDNA and TNF-α, which showed profound increase in their levels at different stages of carcinogenesis.

Conclusion: Our findings suggest that a concaminant increase in various tumor markers like CEA, ctDNA, LDH and TNF-alpha at different stages of carcinogenesis correlates well with the histopathological changes observed at early and late stages of B(a)P induced lung cancer. Aq.Tc successfully improved the various blood markers and decreased the severity of the disease as revealed by histopathological and other parameters. Although AG modulated the above mentioned parameters but Aq.Tc seemed to be much more effective as a chemopreventive agent. The histopathological findings in the present study are in concordance with the biochemical observations and are suggestive of the fact that Aq.Tc and AG have a potential as chemopreventive agents in pulmonary carcinogenesis.

Acknowledgement

We express our heartfelt gratitude to the Department of Biophysics, Panjab University, Chandigarh, India for providing the necessary facilities and assistance to carry out this research work.

Authors' contributions

The idea of the study, its design and interpretation to come to a conclusion were done by AK and VM. However, the experimental procedures were done by VM under the guidance of AK. Both contribute in preparation of the manuscript and agreed publication of the final proof.

Conflict of interests

Authors declare no conflict of interests.

Ethical considerations

Ethical issues have been observed by the authors. The experimental animal studies were approved by the ethical committee, Panjab University, Chandigarh, India (Approval no PU/IAEC/S/15/61 Panjab University, Chandigarh) and were conducted adhering to the Indian National Science Academy Guidelines for the use and care of experimental studies.

Funding/Support

This research was financially supported by the University Grants Commission (UGC) BSR fellowship, New Delhi (India).

References

1. Siegel RL, Miller KD, Jemal A. Cancer statistics, 2016. CA Cancer J Clin. 2016;66(1):7-30. doi: 10.3322/caac.21332.
2. Dela Cruz CS, Tanoue LT, Matthay RA. Lung cancer: epidemiology, etiology, and prevention. Clin Chest Med. 2011;32(4):605-44. doi: 10.1016/j.ccm.2011.09.001.
3. Abdel-Shafy HI, Mansour MSM. A review on polycyclic aromatic hydrocarbons: Source, environmental impact, effect on human health and remediation. Egypt J Petrol. 2016;25(1):107-23. doi: 10.1016/j.ejpe.2015.03.011.
4. Kasala ER, Bodduluru LN, Barua CC, Sriram CS, Gogoi R. Benzo(a)pyrene induced lung cancer: Role of dietary phytochemicals in chemoprevention. Pharmacol Rep. 2015;67(5):996-1009. doi: 10.1016/j.pharep.2015.03.004.
5. Shi X, Liu H, Song Y. Pollutional haze as a potential cause of lung cancer. J Thorac Dis. 2015;7(10):E412-7. doi: 10.3978/j.issn.2072-1439.2015.05.04.
6. Bourgioti C, Chatoupis K, Moulopoulos LA. Current imaging strategies for the evaluation of uterine cervical cancer. World J Radiol. 2016;8(4):342-54. doi: 10.4329/wjr.v8.i4.342.
7. Liu L, Teng J, Zhang L, Cong P, Yao Y, Sun G, et al. The Combination of the Tumor Markers Suggests the Histological Diagnosis of Lung Cancer. Biomed Res Int. 2017;2017:2013989. doi: 10.1155/2017/2013989.
8. Xiang D, Zhang B, Doll D, Shen K, Kloecker G, Freter C. Lung cancer screening: from imaging to biomarker. Biomark Res. 2013;1(1):4. doi: 10.1186/2050-7771-1-4.
9. Yu D, Du K, Liu T, Chen G. Prognostic value of tumor markers, NSE, CA125 and SCC, in operable NSCLC Patients. Int J Mol Sci. 2013;14(6):11145-56. doi: 10.3390/ijms140611145.
10. Mehta S, Shelling A, Muthukaruppan A, Lasham A, Blenkiron C, Laking G, et al. Predictive and prognostic molecular markers for cancer medicine. Ther Adv Med Oncol. 2010;2(2):125-48. doi: 10.1177/1758834009360519.
11. Arora N, Koul A. A 'complex solution' to a 'complex' problem: tackling the complexity of cancer with botanicals. Eur J Cancer Prev. 2014;23(6):568-78. doi: 10.1097/cej.0000000000000045.
12. Sofowora A, Ogunbodede E, Onayade A. The role and place of medicinal plants in the strategies for disease prevention. Afr J Tradit Complement Altern Med. 2013;10(5):210-29.
13. Maresso KC, Tsai KY, Brown PH, Szabo E, Lippman S, Hawk ET. Molecular cancer prevention: Current status and future directions. CA Cancer J Clin. 2015;65(5):345-83. doi: 10.3322/caac.21287.
14. Safarzadeh E, Sandoghchian Shotorbani S, Baradaran B. Herbal medicine as inducers of apoptosis in cancer

treatment. Adv Pharm Bull. 2014;4(Suppl 1):421-7. doi: 10.5681/apb.2014.062.
15. Koul A, Gangar SC, Sandhir V. Pitfalls in journey from traditional to modern medicine. Nat Prod Radiance. 2005;4(1):6-13.
16. Greenwell M, Rahman PK. Medicinal Plants: Their Use in Anticancer Treatment. Int J Pharm Sci Res. 2015;6(10):4103-12. doi: 10.13040/ijpsr.0975-8232.6(10).4103-12.
17. Prakash O, Kumar A, Kumar P, Ajeet A. Anticancer Potential of Plants and Natural Products: A Review. Am J Pharmacol Sci. 2013;1(6):104-15. doi: 10.12691/ajps-1-6-1.
18. Sinha K, Mishra NP, Singh J, Khanuja SPS. *Tinospora cordifolia* (Guduchi), a reservoir plant for therapeutic applications: a review. Indian J Tradit Knowl. 2004;3(3):257-70.
19. Bahadur S, Mukherjee PK, Milan Ahmmed SK, Kar A, Harwansh RK, Pandit S. Metabolism-mediated interaction potential of standardized extract of *Tinospora cordifolia* through rat and human liver microsomes. Indian J Pharmacol. 2016;48(5):576-81. doi: 10.4103/0253-7613.190758.
20. Saha S, Ghosh S. *Tinospora cordifolia*: one plant, many roles. Anc Sci Life. 2012;31(4):151-9. doi: 10.4103/0257-7941.107344.
21. Patni K. The amazing pharmacological properties of *Tinospora cordifolia* - A short review. Int J Ayu Pharm Chem. 2015;4(2):105-29.
22. Handique PJ. In vitro propagation and medicinal attributes of *Tinospora cordifolia*: A review. Austin J Biotechnol Bioeng. 2014;1(5):5.
23. Jagetia GC, Rao SK. Evaluation of the antineoplastic activity of guduchi (*Tinospora cordifolia*) in Ehrlich ascites carcinoma bearing mice. Biol Pharm Bull. 2006;29(3):460-6.
24. Uppuluri S, Ali SL, Nirmala T, Santhi M, Sipai Babu SD. A Review on *Tinospora cordifolia*. International Journal of Current Pharmaceutical Review and Research. 2013;4(2):61-8.
25. Dion C, Chappuis E, Ripoll C. Does larch arabinogalactan enhance immune function? A review of mechanistic and clinical trials. Nutr Metab (Lond). 2016;13:28. doi: 10.1186/s12986-016-0086-x.
26. Shakhtshneider TP, Kuznetsova SA, Zamay AS, Zamay TN, Spivak EA, Mikhailenko MA, et al. New composites of betulin esters with arabinogalactan as highly potent anti-cancer agents. Nat Prod Res. 2016;30(12):1382-7. doi: 10.1080/14786419.2015.1060591.
27. Chaudhari S, Shaikh N. Gaduchi-The Best Ayurvedic Herb. The Pharma Innovation Journal. 2013;2(4):97-102.
28. Nair PK, Rodriguez S, Ramachandran R, Alamo A, Melnick SJ, Escalon E, et al. Immune stimulating properties of a novel polysaccharide from the medicinal plant *Tinospora cordifolia*. Int Immunopharmacol. 2004;4(13):1645-59. doi: 10.1016/j.intimp.2004.07.024.
29. Leyon PV, Kuttan G. Effect of *Tinospora cordifolia* on the cytokine profile of angiogenesis-induced animals. Int Immunopharmacol. 2004;4(13):1569-75. doi: 10.1016/j.intimp.2004.06.015.
30. Tiwari P, Kumar B, Kumar M, Kaur M, Debnath J, Sharma P. Comparative Anthelmintic Activity of Aqueous and Ethanolic Stem Extract of *Tinospora cordifolia*. Int J Drug Dev Res. 2011;3(1):70-83.
31. Mishra R, Kaur G. Aqueous ethanolic extract of *Tinospora cordifolia* as a potential candidate for differentiation based therapy of glioblastomas. PLoS One. 2013;8(10):e78764. doi: 10.1371/journal.pone.0078764.
32. Kokate CK. Pratical Pharmacognosy. New Delhi: Vallabh Prakan; 1994.
33. Sudha G, Priya MS, Rajan-Babu IS, Vadivukkarasi S. In vitro free radical scavenging activity of raw pepino fruit (*Solanum muricatum* Aiton). Int J Curr Pharm Res. 2011;3(2):137-40.
34. Re R, Pellegrini N, Proteggente A, Pannala A, Yang M, Rice-Evans C. Antioxidant activity applying an improved ABTS radical cation decolorization assay. Free Radic Biol Med. 1999;26(9-10):1231-7.
35. Mathew S, Kuttan G. Immunomodulatory and antitumour activities of *Tinospora cordifolia*. Fitoterapia. 1999;70(1):35-43. doi: 10.1016/S0367-326X(98)00017-3.
36. Gupta P, Bansal MP, Koul A. Evaluating the effect of lycopene from Lycopersicum esculentum on apoptosis during NDEA induced hepatocarcinogenesis. Biochem Biophys Res Commun. 2013;434(3):479-85. doi: 10.1016/j.bbrc.2013.03.099.
37. Humanson GL. Animal tissue techniques. 2nd ed. San Fransisco, USA: W.H Freeman; 1961.
38. Bergmeyer HU, Bernt E. Lactate-dehydrogenase, UV-assay with pyruvate and NADH. In: Bergmeyer HU, ed. Methods of Enzymatic Analysis. New York: Academic Press; 1974;2:574-9.
39. Field RW, Withers BL. Occupational and environmental causes of lung cancer. Clin Chest Med. 2012;33(4):681-703. doi: 10.1016/j.ccm.2012.07.001.
40. Farbicka P, Nowicki A. Palliative care in patients with lung cancer. Contemp Oncol (Pozn). 2013;17(3):238-45. doi: 10.5114/wo.2013.35033.
41. Dawson SJ, Tsui DW, Murtaza M, Biggs H, Rueda OM, Chin SF, et al. Analysis of circulating tumor DNA to monitor metastatic breast cancer. N Engl J Med. 2013;368(13):1199-209. doi: 10.1056/NEJMoa1213261.
42. Aoyagi T, Terracina KP, Raza A, Matsubara H, Takabe K. Cancer cachexia, mechanism and treatment. World J Gastrointest Oncol. 2015;7(4):17-29. doi: 10.4251/wjgo.v7.i4.17.
43. Anandakumar P, Kamaraj S, Ramakrishnan G, Jagan S, Devaki T. Chemopreventive task of capsaicin against benzo(a)pyrene-induced lung cancer in Swiss albino mice. Basic Clin Pharmacol Toxicol. 2009;104(5):360-5. doi: 10.1111/j.1742-7843.2009.00387.x.
44. Fulda S, Gorman AM, Hori O, Samali A. Cellular stress responses: cell survival and cell death. Int J Cell Biol. 2010;2010:214074. doi: 10.1155/2010/214074.
45. Ravichandran N, Suresh G, Ramesh B, Manikandan R, Choi YW, Vijaiyan Siva G. Fisetin modulates mitochondrial enzymes and apoptotic signals in benzo(a)pyrene-induced lung cancer. Mol Cell Biochem. 2014;390(1-2):225-34. doi: 10.1007/s11010-014-1973-y.
46. Pendse VK, Dadhich AP, Mathur PN, Bal MS, Madan BR. Anti-inflammatory immunosuppressive and sme related pharmacological actions of the water extract of Neem

Giloe (*Tinospora cordifolia*): A preliminary report. Ind J Pharmacol. 1977;9:221-4.

47. Koul A, Mohan V, Bharati S. Azadirachta indica mitigates DMBA-induced hepatotoxicity: A biochemical and radiometric study. Indian J Biochem Biophys. 2014;51:37-45.
48. Landskron G, De la Fuente M, Thuwajit P, Thuwajit C, Hermoso MA. Chronic inflammation and cytokines in the tumor microenvironment. J Immunol Res. 2014;2014:149185. doi: 10.1155/2014/149185.
49. Wang X, Lin Y. Tumor necrosis factor and cancer, buddies or foes? Acta Pharmacol Sin. 2008;29(11):1275-88. doi: 10.1111/j.1745-7254.2008.00889.x.
50. Anandakumar P, Kamaraj S, Jagan S, Ramakrishnan G, Asokkumar S, Naveenkumar C, et al. Capsaicin inhibits benzo(a)pyrene-induced lung carcinogenesis in an in vivo mouse model. Inflamm Res. 2012;61(11):1169-75. doi: 10.1007/s00011-012-0511-1.
51. Naveenkumar C, Raghunandhakumar S, Asokkumar S, Devaki T. Baicalein abrogates reactive oxygen species (ROS)-mediated mitochondrial dysfunction during experimental pulmonary carcinogenesis in vivo. Basic Clin Pharmacol Toxicol. 2013;112(4):270-81. doi: 10.1111/bcpt.12025.
52. Radhakrishnan VK, Ravikumar V, Shivashangari KS, Kamaraj S, Devaki T. Chemopreventive Role of Lycopene and D-arginine in Benzo (a) Pyrene Induced Lung Cancer with Reference to Lipid Peroxidation, Antioxidant System and Tumor Marker Enzymes. Int J Cancer Res. 2006;2(3):224-33. doi: 10.3923/ijcr.2006.224.233.
53. Kamaraj S, Ramakrishnan G, Anandakumar P, Jagan S, Devaki T. Antioxidant and anticancer efficacy of hesperidin in benzo(a)pyrene induced lung carcinogenesis in mice. Invest New Drugs. 2009;27(3):214-22. doi: 10.1007/s10637-008-9159-7.
54. Koul A, Bala S, Yasmeen, Arora N. *Aloe vera* affects changes induced in pulmonary tissue of mice caused by cigarette smoke inhalation. Environ Toxicol. 2015;30(9):999-1013. doi: 10.1002/tox.21973.
55. Veronesi G, Pelosi G, Sonzogni A, Leon ME, D'Aiuto M, Gasparri R et al. Tumour CEA as predictor of better outcome in squamous cell carcinoma of the lung. Lung Cancer.2005; 48:233–240, doi:10.1016/j.lung can.2004.10.018.
56. Shao Y, Sun X, He Y, Liu C, Liu H. Elevated Levels of Serum Tumor Markers CEA and CA15-3 Are Prognostic Parameters for Different Molecular Subtypes of Breast Cancer. PLoS One. 2015;10(7):e0133830. doi: 10.1371/journal.pone.0133830.
57. Hussein SA, Abdel-Aal SA, Amin A, Khalaf HA. Caspase-3, Bcl-2, p53, CYP1A1 and COX-2 as a potential target in chemoprevention of Benzo (a) pyrene-induced lung carcinogenesis in mice: Role of thymoquinone. Int J Chem Nat Sci. 2016;4(3):430-41.
58. Pathak AK, Bhutani M, Kumar S, Mohan A, Guleria R. Circulating cell-free DNA in plasma/serum of lung cancer patients as a potential screening and prognostic tool. Clin Chem. 2006;52(10):1833-42. doi: 10.1373/clinchem.2005.062893.
59. Gold B, Cankovic M, Furtado LV, Meier F, Gocke CD. Do circulating tumor cells, exosomes, and circulating tumor nucleic acids have clinical utility? A report of the association for molecular pathology. J Mol Diagn. 2015;17(3):209-24. doi: 10.1016/j.jmoldx.2015.02.001.
60. Iba T, Hashiguchi N, Nagaoka I, Tabe Y, Murai M. Neutrophil cell death in response to infection and its relation to coagulation. J Intensive Care. 2013;1(1):13. doi: 10.1186/2052-0492-1-13.

Comparative phytochemical and in vitro antimicrobial activities of the leaf extracts of two medicinal plants growing in North-East, Nigeria

Hamidu Usman*, **Muhammad Awwal Tijjani, Abdulkarim Hassan, Zainab Babagana Aji**

Department of Chemistry, University of Maiduguri, P.M.B. 1069 Maiduguri, Nigeria

ARTICLE INFO

Keywords:
Antimicrobial activity
Phytochemical evaluation
Herbal medicine
Medicinal plants
Punica granatum
Waltheria indica

ABSTRACT

Introduction: The use of plants as medicine is as old as chemistry and common to all societies including the African, notably some parts of Northern Nigeria. Infectious diseases are among the causes of mortality and morbidity in rural areas endemic with hygienic problems in most developing countries including Nigeria. Two plant species with similar ethnomedical reports from different families were used in this study against some microorganisms. Their phytochemicals were also evaluated.
Methods: The leaf samples of *Punica granatum* and *Waltheria indica* were prepared and independently extracted with 80% methanol using maceration technique. The extracts were concentrated to dryness at reduced pressure and then subjected to phytochemical evaluation. Antimicrobial activities were evaluated using hole-in-plate disc diffusion technique.
Results: The phytochemical results of both extracts revealed the absence of anthraquinones. However, both extracts showed the presence of cardenolides, cardiac glycosides, flavonoids, saponins, tannins and terpenoids; while alkaloids were found in *W. indica*. The antimicrobial susceptibility study showed dose-dependent pattern with the highest dose (80 mg/hole) showing inhibition zone of 23.67 ± 0.47 and 23.33 ± 0.47 mm, respectively by *P. granatum* and *W. indica* against *Streptococcus pyogenes* while at 20 mg/hole inhibition was noted as 8.67 ± 0.47 and 7.00 ± 0.00 mm against *Escherichia coli* for *P. granatum* and *W. indica*, respectively.
Conclusion: The findings of this study scientifically support the use of *P. granatum* and *W. indica* in folklore medicine for the cure of infections by microbes.

Implication for health policy/practice/research/medical education:
Waltheria indica showed phytochemicals like cardenolides, cardiac glycosides, flavonoids, saponins, tannins, and terpenoids. However, alkaloids were found in only *W. indica*. The extracts showed dose-dependent broad spectrum antimicrobial activities against the test microorganisms which could be attributed to the secondary metabolites present. Hence both plants might be used as a natural source for preparation of new drugs.

Introduction

Traditional medical practices use the knowledge and belief of involvement of natural products, spiritual therapies and some exercises applied singly or in combination with the cure of man (1). Historically, man has been using various plant parts in prevention and treatment of several diseases (2). In the early 20th century, traditional medicine was regarded as a practice employed by poor society. However, synthetic or biomedical drugs have been doubted by some developed countries; thus giving interest in natural medicines or therapies (3). A plant becomes medicinal only when its biological activity has been ethnomedically reported or scientifically established (4). Depending on the usage, folk medicine may be regarded as traditional medicine, alternative medicine, indigenous medicine, or natural medicine (5). Traditionally, plants have been used as a source for treatment of diseases through secondary metabolites which play a significant role as medicines,

***Corresponding author**: Hamidu Usman,
Email: usmanhamidu@unimaid.edu.ng

flavouring and recreational drug in different parts of the world whose use contributes immensely to the enhancement of primary health care delivery (6,7).

The plant *Punica granatum* Linn. (Lythracea) commonly called pomegranate in English, *"Anar, Anar-ke-per"* in Hindi, *"Anar"* in Urdu, *"Punjabi* and *"Rooman"* in Arabic originated from Iran to the Himalayas in Northern India and found widely distributed the Mediterranean region of Asia, Africa and Europe (8). The rind of the fruit and the bark of the tree are used in the treatment of diarrheoa, dysentery and intestinal parasites, for nose and gum bleeds, toning skin and treating hemorrhoids in ancient Ayurvedic traditional medicine. Its juice is employed as an eye drop to stop the development of cataracts; the seeds and rind are also used as contraceptive and abortifacient. The most abundant phytochemicals in *P. granatum* juice are polyphenols, including the hydrolysable tannins or ellagitannins (9), condensed tannins (10), catechins, gallocatechins and prodelphinidins. The antioxidant property of *Punica granatum* has been reported, previously (11).

Waltheria indica Linn. (Malvaceae) is one of the species of flowering plants in the mallow family which have a tropical distribution. *W. indica* (sleepy morning) commonly called velvet leaf, marsh-mallow, monkey bush, boater bush, leather coat, among other names (12); is abundantly found in West Africa (13). In Nigeria, the plant is locally known as "*hankufa*" or "*hankubah*" in Hausa, "*kori kodi*" in Yoruba, *kafafi*" in Fulani", and "*efu-abe*" in Nupe languages (14). *W. indica* is a plant that has attracted medicinal interest because of its applications in traditional medicine to treat ailments employed as infusion or decoction where febrifugal, purgative, emollient, tonic, analgesic and astringent action is sought (12). The plant is used by Hausas of Northern Nigeria for the treatment of skin diseases, impotency and infertility. It is also used as an aphrodisiac and children's medicine at birth and during teething period (15).

It has been established that infectious diseases especially microbial type constitute a large number of health problems, especially in the developing countries. There is high proliferation of resistance to antimicrobial agents which not only does it result from poor quality drugs manufactured, patient non-compliance and irrational use of antimicrobial agents, but also could be due to mutations within the microbial flora (16). Therefore, the aim of this research was to ascertain the ethnomedical claim by the local populace and to compare the efficacy between the two plant extracts which are locally used here in the treatment of infectious diseases.

Materials and Methods

Sample collection and identification

Fresh leaf sample of *P. granatum* was collected from Gabanni-Babaji Village, Fika Local Government area, Yobe State while *W. indica* was collected from Wadiya Village, Maiduguri Metropolitan Council, Borno State. The plant samples were identified by a taxonomist at Botany section, Department of Biological Sciences, University of Maiduguri, Nigeria. Both plant samples were air-dried at room temperature and freed from twigs and dirt and then ground into coarse-powdered form with wooden mortar and pestle.

Extraction procedure

Two hundred and fifty grams of the powdered plant materials of each sample were independently extracted for 120 hours using 80% methanol in extraction bottle employing maceration technique. The extractives were filtered differently using Whatman No.1. The filtrate was poured into evaporating dish to dryness at reduced temperature and pressure and then kept in a desiccator until use.

Phytochemical screening

Phytochemical screening for the presence or absence of the secondary metabolites such as alkaloids, anthraquinones, cardenolides, cardiac glycosides, flavonoids and saponins were carried out according to the standard procedures as described previously (17-21).

Test for alkaloids

Half gram of the extract was stirred with 5.0 mL of 2 M aqueous hydrochloric acid in a steam bath. 1.0 mL each of the filtrate was separately treated with few drops of Mayer's reagent, Drangendorffs' reagent and Wagner's reagent; appearance of buff-coloured precipitate, orange-red precipitate and a dark-brown precipitate indicated the presence of alkaloid (21).

Test for tannins

Half g of the plant extract was dissolved in 10ml of distilled water and filtered. To 2 ml of the filtrate, few drops of 1% ferric chloride solution was then added. The occurrence of blue-black, green or blue-green precipitate colour indicates the presence of tannins (17).

Test for cardiac glycosides

Liebermann-Burchard's test

To 0.5 g of the extract, 2 mL of acetic anhydride was added. The mixture was cooled in an ice, and then conc. H_2SO_4 was added carefully. Colour development from violet to blue or bluish-green indicates the presence of steroidal ring (20).

Salkowski's test

To 0.5 g of the extract, 2 mL of chloroform was added; followed by conc. H_2SO_4 by the side of the test tube to form a lower layer. The appearance of reddish-brown or yellow colour at the interphase indicates the presence of a steroidal ring (20).

Test for saponins

A small portion of the plant extract was added to distilled water (20 mL) in a 100 mL beaker, boiled and filtered. About 5 mL of the filtrate was shaken vigorously for about 5 minutes. Frothing which persists on warming indicated the presence of saponins (18).

Test for free anthraquinones

About 0.5 g of the plant extract was shaken with 10 mL of benzene and then filtered. Five milliliters of 10% ammonia solution was added to the filtrate. The resultant mixture was shaken. The appearance of pink, red or violent colour at the lower phase indicates the presence of anthraquinones (21).

Test for combined anthraquinones

To 0.5 g of the extract, 10 mL of aqueous H_2SO_4 was added and shaken and transferred while was hot. The filtrate was shaken with 5 mL of benzene. The benzene layer was separated and was added half its own volume with 10% ammonia solution. The presence of pink, red or violet colouration in the ammoniacal phase indicates the presence of combined anthraquinones (21).

Test for flavonoids

Ferric chloride test

To 0.2 g of the extract, 5 mL of water was added, boiled and filtered. To 2 mL of the filtrate, few drops of 10% ferric chloride were added. A green-blue or violet colouration indicates the presence of phenolic hydroxyl group (21).

Shinoda's test

About 0.2 g of the extract was dissolved in 5 mL of ethanol, warmed and then filtered. Few pieces of magnesium chips were added to the filtrate followed by few drops of conc. HCl, a pink, orange or red to purple colouration indicates the presence of flavonoids (19).

Lead acetate test

Exactly 0.5 g of the extract was dissolved in 5 mL of distilled water. Tree milliliters of 10% lead acetate solution were added. The appearance of buff-coloured precipitate indicates the presence of Flavonoids (21).

Test for terpenoids

About 0.2 g of the extract was dissolved in 5 mL of ethanol. One milliliter of acetic anhydride was added, followed by addition of conc. H_2SO_4. The presence of terpenoids in the sample was detected as the colour changes from pink to violet (20).

Test for cardenolides

Keller-Killiani's test

Exactly 0.5 g of the extract was dissolved in 2 mL glacial acetic acid containing a drop of ferric chloride solution. One milliliter of conc. H_2SO_4 was added. The appearance of a brown ring at the interphase shows the presence of digitoxose sugar characteristic of cardenolides (21).

Test for carbohydrates

Molisch's test

Few drops of Molisch's reagent were added to 2 mL of the extract obtained by dissolving in distilled water. To this, 1 mL of conc. H_2SO_4 was added to the side of the test tube. The mixture was allowed to stand for 2 minutes and then diluted with 5 mL distilled water. Formation of red to dull-violet colour at the interphase of the two layers was taken as the positive test (21).

Test for free reducing sugars

Exactly 0.2 g of the extract was dissolved in 5 mL of distilled water and filtered. The filtrate was heated with 5 mL of equal volumes of Fehling's solution A and B formation of a red precipitate of cuprous oxide indicates the presence of reducing sugar's (21).

Test for combined reducing sugars

Exactly 0.2 g of the extract was hydrolyzed by boiling with 5 mL of dilute hydrochloric acid and filtered; the resulting filtrate was neutralized with sodium hydroxide solution. Few drops of Fehling's solution were added and then heated in a water bath for 2 minutes. Formation of reddish-brown precipitate of cuprous oxide indicates the presence of combined reducing sugars (21).

Test organisms

Three strains of gram-positive bacteria used include *Bacillus subtilis, Staphylococcus aureus* and *Streptococcus pyogenes,* Gram-negative were *Escherichia coli, Klebsiella pneumoniae* and *Pseudomonas aeruginosa;* while *Candida albicans* was the only fungal species used in this study. These organisms were clinical isolates obtained from Department of Veterinary Medicine, University of Maiduguri, Maiduguri, Nigeria.

Antimicrobial susceptibility test

The antimicrobial susceptibility test was carried out using the agar plate disc diffusion technique as described by National Committee for Clinical Laboratory Standards (22) and modified by Usman et al (23). The tests were carried out using a stock concentration of 400 mg/mL prepared by dissolving 4 g, 200 mg/mL prepared by dissolving 2 g and 100 mg/mL prepared by dissolving 1 g of the crude extract differently into 10 mL of sterile distilled water. Working volumes was 0.2 mL each of the concentrations prepared and then dispensed into each of the 6 mm bored holes to afford respectively 80, 40 and 20 mg/hole. After incubation, the average diameter of three readings of the clear zone around the hole was recorded as the measure of inhibitory level of the extract against the test bacteria and reported as mean ± SEM. The dilution ratio for gram-positive bacteria and gram-negative bacteria was 1:1000 and 1:5000 respectively using peptone water (23).

Determination of minimum inhibitory concentration

A serial dilution ranging from 100 to 6.25 mg/mL were made. The bacterial strain was cultured in nutrient broth as suspension; 5 ml peptone water was then added. To the suspension, 5 ml of each extract concentration was added to the nutrient broth cultures containing 1.0×10^7 CFU/mL which were seeded into each test tube and then incubated at 37°C for 18-24 hours. Test tube with no turbidity was taken as the MIC value (24).

Determination of minimum bactericidal concentration

Aliquots from the MIC studies were used for the MBC determination. To a solid nutrient agar, a bacterial streak of the suspension from the MIC test tube was made and the procedure repeated all through the required numbers of corresponding isolates. The isolated organism on the nutrient agar was incubated at 37°C for 18-24 hours. After incubation, the plates were observed for bacterial growth; the lowest concentration of the extract required to kill microorganism was considered as the MBC value (24).

Results

The phytochemical screening and antimicrobial activities were conducted on the methanolic leaf extracts of *P. granatum* and *W. indica*. The results of phytochemical screening are presented in Table 1 while the results of antimicrobial susceptibility are shown in Table 2. The minimum inhibitory concentrations (MICs) of the extracts are presented in Table 3; the results for the minimum bactericidal concentrations (MBCs) of the extracts are expressed in Table 4.

Phytochemical screening

The percentage extractive of *W. indica* was 11.43% and of *P. granatum* was 13.83% w/w. Phytoconstituents found in these extracts were cardenolides, cardiac glycosides, flavonoids, saponins, tannins and terpenoids. However, only *W. indica* indicated the presence of alkaloids. More so, both extracts had not any anthraquinones (Table 1).

Antimicrobial susceptibility

The susceptibility pattern of the extract revealed that the highest activity for both extracts was found at the highest concentration of 80 mg/hole with the DIZ values of 23.67±0.47 and 23.33±0.47 mm, respectively for *T. avicceniodes and W. indica against S. pyogenes*. However, the least activities were also recorded as 8.67±0.47 and 7.00±0.00 mm inhibition zone against *E. coli* at 20 mg/hole (Table 2).

Minimum inhibitory concentration

The minimum inhibitory concentration exhibited by *T. avicceniodes* was indicated as 12.5 mg/ml against *K. pneumonia, P. aeruginosa* and *Candida albicans;* while *W. indica* showed inhibition at the same concentration of 12.5 mg/mL against *S. pyogenes* (Table 3).

Table 1. Phytochemical analysis of crude leaf extracts of *Punica granatum* and *Waltheria indica*

S/No.	Phytochemical tests	Plant species	
		P. granatum	*W. indica*
1	Test of alkaloids		
	Preliminary test for alkaloid	-	+
	Confirmatory test for alkaloid	-	+
2	Test of free anthraquinones	-	-
	Test for combined anthraquinones	-	-
3	Test of carbohydrates		
	Molisch's test	+	+
	Test for combined reducing sugars	+	+
	Test of free reducing sugars	-	-
4	Test for Cardiac glycosides		
	Liebermann-Burchard's test	+	-
	Salkowski's test	-	-
5	Test for cardenolides		
	Keller-Killiani's test	+	+
6	Test of saponins glycosides	+	+
7	Test of tannins	+	+
8	Test for flavonoids		
	Ferric chloride test	-	+
	Shinoda's test	+	+
	Lead ethanoate test	+	+
	Sodium hydroxide test	-	+
9	Test of terpenoids	+	+

Key: + = Present, - = Absent

Minimum bactericidal concentration

The results for the minimum bactericidal concentration revealed that the MBC value of 25.0 mg/ml was exhibited by both extracts while *W. indica* was comparatively effective showing MBC value of 12.5 mg/mL against *P. aeruginosa* and *C. albicans* (Table 4).

Discussion

The results of phytochemical screening of leaf extracts of *P. granatum* and *Waltheria indica* indicate the absence of anthraquinones in *P. granatum* as well as in *W. indica* which corroborated to the earlier report by Mohammed et al (15) that no parts of the plants showed the presence of anthraquinones. However, both extracts revealed the presence of cardenolides, cardiac glycosides, flavonoids, saponins, tannins, and terpenoids. Alkaloids were only present in *W. indica* as reported previously (15). These classes of compounds have been reported to be a remedy against many pathogenic consequences and hence, explain their use traditionally for the treatment of different kinds of diseases (25). Secondary metabolites like tannins, terpenoids, alkaloids, and flavonoids have been reported to have *in vitro* antimicrobial properties (26,27).

Table 2 shows the results obtained from the antimicrobial evaluations of the leaf extracts of *P. granatum* and *W. indica*. The susceptibility pattern at concentrations of

Table 2. Antimicrobial susceptibility of the leaf extracts of *Punica granatum* and *Waltheria indica* at different concentrations

Microorganisms	Extract	Concentration of the extract/diameters inhibition zone (mm), mean±SEM		
		80 mg/hole	40 mg/hole	20 mg/hole
Bacillus subtilis	*P. granatum*	18.67±0.47	14.67±0.47	11.00±0.47
	W. indica	17.00±0.00	13.00±0.00	9.33±0.47
Staphylococcus aureus	*P. granatum*	13.67±0.47	10.00±0.00	11.33±4.71
	W. indica	17.67±0.47	13.67±0.47	10.00±0.00
Streptococcus pyogenes	*P. granatum*	23.67±0.47	18.33±0.47	14.00±0.00
	W. indica	23.33±0.47	18.67±0.47	14.33±0.47
Escherichia coli	*P. granatum*	16.67±0.47	11.67±0.47	8.67±0.47
	W. indica	12.00±0.00	9.00±0.00	7.00±0.00
Klebsiella pneumoniae	*P. granatum*	17.00±0.00	12.67±0.47	9.33±0.00
	W. indica	14.66±0.47	10.66±0.47	7.33±0.47
Pseudomonas aeruginosa	*P. granatum*	21.67±0.47	17.67±0.47	14.00±0.00
	W. indica	18.00±0.00	14.00±0.00	10.33±0.47
Candida albicans	*P. granatum*	19.67±0.47	16.33±0.47	12.33±0.47
	W. indica	18.00±0.00	14.33±0.47	10.67±0.47

Table 3. Minimum inhibitory concentrations (MICs) of the crude leaf extract of *Punica granatum* and *Waltheria indica*

Microorganisms	Extract	Concentration (mg/mL)				
		100.0	50.0	25.0	12.5	6.25
Bacillus subtilis	*P. granatum*	-	-*	+	+	+
	W. indica	-	-*	+	+	+
Staphylococcus aureus	*P. granatum*	-*	+	+	+	+
	W. indica	-	-	-*	+	+
Streptococcus pyogenes	*P. granatum*	-	-*	+	+	+
	W. indica	-	-	-	-*	+
Escherichia coli	*P. granatum*	-	-	-*	+	+
Klebsiella pneumonia	*P. granatum*	-	-	-	-*	+
Pseudomonas aeruginosa	*P. granatum*	-	-	-	-*	+
	W. indica	-	-	-*	+	+
Candida albicans	*P. granatum*	-	-	-	-*	+
	W. indica	-	-	-*	+	+

Key: -*= MIC values.

Table 4. Minimum bactericidal concentrations (MBCs) of the crude leaf extract of *Punica granatum* and *Waltheria indica*

Microorganisms	Extract	Concentrations (mg/mL)				
		100.0	50.0	25.0	12.5	6.25
Bacillus subtilis	*P. granatum*	-	-**	+	+	+
	W. indica	-	-**	+	+	+
Staphylococcus aureus	*P. granatum*	-**	+	+	+	+
	W. indica	-	-**	+	+	+
Streptococcus pyogenes	*P. granatum*	-	-	-**	+	+
	W. indica	-	-	-**	+	+
Escherichia coli	*P. granatum*	-**	+	+	+	+
Klebsiella pneumonia	*P. granatum*	-	-**	+	+	+
Pseudomonas aeruginosa	*P. granatum*	-	-**	+	+	+
	W. indica	-	-	-**	+	+
Candida albicans	*P. granatum*	-	-**	+	+	+
	W. indica	-	-	-**	+	+

Key: -** = MBC values.

80 mg/hole of the extract of *P. granatum* and *W. indica* respectively had 23.67±660.47 and 23.33±0.47 mm. The least activity was recorded at the lowest dosage of 20 mg/hole with 8.67±0.47 and 7.00±0.00 mm against *E. coli* for *P. granatum* and *W. indica* respectively. Generally, the activities due by *P. granatum* were considerably higher than that exhibited by *W. indica.* These observations could not be unrelated to the components as well as compositions of the secondary metabolites, even though they almost contained similar phytoconstituents. Moreover, researches have demonstrated the antimicrobial activities of tannins, flavonoids and saponins (28). It was noticed that the only point where *W. indica* exhibited higher activity than *P. granatum* was against *S. aureus.* The activities against gram-negative, gram-positive as well as fungal species corroborated to the earlier findings which revealed that extractives from the plant were capable of inhibiting these groups of microorganisms. These antimicrobial activities against the test microorganisms may be indicative of the presence of broad spectrum antibiotics in both extracts (29).

The zone of inhibition produced by most antibiotic discs against some of the organisms was found to be greater in relation to those activities produced by most organisms under study though not statistically compared to those produced by the extracts. However, the diameters of antibacterial activity zones of inhibition ≥10 mm around the 21 petri dish were considered active (28). The higher activities presented by *P. granatum* could not be unrelated possibly to the concentrations of the phytoconstituents since both had similar compounds.

Punica granatum showed high MICs of 12.5 mg/ml against three organisms (*Klebsiella pneumoniae, Pseudomonas aeruginosa,* and *C. albicans*). *W. indica* on the other hand exhibited good activity against *Streptococcus pyogenes.* Higher MBCs were observed for both extracts against *S. pyogenes* at 25.0 mg/ml which coincide with the work of Deshi et al (30). More so, *W. indica* had the MBC of 25.0 mg/mL on *C. albicans* and *Pseudomonas aeruginosa.*

Conclusion

In conclusion, these comparative studies have revealed the potency of each of the plant towards the test microorganisms studied. Although the overall susceptibility was shown by *P. granatum* but MBC value further expressed that *W. indica* had a very good bactericidal value on *C. albicans, P. aeruginosa* and also on *S. pyogenes.* Therefore, concurring to the earlier findings, it can be surmised that the extracts from *W. indica* can be said with little reservation that it can stand as a choice for the treatment of disease condition afflicted by *S. pyogenes.*

Acknowledgements

The authors wish to acknowledge the technical assistant rendered by Alh. I.A. Gulani.

Authors' contributions

All authors contributed to the study. AH and ZBA acquired data. HU prepared the drafting. HU and MAT revised it critically for important intellectual content and HU submitted it. All read and confirmed the article ready for publication.

Conflict of interests

The authors declared no competing interests exist.

Ethical considerations

Ethical issues (including plagiarism, misconduct, data fabrication, falsification, double publication or submission, redundancy) have been completely observed by the authors.

Funding/Support

This research was financially self-funded and supported by the authors.

References

1. Muazu J, Kaita AH. A review of traditional plants used in the treatment of epilepsy amongst the Hausa/Fulani tribes of northern Nigeria. Afr J Tradit Complement Altern Med. 2008;5(4):387-90.
2. Jamshidi-Kia F, Lorigooini Z, Amini-Khoei H. Medicinal plants: past history and future perspective. J Herbmed Pharmacol. 2018;7(1):1-7. doi: 10.15171/jhp.2018.01.
3. Ansari JA, Inamdar NN. The promise of traditional medicines. Int J Pharmacol. 2010;6(6): 808-12. doi: 10.3923/ijp.2010.808.812.
4. Olaleye MT. Cytotoxicity and antibacterial activity of methanolic extract of *Hibiscus sabdariffa.* J Med Plant Res. 2007;1(1):9-13.
5. Kay MA. Healing with plants in the American and Mexican West. Tucson: University of Arizona press; 1996;19-20.
6. Croteau R, Kutchan TM, Lewis NG. Natural products (secondary metabolites). Biochemistry Molecular Biology Plants. 2000;24:1250-319.
7. Holetz FB, Pessini GL, Sanches NR, Cortez DA, Nakamura CV, Filho BP. Screening of some plants used in the Brazilian folk medicine for the treatment of infectious diseases. Mem Inst Oswaldo Cruz. 2002;97(7):1027-31.
8. Yasoubi P, Barzegar M, Sahari MA, Azizi MH. Total Phenolic Contents and Antioxidant Activity of Pomegranate (*Punica granatum* L.) Peel Extracts. J Agric Sci Technol. 2007;9(1):35-42.
9. Singh RP, Chidambara Murthy KN, Jayaprakasha GK. Studies on the antioxidant activity of pomegranate (*Punica granatum*) peel and seed extracts using in vitro models. J Agric Food Chem. 2002;50(1):81-6.
10. Kamal A, Khan MMR. Phytochemical evolution of some medicinal plants. Ind J Plant Sci. 2014; 3(4):5-8.
11. Chidambara Murthy KN, Jayaprakasha GK, Singh RP. Studies on antioxidant activity of pomegranate (*Punica granatum*) peel extract using in vivo models. J Agric Food Chem. 2002;50(17):4791-5.
12. Burkill HM. Useful plants of West Africa. 2nd ed. Vol. 5.

London, UK: Royal Botanic Gardens, Kew; 2000:248-9.
13. Akobunda IO, Agyaklwa CW. The West African weeds. Ibadan: International Institute of Tropical Agriculture; 1998:406.
14. Hutchinson MJ, Dalziel JM. Flora of West Tropical Africa. Crown Agent for Oversea Government and Administration. London: Mill Bank; 1958:319.
15. Mohammed Z, Shok M, Ilyas N, Musa KY, Yaro AH. Analgesic activity of *Waltheria indica* Linn. Eur J Sci Res. 2007;16(1):6-9.
16. Denyer SP, Hodges NA, Gorman SP. Bacterial resistance to antibiotics and clinical uses of antimicrobial drugs. In: Hugo & Russell's Pharmaceutical Microbiology. 5th ed. Blackwell Publishing; 2004:220-250.
17. Brain KR, Turner TD. The practical evaluation of phytopharmaceuticals. Bristol: Wright Science Technica; 1975.
18. Vishnoi NR. Advanced practical chemistry. Ghaziabad-India: Yikas Publication House, PVT Ltd; 1979:447-9.
19. Markham KR. Techniques of flavonoids identification. New York: Academic Press;1982.
20. Silva LG, Lee IS, Kinghorn DA. Special problem with the extraction of plants. In: Cannell RJP, ed. Natural Products Isolation. New Jersey, USA: Humana Press Inc; 1998:343-364.
21. Trease GE, Evans WC. Pharmacognosy. 15th ed. London: Saunders Publishers; 2002.
22. NCCLS (National Committee for Clinical Laboratory Standards). Methods for Dilution Antimicrobial Susceptibility Tests for Bacteria that Grow Aerobically. Villanova, PA: NCCLS; 1993.
23. Usman H, Haruna AK, Akpulu IN, Ilyas M, Ahmadu AA, Musa YM. Phytochemical and antimicrobial screenings of the leaf extracts of *Celtis integrifolia* Lam. J Trop Biosci. 2005; 5(2):72-76.
24. Pavithra PS, Janani VS, Charamathi KH, Indumathy R, Potala S, Verma RS. Antibacterial activity of plants used in Indian herbal medicine. Int J Green Pharm. 2010;4(1):22-8.
25. Usman H, Osuji JC. Phytochemical and in vitro antimicrobial assay of the leaf extract of *Newbouldia laevis*. Afr J Tradit Complement Altern Med. 2007;4(4):476-80.
26. Cowan MM. Plant products as antimicrobial agents. Clin Microbiol Rev. 1999;12(4):564-82.
27. Usman H, Abdulrahman FI, Ahmed LA, Kaita AH, Khan IZ. Antibacterial effects of cyanogenic glucoside isolated from the stem bark of *Bauhinia rufescens* Lam. Int J Biol Chem Sci. 2013;7(5):2139-50. doi: 10.4314/ijbcs.v7i5.30.
28. Olajuyigbe OO, Babalola AE, Afolayani AJ. Antibacterial and phytochemical screening of crude ethanolic extracts of *Waltheria indica* Linn. Afr J Microbiol Res. 2011;5(22):3760-4. doi: 10.5897/AJMR11.627.
29. Kostova I, Dinchev D. Saponins in *Tribulus terrestris* – chemistry and bioactivity. Phytochem Rev. 2005;4(2):111-37. doi: 10.1007/s11101-005-2833-x.
30. Deshi JJ, Barminas JT, Onwuka J, Dass PM, Maitera O, Muazu I. Antimicrobial efficacy of biosynthesized silver nanoparticles from different solvent extracts of *Waltheria americana* root. J Anal Sci Technol. 2016;7(1):23. doi: 10.1186/s40543-016-0104-7.

26

Larvicidal effects and phytochemical evaluation of essential oils of *Trachyspermum ammi* and *Ziziphora clinopodioides* against larvae *Anopheles stephensi*

Hanieh Torabi-Pour[1*], Mansoureh Shayeghi[2], Hassan Vatandoost[2], Mohammad-Reza Abai[2]

[1]MSc in Medical Entomology, Department of Medical Entomology and Vector Control, School of Public Health, Tehran University of Medical Sciences, Tehran, Iran
[2]Department of Medical Entomology and Vector Control, School of Public Health, Tehran University of Medical Sciences, Tehran, Iran

ARTICLE INFO

Keywords:
Anopheles stephensi
Medicinal plants
Essential oils
Larvicidal effects
Malaria
Iran

ABSTRACT

Introduction: The main purpose of this research was to evaluate larvicidal effects of two native medicinal plants in Iran including seeds of Ajwain (*Trachyspermum ammi*) and leaves and shoots of Blue Mint Bush (*Ziziphora clinopodioides*) against larvae of *Anopheles stephensi*. Their phytochemical compounds of essential oils were also determined using GC-MS method.
Methods: The plants were collected from various regions of the country in the spring of 2013, and the aqueous essential oils were prepared using a Clevenger apparatus. The standard WHO method for anti-larval experiments against third and fourth instar larvae of *A. stephensi* was employed at the Biometric Laboratory next to the Culicidae Insectarium at the School of Public Health of Tehran University of Medical Sciences.
Results: The LC50s (lethal concentrations to kill 50%) and LC90s of the essential oils were 14.26 and 39.54 ppm *T. ammi* and 18.61 and 48.51 ppm for *Z. clinopodioides*. Phytochemical analysis of the essential oils of the tested plants revealed that thymol for *T. ammi* and pulegone for *Z. clinopodioides* had the highest percentage which were 71.989 and 48.609, respectively.
Conclusion: Considering the results of this research, the effective compounds in these essential oils that had larvicidal properties might be used against malaria vectors.

Implication for health policy/practice/research/medical education:
Considering the results of the present research, it seems that the scientific identification of the active ingredients in *Trachyspermum ammi* and *Ziziphora clinopodioides* against larvae *Anopheles stephensi* and utilization of the results of biometric experiments for developing suitable formulations of these active ingredients for controlling pests are necessary.

Introduction

At present, international organizations have restricted the use of toxic chemicals and have started replacing them with less hazardous ones. This has increased interest in natural products and led to discovery and production of less hazardous toxic chemicals including plant-based pesticides by researchers. Essential oils are the most widely known materials that have been tested against insects. The present research studied the larvicidal effects of two native medicinal plants in Iran (Blue Mint Bush and Ajwain) against the main malaria vector in this country (*Anopheles stephensi*). *Ziziphora clinopodioides* belongs to the mint family (Labiatae), grows wild in mountainous regions of central Iran (1), and is a native plant of western and northwestern Iran (2). Based on previous researches, it has various therapeutic effects including antioxidant (3,4), antibacterial (5), antifungal (6), larvicidal properties (7,8). It is also a protector of the digestive system (9), and lowers blood pressure (10). Ajwain is a member of the Umbelliferae family and grows in eastern and southern parts of Iran (1,11). It is also grown in many regions of Egypt, Afghanistan, and India, especially in Bengal (12). The most important reported therapeutic effects reported for it include being an antioxidant, anti-fever,

***Corresponding author**: Hanieh Torabi-Pour,
Email: haniehtorabipour@iran.ir

antimicrobial, anti-spasm, anti-flatulence, sudoriferous, expectorant, antifungal, gastric tonic and diuretic (13). The present research studied larvicidal activities of two medicinal plant species (Ajwain and Blue Mint Bush) against the main malaria vector in Iran (*A. stephensi*), and used logarithmic concentrations of the essential oils of these two plant species under laboratory conditions to determine their larvicidal effects so that, if results were desirable, their use could be recommended as effective larvicides against the main malaria vector in Iran. The phytochemical components of these plants were also determined using GC-MS method.

Materials and methods

Blue Mint Bush plant was collected from Bojnord in Khorasan province and Ajwain plant from Kazeroon in Fars province in the spring of 2013. Their organs were separated and air-dried in the shade, and identified. The physicochemical characteristics of the plants were determined, their compounds were identified, and the effects of their extracts against larvae of *A. stephensi* were studied. Features of the applied apparatus for phytochemical analysis of *Trachyspermum ammi* and *Z. clinopodioides* are shown in Table 1.

Rearing *Anopheles stephensi* larvae

Mosquito larvae were reared and kept in the Culicidae Insectarium of the School of Public Health at 29±2°C, relative humidity of 70±10%, and a photoperiod of 16 hours light, 8 hours dark. Late third instar or early fourth instar larvae of *A. stephensi* were used in antilarval experiments.

Preparing essential oils

A Clevenger apparatus was used for aqueous extraction of the essential oils of the two plant species. The plants were first powdered, about 30 g of the powders were poured in a 1-L flask, about 600 mL of distilled water were added, the Clevenger apparatus was mounted on the flask, and the heater was turned on. After the water boiled and evaporation began, the temperature was kept at a level that the water did not stop boiling (at about 60-80°C) and the heater was turned off. After about 4 hours, the essential oil was collected from the graduated part of the apparatus and poured into a small glass container specifically used for collecting essential oils. The essential oil was dried using anhydrous sodium sulfate and kept in a refrigerator to be used for the experiments.

Table 1. Features of the applied apparatus phytochemical composition of *Trachyspermum ammi* and *Ziziphora clinopodioides*

Apparatus Model GC	Agilent 6890N (USA)
Type of the column	HP-5MS
Column length GC	30 m
Inner diameter of the column	0.25 mm
Thickness of the layer	0.25 µm
Primary oven temperature	40°C
Temperature of the injection location	250°C
The amount of injection	1 µL
Final column temperature	250°C
Injection mode	Split
Type of carrier gas	He
Detector	Mass

Biological (antilarval) tests

The World Health Organization (WHO) method for antilarval biological tests was employed. The mean temperature at the laboratory was kept constant at 28°C, test duration was 24 hours, and 25 larvae were used in each 400 mL beaker. The larvae used for these tests were end of third instar or early fourth instar ones, and chlorine-free water was preferably used. Five concentrations of the insecticide, four replications for each concentration, and two controls are used, and in the control experiments, all materials employed in other experiments were used except the insecticide itself (14).

Preparation of logarithmic concentrations of the essential oils

Essential oils that were obtained from seeds of *T. ammi* and leaves and shoots of *Z. clinopodioides*) were used to conduct biological experiments. Four replications were considered for every concentration of each essential oil. The mortality rate of the larvae after 24 hours of contact with each essential oil was used to evaluate its larvicidal effect. The experiments were performed at the logarithmic concentrations of 5, 10, 20, 40, and 80 ppm for Ajwain and 10, 20, and 40 ppm for Blue Mint Bush with 4 replications for each concentration. The experiments had 2 series of controls (containing 1 mL of ethanol in 249 mL of chlorine-free water). Ajwain essential oil concentration of 80 ppm caused 100% larval mortality and, therefore, the logarithmic concentrations started at 5 ppm and were successively doubled. Blue Mint Bush essential oil concentration of 80 ppm also led to 100% larval mortality and, hence, the logarithmic concentrations started at 10 ppm and were successively doubled. The method for preparing logarithmic concentrations is presented below.

Anti-larval sensitivity test

Similar to the biological tests, the WHO method was employed and the tests were conducted in 400 mL glass beakers. As previously mentioned, logarithmic concentrations of the essential oils were first prepared. Twenty-two 400 mL beakers and twenty-two 50 mL beakers were prepared (4 replications for each concentration, and 2 replications for the control). Using a graduated cylinder, 224 mL of chlorine-free water were added to each 400 mL beaker and 25 mL to each 50 mL beaker. Following that, 25 late third instar or early fourth instar larvae reared in cuvettes (and fed fish meal four hours earlier) were transferred to each 50 mL beaker and, using an insulin syringe, 1 mL of the essential oil with the desired logarithmic concentrations was added to the 400 mL beaker used for that specific concentration and the contents were mixed. In the control beakers, 1 mL of pure ethanol was added instead of the extract. The contents of each 50 mL beaker was then transferred to the related 400 mL beaker and the beaker was covered with a plate, and results of the test were read after 24 hours.

Chemical analysis

Conditions of the applied apparatus for phytochemical analysis of *T. ammi* and *Z. clinopodioides* are shown in Table 2. After the essential oils of the plant species were prepared, they were injected into the GC-MS instrument to analyze the products in the extracts. The GC instrument was a model VARIAN CP-3800 having a VF-5MS column that was 30 m long, had an inner diameter of 0.25 mm, and a film thickness of 0.25 µm. The thermal regime was as follows: oven temperature was initially maintained at 50°C for 1 minute, it was gradually raised to 300°C at 10°/min, and the injection chamber had the temperature of 260°C. Helium was used as the carrier gas at the flow rate of 1 mL/min. The GC instrument used for Blue Mint Bush and Ajwain was a model Agilent 6890N (USA) having an HP-5MS column that was 30 m long and had an inner diameter of 0.25 and a film thickness of 0.25 µm. The initial oven temperature was 40°C, it was gradually raised to 250°C, the injection chamber had a temperature of 250°C, and helium was used as the carrier gas.

Table 2. Conditions of the applied Apparatus for phytochemical analysis of *Trachyspermum ammi* and *Ziziphora clinopodioides*

Initial temperature (°C)	Step 1
Initial time (min)	40
Program rate (°C/min)	1
Final temperature (°C)	3
Final time (min)	250
Split flow (mL/min)	60
Septum purge (mL/min)	25
Flow rate (mL/min)	6
Initial temperature (°C)	1

Statistical analysis

Results of the tests were read after 24 hours as the number of live, dead, and moribund larvae, the number of pupae, and the total number of larvae and pupae. This information was used to draw up mortality tables. LC50s and LC90s of the essential oils were determined and the linear regression equation was estimated with a 95% confidence interval using the probit-analysis method (15). If mortality rate of the control group was less than 5%, the data obtained from the biometric tests were correct, but if mortality rate of the control group was in the 2%-20% range, the data would be corrected using Abbot's formula as follows:

Abbott's formula = (mortality percentage of the test group – mortality percentage of the control group)/ (mortality percentage of the control group) × 100.

Results

Trachyspermum ammi and *Z. clinopodioides* essential oils at 80 ppm caused 100% larval mortality, but this mortality rate declined and approached zero percent at Ajwain concentrations of 5 and 10 ppm, respectively. The LC50s and LC90s were 14.26 and 39.54 ppm for Ajwain and 18.61 and 48.51 ppm for Blue Mint Bush.

Table 3 presents LC50s and LC90s and other statistical data related to biochemical tests on larvicidal effects of the essential oils after the contact time of 24 hours between them and fourth instar larvae of *A. stephensi*.

Linear regression equations for all essential oils are presented in Figures 1 and 2.

GC-MS results concerning the tested essential oils

GC-MS results concerning the tested essential oils are presented in Table 4. Analysis of the essential oils of the tested plant by using the GC-MS method revealed the

Table 3. Lethal concentration 50% and 90% (LC_{50} and LC_{90}) and associated parameters of 24 hours bioassay tests of essential oil of *Trachyspermum ammi* and *Ziziphora clinopodioides* against 3rd-4th instar larvae of *Anopheles stephensi*

Scientific name and family of the plant	Organs of the plant	A	B ± SE	LC_{50} (ppm) ± 95% CI	LC_{90} (ppm) ± 95% CI	χ^2 (Heterogeneity)	χ^2 table (*df*)	*P* value
Trachyspermum ammi (Apiaceae)	Seeds	-3.9130	3.0812 ± 0.234	16.7725 18.6190 20.4846	42.4791 48.5169 57.3649	8.781*	13.816 (2)	0.001
Ziziphora clinopodioides (Labiatae)	Branches and leaves	-2.3913	2.0503 ± 0.574	1.3240 14.0587 49.6484	26.2726 61.2474 79.2400	45.473*	16.266 (3)	0.001

A = y-intercept; B = The slope of the line; SE = standard error; LC50, 95 % CI = Lethal concentration causing 50% mortality and its 95% confidence interval; LC90, 95 % CI = lethal concentration causing 90% mortality and its 95 % confidence interval; *X* 2 = Heterogeneity about the regression line; *P* value = represent heterogeneity in the population of tested.

* No heterogeneity.

compounds that constituted them and their percentages. This information is necessary for purifying the active ingredient and developing the correct formulation of the larvicide (Figures 3 and 4).

Discussion and Conclusion

This research studied the larvicidal effects of essential oils obtained from two plant species against larvae of *A. stephensi* (the main malaria vector in Iran). Both tested essential oils had larvicidal effects against this vector. The essential oils of *T. ammi* and *Z. clinopodioides* at 80 ppm caused 100% mortality of the vector larvae. When the concentrations of the extracts declined, mortality rates decreased and approached zero percent at 5 ppm for Ajwain and at 10 ppm for Blue Mint Bush extracts.
In the biological experiments, the LC50s and LC90s essential oils were 14.26 and 39.54 ppm for *T. ammi* and 18.61 and 48.51 ppm for *Z. clinopodioides.*
In research conducted by Verdian-Rizi in Iran in 2008 on larvicidal effects of Blue Mint Bush against larvae of *A. stephensi* and *C. pipiens*, the LC50s and LC90s were 14.9 and 22.3 ppm and 16.5 and 28.6 ppm, respectively (7). Seo et al carried out a study in 2012 to investigate larvicidal effects of Ajwain essential oil against *Aedes aegypti*. This extract caused 100% mortality of the larvae at 0.1 mg/mL (16). In 2007, Chaubey conducted research on insecticidal effects of Ajwain extract and found that its LC50 for the larval stages of *Tribolium castaneum* was 11.62 mg/mL (17).
In 2009, Pandey et al carried out a study on larvicidal activity of Ajwain seed extract, and of its pure constituent thymol, against *A. stephensi*. They found that thymol was 1.65 times more toxic to fourth instar larvae of *A. stephensi* compared to the extract itself, and the LD50s and LD99s were 48.88 and 105.49 ppm for thymol and 80.44 and 172.12 ppm for the extract (18).
Considering the results of the present research, accurate and scientific identification of the active ingredients in these medicinal plants and use of results in biometric tests seem to be necessary in developing an accurate and suitable formulation for controlling pests. Utilization of larvicidal and repellent effects of these plants can, in general, play a substantial role in preventing diseases transmitted by mosquitoes.

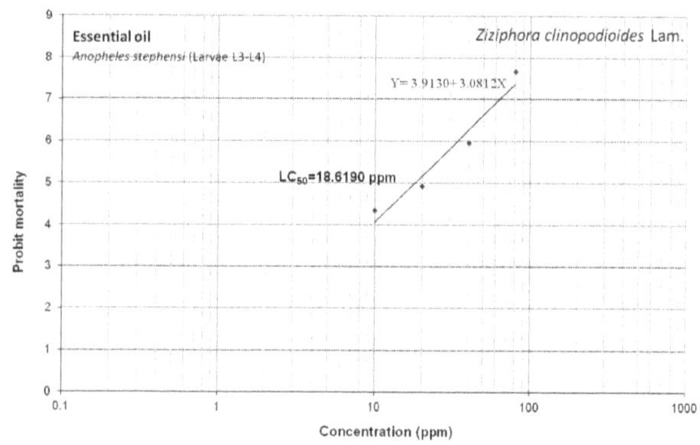

Figure 1. The equation, regression line, and LC_{50} (lethal concentration, 50%) of *Ziziphora clinopodioides* seed essential oil against third- and fourth-instar *Anopheles* stephensi larvae.

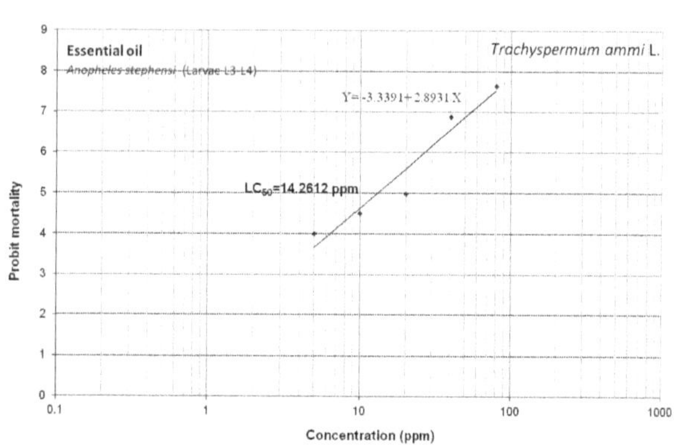

Figure 2. The equation, regression line, and LC50 (lethal concentration, 50%) of *Trachyspermum ammi* seed essential oil against third- and fourth-instar *Anopheles stephensi* larvae.

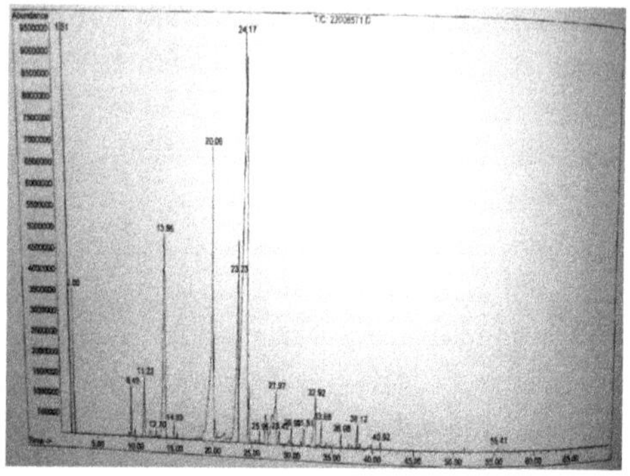

Figure 3. Peaks in the spectrum obtained from GC-Mass of cinnamon plant (*Ziziphora clinopodioides*) essential oil.

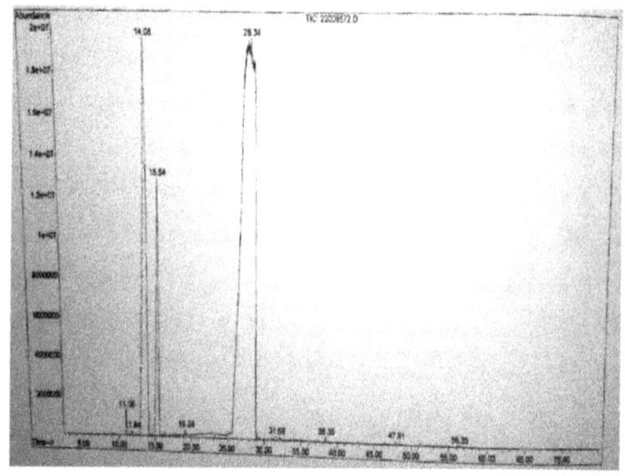

Figure 4. Peaks in the spectrum obtained from GC-Mass of cinnamon plant (*Trachyspermum ammi*) essential oil.

Acknowledgments

The authors of this article appreciate the Department of Medical Entomology and Vector Control of School of Public Health, Tehran University of Medical Sciences for

Table 4. GC-MS results concerning the tested essential oils

The name of the plant	The number of distinguished components of the plant	The percentage of the distinguished components	Main components (high percentage)	Components with larv icidal, Antiparasitic and germicidal properties
Ziziphora clinopodioides	Ethanol	9.497	Pulegone	Limonene
	Pentanal	0.036	p-Menthan-3-one	Carvacrol
	alpha-Thujene	0.090	Ethanol	Sabinene
	alpha-Pinene	0.887	1,8-Cineole	3-Octanol
	Camphene	0.097	Piperitenone	
	Sabinene	1.032	Verbenone	
	beta-Pinene	0.732	Ethanethioic acid, S-phenyl ester	
	beta-Myrcene	0.173		
	3-Octanol	0.166		
	alpha-Terpinene	0.026		
	p-Cymene	0.084		
	1,8-Cineole	9.869		
	cis-Ocimene	0.024		
	gamma-Terpinene	0.230		
	3,8-p-Menthadiene	0.056		
	alpha-Fenchene	0.032		
	trans-2-Caren-4-ol	0.074		
	Limonene	0.573		
	p-Menthan-3-one	14.203		
	p-Menthone	1.152		
	trans-Decalone	0.203		
	Neomenthyl acetate	0.138		
	Citronellol	0.062		
	Pulegone	48.609		
	Carvacrol methyl ether	0.045		
	Piperitone	1.128		
	Bornyl acetate	0.051		
	Menthol acetate	0.149		
	Carvacrol	1.512		
	Verbenone	2.129		
	Piperitenone	2.307		
	Isoeugenol	0.272		
	alpha-Cubebene	0.089		
	beta-Bourbonene	0.228		
	trans-Caryophyllene	0.052		
	Artemeisole	0.311		
	gamma-Elemene	0.059		
	Ethanethioic acid, S-phenyl ester	2.109		
	Sinularene	0.394		
	Caryphyllene oxide	0.087		
	1-p-Menthen-8-yl acetate	0.552		
	Vulgarol A	0.126		
	Visopathulenol	0.137		
	n-Hexadecanoic acid	0.119		
	Pterine	0.023		
	Isophytol	0.079		
Trachyspermum ammi	alpha-Thujene	0.013	Thymol	beta-Pinene
	alpha-Pinene	0.010	p-Cymene	Thymol
	beta-Pinene	0.312	gamma-Terpinene	Carvacrol
	beta-Myrcene	0.108		
	p-Cymene	19.536		
	cis-Ocimene	0.107		
	gamma-Terpinene	7.389		
	Dehydro-p-cymene	0.006		
	Turpentine comphor	0.033		
	Thymol	71.989		
	Carvacrol	0.207		
	trans-Caryophyllene	0.069		
	Caryphyllene oxide	0.013		
	Dillapiole	0.061		
	Fenchyl acetate	0.030		
	p-Menth-3-en-ol	0.022		
	cis-9-Octadecenoic acid	0.027		
	trans-9-Octadecenoic acid	0.055		
	Tetracosane	0.013		

their cooperation during this research.

Authors' contributions

HTP was the main researcher and performed the experiments, MS supervised the research, HV and MRA helped the supervision and preparation of the manuscript. All read and confined the final version of the manuscript for publication.

Conflict of interests

The authors declared no competing interests.

Ethical considerations

Ethical issues in research have been completely observed by the authors.

Funding/Support

Department of Medical Entomology and Vector Control, School of Public Health, Tehran University of Medical Sciences, Tehran, Iran supported the Master's Thesis in which this article was extracted from.

References

1. Amin G. Iranian Traditional Medicinal Plants. 1st ed. Tehran: Deputy of Health and Medical Education; 1991. [Persian].
2. Mozafarian V. Dictionary of Iranian plants names (Latin, English, Farsi). Tehran, Farhange Moaser; 1996.
3. Amiri H. Influence of growth phase on the essential oil composition of *Ziziphora clinopodioides* Lam. Nat Prod Res. 2009;23(7):601-6.
4. Souri E, Amin G, Dehmobed-Sharifabadi A, Nazifi A, Farsam H. Antioxidative activity of sixty plants from Iran. Iran J Pharm Res. 2004;3(1):55-59.
5. Ozturk S, Ercisli S. Antibacterial activity and chemical constitutions of *Ziziphora clinopodioides*. Food Control. 2007;18(5):535-40. doi: 10.1016/j.foodcont.2006.01.002.
6. Khosravi AR, Minooeianhaghighi MH, Shokri H, Emami SA, S MA, Asili J. The potential inhibitory effect of *Cuminum cyminum, Ziziphora clinopodioides* and *Nigella sativa* essential oils on the growth of *Aspergillus fumigatus* and *Aspergillus*. Braz J Microbiol. 2011;42(1):216-24.
7. Verdian-Rizi M. Essential oil composition and biological activity of *Ziziphora clinopodioides* Lam. from Iran. American-Eurasian Journal of Sustainable Agriculture. 2008:2(1):69-71.
8. Lolestani FA. Shayesteh N. Fumigant toxicity of *Ziziphora clinopodioides* (Boiss.)(Lamiaceae) against adults and eggs of *Callosobruchus maculatus* (Fab.)(Coleoptera: Bruchidae). J Biol Sci. 2009;9(1):92-95.
9. Niazmand S, Derakhshan M, Erfanian Ahmadpour M, Hosaeni K. The inhibitory effect of *Ziziphora clinopodioides* Lam. on gastric acid output at basal, vagotomized and vagal stimulated conditions in rat. Iran J Basic Med Sci. 2010;13(2):36-9.
10. Senejoux F, Girard C, Kerram P, Aisa HA, Berthelot A, Bevalot F, et al. Mechanisms of vasorelaxation induced by *Ziziphora clinopodioides* Lam. (Lamiaceae) extract in rat thoracic aorta. J Ethnopharmacol. 2010;132(1):268-73.
11. Zargari E. Medicinal Plants, vol 2. 5th ed. Tehran: Tehran University Publication; 1991. [Persian].
12. Bentley R, Trimen H. Medicinal Plants, vol 2. London: Churchill;1980.
13. Salehi-Sourmaghi MH. Medicinal Plants, vol 2. Tehran: Donyaye Taghzieh Publications; 1998. [Persian].
14. WHO. Instruction for determining the susceptibility or resistance of mosquito larvae to insecticides. Geneva: World Health Organization; 1981.
15. Abbott WS. A method of computing the effectiveness of an insecticide. 1925. J Am Mosq Control Assoc. 1987;3(2):302-3.
16. Seo SM, Park HM, Park IK. Larvicidal activity of ajowan (*Trachyspermum ammi*) and Peru balsam (Myroxylon pereira) oils and blends of their constituents against mosquito, *Aedes aegypti*, acute toxicity on water flea, *Daphnia magna*, and aqueous residue. J Agric Food Chem. 2012;60(23):5909-14.
17. Chaubey MK. Insecticidal activity of *Trachyspermum ammi* (Umbelliferae), *Anethum graveolens* (Umbelliferae) and *Nigella sativa* (Ranunculaceae) essential oils against stored-product beetle *Tribolium castaneum* Herbst (Coleoptera: Tenebrionidae). Afr J Agric Res. 2007:2(11): 596-600.
18. Pandey SK, Upadhyay S, Tripathi AK. Insecticidal and repellent activities of thymol from the essential oil of *Trachyspermum ammi* (Linn) Sprague seeds against *Anopheles stephensi*. Parasitol Res. 2009;105(2):507-12.

Effect of *Boswellia serrata* extract on tissue inflammation and white blood cells responses of spinal cord injury in rat model

Moosa Javdani[1*], **Mojtaba Ahmadi Dastjerdi**[2], **Sadegh Shirian**[3]

[1]Department of Clinical Sciences, Faculty of Veterinary Medicine, Shahrekord University, Shahrekord, Iran
[2]Faculty of Veterinary Medicine, Shahrekord University, Shahrekord, Iran
[3]Department of Pathobiology, Faculty of Veterinary Medicine, Shahrekord University, Shahrekord, Iran

ARTICLE INFO

Keywords
Spinal cord injury
Boswellia serrata
Rat
Inflammation
Traditional medicine

ABSTRACT

Introduction: The severe inflammatory responses that occurs after traumatic spinal cord injury (SCI) is with great strength related to the further tissue damage. As such, developmental strategies have been investigated, aimed at restricting inflammation and encouraging regeneration of injured neural tissue. One of those encouraging strategies is administration of traditional medicinal plants. The current study was conducted to evaluate the neuroprotective effects of *Boswellia serrata* extract on the neuronal tissue inflammation and white blood cells (WBCs) responses in rats with SCI.
Methods: Forty adult female rats were randomly assigned into 2 equal groups as experimental and control groups. Under general inhalation anesthesia, in both groups, SCI was created, at T9-10 level of the column. On the third day after the operation, an oral supplement of *B. serrata* extract was administered to the experimental group at 100 mg/kg/d. The histology of the site of injury and changes in the WBCs were examined in both groups at different pre-surgical and post-surgical times.
Results: The total population of WBCs in the current study was significantly less in the experimental group, compared to the control group at third and fourth weeks of the study which could be related to the anti-inflammatory effects of *B. serrata* extract. Histopathological evaluation of lesion sites confirmed the reduced inflammatory responses in the experimental group compared to the control group ($P < 0.05$).
Conclusion: The decrease in the number of inflammatory cells after oral consumption of *B. serrata* extract and the histopathological results confirm the neuroprotective effects of this extract.

Implication for health policy/practice/research/medical education:
Anti-inflammatory impacts of oral consumption of *Boswellia serrata* extract can control secondary injury associated with SCI.

Introduction

Spinal cord injury (SCI) as a worldwide form of neurological damage can destroy central nervous system of patients, result in high rates of disability and create considerable medical costs (1,2). Trauma is one the most common causes of SCI; therefore, in addition to more than 12 000 subjects that are affected once a year in the United States, many more are influenced in developing countries, additionally (3). Devastating trauma leads to primary injury, by the focal destruction of neural substance and secondary complications that can continue to weeks, and are related to losing strength of blood-spinal cord barrier, neuronal damage, oxidative stress, neuro-inflammation, and ischemic abnormality (4,5).

These problems as a detrimental cascade, can be managed by pharmacological intercessions, but there has been little success or no definite curative therapy in this regard (6). Alternative strategies for SCI interventions such as traditional herbal medicine, with many thousands years history, would be valuable in the prevention and treatment of SCI.

For thousands of years, *Boswellia* species or frankincense has been used for medical reasons. In conventional Asian medicine, *Boswellia* species are a therapeutic element

***Corresponding author**: A Moosa Javdani,
Email: javdani59@gmail.com, m.javdani@sku.ac.ir

applied by diseases of the nervous system; *Boswellia* species were furthermore administrated for the treatment of various diseases of the gastrointestinal tract, and for gynecological plans (7).

Boswellia serrata and its extracts are traditionally used to treat different types of blood disorders, inflammatory health conditions, cardiac debility, and pain (8). There are various scientific investigations about pharmacological actions of *B. serrata*-gum resin. Gummy exudates of *B. serrata* stem bark or its great constituents, boswellic acids possess anti-inflammatory (9,10), anti-cancerous (11) and anti-ulcerous (12) roles.

Boswellia with its neuroprotective activity increases structural development of new nerve networks (13). It also impedes degenerative alternations in the hippocampus, which is the memory-processing region in the brain (14). Therefore, some studies suggest that *B. serrata* and its compounds need to be scientifically investigated in neurophysiology and feasibly for the future handling of neurodegenerative disorders (7,15). Toxicology academic works of *B. serrata* resin directed on animals showed no notable histopathological, genotoxic, and hematological changes after consumption of this resin at doses up to 1000 mg/kg. Furthermore, the adverse effects are insignificant in humans, and occasionally nausea, acid reflux and digestive complaints have been reported in some consumers (16,17).

Based on the above mentioned information, the current study was conducted to evaluate neuroprotective effects of *B. serrata* extract on the neuronal tissues in experimental SCI in rat model.

Materials and Methods

Drug preparation

Boswellia serrata was bought from Iran Darouk Pharmaceutical Co., Iran. After grinding of *B. serrata*, 1000 g of its powder was put in a clean 10-litre flask and mixed with 8 L of 70% ethanol for a period of 48 hours at indoor temperature. The final mixture was then filtered and dried out using a rotary evaporator at a temperature below 50ºC until its volume reduced to 5% of its original volume (18,19). Subsequently, the residual content was kept at refrigerator temperature.

Animals

Forty adult female rats (Sprague-Dawley), weighing approximately 250-300 g were assigned in the current study. The animals were arbitrarily allocated into experimental (n = 20) and control (n = 20) groups. All rats were retained under controlled states at room temperature, with conventional humidity and a 12 h light cycle, and allowed free access to food and water.

Animal model establishment and drug treatment

All rats received premedication regimen subcutaneously (Xylazine 10 mg/kg, Alfasan) and after 10 minutes anesthetized with isoflurane (Terrel Isoflurane; PCC Inc.). Initially, the rats were placed on the operating room table and a midline dorsal area was prepared, surgically. A midline surgical cut was made in skin at level of T8–T11, and the bilateral para-spinal muscles exactly were dissected. In two groups at T9-10 level of column, due to dorsal laminectomy, cord compression as a SCI was made, using aneurysm clip for 60 seconds (20,21).

Hind limb locomotor deficiency and tail paralysis resulted from SCI, confirmed the efficacy of the aneurysm clip compression technique. After exact control of bleeding, paravertebral fascia and skin were sutured in the simple continuous pattern (21).

Manual expression of urinary bladders, twice daily, was performed at the first three days after surgery and additionally all rats received enrofloxacin (2.5 mg/kg; Enrofloxacin 10%; Amineh Gostar Co.), twice daily for five postoperative days, in order to avoid infection. Seventy-two hours later from the cord compression, the experimental group's animals received 100 mg/kg *B. serrata* extract (Daily for 4 weeks), by traditional orogastric gavage.

Histopathological assessment

At different times post-surgery (day 3, 7, 21, and 28), after sacrifice of the rats, a dorsal laminectomy was performed at the total lumbar and thoracic vertebrae levels and spinal cord tissue samples were collected for microscopic examination. The spinal cord samples of all animals in both groups were embedded in paraffin and fixed with 10% buffered formalin for 24 hours. Five μm-thick serial sections were cut from the paraffin blocks, using a microtome and stained with hematoxylin-eosin (H&E) and toluidine blue (TB) for routine histopathological examinations. Histopathological sections were subjected to descriptive analyses, by an experienced Histopathologist, blinded to the groups and study design.

Blood works

In addition, a number of blood samples were accumulated by heart puncture at days 3, 7, 21, and 28, postoperatively, just before sacrificing of the rats, and total and differential White blood cell (WBC) count, and neutrophil/lymphocyte ratios (N/L ratio) were evaluated.

Statistical analysis

The mean of the measured parameters (mean ± SEM) were compared between the control and experimental groups, using an independent *t* test. Data changes in each group were analyzed, using the ANOVA test. $P<0.05$ was regarded as statistically significant.

Results

Histopathological assessment and cell counts

Histological changes in both control and experimental groups at third day post-operation revealed apparent

hemorrhage and severe inflammation at the injured site (Figure 1).
Neural tissue sections from the control group in first week post-injury showed extensive necrosis with inflammation and obvious hemorrhagic area but less than third day post-operation. Necrotic and degenerated neurons observed at the injured site (Figure 2).
Histological features of animals in experimental group in first week after surgery indicated degenerated and necrotic neurons with moderate hemorrhage and inflammation at the lesion site (Figure 3).
During the third week, mild to severe hemorrhage and inflammation, accompanied with notable neuronal necrosis were observed in the control group (Figure 4), while considerable reduction in inflammation and hemorrhage also with total necrosis of gray matter of cord were noticed in the experimental group (Figure 5).
At 28th day post-injury in the control group, minimal hemorrhage, and mild inflammation were noted, while neuronal necrosis in both gray and white matter was observed (Figure 6). However, in the experimental group, the smallest amount of inflammation and hyperemia accompanied with little necrotic neuronal zones was detected at the lesion site (Figure 7). In sum, descriptive data revealed a considerabe decrease in inflammation and hemorrhage, during the third and fourth weeks, in the experimental group, compared to the control group.

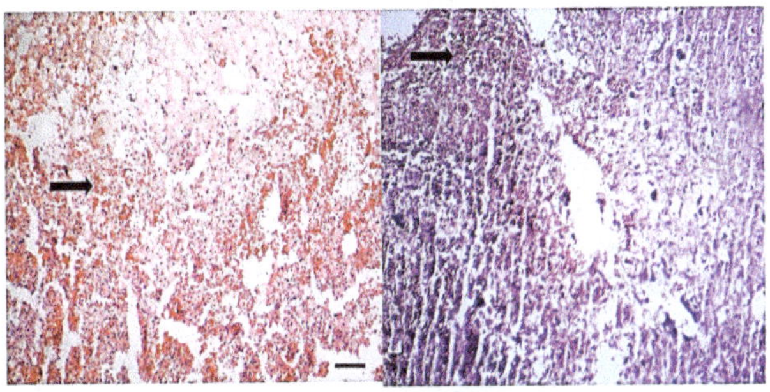

Figure 1. Day 3 of post-operation in both groups; severe hemorrhage (arrow) around the lesion; H&E stain (left), TB stain (right); scale bar =56 μm

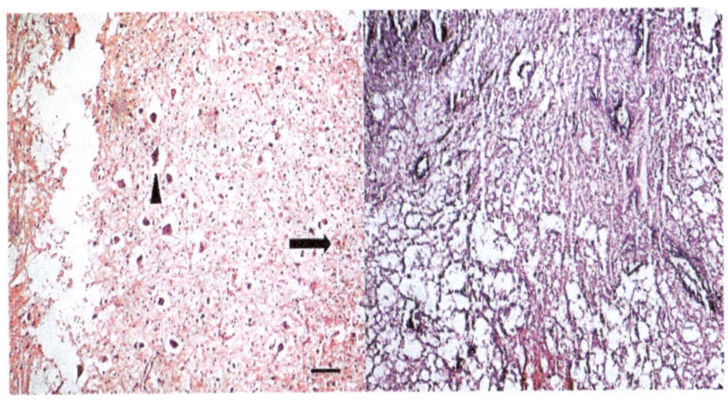

Figure 2. Histological structures in the control group at 1st week after surgery; Inflammation and obvious hemorrhage (arrow) with neuronal necrosis (arrowhead) at the lesion site. H&E stain (left fig.), TB stain (right fig.); scale bar= 56 μm

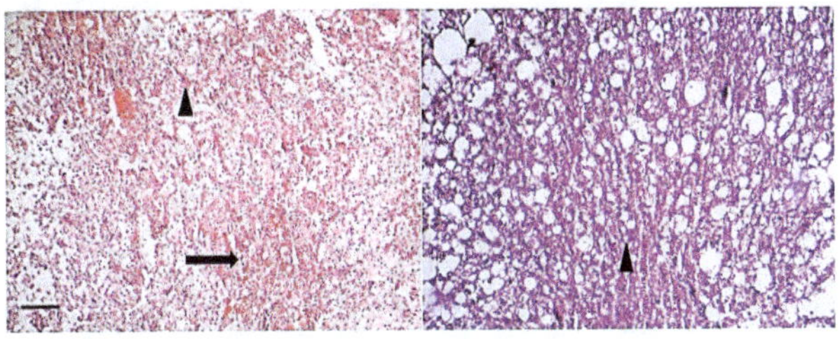

Figure 3. Histological features in the experimental group at first week after surgery; moderate inflammation and hemorrhage (arrow) and necrosis (arrowhead) around the injured site; H&E stain (left), TB stain (right); scale bar= 56 μm.

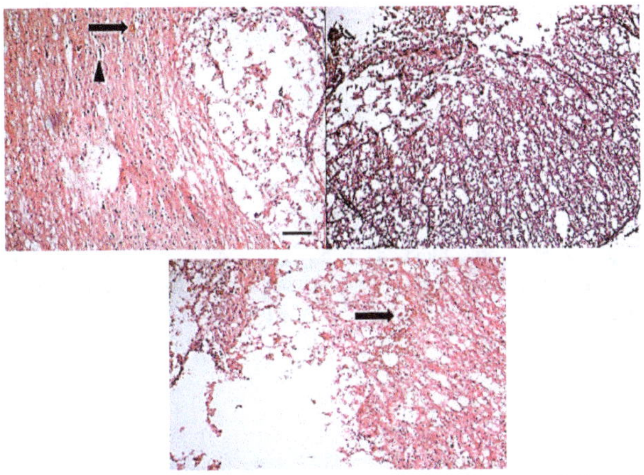

Figure 4. Histopathological changes in the control group at 3rd week after operation; Hemorrhage (arrow) and inflammation accompanied with neuronal necrosis (arrowhead) in the defected site; H&E stain (left and below), TB stain (right); scale bar= 56 μm.

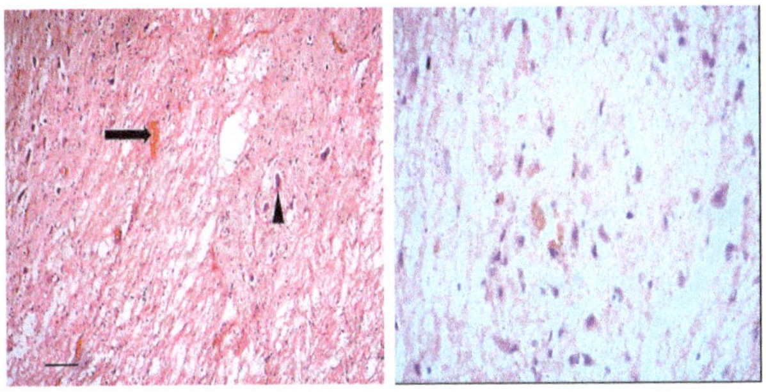

Figure 5. Histopathological findings in the experimental group at 3rd week post-surgery; hemorrhage (arrow) and neuronal necrosis (arrowhead) in the vicinity of the lesion; H&E stain (both figs.); scale bar =56 μm.

Leukogram analysis

Mean (±SEM) of the total Wright-Giemsa stained white blood cell (tWBC) of the different times, in both groups are delineated in Figure 8. There was no significant difference between this parameter in day 3 and week 1 of the study ($P > 0.05$). Analyzed data revealed a significant decrease in tWBC, during the third and fourth weeks, in the experimental group, compared to the control group ($P < 0.05$).
Figures 9 to 11 show neutrophils, lymphocyte, and

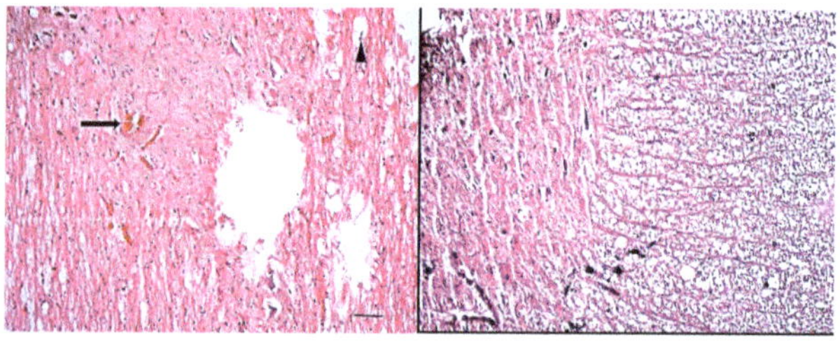

Figure 6. Histological findings in the control group at 4th week after surgery; Neuronal necrosis (arrowhead) and hemorrhage (arrow) at the lesion site; H&E stain (left), TB stain (right); scale bar= 56 μm.

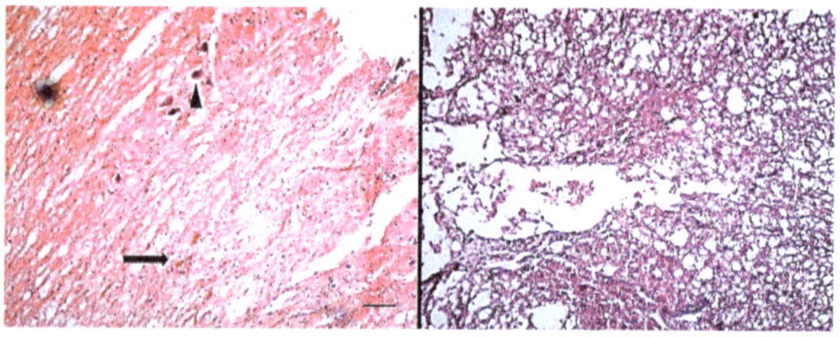

Figure 7. Histological findings in the experimental group at 4th week after surgery; minimal hyperemia (arrow) and mild inflammation with necrotic neurons (arrowhead); H&E stain (left), TB stain (right); scale bar= 56 μm.

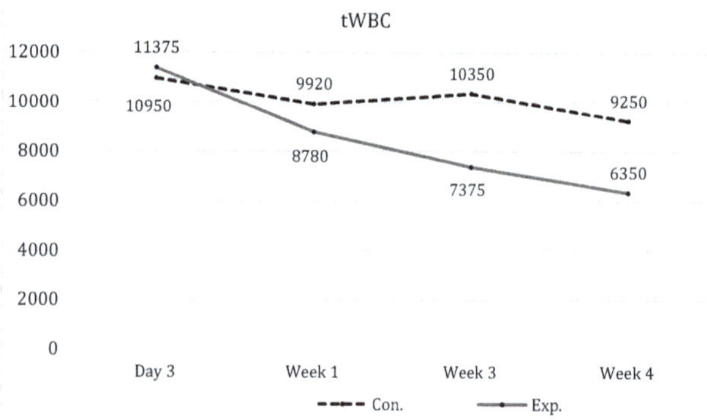

Figure 8. tWBC (10^6/L) changes during the various times in both groups; tWBC: total White Blood Cell; Con.: Control group, Exp.: Experimental group.

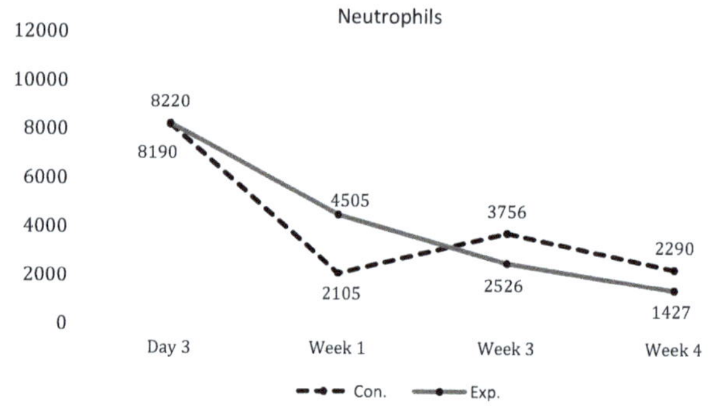

Figure 9. Neutrophils (10^6/L) changes during the different times in both groups; Con.: Control group, Exp.: Experimental group.

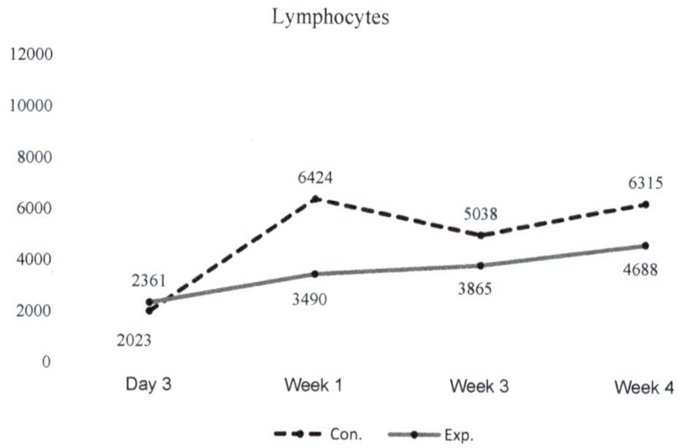

Figure 10. Lymphocyte (10^6/L) changes during the different times in both groups. Con.: Control group, Exp.: Experimental group.

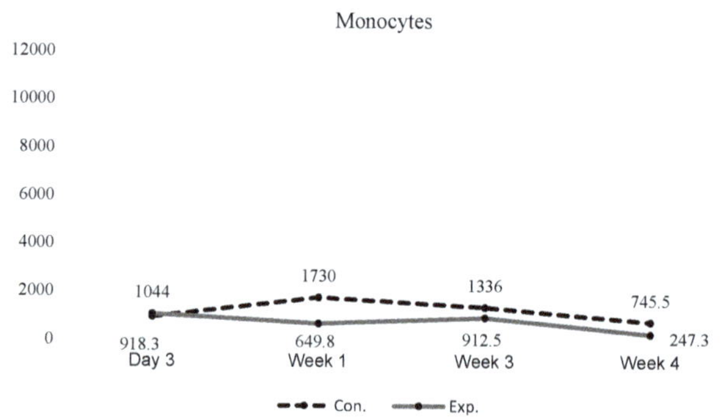

Figure 11. Monocyte (10^6/L) alternations at the different times in the control and experimental groups; Con.: Control group, Exp.: Experimental group.

monocyte changes during the different times of the current study in the control and experimental groups. There were significant differences between mean (±SEM) of the neutrophils in week 1 and week 4 of the study ($P > 0.05$).

The analyzed results revealed a significant reduction between the mean (±SEM) of lymphocyte, between the control and experimental groups in day 3 and week 4 after operation. Twenty-eight days after surgery, the mean (±SEM) of monocyte showed remarkable differences ($P = 0.02$), between both groups. Evaluation of N/L ratio in the 2 groups demonstrates significant difference during weeks 1 and 4.

The presented figures delineated alternations of inflammatory cells (lymphocytes, neutrophils, and monocytes), at different times, in the control and experimental groups. These figures show noticable decrease of neutrophils over the 7 days after spinal injury ($P < 0.05$), resulting in an obvious decrease of tWBC due to surgery.

Discussion

Over the past few years, the extent of herbal extracts utilization with neuroprotective activities, such as *Boswellia* species in biological needs have been widened.

For that reason, the contemporary study was conducted to decrease the inflammation and also to promote myelination associated with oral medication of *B. serrata* extract, in the rat suffered from compressive SCI. Twenty-eight days administration of this extract in the affected adult female rats, showed interesting findings that the extract could limit secondary complications following SCI.

Trauma, as a mechanical damage, compresses the spinal cord and disfigures the cord vessels and produces hemorrhage at the contusion site, and after a period of time induces edema and regional ischemia (22,23).

Secondary complications will happen after few minutes and move forward several weeks following SCI, and the correlated events, such as inflammation, gliosis, and neuronal degeneration cause severe functional abnormalities. Post-traumatic inflammatory environment has associated with active microglia and astrocytes, and as well penetrated macrophages, which strongly make it possible to develop secondary damages. The angiogenic reactions and reconstruction of vessels increase secondary injuries. Therefore, restriction of secondary injuries leads to limiting of neurodegeneration, and subsequently functional recovery attains more rapid (22,24). SCI induces immune depression syndrome, which is due to disturbance of the sympathetic nervous system and impairment of the immune system function (25).

Additionally, general inflammatory responses, because of SCI, persuade an increase of inflammatory cells into the circulation and secondary tissues, activation of immune cells, and pro-inflammatory cytokine secretion, all of which intervene with the pathogenesis of various organs after SCI (22). Evaluated leukograms in the current experiment revealed a significant decrease in total WBCs and neutrophils during the third and fourth weeks, in the experimental group, compared to the control group. Furthermore, histological sections during these weeks confirmed notable reduction of inflammation in the experimental group in comparison to the control group. The advantage of N/L ratio is related to anticipation of systemic inflammation and stress (26,27). In fact, it is index of a disorganized cell-mediated immunity, related to the systemic inflammation (28). Our data showed a notable decrease of N/L ratio in the experimental and control groups that is related to significant increase of neutrophils at the day 7. There was no significant difference between two groups about this value in various times.

An interesting point to consider is that the total population of WBCs in the current study was significantly less in the experimental group, compared to the control group at third and fourth weeks of the study which is related to the anti-inflammatory effects of *B. serrata* extract. Histopathological evaluation of lesion sites confirmed this desirable effect. Similar other studies, our data reveal that neutrophils are needed for encouraging functional recovery after spinal cord damage. They are initial inflammatory cells which appear at the lesion site and act by different mechanisms, such as releasing angiogenic factors, to induce inflammation-mediated tissue remodeling (29,30).

We did not find any studies that investigate effects of *B. serrata* extract on the neuronal cells in traumatic SCI. A few available studies just evaluated effects of this medicine herb on the brain. Resins of *Boswellia* species act as a natural anti-inflammatory product that has been administrated in some centuries (9).

Several found compounds of *Boswellia* have effects on the immune system in different routes. Boswellic acids, beta-boswellic acid (BA), 3-acetyl-beta-boswellic acid (ABA), 11-keto-boswellic acid (KBA) and 3-acetyl-11-keto-beta-boswellic (AKBA), are named as the major ingredients of *B. serrata* (31). AKBA, as a potent component of extract of *B. serrata*, move across the blood brain barrier (32) and is able to inspire its anti-inflammatory effects. Boswellic acids (AKABA) inhibit 5-lipoxygenase enzyme so suppress leukotriene biosynthesis. It has been revealed that boswellic acid decreases some interleukins (1, 2, 4, 6, 10, 12) and IFN$^{\gamma}$, induces down regulation of Tumor necrosis factor (TNFα), and puts down WBC migration. Also, *B. serrata* suppresses mast cell degranulation and induction of monocytes and macrophages and inhibits pathways of complement directly or indirectly (33).

It has been reported that boswellic acids through activating protein kinase-C, is effective in learning and memory storage and cause synaptic plasticity in the hippocampus (34,35). Another identified constituent in *Boswellia* resin is incensole-acetate, which shows anti-inflammatory activities on the central nervous system (CNS) and has been shown antianxiety and in addition anti-depression impacts. Previous studies have revealed that incensole-acetate holds back degenerative changes in the hippocampus by increase of calcium influx and releasing of calcium dependent-neurotransmitters in the brain (13,14,36). So, it seemed that *Boswellia serrata* extract by inhibition of different enzymes of the arachidonic acid cascade including lipoxygenases and cyclooxygenases potentially are able to control secondary injuries of compressed spinal cord. Therefore, evaluation of these enzymes in the future is recommended.

Conclusion

Examined histologic sections and analyzed systemic WBC alternations in the experimental group of the present study confirmed anti-inflammatory effects of oral consumption of *Boswellia serrata* extract in the rats suffered traumatic spinal cord damage.

Authors' contributions

MJ conducted the full work and performed the experiments. MAD participated in the clinical and laboratory processes. SS gave histopathological support. All authors have read and approved the submission of this paper.

Conflict of interests

The authors declare that there are no conflicts of interest associated with this manuscript.

Ethical considerations

All investigational procedures used in this study were reviewed and approved by the Council of Department of Veterinary Clinical Sciences of the Shahrekord University (170-572).

Funding/Support

None.

References

1. Ackery A, Tator C, Krassioukov A. A global perspective on spinal cord injury epidemiology. J Neurotrauma. 2004;21(10):1355-70. doi: 10.1089/neu.2004.21.1355.
2. van den Berg ME, Castellote JM, Mahillo-Fernandez I, de Pedro-Cuesta J. Incidence of spinal cord injury worldwide: a systematic review. Neuroepidemiology. 2010;34(3):184-92; discussion 92. doi: 10.1159/000279335.
3. Devivo MJ. Epidemiology of traumatic spinal cord injury: trends and future implications. Spinal Cord. 2012;50(5):365-72. doi: 10.1038/sc.2011.178.
4. Anwar MA, Al Shehabi TS, Eid AH. Inflammogenesis of secondary spinal cord injury. Front Cell Neurosci. 2016;10:98. doi: 10.3389/fncel.2016.00098.
5. Hausmann ON. Post-traumatic inflammation following spinal cord injury. Spinal Cord. 2003;41(7):369-78. doi: 10.1038/sj.sc.3101483.
6. Wyndaele M, Wyndaele JJ. Incidence, prevalence and epidemiology of spinal cord injury: what learns a worldwide literature survey? Spinal Cord. 2006;44(9):523-9. doi: 10.1038/sj.sc.3101893.
7. Hamidpour R, Hamidpour S, Hamidpour M, Shahlari M. Frankincense (rǔ xiāng; *Boswellia* species): from the selection of traditional applications to the novel phytotherapy for the prevention and treatment of serious diseases. J Tradit Complement Med. 2013;3(4):221-6. doi: 10.4103/2225-4110.119723.
8. Paranjpe P. S΄allaký – *Boswellia serrata*. In: Indian Medicinal Plants – Forgotten Healers: A Guide to Ayurvedic Herbal Medicine. Delhi: Dehli Chaukhamba Sanskrit Pratishthan Publishers; 2001:233-4.
9. Ammon HP. Boswellic acids in chronic inflammatory diseases. Planta Med. 2006;72(12):1100-16. doi: 10.1055/s-2006-947227.
10. Shen T, Lou HX. Bioactive constituents of myrrh and frankincense, two simultaneously prescribed gum resins in Chinese traditional medicine. Chem Biodivers. 2008;5(4):540-53. doi: 10.1002/cbdv.200890051.
11. Upaganlawar A, Ghule B. Pharmacological activities of *Boswellia serrata* Roxb. - mini review. Ethnobotanical Leaflets. 2009;13(6):766-74.
12. Singh S, Khajuria A, Taneja SC, Khajuria RK, Singh J, Johri RK, et al. The gastric ulcer protective effect of boswellic acids, a leukotriene inhibitor from *Boswellia serrata*, in rats. Phytomedicine. 2008;15(6-7):408-15. doi: 10.1016/j.phymed.2008.02.017.
13. Moussaieff A, Shein NA, Tsenter J, Grigoriadis S, Simeonidou C, Alexandrovich AG, et al. Incensole acetate: a novel neuroprotective agent isolated from *Boswellia carterii*. J Cereb Blood Flow Metab. 2008;28(7):1341-52. doi: 10.1038/jcbfm.2008.28.
14. Ring RH, Alder J, Fennell M, Kouranova E, Black IB, Thakker-Varia S. Transcriptional profiling of brain-derived-neurotrophic factor-induced neuronal plasticity: a novel role for nociceptin in hippocampal neurite outgrowth. J Neurobiol. 2006;66(4):361-77. doi: 10.1002/neu.20223.
15. Hosseini Sharifabad M, Esfandiary E. A morphometeric study on CA3 hippocampal field in young rats following maternal administration of *Boswellia serrata* resin during gestation. Iran J Basic Med Sci. 2007;10(3):176-82. doi: 10.22038/ijbms.2007.5292.
16. Singh GB, Atal CK. Pharmacology of an extract of salai guggal ex-*Boswellia serrata*, a new non-steroidal anti-inflammatory agent. Agents Actions. 1986;18(3-4):407-12.
17. Sharma R, Singh S, Singh GD, Khajuria A, Sidiq T, Singh SK, et al. In vivo genotoxicity evaluation of a plant based antiarthritic and anticancer therapeutic agent boswelic acids in rodents. Phytomedicine. 2009;16(12):1112-8. doi: 10.1016/j.phymed.2009.06.009.
18. Siahpoosh A, Mehrpeyma M. Antioxidant effects of *Albizia lebbek* and *Prosopis julifora* barks. Int J Biosci. 2014;5(9):273-84.
19. Majdinasab N, Siahpush A, Mousavinejad SK, Malayeri A, Sajedi SA, Bizhanzadeh P. Effect of *Boswellia serrata* on cognitive impairment in multiple sclerosis patients. J Herb Med. 2016;6(3):119-27. doi: 10.1016/j.hermed.2016.05.003.
20. Onifer SM, Rabchevsky AG, Scheff SW. Rat models of traumatic spinal cord injury to assess motor recovery. Ilar j. 2007;48(4):385-95.
21. Erbayraktar Z, Gokmen N, Yilmaz O, Erbayraktar S. Experimental traumatic spinal cord injury. Methods Mol Biol. 2013;982:103-12. doi: 10.1007/978-1-62703-308-4_6.
22. Sun X, Jones ZB, Chen XM, Zhou L, So KF, Ren Y. Multiple organ dysfunction and systemic inflammation after spinal cord injury: a complex relationship. J Neuroinflammation. 2016;13(1):260. doi: 10.1186/s12974-016-0736-y.
23. Ropper AH. Traumatic injuries of the head and spine. In: Braunwald E, Fauci AS, Kasper DL, Hauser SL, Longo DL, Jameson JL, eds. Harrison's Principles of Internal Medicine. New York: McGraw-Hill; 2001:2441-2.
24. Profyris C, Cheema SS, Zang D, Azari MF, Boyle K, Petratos S. Degenerative and regenerative mechanisms governing spinal cord injury. Neurobiol Dis. 2004;15(3):415-36. doi: 10.1016/j.nbd.2003.11.015.
25. Lucin KM, Sanders VM, Jones TB, Malarkey WB, Popovich PG. Impaired antibody synthesis after spinal cord injury is level dependent and is due to sympathetic nervous system dysregulation. Exp Neurol. 2007;207(1):75-84. doi: 10.1016/j.expneurol.2007.05.019.
26. Zahed NS, Karimi Mahali Z. Evaluation of cutoff point and power of neutrophil to lymphocyte ratio in diagnosing chronic inflammation in end-stage renal disease (ESDR)

patients. Medical Journal of Mashhad University of Medical Sciences. 2015;58(6):289-94.
27. Al-Hussain F, Alfallaj MM, Alahmari AN, Almazyad AN, Alsaeed TK, Abdurrahman AA, et al. Relationship between neutrophil-to-lymphocyte ratio and stress in multiple sclerosis patients. J Clin Diagn Res. 2017;11(5):Cc01-cc4. doi: 10.7860/jcdr/2017/24388.9764.
28. McMillan DC. Systemic inflammation, nutritional status and survival in patients with cancer. Curr Opin Clin Nutr Metab Care. 2009;12(3):223-6. doi: 10.1097/MCO.0b013e32832a7902.
29. Schruefer R, Lutze N, Schymeinsky J, Walzog B. Human neutrophils promote angiogenesis by a paracrine feedforward mechanism involving endothelial interleukin-8. Am J Physiol Heart Circ Physiol. 2005;288(3):H1186-92. doi: 10.1152/ajpheart.00237.2004.
30. Neirinckx V, Coste C, Franzen R, Gothot A, Rogister B, Wislet S. Neutrophil contribution to spinal cord injury and repair. J Neuroinflammation. 2014;11:150. doi: 10.1186/s12974-014-0150-2.
31. Jauch J, Bergmann J. An efficient method for the large-scale preparation of 3-o-acetyl-11-oxo-β-boswellic acid and other boswellic acids. European J Org Chem. 2003;2003(24):4752-6. doi: 10.1002/ejoc.200300386.
32. Kruger P, Daneshfar R, Eckert GP, Klein J, Volmer DA, Bahr U, et al. Metabolism of boswellic acids in vitro and in vivo. Drug Metab Dispos. 2008;36(6):1135-42. doi: 10.1124/dmd.107.018424.
33. Ammon HP. Modulation of the immune system by *Boswellia serrata* extracts and boswellic acids. Phytomedicine. 2010;17(11):862-7. doi: 10.1016/j.phymed.2010.03.003.
34. Nguyen PV, Woo NH. Regulation of hippocampal synaptic plasticity by cyclic AMP-dependent protein kinases. Prog Neurobiol. 2003;71(6):401-37. doi: 10.1016/j.pneurobio.2003.12.003.
35. Alkon DL, Sun MK, Nelson TJ. PKC signaling deficits: a mechanistic hypothesis for the origins of Alzheimer's disease. Trends Pharmacol Sci. 2007;28(2):51-60. doi: 10.1016/j.tips.2006.12.002.
36. Guyton AC, Hall JE. Text Book of Medical Physiology. Philadelphia: Saunders; 2011:751-2.

Phytochemical, nutraceutical and antioxidant studies of the aerial parts of *Daucus carota* L. (Apiaceae)

Emmanuel Ayodeji Ayeni[1]*, Ahmed Abubakar[1], Garba Ibrahim[1], Vallada Atinga[2], Zainab Muhammad[1]

[1]Department of Pharmacognosy and Drug Development, Ahmadu Bello University Zaria, Nigeria

[2]Department of Pharmacognosy and Drug Development, Gombe State University, Gombe, Nigeria

ARTICLE INFO

Keywords:
Daucus carota
Carrot
Proximate
Antioxidant
Spectrophotometry

ABSTRACT

Introduction: Carrot is a rich source of anthocyanins, carotenoids, vitamins A, B and C. The aerial parts are used as livestock feed in some parts of Northern Nigeria with little or no scientific evidence of its nutritional potential. This study established the phytochemical, nutritional and antioxidant potentials of carrot aerial parts.
Methods: The proximate and elemental analyses of the aerial parts were determined using Association of Official Analyst Chemist (AOAC) method and 2,2-diphenyl-1-picrylhydrazyl (DPPH) method for quantification of antioxidant properties in the crude extracts.
Results: The preliminary phytochemical screening revealed presence of steroid/triterpenes, flavonoids, tannins and saponins in ethylacetate and methanol crude extracts. The proximate analysis revealed crude protein (14.59%), lipid (10.37%), fibre (9.07%), carbohydrate (51.81%), moisture (10.23%) and the ash content (12.99%). The aerial parts were rich in P (11.00 mg/L), Na (5.38 mg/L), Fe (3.19 mg/L), K (2.25 mg/L), Ca (2.02 mg/L), Mn (1.15 mg/L), Mg (1.02 mg/L), As (0.83 mg/L), Se (0.40 mg/L), Zn (0.26 mg/L), Cu (0.13 mg/L), Cd (-0.02 mg/L), Cr (0.02 mg/L), Ni (0.17 mg/L) and Pb (0.04 mg/L). The antioxidant activity showed that ethylacetate and methanol extracts had EC50 of 86.89 ug/mL and 166.79 ug/mL, respectively.
Conclusion: *Daucus carota* aerial parts are rich in nutritional compositions and may be used as livestock feed supplements and also as vegetables for mankind. Its utilization could be incorporated in daily diets and boost food security in developing countries.

Implication for health policy/practice/research/medical education:
This study confirms the requisite for continuous search of rich edible foods in achieving zero hunger among developing countries. It looked inward in alternative sources of sustenance through conversion of peels from fruits, vegetables and other values added products into production of essential oils, nutraceuticals, food additives and its prospect in boosting food security in developing countries with significant poverty indices.

Introduction

Natural products especially from plants have led to drug developments (1). It is well-known that plants are the main sources of food, clothing, shelter, herbal beverages and drugs in health care management including Nigeria (2,3). The World Health Organization (WHO) established that over 68% of the world population solely depends on medicinal plant to meet their health demands (4). Natural products especially from plant are always and readily available, inexpensive and utilizations are relevant to people cultures and origins (5). This expresses the potential of medicinal plants in achieving and attaining the global statutory quotes of health for all.

Antioxidant activities in plants have been contributed in delaying, preventing and removing the oxidative damages to target molecules (6). Such oxidative processes are dangerous for all living cells, especially those in proximity to sites where active oxygen is released by photosynthesis (7).

Carrot (*Daucus carota* L.) belongs to the family of Apiaceae (8). It is one of the edible root plants and a rich source of anthocyanins, carotenoids (α, β, λ carotene), vitamins A, B and C (8). All the parts of *D. carota* have been used traditionally as aphrodisiac, diuretic, antidiabetic, muscle and back pain reliever. Also the hot water extract of the leaf is taken orally as a uterine stimulant during

Corresponding author: Emmanuel Ayodeji Ayeni,
Email: ayeniemmanuel91@yahoo.com

parturition and has abortifacient potentials (9). Generally, some of the species possess antimicrobial activities and have been used in flavoring of alcoholic beverages (9). Commonly, the plants in Apiaceae family are known to possess antioxidant and anti-inflammatory activities, used in treating infections, respiratory ailments and have hepatoprotective activities (10). In Nigeria, carrot is called *Karas* among the Hausa, *Karoti* or *Atoka* in Yoruba and *Karotu* in Igbo (11). However, the *D. carota* aerial parts are usually thrown away after harvesting or after eating the edible root part and in some parts of Northern Nigeria the aerial part is used as components of livestock feed. The aim of the study is to establish the phytochemicals, nutritional and antioxidant potentials of the *D. carota* aerial parts and suggest its possible utilizations as vegetable.

Materials and Methods

Collection, identification and preparation of plant material

The aerial parts of *D. carota* were collected from carrot sellers in Samaru market, Sabon Gari Local Government Area, Zaria, Nigeria. The whole plant (root inclusive) was identified by Mallam Namadi Sanusi, a Taxonomist in the Department of Botany, Ahmadu Bello University, Zaria and the voucher specimen was obtained and deposited in the herbarium unit (No: 12034) for future references. The foreign materials in the plant samples were removed, air dried for 5-6 days, pulverized and stored in a cleaned polythene bag for further use.

Extraction of *Daucus carota* aerial parts

The plant materials were successively extracted by cold maceration based on solvents polarity using n-hexane, ethyl-acetate and methanol, respectively (12).

Chemicals and solvents

All chemicals and reagents were of analytical grades (Sigma Aldrich, Lagos distributor, Nigeria). The instruments used included atomic emission spectrophotometer (MP-AES), flame emission spectrophotometer (A-Analyst-700) all from Agilent Company LTD and HACH Spectrophotometry (DR/4200) was used for phosphorus determination. All instruments were calibrated to standard before use.

Preliminary phytochemical screening of *Daucus carota* aerial parts

The n-hexane, ethyl acetate and methanol extracts of the plant aerial parts were subjected to preliminary phytochemical screening using standard methods for qualitative analysis of phytochemicals present in *D. carota* aerial parts (13).

Test for saponins

i. Frothing test: About 0.5 g of the extracts was shaken with water in a test tube followed by warming on a water bath. Frothing which persisted on warming was taken as an evidence for the presence of saponins.
ii. Hemolysis test: 2 mL of sodium chloride (1.8% solution in distilled water) was added to two test tubes A and B. Then, 2 mL of distilled water was added to test tube A, 2 mL of the extract was added to test tube B. Five drops of blood were added to each tube and the tubes were inverted gently to mix the contents. Hemolysis in tube B containing the extract but not in tube A (i.e. control), indicated the presence of saponins in the extract.

Test for steroid/triterpenes

i. Lieberman-Buchard test: A small portion of each extract was dissolved in chloroform. Then, volume of acetic anhydride was added, followed by concentrated sulphuric acid down the side of the test tube. The mixture was observed for the presence of a brown ring at the interphase which indicated the presence of triterpenes.
ii. Salkowski test: A small amount of each extract was dissolved in 1 mL chloroform and 1 mL of concentrated sulphuric acid was added down the side of the test tube. Formation of red coloration at the interphase was observed as an indication of presence of sterols.

Test for flavonoids

i. Shinoda test: About 0.5 g of each extract was dissolved in 5 mL of 95% ethanol, warmed and filtered. Three pieces of magnesium chips were added followed by five drops of concentrated hydrochloric acid. Pink or slight orange color indicated the presence of flavonoids.
ii. Sodium hydroxide test: Few quantities of each extract were dissolved in water and filtered; 2 mL of 10% aqueous sodium hydroxide solution was added. In the solution, the presence of yellow color, a change in color from yellow to colorless on addition of dilute hydrochloric acid, indicated and confirmed the presence of flavonoids.

Test for Tannins

i. Ferric chloride test: 0.5 g of each extract was stirred with 10 mL distilled water and filtered. Two drops of 1% ferric chloride solution was added to 2 mL of the filtrate. Formation of a blue-black color indicated the presence of tannins.
ii. Lead sub-acetate test: To a small quantity of each extract, three drops of lead sub-acetate solution were added. The solution observed the presence of green precipitate which confirmed the presence of tannins.

Test for alkaloids

About 0.5 g of each extract was stirred with 5 mL of 1%

aqueous hydrochloric acid in a water bath and filtered. Ammonia solution was added to the filtrate until it is basic, then chloroform was added, gently shaken to allow separation. The chloroform layer was collected and dilute HCl was added, gently shaken to allow separation and the aqueous layer was divided into three portions.

i. To the first portion, few drops of freshly prepared Dragendorff reagent was added and observed for formation of orange to brownish precipitates.
ii. To the second portion, one drop of Mayer's reagent was added and observed for formation of white to yellowish or cream color precipitates.
iii. To the third portion, 1 mL of Wagner's reagent was added to give a brown or reddish or reddish-brown precipitates, which indicated the presence of alkaloids.

Test for anthraquinone

i. Borntrager's test: The extracts were shaken with 10 mL of chloroform, the content of each extract was filtered and 5 mL of 10% ammonia solution was added to the filtrate, the mixture was shaken. Pink or slight red colour in the upper part of the aqueous layer indicated the presence of free anthraquinone.
ii. Modified Bontrager's test: The extracts were boiled with 10 mL of aqueous sulphuric acid and filtered hot. The filtrate, after cooling to room temperature, was shaken with 5 mL chloroform, the chloroform layer was separated and to half of its volume, 10% ammonium hydroxide was added. A pink, red or violet coloration in the ammonia phase (lower phase) indicated the presence of combined anthraquinone or anthraquinone derivatives.

Test for cardiac glycosides

i. Keller-Kiliani test: 0.5 g of each extract was dissolved in 2 mL of glacial acetic acid containing one drop of ferric chloride solution. Then 1 mL of concentrated sulphuric acid was added, gently. Brown ring obtained at the interphase indicated the presence of deoxy sugar characteristic of cardenolides.
ii. Kedde's test: Few drops of 2% solution of 3, 5-dinitrobenzoic acid in 95% alcohol were added to small portion of filtrate. A solution of 5% sodium hydroxide was also added to make the solution alkaline appearance. The presence purple-blue colour indicated the presence of cardenolides and the absence confirmed absence of cardenolides.

Thin Layer Chromatography profiles of the aerial parts extracts

Thin layer chromatography (TLC) of stationary phase (Silica Gel 60 F_{254}) pre-coated plates (Merck, Germany) of 0.25 mm thickness was used. The spotting was done manually and the TLC aluminum plates were developed at room temperature in ascending order of chromatography technique inside saturated solvents chromatographic tank. Separations were observed moving from the solvent baseline to the solvent front in the chromatographic tank. The chromatograms were allowed to dry and then observed under iodine tank before spraying with P-anisaldehyde as general spraying agent and placed in the oven at 120°C for 2 minutes (14). The best solvent used was hexane:ethylacetate (9:1) while hexane:ethylacetate (5:5) was used for the ethylacetate extract and butanol:acetic acid:water (8:1:1) was used to develop the methanol extract. The R_f values of each spot observed were calculated and the chromatograms were photomicrograph.

Determination of proximate analyses

The proximate analysis of the aerial parts was carried out to know the nutritional proportion of carbohydrates, fats (lipid), crude proteins, moisture and ash contents using Association of Official Analytical Chemists (AOAC) method. Percentages were used for result presentation and all samples were replicated three times for statistical analysis alongside with their standard deviation (15).

Determination of elemental analysis of *Daucus carota* aerial parts

Acid digestion of the samples: 0.5 g of the *D. carota* aerial parts was weighed into 10 different beakers each of 50 mL, to which 6 mL of a mixture of perchloric acid ($HClO_4$) and nitric acid (HNO_3) in 1:5 ratio were added. The 10 beakers used were placed in an open space for 2 hours and a mixture of hydrochloric acid (HCl) and nitric acid (HNO_3) in 1:1 ratio was added to each beaker. It was kept on a hot plate at 300°C for 4 hours. After the contents of beakers dried, 5 mL of HCl was added to each beaker and was kept on the hot plate until the entire liquid content in the beakers evaporated. Then, 5 mL of de-ionized water was added to each beaker and the solutions were poured in sterile bottles and tested for the quantification of the metals (16,17). The concentrations of Fe, Mg, Zn, Cu, K and Na were read using the flame atomic spectrophotometer (AA-500-model). HACH Spectrophotometry (DR/4200) was used for phosphorus determination and Atomic Emission Spectrophotometer (A-ES- Agilent Company) was used for other elements detected.

The antioxidant activities of the extracts were carried out according to an established method (18,19). The antioxidant effective concentrations were compared with gallic acid as the positive control.

Statistical analysis

All results are presented in tables and figures. The mean and standard deviation (SD) were in three replicates and analyzed using the Statistical Package for Social Sciences (SPSS version 20.0 Chicago).

Results

The preliminary phytochemical screening in the n-hexane, ethylacetate and methanol extracts revealed the absence of alkaloids, cardiac glycosides and anthraquinone while steroids/triterpenes was present. The ethyl acetate and methanol extracts showed the presence of saponins, flavonoids and tannins (Table 1).

The proximate composition revealed that the aerial part contained carbohydrate (51.81%), crude protein (14.59%), lipid (10.37%), fibre (9.07%), moisture content (5.67%) and ash content (11.60%), respectively (Table 2).

The antioxidant activity showed that ethylacetate and methanol extracts had EC_{50} of 86.89 mol/L and 166.79 mol/L, respectively (Table 3).

The aerial parts were rich in macro and trace elements including, P (11.00 mg/L), Na (5.38 mg/L), Fe (3.19 mg/L), K (2.25 mg/L), Ca (2.02 mg/L), Mn (1.15 mg/L), Mg (1.02 mg/L), As (0.83 mg/L), Se (0.40 mg/L), Zn (0.26 mg/L), Cu (0.13 mg/L), Cd (-0.02 mg/L), Cr (0.02 mg/L), Ni (0.17 mg/L) and Pb (0.04 mg/L) (Figure 1).

The n-hexane extract showed 11 spots alongside with R_f values of 0.09, 0.17, 0.23, 0.36, 0.40, 0.46, 0.50, 0.57, 0.60, 0.79 and 0.91, the ethylacetate extract showed seven spots with R_f values of 0.16, 0.28, 0.65, 0.81, 0.88, 0.90 and 0.91 while the methanol extract showed thirteen spots along side with R_f values of 0.16, 0.24, 0.29, 0.36, 0.42, 0.47, 0.51, 0.54, 0.57, 0.63, 0.66, 0.76 and 0.81 respectively (Figure 2).

Table 1. Preliminary phytochemical screening of *Daucus carota* aerial part

Phytochemical constituents	NDCA	EDCA	MDCA
Alkaloids			
Dragendorf test	-	-	-
Wagner's test	-	-	-
Mayers test	-	-	-
Cardiac glycosides			
Keller-killani	-	-	-
Keddes test	-	-	-
Saponins			
Frothing test	-	+	+
Haemolysis test	-	+	+
Flavonoids			
Shinodas test	-	+	+
Lead acetate test	-	+	+
Anthraquinones			
Bontragers test	-	-	-
Modified bontragers test	-	-	-
Tannins			
$Fecl_3$	-	+	+
Lead acetate test	-	+	+
Steroid/triterpenes			
Liberman buchard	+	+	+
Salkwoski test	+	+	+

Key: (-) Absent; (+) Present

NDCA, n-hexane extract; EDCA, ethylacetate extract; MDCA, methanol extract.

Discussion

The results of the phytochemical screening showed various classes of the secondary metabolites in the *D. carota* aerial parts (Table 1). The n-hexane, ethylacetate and methanol extracts revealed the absence of alkaloids, cardiac glycosides and anthraquinone while steroids/triterpenes were present in the extracts. However, the steroids/triterpenes may be investigated for possible pharmacological activities such as antioxidant and anti-inflammatory properties. The ethylacetate and methanol extracts showed the presence of saponins, flavonoids and tannins (Table 1) which indicated its potential as antioxidant, antimicrobial, hepatoprotective and anti-inflammatory properties. The TLC which is a simple and cheap method for detection of plant active constituents revealed the various degree of separation and richness of the extracts.

The proximate analysis (Table 2) showed the nutritional potentials of the *D. carota* aerial parts such as the moisture

Table 2. Proximate analysis of *Daucus carota* aerial parts

Parameters	%Moisture	%Carbohydrate	% Crude fibre	%Crude protein	% Crude lipid	%Ash content
Values	10.23±0.01	51.81±0.65	9.07±0.38	14.59±1.00	10.37±0.55	12.99±0.05

Values are means ± standard deviation (SD) of triplicate samples.

Table 3. Percentage of antioxidant activity of different extracts in the *Daucus carota* aerial parts

Concentration	Hexane extracts	Ethyl acetate extracts	Methanol extracts	Gallic acid (Positive control)
250 µg/mL	-8.30±1.56	85.21±2.14	82.86±19.78	75.00±2.00
125 µg/mL	-17.47±4.56	32.75±1.85	62.39±17.98	58.00±3.10
50 µg/mL	-25.78±4.00	2.10±0.47	20.65±5.77	40.00±5.00
25 µg/mL	-27.92±4.79	-12.99±2.86	16.80±0.15	20.00±0.00
10 µg/mL	-28.34± 2.47	-21.66±1.37	13.03±0.12	15.00±4.00
5 µg/mL	-34.72±0.27	-27.66±3.57	7.56±0.36	12.00±0.90
EC_{50}	490.74	86.29	166.79	211.14

Values (%) are means ± standard deviation (SD) of three determinations.

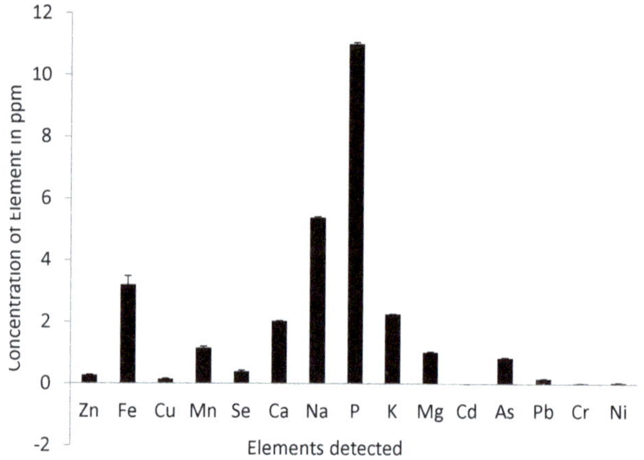

Figure 1. Elemental composition in the aerial parts of *Daucus carota*.

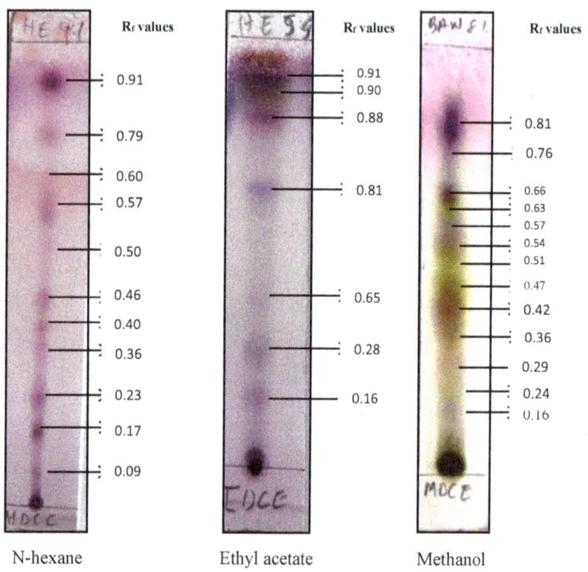

Figure 2. Chromatogram of the *Daucus* carota aerial parts extracts.

content (10.23%), carbohydrate (51.81%), crude protein (14.59%), crude fibre (9.07%), lipid content (10.37%) and ash content (12.99%) which shows that it could be good source of food and may contribute to daily nutritional requirement of a person (20-22). This result is comparable to other findings on proximate and mineral compositions of some leafy vegetables consumed in Nigeria and nutraceutical potential of some fruits peels as sources of vegetables (21,23,24). Fifteen mineral elements detected (Figure 1) showed that *D. carota* aerial parts contain macro and trace elements that could function during muscle contraction, bone formations, growth, metabolism, osmotic balance, regulatory processes activation and other organic bimolecular activities. The presence of heavy metals such as As, Ni, Cd, Pb and Cr could be attributed to the toxic components but with the use of good agricultural practices, lower use of chemicals and fertilizer, the toxic components might be prevented or reduced without any harmful effects when ingested over a long period of time (25).

The antioxidant activity of the *D. carota* aerial parts (Table 3) showed that ethylacetate and methanol extracts had the best antioxidant activity with the EC_{50} (86.89 ug/mL and 166.79 ug/mL) respectively. Both ethyl acetate and methanol extracts had dose dependent antioxidant activity probably because of their phenolic constituents in the aerial parts (26,27). The antioxidant activity in the extracts may be explored for further pharmacological activities.

Conclusion

Daucus carota aerial parts are rich in nutrients that could be used as livestock feed supplements and vegetables for mankind. Its utilization could be incorporated in daily diets and boost food security in developing countries with significant poverty indices. However, its further pharmaceutical utilization and toxicity should be investigated for safety.

Authors' contributions

EA, AA and IG conceived the idea and designed the study. VA and MZ assisted during the literature search and preparation of the manuscript. All authors read the manuscript and confirmed the publication for final version.

Conflict of interests

The authors declare no conflict of interest.

Ethical considerations

Ethical issues have been observed by the authors.

Funding/Support

This research had no financial support.

References

1. Cragg GM, Newman DJ. International Collaboration in Drug Discovery and Development from Natural Sources. Pure Appl Chem. 2005;77(11):1923-42. doi: 10.1351/pac200577111923.
2. Elujoba AA, Odeleye OM, Ogunyemi CM. Traditional Medicine Development from Medical and Dental Primary Health Care Delivery System in Africa. Afr J Tradit Complement Altern Med. 2005;2(1):46-61
3. Etkin NL. Edible Medicine: An Ethnopharmacology of Food. Teuson: University of Arizona Press; 2007:201-20.
4. World Health Organization. Traditional Medicine. WHO Fact Sheet No. 134. Geneva: WHO; 2003.
5. Sofowora A. Medicinal Plants and Traditional Medicine in Africa. Ibadan, Nigeria: Spectrum books Ltd; 1993:191-289.
6. Halliwell B. Free radicals, antioxidants, and human disease: curiosity, cause, or consequence? Lancet. 1994;344(8924):721-4. doi: 10.1016/S0140-6736(94)92211-X.

7. Shebis Y, Iluz D, Kinel-Tahan Y, Dubinsky Z, Yehoshua Y. Natural antioxidants: function and sources. Food Nutr Sci. 2013;4(6):643-9. doi: 10.4236/fns.2013.46083.
8. Bao B, Chang KC. Carrot juice color, carotenoids, and nonstarchy polysaccharides as affected by processing conditions. J Food Sci. 1994;59(6):1155-8. doi: 10.1111/j.1365-2621.1994.tb14665.x.
9. Ross IA. Medicinal Plants of the World, volume 3, Chemical Constituents, Traditional and Modern Uses. New Jersey: Humana Press Inc; 2005.
10. Kataria D, Chahal KK, Kaur P, Kaur R. Carrot plant-A potential source of high value compounds and biological activities: A review. Proceedings of the Indian National Science Academy. 2016;82(4):1237-48. doi: 10.16943/ptinsa/2016/48573.
11. Ayeni EA, Ahmad A, Ibrahim G, Vallada A. Pharmacognostic evaluation of *Daucus carota* Linn. leaf (Apiaceae). Journal of Pharmacognosy and Phytochemistry. 2017;6(5):2400-5.
12. Brain DR, Tuner TD. Extraction procedures. In: The Practical Evaluation of Phytopharmaceuticals. UK, Bristol; 1975:1-107.
13. Harborne ZB. Phytochemical methods: A Guide to Modern Techniques of Plant Analysis. 3rd ed. London: Chapman and Hall Press; 2009:1-283.
14. Stahl E. Thin Layer Chromatography: A laboratory handbook. New Delhi, India: Springer India Private Limited; 2005:1041.
15. AOAC. Official Methods of Analysis of the Association of Analytical Chemists International. 18th ed. Gaithersburg, MD, USA: AOAC; 2005.
16. Idoko O, Emmanuel S, Aguzue O, Fausat A, Osuagwu I, Asuquo T. Phytochemical sreening, proximate analysis and mineral composition of some leafy vegetables consumed in Nigeria. Int J Adv Chem. 2014;2(2):175-7. doi: 10.14419/ijac.v2i2.3514.
17. Mgbemena NM, Obodo GA. Comparative Analysis of Proximate and mineral composition of *Moringa oleifera* root, leave and seed obtained in Okigwe Imo State, Nigeria. J Mol Stud Med Res. 2016;1(2):57-62. doi: 10.18801/jmsmr.010216.07.
18. Akinmoladun AC, Ibukun EO, Afor E, Obuotor EM, Farombi EO. Phytochemical constituent and antioxidant activity of extract from the leaves of Ocimum gratissimum. Sci Res Essays. 2007;2(5):163-6.
19. Mensor LL, Menezes FS, Leitao GG, Reis AS, dos Santos TC, Coube CS, et al. Screening of Brazilian plant extracts for antioxidant activity by the use of DPPH free radical method. Phytother Res. 2001;15(2):127-30. doi: 10.1002/ptr.687.
20. Asaolu SS, Adefemi OS, Oyakilome IG, Ajibulu KE, Asaolu MF. Proximate and Mineral Composition of Nigerian Leafy Vegetables. J Food Res. 2012;1(3):214-8. doi: 10.5539/jfr.v1n3p214.
21. Imran M, Talpur FN, Jan MI, Khan A, Khan I. Analysis of nutritional components of some wild edible edible plants. J Chem Soc Pak. 2007;29(5):500-5.
22. FAO/WHO. Vitamin and mineral requirements in human nutrition. Bangkok, Thailand: FAO/WHO; 1998.
23. Akindahunsi AA, Salawu SO. Phytochemical screening and nutrient-anti-nutrient composition of selected tropical green leafy vegetables. Afr J Biotechnol. 2005;4(6):497-501.
24. FD Romelle, Ashwini-Rani P, RS Manohar. Chemical composition of some selected fruit peels. Eur J Food Sci Technol. 2016;4(4):12-21.
25. Soetan KO, Oyewole OE. The need for adequate processing to reduce the anti-nutritional factors in plants used as human foods and animal feeds: A review. Afr J Food Sci. 2009;3(9):223-32.
26. Sudewi S, Wahyuono S, Astuti P. Isolation and identification of free radicals scavenger from *Daucus carotal* leaves. Traditional Medicine Journal. 2014;19(3):142-8.
27. Mohammedi H, Mecherara-Idjeri S, Foudil-Cherif Y, Hassani A. Chemical composition and antioxidant activity of essential oils from Algerian *Daucus carota* L. subsp. Carota aerial parts. Journal of Essential Oil Bearing Plants. 2015;18(4):873-83. doi: 10.1080/0972060X.2015.1010596.

Portulaca oleracea seeds extract does not prevent dexamethasone-induced hypertension in rats

Leila Safaeian[1*], Bahar Baniahmad[2], Zahra Esfandiari[3], Sayed Ali Alavi[4]

[1]Department of Research and Development, Vice Chancellery for Food and Drug, Department of Pharmacology and Toxicology, School of Pharmacy and Pharmaceutical Sciences, Isfahan University of Medical Sciences, Isfahan, Iran
[2]Department of Pharmacology and Toxicology, Isfahan Pharmaceutical Sciences Research Center, School of Pharmacy and Pharmaceutical Sciences, Isfahan University of Medical Sciences, Isfahan, Iran
[3]Department of Research and Development, Vice-Chancellery for Food and Drug, Isfahan University of Medical Sciences, Isfahan, Iran
[4]Hakiman Shargh Investigative Corporation, Isfahan Science and Technology Town, Isfahan, Iran

ARTICLE INFO

Keywords:
Portulaca oleracea
Hypertension
Dexamethasone

ABSTRACT

Introduction: *Portulaca oleracea* is used as a nutritional and medicinal plant. The aim of this study was to assess the effect of hydroalcoholic extract of *P. oleracea* seeds in dexamethasone -induced hypertension in rats.
Methods: For induction of hypertension, dexamethasone (30 μg/kg/d, subcutaneously) was administered for 14 days. Animals received *P. oleracea* extract as a pretreatment at various doses of 100, 200 and 400 mg/kg/d orally from 4 days before dexamethasone administration and during the test period. Systolic blood pressure (SBP) and heart rate were measured using tail-cuff method. The weight of thymus gland was estimated as a marker of glucocorticoid activity.
Results: Dexamethasone injection significantly increased SBP ($P < 0.001$) while decreased the body and thymus weights ($P < 0.05$ and $P < 0.001$, respectively). Oral administration of *P. oleracea* could not prevent rising in SBP and decreasing in thymus weight. It also increased heart rate in hypertensive rats at the dose of 400 mg/kg/d ($P < 0.05$).
Conclusion: The results of this study revealed that hydroalcoholic extract of *P. oleracea* seeds aggregates hypertension in dexamethasone-induced hypertensive rats. Hence, it should be used with caution in hypertensive patients receiving glucocorticoids.

Implication for health policy/practice/research/medical education:
The results of this study revealed that hydroalcoholic extract of *P. oleracea* seeds aggregates hypertension in dexamethasone-induced hypertensive rats. Therefore, it is recommended that its using be avoided in hypertensive patients receiving glucocorticoids.

Introduction

Hypertension or high blood pressure is a common global health problem. According to the statistical report of the World Health Organization (WHO) in 2015, about 24.0% of male and 20.5% of female subjects suffer from high blood pressure worldwide. There is also a high prevalence of hypertension in Iran and this vascular disease affects 24.1% of Iranian male and 23.3% of Iranian female subjects above 18 years old (1). Hypertension is an important cause for dangerous disorders in major end-organs such as ischemic heart diseases, stroke and renal failure (2). The early diagnosis of hypertension and its medical treatment along with a change in life style would be associated with a decline in the risk of cardiovascular events (3). However, high blood pressure is properly managed only in less than 30% of patients and many people complain of side effects of conventional antihypertensive drugs (4). Recent studies have reported the preventive and helpful effects of various herbal medicines in cardiovascular diseases including hypertension (5).

Portulaca oleracea L. commonly known as purslane belongs to the Portulacea family. This annual succulent herb is growing throughout the Old World and used as a salad and vegetable in many countries (6). Wide

***Corresponding author**: Leila Safaeian,
Email: leila_safaeian@pharm.mui.ac.ir

range of pharmacological properties has been reported for various extracts of *P. oleracea* including antioxidant, antibacterial, hepatoprotective, analgesic, muscle relaxant, anti-inflammatory, bronchodilatory, antihyperglycemic, antihyperlipidemic and anticancer activities (6-11). Some investigations have proposed the potential of this herbal medicine for protection against cardiovascular diseases (12).

In this study, an attempt was made to determine the effect of hydroalcoholic extract of *P. oleracea* seeds in dexamethasone-induced hypertension in rats.

Methods

Animals

Male Wistar rats weighing 180 to 220 g were randomly selected from the animal house of the School of Pharmacy and Pharmaceutical Sciences (Isfahan, Iran). The animals were kept under standard laboratory conditions including 12 h light/12 h dark cycle and room temperature of 20-25°C with free access to water and standard animal diet.

Chemicals

Captopril was purchased from Tehran Darou Pharmaceutical Co. (Tehran, Iran) and dexamethasone was obtained from Darou Pakhsh Pharmaceutical Co. (Tehran, Iran).

Plant material and preparation of the extract

The *P. oleracea* seeds were purchased from a local market of medicinal plants in Isfahan, Iran, and authenticated by Dr Ghaemmaghami (Department of Biology, School of Science, University of Isfahan). A voucher specimen (No. 1891) was deposited at the Herbarium of the School of Pharmacy and Pharmaceutical Sciences, Isfahan, Iran. For the preparation of hydroalcoholic extract, the powdered seeds of plant were extracted with ethanol (70%), using maceration method for 72 hours at room temperature. After completion of extraction (3 times), the solvent was removed by a rotary evaporator under low pressure at 50°C to yield a viscous residue. The obtained extract was stored at -20°C.

Experimental design

For induction of hypertension, dexamethasone (30 μg/kg/d) was injected subcutaneously (s.c.) in rats for 14 days, and the control group received daily s.c. injection of normal saline (1 mL/kg). In this prevention study, animals received *P. oleracea* seeds extract (100, 200 and 400 mg/kg) or captopril (40 mg/kg, an antihypertensive agent as a reference drug) orally using an intra-gastric tube from 4 days before dexamethasone administration and during the test period (days 1-18). Six rats were used in each group. All animals were weighted on alternate days. At the end of the experiment, the rats were sacrificed under ether anesthesia and the thymus glands were isolated. The weight of thymus was measured and expressed as milligrams per 100 g body weight. Decline in thymus weight was considered as a marker of glucocorticoid activity (13,14).

Measurement of systolic blood pressure and heart rate

The systolic blood pressure (SBP) and heart rate were recorded by non-invasive tail-cuff method (AD Instrument PowerLab Data Acquisition System, Australia) at the first and last days of the experiment in conscious rats. Ten minutes before measurements, each animal was restrained in a heated chamber at 38±1°C. A training period of 1 week was established before the experiment to allow the rats become adapted to the procedure. Five measurements of blood pressure and heart rate were taken for each rat and their averages were used to obtain the mean values.

Statistical analysis

All values were shown as the mean ± standard error of mean (SEM). For statistical evaluation, one-way analysis of variance (ANOVA) followed by Tukey post hoc test was used (SPSS software version 18.0). Differences with a value of $P< 0.05$ were considered to be significant.

Results

Effect of *Portulaca oleracea* seeds extract on blood pressure

Administration of dexamethasone significantly increased SBP from 116.3 ± 2.7 to 152.6 ± 3.6 mmHg ($P< 0.001$) compared to the normal control group (122. 5 ± 1.5 mm Hg). Captopril caused a significant decrease in SBP ($P < 0.001$) but pretreatment with *P. oleracea* seeds extract could not prevent the increase in SBP (Figure 1).

Effect of *Portulaca oleracea* seeds extract on heart rate

As shown in Figure 2, heart rate was not significantly changed after administration of dexamethasone, captopril or *P. oleracea* seeds extract at the doses of 100 and 200 mg/kg. However, treatment with 400 mg/kg of *P. oleracea* seeds extract caused a significant increase in rats heart

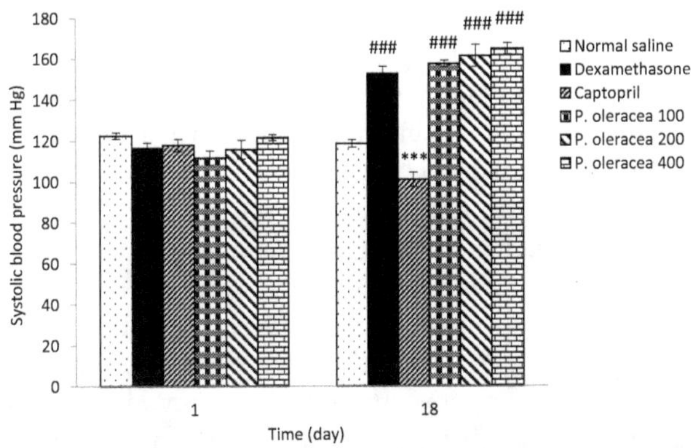

Figure 1. Effects of *P. oleracea* seeds extract and captopril (40 mg/kg) on systolic blood pressure in dexamethasone-induced hypertensive rats. Values are means ± SEM for six rats. ###P <0.001 versus normal saline group, and ***P < 0.001 versus dexamethasone group.

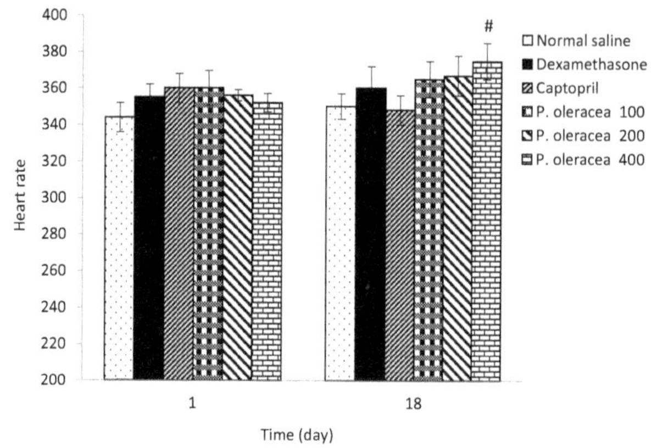

Figure 2. Effects of *P. oleracea* seeds extract and captopril (40 mg/kg) on heart rate in dexamethasone-induced hypertensive rats. Values are means ± SEM for six rats. #P < 0.05 versus normal saline control group.

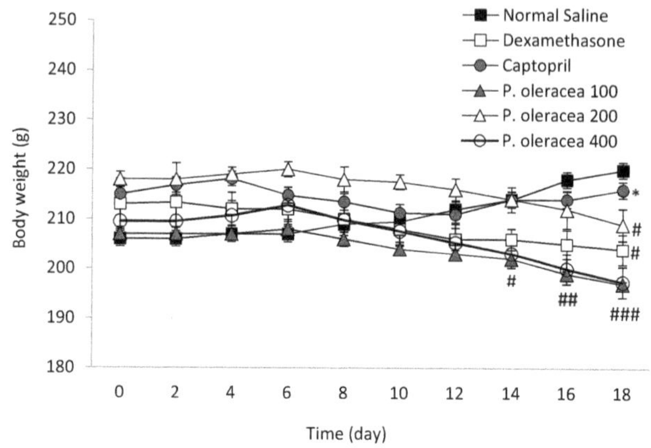

Figure 3. Effects of *P. oleracea* seeds extract and captopril (40 mg/kg) on body weight in dexamethasone-induced hypertensive rats. Values are means ± SEM for six rats. #P < 0.05, ##P < 0.01 and ###P < 0.001 versus normal saline control group and *P < 0.05 versus dexamethasone group.

rate compared to the normal control group (P <0.05).

Effect of *Portulaca oleracea* seeds extract on body weight
Dexamethasone injection caused a significant decrease in body weight in hypertensive animals compared to normal control group (P <0.05). Administration of *P. oleracea* seeds extract significantly increased weight loss at all doses. However, captopril could prevent body weight loss induced by dexamethasone (P <0.05, Figure 3).

Effect of *Portulaca oleracea* on thymus weight
Administration of dexamethasone significantly reduced the thymus gland weight as a marker of glucocorticoid activity in hypertensive rats (P < 0.001). Treatment with *P. Oleracea* seeds extract and captopril could not prevent the thymus weight decline (Figure 4).

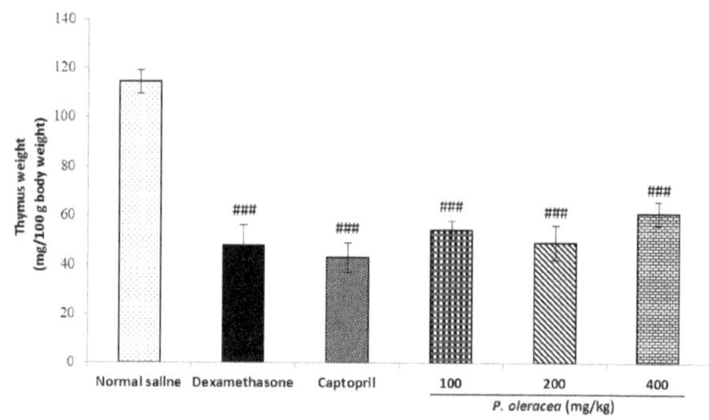

Figure 4. Effects of *P. oleracea* seeds extract and captopril (40 mg/kg) on thymus weight in dexamethasone-induced hypertensive rats. Values are means ± SEM for six rats. ###P < 0.001 versus normal saline control group

Discussion

The present study investigated the effect of hydroalcoholic extract of *P. oleracea* seeds on blood pressure in the animal model of dexamethasone-induced hypertension in rats. The results showed that oral administration of *P. Oleracea* seeds extract could not prevent rising in SBP.

Chronic use of dexamethasone leads to hypertension through various mechanisms including increased activity of cardiovascular regulating systems such as sympathetic, renin-angiotensin and endothelin systems and changing in hemodynamic status (15). Augmented sensitivity and reactivity to angiotensin II and norepinephrine and subsequently increased vascular resistance have been defined following dexamethasone administration (16). The roles of oxidative stress and over-production of reactive oxygen species (ROS) through nicotinamide adenine dinucleotide phosphate (NAPDH) oxidase pathway and nitric oxide (NO) deficiency have also been implicated in the pathophysiology of glucocorticoid-induced hypertension (17). Some antioxidant agents and herbal medicines have been able to prevent and reduce hypertension from dexamethasone in various investigations (18). The hydroalcoholic extract of stems and green leaves of *P. oleracea* has been reported to have antihypertensive activity with negative ionotropic and chronotropic effects (19). Phytochemical analysis of *P. oleracea* demonstrated the presence of flavonoids, terpenoids, coumarins, alkaloids, sterols and various nutrients including calcium, magnesium, thiamin, riboflavin, nicotinic acid, vitamin C, carotene, vitamin E, fatty acids, omega-3, linolenic acid, oxalic acid and others (20,21). Its aerial parts are also rich in potassium ions elucidating the muscle relaxant effect of *P. oleracea* (8). There are also valid documents for the presence of biologically active catecholamines including noradrenaline, dopamine and L-dopa in *P. oleracea*. Large concentrations of noradrenaline in the fresh plant have been reported as 2.5 mg/g which is probably larger than that of extractable amount from the mammalians suprarenal glands (22). These neurotransmitters may be responsible for increasing blood pressure in this model of hypertension in which dexamethasone intensifies the reactivity to vasopressor effects of catecholamines.

There is no accurate data for toxicity profile of seeds

of *P. oleracea*, however Musa and coworkers reported moderate toxicity and LD50 about 1853-1875 mg/kg for methanolic extract of *P. oleracea* (23). There are some reports for the alteration in oxalic acid content in *P. oleracea* extract based on the nitrogen concentration and nitrate/ammonium ratio in the nutrient solutions (24). Toxic level of plasma oxalate has been associated with atherogenic activity through increasing the intracellular calcium concentration in endothelial cells and inhibition of endothelial proliferation (25). Although *P. oleracea* extract at the dose of 400 mg/kg has been used in some studies (26), but it seems that the lower doses would have the better safety profile with minor adverse effects.

The results of the present study also showed increasing in weight loss after administration of *P. oleracea* seeds extract in dexamethasone-induced hypertensive rats. The hypolipidemic effect and reducing body weight gain have been reported for *P. oleracea* in animal models of hyperlipidemia. Different biochemicals such as polyphenols, phytosterols, alkaloids and saponins may be responsible for antihyperlipidemic effect of this plant through decreasing food intake, increasing gastrointestinal motility, promoting insulin sensitivity, regulating the cell energy metabolism or reducing free fatty acids, reducing cholesterol absorption through interfering with its enterohepatic circulation and increasing cholesterol fecal excretion (11,27).

Conclusion

The results of this study revealed that hydroalcoholic extract of *P. oleracea* seeds could not prevent dexamethasone-induced hypertension. The presence of high amounts of catecholamines in this extract and increasing reactivity to vasopressor effects of catecholamines in dexamethasone-induced hypertension may be accountable for increasing blood pressure in this animal model of hypertension.

Authors' contributions

All authors made substantial contributions to conception and design, and/or acquisition of data, and substantially to the writing of the manuscript. All authors read the final version and confirmed the manuscript publication.

Conflict of interests

The authors declare no conflicts of interest. The authors alone are responsible for the content of the paper.

Ethical considerations

All procedures were approved by the ethics committee of Isfahan University of Medical Sciences (IR.MUI.REC.1395.2.104).

Funding/Support

This study was financially supported by a research project No. 295104 from Isfahan University of Medical Sciences, Isfahan, Iran.

References

1. WHO. World health statistics. Geneva, Switzerland: WHO; 2015.
2. Kearney PM, Whelton M, Reynolds K, Muntner P, Whelton PK, He J. Global burden of hypertension: analysis of worldwide data. Lancet. 2005;365(9455):217-23. doi: 10.1016/s0140-6736(05)17741-1.
3. Hansson L, Zanchetti A, Carruthers SG, Dahlof B, Elmfeldt D, Julius S, et al. Effects of intensive blood-pressure lowering and low-dose aspirin in patients with hypertension: principal results of the hypertension optimal treatment (HOT) randomised trial. HOT Study Group. Lancet. 1998;351(9118):1755-62.
4. Evans RG, Kett MM, Shweta A, Fitzgerald SM, Denton KM, Eppel GA, et al. New physiological targets within the kidney for antihypertensive therapy. Drug Design Reviews Online. 2005;2(2):167-78. doi: 10.2174/1567269053202651.
5. Safaeian L, Ghannadi A, Javanmard SH, Vahidian MH. The effect of hydroalcoholic extract of *Ferula foetida* stems on blood pressure and oxidative stress in dexamethasone-induced hypertensive rats. Res Pharm Sci. 2015;10(4):326-34.
6. Elkhayat ES, Ibrahim SR, Aziz MA. Portulene, a new diterpene from *Portulaca oleracea* L. J Asian Nat Prod Res. 2008;10(11-12):1039-43. doi: 10.1080/10286020802320590.
7. Chan K, Islam MW, Kamil M, Radhakrishnan R, Zakaria MN, Habibullah M, et al. The analgesic and anti-inflammatory effects of *Portulaca oleracea* L. subsp. Sativa (Haw.) Celak. J Ethnopharmacol. 2000;73(3):445-51.
8. Habtemariam S, Harvey AL, Waterman PG. The muscle relaxant properties of Portulaca oleracea are associated with high concentrations of potassium ions. J Ethnopharmacol. 1993;40(3):195-200.
9. Malek F, Boskabady MH, Borushaki MT, Tohidi M. Bronchodilatory effect of *Portulaca oleracea* in airways of asthmatic patients. J Ethnopharmacol. 2004;93(1):57-62. doi: 10.1016/j.jep.2004.03.015.
10. Lee AS, Lee YJ, Lee SM, Yoon JJ, Kim JS, Kang DG, et al. *Portulaca oleracea* ameliorates diabetic vascular inflammation and endothelial dysfunction in db/db Mice. Evid Based Complement Alternat Med. 2012;2012:741824. doi: 10.1155/2012/741824.
11. Pragda SS, Kuppast IJ, Mankani KL, Ramesh L. Evaluation of antihyperlipidemic activity of leaves of *Portulaca oleracea* Linn against dexamethasone induced hyperlipidemia in rats. Int J Pharm Pharm Sci. 2012;4(4):279-83.
12. Chen T, Wang J, Li Y, Shen J, Zhao T, Zhang H. Sulfated modification and cytotoxicity of *Portulaca oleracea* L. polysaccharides. Glycoconj J. 2010;27(6):635-42. doi: 10.1007/s10719-010-9307-0.
13. Simopoulos AP, Norman HA, Gillaspy JE, Duke JA. Common purslane: a source of omega-3 fatty acids and antioxidants. J Am Coll Nutr. 1992;11(4):374-82.
14. Safaeian L, Ghasemi-Dehkordi N, Javanmard SH, Namvar H. Antihypertensive and antioxidant effects of a hydroalcoholic extract obtained from aerial parts of *Otostegia persica* (Burm.) Boiss. Res Pharm Sci. 2015;10(3):192-9.
15. Ong SL, Zhang Y, Whitworth JA. Mechanisms of dexamethasone-induced hypertension. Curr Hypertens Rev. 2009;5(1):61-74. doi: 10.2174/157340209787314315.
16. Russo D, Fraser R, Kenyon CJ. Dexamethasone therapy selectively increases the sensitivity to noradrenaline

of the rat mesenteric circulation. J Hypertens Suppl. 1989;7(6):S126-7.

17. Zhang Y, Croft KD, Mori TA, Schyvens CG, McKenzie KU, Whitworth JA. The antioxidant tempol prevents and partially reverses dexamethasone-induced hypertension in the rat. Am J Hypertens. 2004;17(3):260-5. doi: 10.1016/j.amjhyper.2003.11.004.
18. Safaeian L, Hajhashemi V, Haghjoo Javanmard S, Sanaye Naderi H. The effect of protocatechuic acid on blood pressure and oxidative stress in glucocorticoid-induced hypertension in rat. Iran J Pharm Res. 2016;15(Suppl):83-91.
19. Parry O, Okwuasaba F, Ejike C. Effect of an aqueous extract of *Portulaca oleracea* leaves on smooth muscle and rat blood pressure. J Ethnopharmacol. 1988;22(1):33-44.
20. Kamil M, Jayaraj AF, Ahmad F, Gunasekhar C, Thomas S, Habibullah M, Chan K. Chemical standardization of *Portulaca oleracea* V. Sativa. J Pharm Pharmacol. 1998; 50(59):259-263.
21. Rasheed AN, Afifi FU, Shaedah M, Taha MO. Investigation of the active constituents of *Portulaca oleraceae* L. (Portulacaceae) growing in Jordan. Pak J Pharm Sci. 2004;17(1):37-45.
22. Yue ME, Jiang TF, Shi YP. Simultaneous determination of noradrenaline and dopamine in *Portulaca oleracea* L. by capillary zone electrophoresis. J Sep Sci. 2005;28(4):360-4. doi: 10.1002/jssc.200400045.
23. Musa KY, Ahmed A, Ibrahim G, Ojonugwa OE, Bisalla M, Musa H, et al. Toxicity studies on the methanolic extract of *Portulaca oleracea* L. (Fam. Portulacaceae). J Biol Sci. 2007; 7(7):1293-95. doi: 10.3923/jbs.2007.1293.1295.
24. Fontana E, Hoeberechts J, Nicola S, Cros V, Battista Palmegiano G, Giorgio Peiretti P. Nitrogen concentration and nitrate/ammonium ratio affect yield and change the oxalic acid concentration and fatty acid profile of purslane (*Portulaca oleracea* L.) grown in a soilless culture system. J Sci Food Agric. 2006;86(14):2417-24. doi: 10.1002/jsfa.2633.
25. Recht PA, Tepedino GJ, Siecke NW, Buckley MT, Mandeville JT, Maxfield FR, et al. Oxalic acid alters intracellular calcium in endothelial cells. Atherosclerosis. 2004;173(2):321-8. doi: 10.1016/j.atherosclerosis.2003.11.023.
26. Martins WB, Rodrigues SA, Silva HK, Dantas CG, Junior Wde L, Filho LX, et al. Neuroprotective effect of Portulaca oleracea extracts against 6-hydroxydopamine-induced lesion of dopaminergic neurons. An Acad Bras Cienc. 2016;88(3):1439-50. doi: 10.1590/0001-3765201620150574.
27. El-Newary SA. The hypolipidemic effect of *Portulaca oleracea* L. stem on hyperlipidemic Wister Albino rats. Annals Agricultural Sciences. 2016;61(1):111-24. doi: 10.1016/j.aoas.2016.01.002.

A significant antihypertensive effect of *Holarrhena floribunda* supported by an exploratory phytochemical study

Kafui Kpegba[1], Etonam Tété Kondo[1], Oudjaniyobi Simalou[1*], Komlatsè Togbenou[2], Pakoupati Boyode[1], Outéndé Toundou[1], Nagba Yendoubé Gbandjaba[1], Amegnona Agbonon[2], Messanvi Gbeassor[2]

[1]Laboratoire de Chimie Organique et des Substances Naturelles (Lab COSNat), Faculté des Science, Université de Lomé, 01 BP 1515 Lomé 01, Lomé-Togo
[2]Laboratoire de Physiologie et de Pharmacologie, Faculté des Science, Université de Lomé ; 01 BP 1515 Lomé 01, Lomé-Togo

ARTICLE INFO

Keywords:
Holarrhena floribunda
Phytochemical screening
Antioxidant activity
Antihypertensive activity

ABSTRACT

Introduction: *Holarrhena floribunda* (G.Don) T.Durand & Schinz is a tree that can grow up to 25 m with white latex in its organs. The bark of this plant is commonly used in traditional medicine to treat dysentery, diarrhea, diabetes, malaria, and high blood pressure. In this study, phytochemical groups were widely investigated on trunk bark as well as on leaves of *H. floribunda* harvested in Danyi (Togo). Antioxidant activity and antihypertensive properties of the plant extracts were also evaluated on sound guinea pigs.
Methods: The hydro-ethanolic extract of the trunk bark was prepared and antioxidant activity was evaluated via the DPPH radical-scavenging and the ferric-reducing antioxidant power (FRAP) methods, and via the determination of the total phenolics content. This hydro-ethanolic extract was used to assess the plant extract effect on blood pressure of sound guinea pigs.
Results: So, phytochemical screening revealed that *H. floribunda* contained most of the phytochemical groups. The 50% inhibitive concentration of that extract by DPPH was 29.80 ± 0.001 µg/mL. The equivalent of Fe^{2+} by FRAP was 1009.9 ± 0.6 µmol/g of dry extract. The content of phenolic compounds was 139 ± 0.053 mg GAE (gallic acid equivalents)/g of dry extract. Intravenous injection of the extract (10, 20, 40, 80 mg/kg) via the invasive method in guinea pigs under normal strain caused a decrease in diastolic blood pressure, systolic blood pressure, and so in mean arterial pressure (MAP) by dose cumulative and time-dependent.
Conclusion: The results show that hydro-ethanolic extract of *H. floribunda* trunk bark has antihypertensive and antioxidant properties. This might be the reason for the use of that extract for the treatment of hypertension in traditional medicine.

Implication for health policy/practice/research/medical education:
Holarrhena floribunda trunk bark exhibited antihypertensive and antioxidant properties, supporting its use for the treatment of hypertension in traditional medicine. So, more investigations are needed for identification of the active compounds in *Holarrhena floribunda* ethanolic extract involved in antioxidant and antihypertensive activities.

Introduction

Cardiovascular diseases (CVD) are pathologies that affect the heart and blood vessels. They are the main cause of deaths in the world (1). More than three-quarters of deaths in low- and middle-income countries are due to CVD (2). In Togo, the situation of CVD is of great concern while their incidence is not fully known (3). Risk factors for CVD include poor nutrition and physical inactivity, smoking, oxidative stress, heavy drinking, diabetes, hyperlipidemia, and hypertension. Indeed, hypertension is a chronic pathology that constitutes a real public health problem with a global prevalence in the world for adults estimated at 26.4% in 2000 (972 million people including 639 million in resource-limited countries) and could reach 29% by 2025 (1.56 billion of peoples) (4). The conventional treatments of hypertension require synergy of several

***Corresponding author**: Oudjaniyobi Simalou,
Email: jacobsimalou@yahoo.fr

classes of antihypertensive agents; even so none of those treatments definitely cured this pathology. Moreover, the high cost when facing the treatment of hypertension with conventional drugs makes it hardly affordable for common peoples. For that, common people prefer using traditional medicines. Indeed, some studies have shown the positive effects of antioxidants from plants as good agents for the prevention of hypertension diseases (5). It is known that several plants are used in traditional medicine to treat high blood pressure (6). *Holarrhena floribunda* is one of those species which natural ecological zone covers many African countries namely Togo, Senegal, Guinea-Bisseau, Guinea, Mali; Burkina Faso, Sierra Leonne, Liberia, Ivory Coast, Ghana, Benin, Nigeria, Chad, Cameroon, Gabon, Congo, Central Africa. The many uses of *H. floribunda* in traditional medicine in those African countries include the treatment of dysentery, diarrhea, fever, snake bite, infertility, venereal disease, diabetes, hypertension, and malaria (7,8). So, the present study aimed mainly the assessment of the antihypertensive effects of the ethanolic extract of the trunk bark of *H. floribunda*. For that, the phytochemical groups of the leaves and the trunk bark were firstly investigated. Then, the anti-radical activity and the effect on the blood pressure of normal strained guinea pigs of the trunk bark hydro-ethanolic extract were evaluated.

Materials and Methods

General information

Optical densities (absorption spectra) were determined on a Shimadzu UV-1601PC spectrophotometer. Samples were weighted using a Sartorius lab instruments balance with maximum weight of 1000 ± 0.01 g. Evaporation was carried out on an R-100 BÜCHI Rotavapor. An electric shredder and a transducer connected to Biopac System (Model MP100, Harvard Apparatus) allowed the assessment of extract effects on sound guinea pigs blood pressure. Analytical grade solvents and all others materials were used as received.

Phyto-constituents characterization

Phytochemical screening refers to all methods and techniques for the detection of active chemical groups in the plant. In this study, the whole phytochemical screening was performed according to standard methods described by Badiaga et al (9). So, the presence of alkaloids has been revealed by Mayer or Dragendorff's reagent. STIANSY reagent or 1% ferric chloride was used to characterize tannin derivatives. Flavonoids derivatives and buffy anthocyanins were evidenced by the cyanidine reaction (SHINODA reagent). Quinone compounds were evidenced by the Bornträger reaction. The detection of sterols and triterpenes were possible with Liebermann-Burchard reaction. Cardiotonic glycosides were revealed when green or purple color came out after adding the acetic and sulfuric acid in chloroformic extract. The appearance of a flaky precipitate revealed the presence of mucilages. Saponosides were characterized by their foaming power. Reducing constituents were characterized using A and B Fehling liquors. The anthracites derivatives were revealed using a 50% ammonia solution.

Biological materials

The bark of the trunk and the leaves of *H. floribunda* were harvested in March 2015 at Danyi Mountain in the plateaus region (Zone IV) of Togo. The plant is locally called "Afèkèti" or "Kpomiti" in "Ewé". It was (the plant species) identified by the Herbarium of "Université de Lomé" (TOGO; TOGO02074) and previously registered under the identification number 1987/03 by K. Akpagana (K. Akpagana, #1522). The plant samples were left at room temperature for two weeks. After this drying process, the samples were reduced in powder using a lab scale grinder. Hydro-ethanolic extract of the trunk was prepared to assess pharmacological effects of *H. floribunda* on guinea pigs under normal blood pressure (systolic blood pressure $\leq$120 mm Hg) weighting about 400-550 g. They were bought in Gbonsimé market in Lomé city (Togo) and placed at animal house of the Laboratory of physiology and pharmacology of natural products of the Faculty of Sciences, "Université de Lomé" (Togo), for a week before the experiments. These guinea-pigs had free access to water and were fed with fresh grass.

Cardiovascular effects assessment via bloody method

The so-called direct bloody method is an invasive technique for measuring blood pressure using a catheter introduced into the carotid artery of an anesthetized animal (10). The measurement of invasive pressure presents some advantages, notably the beat-by-beat tracking of blood pressure and the achievement of a very precise pressure even at very low extent. The invasive pressure was measured using a transducer (connected to the catheter) with an ultra-sensitive membrane capable of converting the slightest mechanical variations of the animal's blood pressure into electrical signals. The recording of the cardiovascular parameters was done according to this method exhaustively described previously (11). The guinea pig, anesthetized intraperitoneally with 20% of urethane (ethyl carbamate) at a dose of 1 g/kg (that is 1 mL/200 g body weight), was placed in supine position (12). The jugular vein and the carotid artery were exposed, dissected, and then intubated towards the heart using fine polyethylene catheters.

The catheter of the jugular vein connected to one syringe and that of the carotid artery linked to a pressure sensor connected to a transducer were used to visualize the hemodynamic parameters such as the systolic blood pressure (SBP, mm Hg) and the diastolic blood pressure (DBP, mm Hg). Those two types of blood pressure correspond to the maximum and the minimum pressures, respectively. Mean arterial pressure (MAP, mmHg) does not an arithmetic average of SBP and DBP, because blood pressure values in the arteries are more closed to DBP value for a long time. For that, the average pressure was obtained from the following stated Pelletier' relation (13):

$$MAP = DBP + \frac{(SBP - DBP)}{3}$$

After stabilization of the cardiovascular parameters for about 45 minutes, the extracts of *H. floribunda* at cumulative doses of 10; 20; 40; 80 mg/kg (taking into account the toxicity studies of *H. floribunda* by Bogne et al (14) and Antwi (15)) were administered intravenously through the syringe connected to catheter of the jugular vein of a guinea pig under normal blood pressure. The NaCl solution (9‰) containing 10% of heparin was injected at a rate of 1 mL/1000 g via this jugular vein to prevent blood from clotting. The decrease rate in MAP was calculated using the following relation:
$\% \Delta MAP = ((MAP_i - MAP_f) \times 100) / (MAP_i)$
With i = initial; f = final

Determination of total phenols and polyphenolic antioxidants
The determination of total phenols content is an in vitro colorimetric assay based on the ability to reduce the Folin-Ciocalteu reagent (FCR) (16) which is a yellow acid solution consisting of a mixture of phosphotungstic and phosphomolybdic polyheterocyclic acids. In a basic medium, the FCR oxidizes the hydroxyl groups of polyphenolic compounds giving a blue coloration. This determination was carried out according to the method described by Al-Farsi et al (17). A mixture consisting of 100 µL of extract in methanol at 1 mg/mL and 750 µL of the FCR 10 times diluted was prepared. After stirring for 5 minutes, 750 µL of a saturated sodium carbonate (Na_2CO_3) solution at 60 g/L was added. The obtained solution was incubated for 90 minutes at room temperature in the darkness. The absorption spectra (optical densities) were recorded with respect to a blank at 725 nm using a UV-visible spectrophotometer. Referring to the calibration regression equation established with gallic acid in a concentration range of 0-500 µg/mL (Figure 1), the content of polyphenols in the extract was determined. The test was performed in triplicate. The following formula was used to calculate the total phenol contents expressed in mg Equivalent of Gallic Acid (EGA) over 1 g of dry extract:

$$Polyphenol\ content\ (EAG\ par\ g) = \frac{Rec.Conc \times Dil.Fact \times Vo}{sampl.mass}$$

Rec.Conc: recorded concentration; Dil.Fac: dilution factor; Vo: initial volume; Sampl.mass: masse of the sample.

Free DPPH• radical trapping activity
The antiradical activity was determined using the method described by Brand-Williams et al (18), modified by Agbonon et al (19). This method relies on the trapping of the stable free radical DPPH in the presence of antioxidant molecules.
The DPPH solution of about 10^{-4} mol/L was prepared (about 1 to 2 hours in advance) by making soluble the pure DPPH in methanol so that the solution exhibited an optical density between 0.787 and 0.788 at 517 nm. A range of concentrations (1 to 50 µg/mL) of *H. floribunda* extract or quercetin solutions was prepared in methanol. A volume of 250 µL of each of those prepared solutions was added to 1.5 mL of the DPPH solution ($C = 10^{-4}$ mol/L), the mixture was homogenized and incubated at room temperature for 30 minutes. The optical density was then recorded at 517 nm using a UV-visible spectrophotometer. The control was recorded under the same conditions. The inhibition percent (%I) of the DPPH was calculated according to the following formula:

$$\%I = 100 \times \frac{ODc - ODs}{ODc}$$

ODc: Optical Density of the control; OD: Optical Density of the sample (extract or quercetin).
The anti-radical power was defined as the concentration of extract needed to induce the reduction of 50% of the free radical DPPH (IC_{50}). The IC_{50} value was calculated by the linear regression method shown in Figure 2: %I = f (concentration) = ***a*x + *b***, with ***a*** and ***b*** constants and **x** a concentration; %I = 50% = f (IC_{50}). Standard deviations were calculated from three sets of experiments. The IC_{50} value depends on the nature of the sample and the final residual concentration of the DPPH.

Antioxidant power by the FRAP
The ferric ion reducing antioxidant power (FRAP) method consists of reducing ferric ions from the ferric tripyridyltriazine complex (Fe^{3+}-TPTZ) to ferrous ions under a low pH and temperature of about 37°C. The change in absorbance at 593 nm is directly associated with

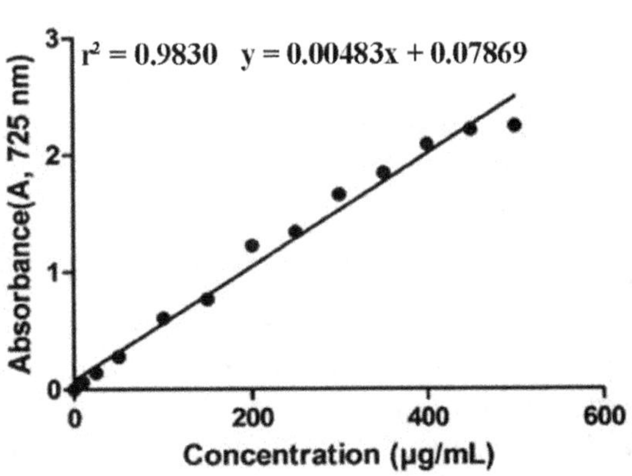

Figure 1. Calibration graph of gallic acid.

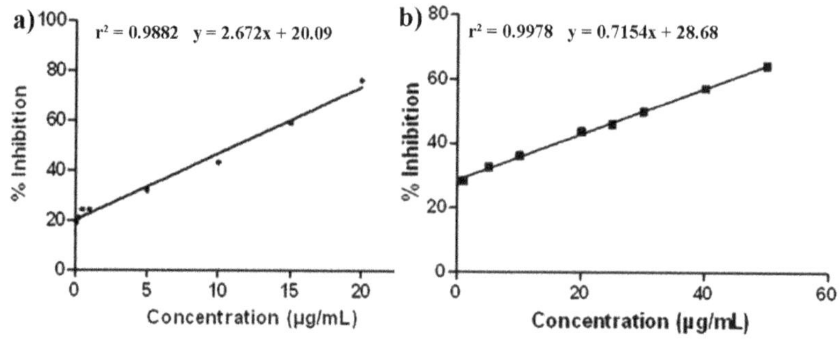

Figure 2: a) Linear regression line of quercetin, b) Linear regression line of *Holarrhena floribunda* extract with DPPH

the combined reducing power of all antioxidant molecules present in the reaction mixture (20).

For that, freshly prepared 1980 µL FRAP solution consisting of 25 mL acetate buffer (pH = 3.6), 2.5 mL TPTZ at 10 mmol/L in HCl 40 mmol/L, and 2.5 mL of $FeCl_3.6H_2O$ at 20 mmol/L, was added to 15 µL of the extract solution. The optical densities of samples and blank at 593 nm were recorded using a UV-visible spectrophotometer. A calibration range was established from different concentrations (0 to 2000 µmol/L) of $FeSO_4.7H_2O$ in methanol. Referring to the regression equation of the calibration established with $FeSO_4.7H_2O$ (Figure 3), the content of polyphenols in the extract was determined and expressed in µmol of Fe^{2+} equivalent per gram of extract. The test was performed in triplicate from which the standard deviations were calculated. The concentration (content of polyphenols) of the stock solution was obtained using the following formula:

$$FRAP\ value\ (\mu mol\ equivalent\ Fe^{2+}\ per\ g) = \frac{Rec.Conc \times Dilut.Fact \times Vo}{Sampl.Mass}$$

Rec.Conc: recorded concentration; Dilut.Fact: dilution factor; Vo: volume of the stock solution; Sampl.mass: mass of the sample.

Statistical processing

Data were expressed as means ± standard deviation (SD) of experiments performed in triplicate or in quintuplicate according to the test. The values were analyzed by analysis of variance (ANOVA) test, followed by Tukey's multiple comparison tests using GraphPad Prism 5.00. The statistical significance between results for different samples and between results for samples and controls were set at $P<0.05$.

Results

Phytochemical screening of *Holarrhena floribunda*

In order to investigate the phytochemical composition of *H. floribunda*, infusion, maceration, and decoction were used and many extracts obtained. For that, the leaves and bark of trunk powder samples were firstly subjected to infusion and decoction. The similar powder samples were then macerated in many organic solvents (ethanol, chloroform, hydrochloric acid, ethyl acetate, and petroleum ether). The various phytochemical groups detected in infused and decocted samples are recorded on the Table 1, and those from the maceration are drawn up in Table 2.

From infusion method (Table 1), one can see that anthocyanins were not detected. In the same time, tannins (catechics and gallic), saponosides, and flavonoids have been detected. From the decocted phases, the leuco-anthocyanins, saponosides, mucilages, flavonoids, and reducing compounds were revealed in the two parts. Moreover, foam index performed on the decocted phase was 500 in the leaves against 333.33 in the trunk bark. In macerated samples and when using some specific tests, various phytochemical compounds were detected (Table 2). So, only alkaloids and saponosides were detected in ethanol while cardiotonic heterosides, c-heteroside, and o-heteroside anthracenic were found in chloroformic macerated phases. Alkaloids were found in hydrochloric acid; sterols and terpenes in ethyl acetate, and free quinones in petroleum.

Anti-radical activity by DPPH, antioxidant power by FRAP and total phenol content

Based on the calibration regression equation established in Figure 1, the total phenol content (in equivalent of gallic acid per gram of dry extract) of the trunk bark hydro-ethanolic extract was 139±0.053 mg EGA/g dry

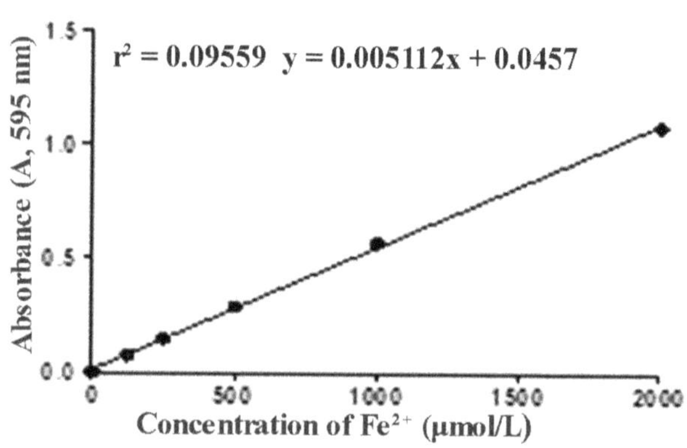

Figure 3. Calibration curve of $FeSO_4.7H_2O$

Table 1. Chemical groups detected in infuse and decocted powders of the leaves and the bark of the trunk

Extraction method	Phyto-constituents	Leaves	Trunk bark
Infusion	Tannins	+	+
	Catechic tanins	+	+
	Gallic tannins	+	+
	Saponosides	+	+
	Flavonoids	+	+
	Anthocyanins	-	-
Decoction	Leuco-anthocyanins	+	+
	Saponosides	+	+
	Foam Index	500	333.33
	Mucilages	+	+
	Flavonoids	+	+
	Reducing compounds	+	+

+: Detected; -: Not detected.

Table 2. Phyto-constituents from different macerated phases of leaves and trunk bark

Extraction method	Phytoconstituents	Leaves	Bark of the trunk
Maceration in ethanol	Alkaloids	+	+
	Saponosides	+	+
Maceration in $CHCl_3$	Cardiovascular heterosides	+	+
	Free anthracenic	-	-
	Anthra.O-heterosides	+	+
	Anthra.C-heterosides	+	+
Maceration in HCl	Alkaloids	+	+
Maceration in ethyl acetate	Sterols and terpenes	+	+
Maceration in petroleum ether	Free quinones	+	+

+: Detected; -: Not detected.

extract. The antioxidant activity of the same extract was evaluated by the DPPH and the FRAP methods. The DPPH test allows getting the anti-radical activity. Indeed, it is known that an extract is more antioxidant if its IC_{50} is lower. From Table 3, the IC_{50} of this extract is 29.80±0.001 µg/mL while that of quercetin is 11.19±0.23 µg/mL. The reducing power assessed by the FRAP method gave the value of 1009.9 ± 0.6 µmol Equivalent Fe^{2+}/g (Table 3). Furthermore, the kinetics of the reduction of DPPH under different concentrations of the extract was monitored. As shown in Figure 4, the decrease in absorbance is more pronounced for large concentrated sample. The kinetic profiles are dependent on the concentration of the extract. Close observation shows that the extract reacted quickly with the DPPH reaching a steady state in about 5 minutes.

Assessment of the extract effect on guinea-pigs blood pressure

Intravenous injection of the hydro-ethanolic extract (by cumulative dose in the order of 10; 20; 40; 80 mg/kg) resulted in immediate decreases in mean arterial pressure (MAP) of normal strained guinea pigs (Figures 5 and 6). Indeed, a few seconds after injection of 10 mg/kg of the prepared dose, MAP decreased from 82.734 mm Hg to 65.067 mm Hg, which is an immediate and significant decrease of about 21.35%. Then, the pressure rose to hit the initial value in about 10 minutes later. Administering the dose of 20 mg/kg resulted in a sharp and significant decrease in MAP of about 27.86%; 15 minutes later, the MAP rose and stabilized at about 70.6 mm Hg. The 40

Table 3. Results of DPPH and FRAP tests

Sample	IC50±SD (µg/mL)	FRAP Equi.Fe^{2+} (µmol/g)
Extract	29.80±0.001	1009.9±0.6
Quercetin	11.19±0.23	-

Values are expressed as means ± standard deviation (SD) (n = 3).

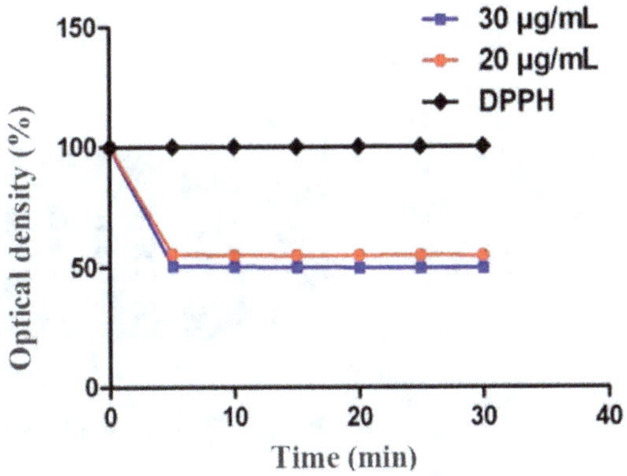

Figure 4. Kinetics of the reduction of the DPPH alone (black), DPPH with 20 µg/mL of *Holarrhena floribunda* extract (red), and DPPH with 30 µg/mL of *Holarrhena floribunda* extract (blue).

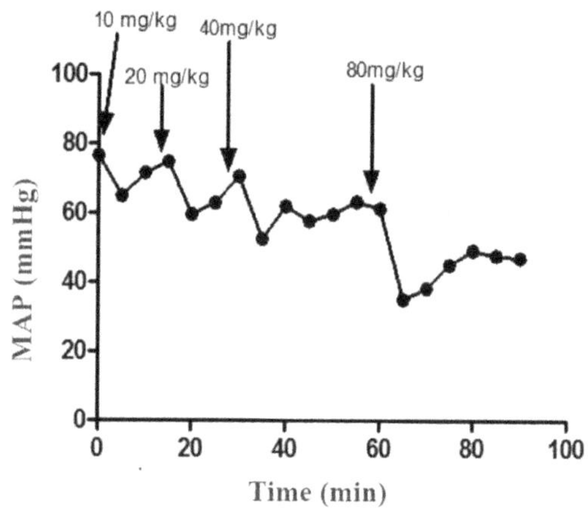

Figure 5. Effect of dose-response of *Holarrhena floribunda* extract on MAP.

mg/kg dose resulted in a sharp and significant decrease in MAP of about 36.41%; 20 minutes later the MAP rose and steadied at about 61.33 mm Hg. When 80 mg/kg was injected, a drastic and significant drop in MAP of about 57.68% was observed, 20 minutes later, the MAP rose slowly and steadied at about 47.67 mm Hg. It should be noted that the physiological solution of NaCl 9% with 10% of heparin had no significant effect on MAP (a variation of 0.025% has been obtained).

Discussion

First of all, the results of phytochemical screening of the leaves and the trunk bark confirmed the previous works of Badmus et al (21) and of Gnangoran et al (22). Indeed, most of the metabolites found in the current study possess significant pharmacological properties, including analgesics, anesthetics, antibiotics, and anti-cancer (23). For instance, plants containing flavonoids are known as potent antioxidants, antiradicals, diuretics, purgatives, disinfectants, analgesics, anti-inflammatories, antipyretics, and antispasmodics (24).

The revealed antioxidant properties (Table 3) of the hydro-ethanolic extract of the trunk bark of *H. floribunda* could have beneficial effects on the preventive treatment of CVD. Indeed, antioxidants have the ability to trap and inhibit the formation of free radicals. Flavonoids as antioxidants have effects on veins and arteries by decreasing permeability and increasing capillary resistance (23). It is known that the regular feeding of fruits and vegetables decreases the risk of developing CVD (25), as they contain antioxidants. According to the total polyphenols content and the screening study, the antioxidant properties might be mainly due to the presence of polyphenolic compounds such as tannins, flavonoids, and leuco-anthocyanins. Polyphenols are known as antioxidants and include five main families, namely phenolic acids, phenolic alcohols, flavonoids, tannins, and lignans (26). This work confirms that of Badmus et al (21) who showed that the leaves of *H. floribunda* possess antioxidant activity. Moreover, according to N'guessan et al (27), the anti-radical capacity is often correlated with the total polyphenols content of plant extracts. The result of the kinetics of the reduction obtained in the current study (Figure 4) is similar to those of Popovici et al (28). These observations show that the hydro-ethanolic extract of *H. floribunda* bark exhibited strong anti-radical efficiency.

The fall in MAP was based on the administered dose (Figures 5 and 6). Intravenous injection of the hydro-ethanolic extract of *H. floribunda* induced a significant decrease in DBP, in SBP, and thus in MAP. It should be noted that the dose of 40 mg/kg was seen as a best one (induce a better effect) because the return back effect under this dose is not only very slow but also weak. These results are somewhat similar to those obtained on the extracts of *Bidens pilosa* by Dimo et al (29) and Kouakou et al (30), and might be due to the presence of polyphenols, alkaloids, and saponosides in the current extract. The extract of *H. floribunda* therefore exhibits antihypertensive (hypothensive) effects, as shown in similar studies (12,31). Indeed, similar development has been obtained by Titrikou et al (12) on the extracts

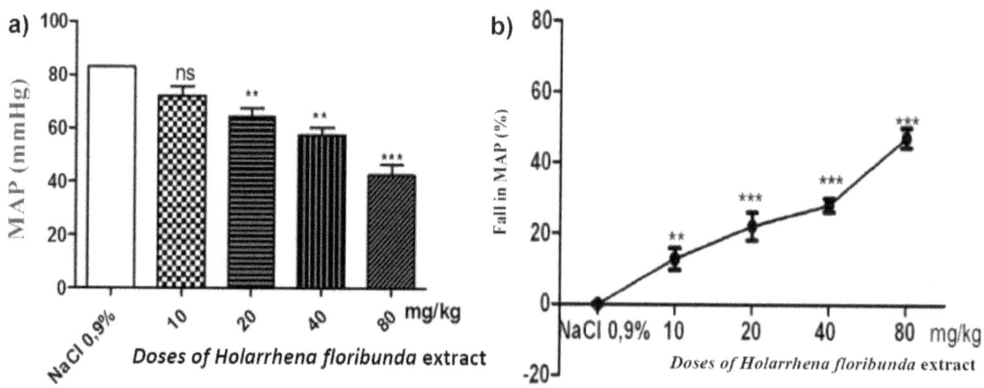

Figure 6. a) MAP of normal guinea pigs development under NaCl 9‰ and doses of *Holarrhena floribunda* extract 15 minutes after injection; b) Impact of NaCl 9‰ and extract of *Holarrina floribunda* on fall in MAP of normal guinea pigs. Each point represents an average ± SD (standard deviation). With n = 5, **P* < 0,05; ***P* < 0,01 and ****P* < 0,001 significantly different compared to the initial value of the MAP.

of *Biophytum petersianum* and Etou et al (31) on the extracts of *Lippia multiflora*. Furthermore, the possible mechanisms involved in this positive effect (hypothensive) could be an inhibition of orthosympathetic activity or a decrease in oxidative stress. Indeed, an increase in oxidative stress is observed in hypertensive patients (32). The polyphenols content in this extract might play a key role in inhibiting the action of activated oxygen species. Moreover, the antidiabetic activity of *H. floribunda* (22) might also have positive preventive effects, by improving the insulin sensitivity.

Conclusion

This study showed the presence of various active phytochemical groups in the bark of the trunk and the leaves of *H. floribunda* specimen of the Zone IV of Togo. So, the phytochemical screening revealed alkaloids, tannins (catechics, gallic), flavonoids, leuco-anthocyanins, saponosides, free quinones, anthrax C- and O-heterosides), reducing compounds, mucilages, cardiotonic heterosides, sterols, and terpenoids in the two parts of *H. floribunda*. The hydro-ethanolic extract of the trunk bark of *H. floribunda* exhibited in vitro antioxidant activity and in vivo antihypertensive effect. The two observations might prove the use of *H. floribunda* extract in traditional medicine against cardio-cardiovascular diseases. However, further study might be envisaged in order to elucidate the mechanism of action of the observed effects. This could provide strong pharmacological arguments that converge in favor of the use of *H. floribunda* as an alternative treatment against high blood pressure (hypertension). In the same way, it might be very interesting to carry out a more thorough phytochemical study in the hope of isolating some active principles responsible for this hypotensive activity.

Author Contributions

KK, ETK, and OS conducted the full work. PB, OT, and NYG participated in the writing process. KT, AA, and MG gave technical support via the availability and the using of the Biopac System Apparatus. They also participated in the writing process. All authors have approved the submission of this paper.

Conflict of interests

Authors declare no conflict of interests.

Ethical considerations

The project was done with consideration of ethical issues and obtaining license from the ethics committee of local institute (Université de Lomé in Togo has a branch of National Ethic Committee that approved the experimental protocols using World Health Organization guidelines for the care and use of laboratory animals). Also, the general care of the experimental animals used for this study was done in compliance with the Animal Welfare Act.

Acknowledgements

The authors are grateful to Laboratory of Botany and Plant Ecology of the Faculty of Sciences, "Université de Lomé" (Togo), especially to his head Professor Koffi Akpagana, for the help in identification of the plant.

References

1. Gaziano T. Prevention and treatment of chronic diseases in developing countries, Population Division of United Nations, Department of Economic and Social Affairs. Expert Paper No. 2011/2, 2011.
2. WHO. Maladies cardiovasculaires. http://www.who.int/mediacentre/factsheets/fs317/fr/. Accessed January 2015.
3. National Program for the Fight against Non-Transmissible Diseases-TOGO (PNMNT-TOGO). Integrated strategic plan for non-transmissible diseases for 2012-2015. PNMNT-TOGO; 2012.
4. Kearney PM, Whelton M, Reynolds K, Muntner P, Whelton PK, He J. Global burden of hypertension: analysis of worldwide data. Lancet. 2005;365(9455):217-23. doi: 10.1016/s0140-6736(05)17741-1.
5. Girouard H, Chulak C, LeJossec M, Lamontagne D, de Champlain J. Chronic antioxidant treatment improves sympathetic functions and beta-adrenergic pathway in the spontaneously hypertensive rats. J Hypertens. 2003;21(1):179-88. doi: 10.1097/01.hjh.0000045536.21915.1a.
6. Asgary S, Sahebkar A, Afshani MR, Keshvari M, Haghjooyjavanmard S, Rafieian-Kopaei M. Clinical evaluation of blood pressure lowering, endothelial function improving, hypolipidemic and anti-inflammatory effects of pomegranate juice in hypertensive subjects. Phytother Res. 2014;28(2):193-9. doi: 10.1002/ptr.4977.
7. Arbonnier M. Arbres, arbustes et lianes des zones sèches d'Afrique de l'Ouest. Cirad, Mnhn, Uicn, 573p, 2002.
8. Arbonnier M. Arbres, arbustes et lianes des zones sèches d'Afrique de l'Ouest. http://www.quae.com/en/r1281-arbres-arbustes-et-lianes-des-zones-seches-d-afrique-de-l-ouest.html. 2009. Accessed 13 March 2009.
9. Badiaga M. Etude ethnobotanique, phytochimique et activités biologiques de *Nauclea latifolia* Smith, une plante médicinale africaine récoltée au Mali. PhD thesis, University of Blaise Pascal - Clermont-Ferrand II, 2011. NNT:2011CLF22187.
10. Van Vliet BN, Chafe LL, Antic V, Schnyder-Candrian S, Montani JP. Direct and indirect methods used to study arterial blood pressure. J Pharmacol Toxicol Methods. 2000;44(2):361-73.
11. Ngelefack TB, Mekhfi H, Dimo T, Afkir S, Nguelefack-Mbuyo EP, Legssyer A, et al. Cardiovascular and anti-platelet aggregation activities of extracts from Solanumtorvum (Solanaceae) fruits in rat. J Complement Integr Med. 2008;5(1):1-11. doi: 10.2202/1553-3840.1105.
12. Titrikou S, Eklu-Gadegbeku K, Aklikokou KA, Gbeassor M. Effets de Biophytum petersianum (Oxalidaceae) sur la pression artérielle chez le rat Wistar. [Effects of Biophytum petersianum (Oxalidaceae) on arterial blood pressure in

Wistar rats]. Phytotherapie. 2008;6(4):215-8. doi: 10.1007/s10298-008-0321-3.

13. Pelletier A. Origine métabolique et effets des nucléotides extracellulaires sur le système circulatoire du cobaye. Méd Trad Afr. 1998;17(1):1-9.
14. Bogne KP, Penlap BV, Mbofung CM, Etoa FX. Acute and subacute toxicity of the methanol extract from *Holarrhena floribunda* G. Don (Apocynaceae). Euro J Exp Biol. 2012;2(4):1284-8.
15. Antwi S. Evaluation of the anti-inflammatory effects of the hydroethanolic extract of *Holarrhena floribunda* in Murine Models of inflammation [Master Thesis]. Kumasi : Kwame Nkrumah University of Science and Technology (Ghana); 2015.
16. Singleton VL, Orthofer R, Lamuela-Raventos RM. Analysis of total phenols and other oxidation substrates and antioxidants by means of Folin-Ciocalteu Reagen. Methods Enzymol. 1999;299C(1):152-78. doi: 10.1016/S0076-6879(99)99017-1.
17. Al-Farsi M, Alasalvar C, Morris A, Baron M, Shahidi F. Comparison of antioxidant activity, anthocyanins, carotenoids, and phenolics of three native fresh and sun-dried date (*Phoenix dactylifera* L.) varieties grown in Oman. J Agric Food Chem. 2005;53(19):7592-9. doi: 10.1021/jf050579q.
18. Brand-Williams W, Cuvelier ME, Berset C. Use of a free radical method to evaluate antioxidant activity. LWT - Food Sci Technol. 1995;28(1):25-30. doi: 10.1016/S0023-6438(95)80008-5.
19. Agbonon A, Gbeassor M. Hepatoprotective Effect of *Lonchocarpus sericeus* Leaves in CCl4- Induced Liver Damage. J Herbs Spices Med Plants. 2009;15(2):216-26. doi: 10.1080/10496470903139512.
20. Benzie IF, Strain JJ. The ferric reducing ability of plasma (FRAP) as a measure of "antioxidant power": the FRAP assay. Anal Biochem. 1996;239(1):70-6. doi: 10.1006/abio.1996.0292.
21. Badmus JA, Ekpo OE, Rautenbach F, Marnewick JL, Hussein AA, Hiss DC. Isolation and antioxidant activity of flavonoids from *Holarrhena floribunda* (G.don) leaves. Acta Biochim Pol. 2016;63(2):353-8. doi: 10.18388/abp.2015_1178.
22. Gnangoran BN, N'guessan BB, Amoateng P, Dosso K, Yapo AP, Ehile EE. Hypoglycemic activity of ethanolic leaf extract and fractions of *Holarrhena floribunda* (Apocynaceae). J Med Biomedical Sci. 2012;1(3):46-54.
23. Bruneton J. Pharmacognosie, Plantes Médicinales. Paris: Lavoisier Technique et Documentation; 1999:405.
24. Ngene JP, Ngoule CC, Pouka Kidik CM. Importance dans la pharmacopée traditionnelle des plantes à flavonoïdes vendues dans les marchés de Douala est (Cameroun). J Appl Biosci.2015;88:8194-210. doi: 10.4314/jab.v88i1.6.
25. Hertog MG, Feskens EJ, Hollman PC, Katan MB, Kromhout D. Dietary antioxidant flavonoids and risk of coronary heart disease: the Zutphen Elderly Study. Lancet. 1993;342(8878):1007-11.
26. Saloufou K. Teneur en composés phénoliques et pouvoir Antioxydant des extraits de cinq plantes Médicinales de la flore togolaise [Master thesis]. Lomé : Université de Lomé; 2013.
27. N'guessan JD, Zirihi GN, Kra AKM, Kouakou K, Djaman AJ, Guede-Guina F. Free radical scavenging activity, flavonoid and phenolic contents of selected Ivoirian plants. International Journal of Natural and Applied Sciences. 2007;3(4):425-9. doi: 10.4314/ijonas.v3i4.36155.
28. Popovici C, Saykova I, Tylkowski B. Evaluation de l'activité antioxydant des composés phénoliques par la réactivité avec le radical libre DPPH. Revue de Génie Industriel. 2009;4:25-39.
29. Dimo T, Nguelefack TB, Tan PV, Yewah MP, Dongo E, Rakotonirina SV, et al. Possible mechanisms of action of the neutral extract from *Bidens pilosa* L. leaves on the cardiovascular system of anaesthetized rats. Phytother Res. 2003;17(10):1135-9. doi: 10.1002/ptr.1132.
30. Kouakou LK, Traore F, Abo JCK, Ehile EE. Effets pharmacologiques d'un extrait aqueux de *Bidens pilosa* L.(Asteraceae) sur le système cardiovasculaire de mammifères. [Pharmacological effects of an aqueous extract of Bidens pilosa L. (Asteraceae) on the cardiovascular system of mammals]. Afrique Science. 2007;3(2):284-304. doi: 10.4314/afsci.v3i2.61275.
31. Etou-Ossibi AW, Elion-Itou RD, Nzonzi J, Nsonde Ntandou GF, Dimo T, Ouamba JM, et al. Effets de l'extrait aqueux de *Lippia multiflora* Moldenke (Verbenaceae) sur la pression artérielle, la fréquence cardiaque et les ondes de l'électrocardiogramme chez le rat normotendu. [Effects of aqueous extract of *Lippia multiflora* Moldenke (Verbenaceae) on the blood pressure, the heart rate and onelectrocardiogramwaves at the normotensive rat]. Revue CAMES-Série Pharm Méd Trad Afr. 2014;17(1):1-9.
32. Rodrigo R, Prat H, Passalacqua W, Araya J, Guichard C, Bachler JP. Relationship between oxidative stress and essential hypertension. Hypertens Res. 2007;30(12):1159-67. doi: 10.1291/hypres.30.1159.

The effect of hydroalcoholic extract of *Crataegus monogyna* on hyperglycemia, oxidative stress and pancreatic tissue damage in streptozotocin-induced diabetic rats

Saeid Valipour Chahardahcharic[1], **Mahbubeh Setorki**[1*]

[1]Department of Biology, Izeh Branch, Islamic Azad University, Izeh, Iran

ARTICLE INFO

Keywords:
Crataegus monogyna
Diabetes mellitus
Stress oxidative
Rat

ABSTRACT

Introduction: Diabetes mellitus is one of the most common metabolic diseases that causes damage to different tissues through oxidative stress. The aim of this study was to evaluate the effect of hydroalcoholic extract of *Crataegus monogyna* on oxidative stress, hyperglycemia and pancreatic tissue damage in diabetic rats.
Methods: In this experimental study, 40 male Wistar rats were equally divided into 5 groups including control (normal saline), diabetic control (streptozotocin), intervention (streptozotocin plus *C. monogyna* extract at doses of 100, 200 and 400 mg/kg). After treatment, serum levels of malondialdehyde (MDA), Ferric reducing ability of plasma (FRAP) and glucose were determined. Histological sections of the pancreas were also prepared for histological examination.
Results: Treatment of diabetic rats with *C. monogyna* extract significantly reduced blood glucose level ($P<0.05$). Compared with control group MDA was increased and TCA was decreased in diabetic rats ($P<0.05$). Treatment of diabetic rats with *C. monogyna* extract significantly increased TCA and reduced MDA ($P<0.05$). In the pancreas of diabetic rats, degeneration of pancreatic acinar cells and formation of dermato space, damage of lobules and Acinii and edema were observed and treatment with *C. monogyna* extract ameliorated them.
Conclusion: The results confirm the role of *C. monogyna* extract in the treatment of hyperglycemia, stress oxidative indices and pancreatic tissue damage in diabetic rats. Therefore, it might be beneficial in diabetic patients.

Implication for health policy/practice/research/medical education:
The results confirm the role of *C. monogyna* extract in treatment of hyperglycemia, oxidative stress indices and pancreatic tissue damage in diabetic rats. Therefore, it might be beneficial in diabetic patients.

Introduction

One of the most common diseases of the body's endocrine system is diabetes, which prevalence is increasing in human societies. There are two main types of diabetes. In type I diabetes, the degradation of beta cells in the pancreas leads to defective insulin production. In type II diabetes, there is a progressive body's resistance to insulin, which may ultimately lead to the destruction of pancreatic beta cells and the complete defect in the synthesis of insulin (1). In type II diabetes, which account for 90%-95% of diabetic cases, genetic factors, obesity, and dementia play important roles in developing the disease (2). It is estimated that more than 3.6% of the world's population currently have diabetes mellitus (3). Diabetes mellitus is characterized with symptoms such as hyperglycemia, polyuria, polydipsia, polyphagia, and the appearance of glucose in the urine. In long terms, it will be associated with serious and irreversible complications such as retinopathy, nephropathy, neuropathy, and vascular injuries (4).

In diabetes mellitus, the oxidative stress caused by chronic hyperglycaemia plays a major role in the progression of the disease and the appearance of related symptoms. The oxidative stress in the cells and tissues originates from the increased production of reactive oxygen species (ROS) or the reduced potential for antioxidant defense (5). Several hypotheses have been introduced to explain the increase

***Corresponding author**: Mahbubeh Setorki,
Email: doctor.setorgi@gmail.com

in the ROS production during diabetes, including glucose autoxidation, non-enzymatic and progressive glycosylation of proteins, increased ultimate glycemic products and the polyol metabolism pathway. The formation of free radicals causes the destruction of cells vital macromolecules, peroxidation of membrane lipids, and ultimately the cell damage (4). Streptozotocin (STZ) is an antibiotic produced by *Streptomyces achromogenes*, and is usually used to induce diabetes in the experimental models. Hyperglycemia and oxidative stress play an important role in the etiology and pathology of STZ-induced complications (6). Through increasing the production of free radicals and ROS, STZ causes the DNA cleavage and methylation in the pancreatic beta cells (7). The STZ also discharges nicotinamide adenine dinucleotide (NAD) in the insulin-making cells of the Islets of Langerhans (8). Due to the role of oxidative stress in the pathogenesis and etiology of diabetes, the researchers have nowadays focused on the use of compounds with antioxidant activity and the potential of free radicals removal to prevent the damage and degeneration of the pancreatic beta cells in the diabetic models (6).

Nowadays, the researchers' attention has focused on the use of natural compounds with multiple antioxidant, anti-inflammatory, anti-hyperlipidemia, and hepatoprotective activities for the management of diabetes-related disorders (10). Common hawthorn (*Crataegus monogyna*) is the name of a species of Hawthorn (*Crataegus*) species. It is a native ornamental herb of Europe, North-West Africa and West Asia and is an invasive species (11). Common hawthorn has dark red small fruits called haw, which ripen in the mid-autumn and are used for medical purposes and also as a condiment in some foods like jellies, jams, and syrups (12). Scientific evidence has shown that the common hawthorn fruit has anti-oxidant and strong inhibiting activity on free radicals due to the presence of various bioactive compounds such as epicatechin, hyperoside, quercetin, vitexin, coumarin, and chlorogenic acid (12,13). These compounds have numerous pharmacological neuroprotective, hepatoprotective, and cardioprotective effects (10,12). In addition, the common hawthorn fruit has tonic effects on the heart (12). Several studies have shown that the common hawthorn can reduce some cardiovascular risk factors such as high blood pressure, hypocholesterolemia, and hyperlipidemia (14,15). Thus, the aim of this study was to evaluate the effect of hydro-alcoholic extract of common hawthorn on hyperglycemia and oxidative stress in streptozotocin-induced diabetic rats.

Material and Methods

Extraction

The common hawthorn plant was purchased from an authentic attar. After scientific and systematic confirmation, 1 kg of dried fruit without kernel was powdered and placed into a beaker. Subsequently, an adequate amount of 70% methanol solution was added to completely cover the powdered particles. Then, it was placed on a shaker for 2 days at room temperature. The resulting mixture was filtered and the solvent was separated by a rotary. The resulted extract was then dried completely at 37°C in the incubator and used for the preparation of the required concentrations. The extract was stored in the freezer -20°C (16).

Laboratory animals

The tested animals were male Wistar rats weighing 250-300 g. The animals were kept in appropriate temperature conditions (22 ± 2°C) under 12 hours of light (from 8 to 20) and 12 hours of dark with free access to similar water and food at the animal nest of Islamic Azad University, Izeh Branch. The tests on animals were done based on the Ethics of Working with laboratory animals approved by the Ethics Committee at the Deputy of Research and Technology of Islamic Azad University. To perform the study, we used the rats that their serum glucose levels were less than 130 mg/dL in normal and fasting conditions (17). To do the test, a drop of blood was taken from the rat's tail and the blood glucose levels were determined using a glucometer device. To induce diabetes in the rats, the STZ was administered as 60 mg/kg single dose intraperitoneally as solution in the physiologic cold saline. Following 72 hours of the STZ injection and after observing the symptoms of diabetes (increased blood glucose levels to more than 250 mg/dL and polydipsia) (17), the treatment with the extract was done for 3 weeks daily and intraperitoneally. The rats were divided into five groups (n = 8). The control group included healthy rats that received normal saline as intraperitoneal injection for 3 weeks. The negative control group included untreated diabetic rats that received normal saline for 3 weeks. The treated diabetic groups received the common hawthorn extract at doses of 100, 200, and 400 mg/kg for 3 weeks (18,19). After 3 weeks, the rats were kept for 12 hours in a fasting condition. They were then anaesthetized by chloroform and blood samples were taken from their hearts. The serum was isolated from the blood samples by centrifugation and transferred to the laboratory for performing biochemical tests (20). The pancreatic tissue was also prepared for histological examination.

Serum glucose measurement

At the end of the study, the samples were transferred to the laboratory. The serum specimens were separated from the blood samples. Then, using the commercial kits of Pars Azmoon Company (Tehran, Iran) and an Autoanalyzer (Biotecnica BT-3000), the blood glucose levels were determined.

Malondialdehyde measurement

A volume of 100 μL of the serum sample and 1.5 mL of 20% acetic acid were added to the test tubes with 1.5 mL of 0.8% thiobarbituric acid (TBA), 200 uL of 8.1% sodium dodecyl sulfate (SDS) and 700 μL of distilled water. The tubes were placed in a boiling water bath for 60 min. Then, 1 mL of distilled water and 5 ml of butanol/pyridine were added to the specimens, which were then centrifuged and the light absorbance rates of the supernatants were measured at 532 nm (21).

Ferric reducing ability of plasma

The ferric reducing ability of plasma (FRAP) method was used to measure the antioxidant capacity of the serum. The FRAP work solution was prepared by using 10 ml of acetate buffer (0.25 M) (pH = 3.6), 5 ml of 10 mM TPTZ (prepared in the 40 mM HCl) and 2.5 mL of 20 mM of $FeCl_3(6H_2O)$. Then, 25 μL of the serum sample was mixed with 1.5 ml of the FRAP solution and placed at 37°C for 10 minutes. Subsequently, the optical absorption was recorded at a wavelength of 593 nm (21).

Histological studies

The pancreatic tissue of rats was fixed in the 10% buffered formalin solution and paraffin embedded. The 3-5 μm sections were placed on glass slides, which paraffin was removed and watered again. The slides were stained with hematoxylin and eosin (E & H) for microscopic examination (22).

Statistical analysis

The resulting data were analyzed by SPSS software version 21. Considering that the obtained results were quantitative, the assumption of normal distribution of the frequency of data was confirmed by the Kolmogorov-Smirnov non-parametric test ($P>0.05$). The data were also analyzed by one-way ANOVA and the post hoc least significant difference (LSD) tests. Also, the results obtained were reported together with the corresponding statistical calculations as mean ± SEM. In all cases, the difference between groups was considered significant with $P < 0.05$.

Results

The results of blood glucose levels in the experimental groups are shown in Figure 1. According to the results, the mean blood glucose levels in the STZ-receiving rats showed a significant increase compared with the control group. In addition, the treatment with doses of 100, 200, and 400 mg/kg of the common hawthorn extract caused a significant decrease of the mean values compared to the diabetic group.

The serum FRAP decreased significantly in the untreated diabetic rats compared to the control group rats ($P<0.001$) and treatment with doses of 100, 200, and 400 mg/kg of common hawthorn extract ($P<0.001$) significantly increased the FRAP levels compared to the diabetic group (Figure 2). The administration of STZ to rats significantly increased the serum MDA levels ($P<0.001$)

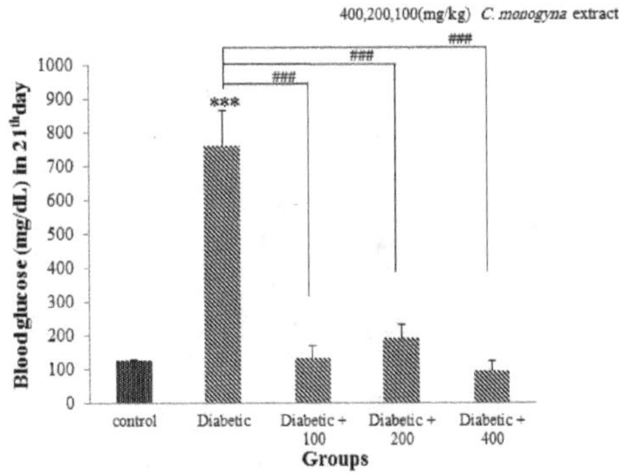

Figure 1. Comparison (mean ± SEM) of blood glucose levels in the control, diabetic, diabetic treated with different doses of common hawthorn extract (Sign * indicates a significant difference with the control group ($P < 0.001$), sign # represents a significant difference with the diabetic group ($P < 0.001$ and $P < 0.05$).

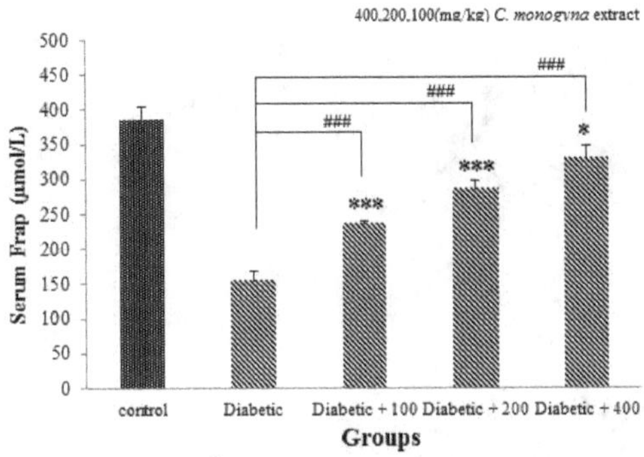

Figure 2 Comparison (mean ± SEM) of FRAP levels in the control, diabetic, diabetic treated with different doses of common hawthorn extract (Sign * indicates a significant difference with the control group ($P < 0.001$), sign # represents a significant difference with the diabetic group ($P < 0.001$ and $P < 0.05$)

and treatment with doses of 100, 200, and 400 mg/kg of common hawthorn extract significantly decreased the MDA levels compared to the diabetic group ($P<0.001$, $P<0.05$, Figure 3).

The results of histological studies of the rats' pancreas are shown in Figure 4. In the rats of the control group, the acinar cells had a normal appearance and no necrosis or degenerative changes were observed. In the pancreas of untreated diabetic rats, the degeneration of Acini and the creation of dermatome space, the brittleness of the lobules and the Acini, and edema were observed. The histological examination of the pancreatic tissue in the diabetic rats treated with common hawthorn extract at a dose of 100 mg/kg indicated the health of the acini cells and the lobules and there were no other pathologic changes except for a brief hyperemia. In the diabetic groups treated with common hawthorn extract at doses of 200 and 400 mg/kg, the Acini had a normal appearance and no necrosis and degenerative changes were seen (Figure 4).

Discussion

In this study, which was performed to examine the effect

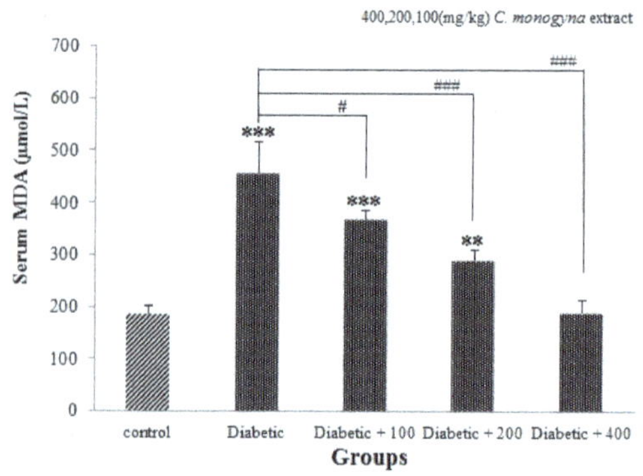

Figure 3. Comparison (mean ± SEM) of MDA levels in the control, diabetic, diabetic treated with different doses of common hawthorn extract (Sign * indicates a significant difference with the control group ($P < 0.001$), sign # represents a significant difference with the diabetic group ($P < 0.001$ and $P < 0.05$).

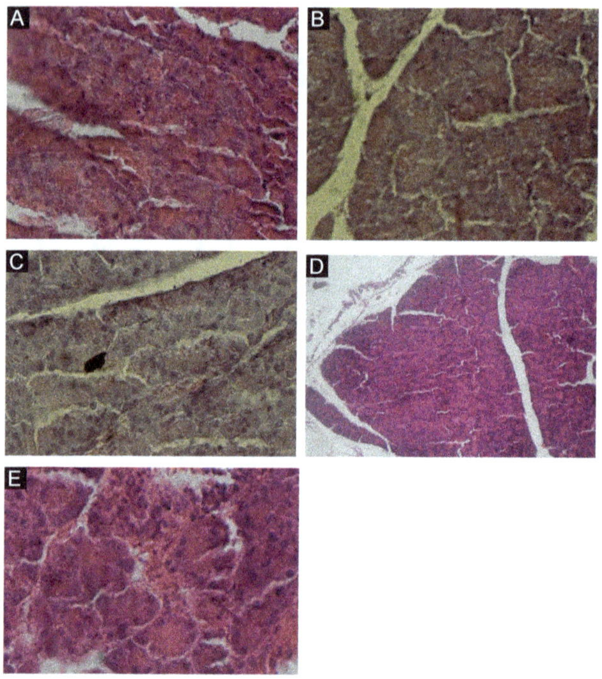

Figure 4. Pancreatic tissue sections of the control group (A), diabetic (B), diabetic recipient of a dose of 100 mg/kg of common hawthorn extract (C), diabetic recipient of 200 mg/kg of common hawthorn extract (D), and the diabetic recipient of 400 mg/kg of common hawthorn extract (E). (H&E staining); x40 magnification.

of common hawthorn extract on hyperglycemia, oxidative stress, and pancreatic tissue damage in the STZ-diabetic rats, administration of STZ resulted in a significant increase in the serum glucose and malondialdehyde levels and a significant reduction in the serum antioxidant capacity. Consistent with the results of this study, hyperglycemia and the increased lipid peroxidation in the serum, liver, kidney, and pancreas have been reported in a number of studies following the treatment of rats with STZ (6,16). In other studies, the decreased activity of antioxidant enzymes and reduced levels of endogenous antioxidants have been reported in STZ-induced diabetic rats (6).

STZ is widely used to induce experimental diabetes in the animal models (6). STZ is removed by beta-pancreatic cells via GLUT2 receptors, through which, enters these cells and causes tissue damage (4). The mechanism by which STZ leads to diabetes is not well known. However, it is believed that active oxygen species, including hydroxyl radicals play an important role in causing STZ-induced cell injury (7). STZ is an unstable molecule that accumulates in the pancreatic beta cells and its decomposition produces carbonium radicals. The carbonium radicals are highly reactive and cause direct or indirect toxic effects on the endothelium of the islets of Langerhans with increasing ROS production (23), leading to DNA fragmentation and DNA methylation of the pancreatic beta cells (24,25). It is also found that STZ causes inflammation through infiltration of mononuclear cells in the islets of Langerhans and ultimately damage the beta cells of the pancreas (26). In addition, studies have shown that nitric oxide (NO) produced by STZ plays a major role in causing damage to the beta cells in the pancreas (27). The increased serum nitric oxide is seen in the STZ-exposed rats (6) and the use of inducing nitric oxide synthase enzyme inhibitors (iNOS), like the LNG-mono-methyl arginine (NMMA) and aminoguanidine, decreases hyperglycemia and prevents the destruction of the Langerhans islets by STZ (28,29). It has also been observed that the oxidative destruction of DNA caused by STZ in the islets of Langerhans is decreased by NMMA and nicotinamide (30). In the present study, the increased serum MDA as the lipid peroxidation index and pancreatic tissue damage in diabetic rats confirmed the damage caused by STZ and the resulting free radicals.

In the present study, we observed that the treatment of STZ-receiving rats by different doses of common hawthorn extract significantly decreased the blood glucose levels and improved the tissue damage of the pancreas. The common hawthorn extract also increased the serum antioxidant capacity and reduced the levels of MDA. Therefore, one can state that the common hawthorn extract represents protective effects against hyperglycemia and tissue damage of the pancreas in the diabetic rats due to antioxidant activity and reducing lipid peroxidation. Based on the studies done in the laboratory environment, the common hawthorn extract indicates a high antioxidant activity in inhibiting hydroxyl and superoxide free radicals (31-33). In hypercholesterolemic rats, the common hawthorn extract has reduced the lipids peroxidation and increased the antioxidant capacity (34). The antioxidant activity of the common hawthorn extract has been attributed to the presence of various bioactive compounds such as epicatechin, hyperoside, quercetin, vitexin, coumarin, and chlorogenic acid (12,13). One study found that quercetin reduces peroxidation of lipids, forms NO, and increases the activity of antioxidant enzymes in the STZ-induced diabetic rats. The researchers concluded that quercetin protects the pancreatic beta cells against

STZ's destructive effects by reducing the oxidative stress parameters (6). Coumarin has also shown protective effects against hyperglycemia and the tissue damage in the liver (35). In addition, epicatechin has increased the activity of antioxidant enzymes and decreased the peroxidation of lipids in the STZ-induced diabetic rats (36). These results are consistent with the results of this study.

Conclusion

The results of this study showed that the doses of common hawthorn extract used in the diabetic rats reduce the blood glucose levels and prevent the pancreatic tissue damage, which seem to be due to the strengthening of the antioxidant defense and the reduction of lipids peroxidation.

Acknowledgments

This article is a result of the research results in the Department of Biology at Islamic Azad University, Izeh Branch. Hereby, the authors of the article would like to appreciate the Deputy of Research and Technology of Islamic Azad University, Izeh Branch for providing the proper laboratory conditions to perform this research project.

Authors' contributions

MS: Statistical analysis, data interpretation, manuscript preparation. SVC: Data collection, design of the study, literature search, funding collection. The authors read and confirmed publication of the manuscript.

Conflict of interest

The authors declare that there is no Conflict of interest.

Ethical considerations

The protocol was approved by the Vice-Chancellor of Islamic Azad University. The ethical issues (including plagiarism, misbehavior, data provision, forgery, duplicate release or submission, redundancy) were fully observed by the authors.

Funding/Support

This research was financially supported by Azad University of Izeh, Iran.

References

1. Classification and diagnosis of diabetes mellitus and other categories of glucose intolerance. National Diabetes Data Group. Diabetes. 1979;28(12):1039-57.
2. Colditz GA, Willett WC, Rotnitzky A, Manson JE. Weight gain as a risk factor for clinical diabetes mellitus in women. Ann Intern Med. 1995;122(7):481-6.
3. King H, Rewers M. Global estimates for prevalence of diabetes mellitus and impaired glucose tolerance in adults. WHO Ad Hoc Diabetes Reporting Group. Diabetes Care. 1993;16(1):157-77.
4. Eleazu CO, Eleazu KC, Chukwuma S, Essien UN. Review of the mechanism of cell death resulting from streptozotocin challenge in experimental animals, its practical use and potential risk to humans. J Diabetes Metab Disord. 2013;12(1):60. doi: 10.1186/2251-6581-12-60.
5. Baynes JW. Role of oxidative stress in development of complications in diabetes. Diabetes. 1991;40(4):405-12.
6. Coskun O, Kanter M, Korkmaz A, Oter S. Quercetin, a flavonoid antioxidant, prevents and protects streptozotocin-induced oxidative stress and beta-cell damage in rat pancreas. Pharmacol Res. 2005;51(2):117-23. doi: 10.1016/j.phrs.2004.06.002.
7. Szkudelski T. The mechanism of alloxan and streptozotocin action in B cells of the rat pancreas. Physiol Res. 2001;50(6):537-46.
8. Schein PS, Cooney DA, McMenamin MG, Anderson T. Streptozotocin diabetes--further studies on the mechanism of depression of nicotinamide adenine dinucleotide concentrations in mouse pancreatic islets and liver. Biochem Pharmacol. 1973;22(20):2625-31.
9. Nasri H, Rafieian-Kopaei M. Protective effects of herbal antioxidants on diabetic kidney disease. Journal of Research in Medical Sciences. 2014;19(1):82-3.
10. Kirakosyan A, Seymour E, Kaufman PB, Warber S, Bolling S, Chang SC. Antioxidant capacity of polyphenolic extracts from leaves of *Crataegus laevigata* and *Crataegus monogyna* (Hawthorn) subjected to drought and cold stress. J Agric Food Chem. 2003;51(14):3973-6. doi: 10.1021/jf030096r.
11. Sallabanks R. Fruit fate, frugivory, and fruit characteristics: a study of the hawthorn, *Crataegus monogyna* (Rosaceae). Oecologia. 1992;91(2):296-304. doi: 10.1007/bf00317800.
12. Barros L, Carvalho AM, Ferreira IC. Comparing the composition and bioactivity of *Crataegus monogyna* flowers and fruits used in folk medicine. Phytochem Anal. 2011;22(2):181-8. doi: 10.1002/pca.1267.
13. Bahorun T, Aumjaud E, Ramphul H, Rycha M, Luximon-Ramma A, Trotin F, et al. Phenolic constituents and antioxidant capacities of *Crataegus monogyna* (Hawthorn) callus extracts. Nahrung. 2003;47(3):191-8. doi: 10.1002/food.200390045.
14. Chang WT, Dao J, Shao ZH. Hawthorn: potential roles in cardiovascular disease. Am J Chin Med. 2005;33(1):1-10. doi: 10.1142/s0192415x05002606.
15. Salehi S, Long SR, Proteau PJ, Filtz TM. Hawthorn (*Crataegus monogyna* Jacq.) extract exhibits atropine-sensitive activity in a cultured cardiomyocyte assay. J Nat Med. 2009;63(1):1-8. doi: 10.1007/s11418-008-0278-4.
16. Sowndhararajan K, Kang SC. Free radical scavenging activity from different extracts of leaves of *Bauhinia vahlii* Wight & Arn. Saudi J Biol Sci. 2013;20(4):319-25. doi: 10.1016/j.sjbs.2012.12.005.
17. Nayak SB, Pereira PL, Maharaj D. Wound healing activity of Carica papaya L. in experimentally induced diabetic rats. Indeian Journal of Experimental Biology. 2007;45 (8):739-743.
18. Chowdhury SS, Islam MN, Jung HA, Choi JS. In vitro antidiabetic potential of the fruits of *Crataegus pinnatifida*. Res Pharm Sci. 2014;9(1):11-22.
19. Shalizar Jalali A, Hasanzadeh S. *Crataegus monogyna* fruit aqueous extract as a protective agent against doxorubicin-

induced reproductive toxicity in male rats. Avicenna J Phytomed. 2013;3(2):159-70.

20. Srivastava A, Shivanandappa T. Hepatoprotective effect of the root extract of *Decalepis hamiltonii* against carbon tetrachloride-induced oxidative stress in rats. Food Chem. 2010;118(2):411-7. doi: 10.1016/j.foodchem.2009.05.014.
21. Zahedi M, Hojjati MR, Fathpour H, Rabiei Z, Alibabaei Z, Basim A. Effect of Rheum Ribes Hydro-Alcoholic Extract on Memory Impairments in Rat Model of Alzheimer's Disease. Iran J Pharm Res. 2015;14(4):1197-206.
22. Ashraf H, Zare S, Farnad N. The effect of aqueous extract of barberry fruit on liver damage in streptozotocin - induced diabetic rats. J Shahrekord Univ Med Sci. 2014;15(6):1-9.
23. Jang YY, Song JH, Shin YK, Han ES, Lee CS. Protective effect of boldine on oxidative mitochondrial damage in streptozotocin-induced diabetic rats. Pharmacol Res. 2000;42(4):361-71. doi: 10.1006/phrs.2000.0705.
24. Yamamoto H, Uchigata Y, Okamoto H. Streptozotocin and alloxan induce DNA strand breaks and poly(ADP-ribose) synthetase in pancreatic islets. Nature. 1981;294(5838):284-6.
25. Takasu N, Komiya I, Asawa T, Nagasawa Y, Yamada T. Streptozocin- and alloxan-induced H2O2 generation and DNA fragmentation in pancreatic islets. H2O2 as mediator for DNA fragmentation. Diabetes. 1991;40(9):1141-5.
26. Like AA, Rossini AA. Streptozotocin-induced pancreatic insulitis: new model of diabetes mellitus. Science. 1976;193(4251):415-7.
27. Kaneto H, Fujii J, Seo HG, Suzuki K, Matsuoka T, Nakamura M, et al. Apoptotic cell death triggered by nitric oxide in pancreatic beta-cells. Diabetes. 1995;44(7):733-8.
28. Lukic ML, Stosic-Grujicic S, Ostojic N, Chan WL, Liew FY. Inhibition of nitric oxide generation affects the induction of diabetes by streptozocin in mice. Biochem Biophys Res Commun. 1991;178(3):913-20.
29. Corbett JA, McDaniel ML. The Use of Aminoguanidine, a Selective iNOS Inhibitor, to Evaluate the Role of Nitric Oxide in the Development of Autoimmune Diabetes. Methods. 1996;10(1):21-30.
30. Bedoya FJ, Solano F, Lucas M. N-monomethyl-arginine and nicotinamide prevent streptozotocin-induced double strand DNA break formation in pancreatic rat islets. Experientia. 1996;52(4):344-7.
31. Bahorun T, Trotin F, Pommery J, Vasseur J, Pinkas M. Antioxidant activities of *Crataegus monogyna* extracts. Planta Med. 1994;60(4):323-8. doi: 10.1055/s-2006-959493.
32. Bernatoniene J, Masteikova R, Majiene D, Savickas A, Kevelaitis E, Bernatoniene R, et al. Free radical-scavenging activities of *Crataegus monogyna* extracts. Medicina (Kaunas). 2008;44(9):706-12.
33. Ruiz-Rodriguez BM, de Ancos B, Sanchez-Moreno C, Fernandez-Ruiz V, Sanchez-Mata Mde C, Camara M, et al. Wild blackthorn (*Prunus spinosa* L.) and hawthorn (*Crataegus monogyna* Jacq.) fruits as valuable sources of antioxidants. Fruits. 2014;69(1):61-73. doi: 10.1051/fruits/2013102.
34. Rezaei-Golmisheh A, Malekinejad H, Asri-Rezaei S, Farshid AA, Akbari P. Hawthorn ethanolic extracts with triterpenoids and flavonoids exert hepatoprotective effects and suppress the hypercholesterolemia-induced oxidative stress in rats. Iran J Basic Med Sci. 2015;18(7):691-9.
35. Pari L, Rajarajeswari N. Efficacy of coumarin on hepatic key enzymes of glucose metabolism in chemical induced type 2 diabetic rats. Chem Biol Interact. 2009;181(3):292-6. doi: 10.1016/j.cbi.2009.07.018.
36. Quine SD, Raghu PS. Effects of (-)-epicatechin, a flavonoid on lipid peroxidation and antioxidants in streptozotocin-induced diabetic liver, kidney and heart. Pharmacol Rep. 2005;57(5):610-5.

Effect of garlic (*Allium sativum*) on male fertility

Hadis Musavi[1], Malihe Tabnak[2], Farzaneh Alaei Sheini[3], Maryam Hasanzadeh Bezvan[4], Fardin Amidi[5], Mojtaba Abbasi[6*]

[1]Department of Biochemistry, Faculty of Basic Science, Razi University Kermanshah, Kermanshah, Iran
[2]Department of Basic Sciences, East Tehran Branch, Islamic Azad University, Tehran, Iran
[3]Department of Biology, Shahrekord Branch, Islamic Azad University, Shahrekord, Iran
[4]Department of Microbiology, Shahr-e-Qods Branch, Islamic Azad University, Tehran, Iran
[5]Department of Anatomy, School of Medicine, Tehran University of Medical Sciences, Tehran, Iran
[6]Veterinary Medicine, Faculty of Veterinary Medicine, Shahrekord Branch, Islamic Azad University, Shahrekord, Iran

ARTICLE INFO

Keywords:
Garlic
Allium sativum
Fertility
Infertility
Spermatogenesis
Medicinal plants

ABSTRACT

Introduction: Fertility in men mainly depends on the number, quality, motility, and morphology of the sperms, and disruption of each of these factors leads to infertility. A large number of couples suffer from infertility problems. Among the various therapies, medicinal herbs are used in many countries to treat male infertility. Current systematic review was conducted to study the effects of garlic on male fertility.
Methods: The information of this systematic review was collected by searching the key words: treatment, fertility, infertility, male, herbal medicine, garlic, Allium sativum, medicinal plant, sperm, sex hormones, testis and spermatogenesis in international databases such as: Web of Science (ISI), PubMed, Scopus and Embase until March 2018. This study was conducted in accordance with the PRISMA statement for systematic reviews and meta- analysis. and the SYRCLE risk of bias tool was used for qualitative assessment.
Results: A total of 18 experimental studies were included in the study. Thirteen studies evaluated garlic and 5 studies compared garlic effect with adriamycin, titanium dioxide, furan, vitamin E, N-acetylcysteine and cadmium. All studies were conducted in in vivo condition. The results of the studies indicated the potential effect of garlic on enhancing fertility and spermatogenesis, increasing the level of testosterone and improving the testicular structure.
Conclusion: Garlic can increase fertility probably due to its antioxidant properties. However, more clinical trials are recommended.

Implication for health policy/practice/research/medical education:
This article presented useful information about garlic, especially on fertility and reproduction system which could help pharmacists and scientists in the provision of new drugs.

Introduction

Failure to have a child is an unpleasant event in the lives of infertile people (1). Inability to become pregnant after one year of regular intercourse, without using contraception, is defined as infertility (2). About 30%-50% of the causes of infertility are related to male problems (3). Each day, the number of medical reports about the extent of infertility in the world increases, according to a systematic review in this regard, about 48.5 million couples around the world affected by this problem (4). The total mean of infertility in Iran is estimated about 11%-19%, which is more in the age group of 20-39 years (5). Infertility is a multi-parameter phenomenon with a wide range of factors that affects spermatogenesis and sperm quality (6). Spermatogenesis is a process in which male sex cells are produced and the disorder in each of these stages can cause infertility (7). Fertility in men depends largely on the number, quality, motility, and morphology of the sperm, and the disruption of each of these factors leads to infertility in men (3). Infertility, as a psychological crisis, imposes a lot of stress on infertile couples and in different ways threatens their mental health. The most

***Corresponding author**: Mojtaba Abbasi,
Email: Dr_Abbasi_m@yahoo.com

emotional and psychological problems of infertile couples are disappointment, frustration, fear and anxiety, and are less associated with anger and aggression. However, the rate of divorce and remarriage among infertile couples has risen. In addition to mental problems, the economical treatment of infertility imposes a relative high cost on infertile couples (8).

Nowadays, various methods are used to treat infertility, including: hormone therapy, surgical procedures, assisted reproductive technology (ART) that include in vitro fertilization (IVF), intra uterine insemination (IUI), zygote intrafallopian transfer (ZIFT), gamete intrafallopian transfer (GIFT), intracytoplasmic sperm injection (ICSI) and third-party fertilization (donation eggs, donation sperm, uterus, and donated embryos) (9).

ART is one of the costly treatments among infertile couples, but many people are not able to do so because financial problems, and surgical procedures have a lot of stress and complications for the family, and in addition they are expensive (8). Hormone therapy is also prohibited in some people, and in many people with impaired hypothalamic-pituitary-gonadal axis function, this treatment is not responsive therefore, due to individual and social problems caused by infertility, couples always try to find low-cost, safe and effective treatments (10). Regarding the problems that have been observed among couples and the high costs of medical interventions, people have turned to complementary medicine (11). Among different therapeutic methods, herbs are used in many countries to treat male infertility (1,12,13). Plants are more affordable and accessible than invasive and chemical treatments (14). Medicinal herbs with high antioxidant properties are used to treat sperm abnormalities, sexual dysfunction, erectile and ejaculatory disorders (1,15). Among the plants that improve male fertility, celery (16), fennel (17), black seed (18), German chamomile (19), saffron (20), *Fumaria parviflora* (21), *Origanum vulgare* (22) and carrot (23) can be mentioned. Some plants change the number and motility of the sperm by changing sex hormones. Other plants with androgenic properties affect the hypothalamus-pituitary axis and increase sex hormones (24). Garlic with its antioxidant properties, have been shown to increase the weight of the epididymis, seminal vesicles and increases the number of sperms (25). Garlic is one of the most potent and most prominent species of plants, which is a part of the onion family (7). Garlic has been known since 5000 years ago. In ancient times, Babylonians, Egyptians, Vikings, Chinese, Greeks, Romans and Hindus used garlic (26). In 3000 BC garlic was used for heart disease, arthritis, uterine disease, pulmonary disease, skin diseases, diarrhea, headache, wound healing and tumor (27,28). It is native to Western Asia, also found in most regions of Iran, especially in the northern regions (29). The perennial plant, has a height of 100-300 cm, has flowers in pink or green (16). It is used

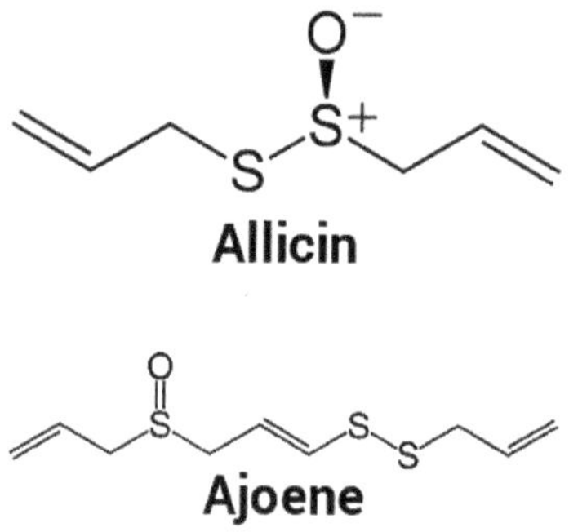

Figure 1: The main compounds of garlic.

commonly as a medicinal herb and food flavor, and it is one of the herbs that have a long history of medical uses (30). Garlic contains many compounds, including vitamins B2, B6, B1, A and C, a lot of antioxidants, flavonoids, sulfur compounds and allicin (7). Allicin (dialkly thiosulfinate) plays a key role in the garlic medicinal properties, however, this compound is not found in fresh garlic, and made by action of allinase on alliin (S-alkyl-l-cysteine sulfoxide). Ajoene is another important compound in garlic (Figure 1) (31). Garlic protects the liver and has anticholesterolemic, antithrombotic, antihypertensive and antimicrobial activity (30), and consumption of garlic acts like insulin receptor and reduces glucose levels in diabetic patients (3). Solving infertility problem is a fundamental issue in every community's health system. Considering the complications and limitations of chemical drugs and surgical procedures, and according to the mentioned therapeutic effects of garlic, this systematic review was conducted to investigate the effects of garlic on male fertility.

Methods

Study protocol

Current systematic review was reported in accordance with PRISMA (Preferred Reporting Items for Systematic Reviews and Meta-analyses) guidelines (32). In this study, the search process was done aimed to find studies in English without time limitations.

Search strategy

Data were collected by searching the key words: treatment, fertility, infertility, male, herbal medicine, *garlic*, medicinal plant, sperm, sex hormones and spermatogenesis in international databases such as: Web of Science (ISI), PubMed, Scopus and Embase until March 2018.

Inclusion criteria

- To conduct experimental studies or clinical trials
- Randomization in studies
- Evaluation of fertility, spermatogenesis or male sex hormones
- Mentioning of ethical considerations in articles

Exclusion criteria
- Absence of proper sampling method in studies
- Evaluation of fertility in female, not male, samples
- Not mentioning moral considerations

Selection of studies and data extraction
The articles' information was reviewed independently by two authors based on inclusion and exclusion criteria. Finally, both of authors classified the information and, in cases that the information was inconsistent, the comments of the third author were used. The information obtained from the articles was entered into the checklist considering the quality approval of the articles. The checklist contained: author's name, year of the study, type of study, molecular change, type of sample, type of administration, dosage, part of plant and period of extract administration. SYRCLE risk of bias tool was used for assessment of the quality. This tool is an advanced and improved model of the past quality assessment tools that is specific to animal and pre-clinical studies (33) and solve some of defects of the previous tools that was related to clinical trials.

Results
In the first stage of search, 980 articles were found. After removing duplicates and unrelated articles, 18 experimental studies included in this systematic review (Figure 2).
Thirteen studies evaluated garlic and 5 studies compared garlic effects with other drugs. A study compared aged garlic extract with adriamycin, a study compared aged garlic extract with titanium dioxide, a study compared garlic oil extract with furan, a study compared garlic blue extract with vitamin E and N-acetyl cysteine and a study compared garlic extract and onion with cadmium.
Qualitative assessment showed that most studies were in high risk for bias. In most of these studies, randomization in animal housing, randomization in sampling, researcher and statistical analyzers blinding were not me n tioned clearly (Table 1).
In 10 studies garlic extract was prescribed as crude plant and powder for animals. The maximum sample size was 62 mice and the lowest sample size was 10 mice that were examined in experimental studies. All studies were conducted in the in vivo condition. The control group received distilled water, normal saline or powder containing starch, and the treatment group received aged garlic extract, adriamcyin, titanium dioxide, garlic oil, N-acetylcyseinne, vitamin E, cadmium, cooked garlic or garlic juice. The treatment period varied from 7 to 120 days and complications such as impaired spermatogenesis, apoptosis, abnormal sperm, decreased sperm motility, seminal vesicle disorder, increased blood cholesterol, leukocytosis, decreased testicular weight, decreased Leydig cells, increased prostate weight and increased cortisol were mentioned in the studies. All of these complications were reported as chemical substances toxicity. Further information is presented in Table 2.

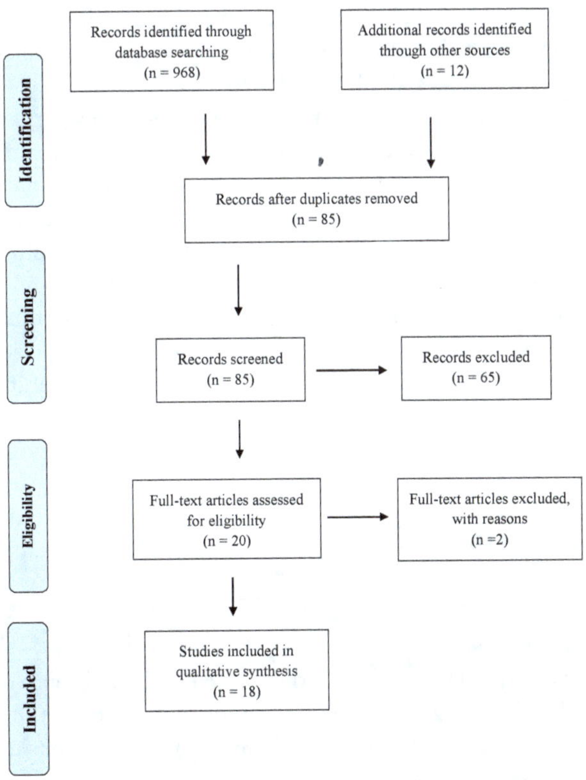

Figure 2. Trend of screening and choosing articles based on PRISMA guidelines.

Discussion
The present study was a systematic review of the effects of garlic on fertility. In general, in this paper, 18 studies were reviewed. Thirteen studies were conducted on the effect of garlic on fertility treatment. Due to the lack of side effects, as well as containing flavonoids, vitamins, fructose and sulfur compounds, garlic can help with neutralizing free radicals (1). Sulfur compounds in garlic, with a direct effect on the metabolism of cytochrome P450 and glutathione -s-transferase, have a protective effect on spermatogenesis. In addition to sulfur compounds, garlic has antioxidant properties and can increase fertility by reducing lipid peroxidation (32). Given the above mentioned factors, garlic is recommended for the treatment of infertility. In a study by Asadpour et al it was indicated that garlic has antioxidant activity due to presence of vitamin E, which prevents oxygen peroxide (49). Also, the results of the study by Nasr showed that garlic antioxidant properties can reduce the toxicity of harmful drugs on the testes and increase the spermatogenesis and fertility in men (35).
In the study by Akabawy and Sherif, it was concluded that garlic inhibited caspase-3 and cytochrome P450 2E1 (CYP2E1) enzymes, which had a toxic effect on the testes and, by decreasing these two enzymes, improved the testicular performance and spermatogenesis (37).

Table 1. Risk of bias for animal studies, using the SYRCLE risk of bias tool

Study	1 Selection bias 1	2 Selection bias 2	3 Selection bias 3	4 Performance bias 1	5 Performance bias 2	6 Detection bias 1	7 Detection bias 2	8 Attrition bias	9 Reporting bias	10 Other potential bias
Hajiuon (34)	x	✓	✓	؟	X	؟	X	؟	✓	✓
Nasr (35)	✓	✓	✓	؟	X	X	؟	✓	✓	✓
Abu Zeid et al (36)	✓	✓	✓	؟	؟	؟	؟	✓	✓	✓
El-Akabawy and El-Sherif (37)	✓	✓	✓	؟	؟	x	؟	✓	✓	✓
Abdelmalik (38)	✓	✓	x	؟	X	؟	X	؟	✓	✓
Ouarda and Abdennour (39)	؟	✓	؟	؟	؟	؟	؟	؟	✓	؟
Ghalehkandi (40)	✓	✓	؟	؟	X	؟	؟	؟	✓	✓
Bahrami et al (7)	✓	✓	✓	؟	؟	؟	؟	x	✓	؟
Safaei et al (41)	✓	؟	✓	؟	؟	✓	؟	؟	؟	؟
Ola-Mudathir et al (42)	✓	✓	✓	✓	؟	؟	؟	؟	✓	✓
Omotoso et al (25)	✓	✓	✓	؟	؟	؟	؟	؟	✓	✓
Nahdi et al (43)	✓	✓	؟	؟	؟	؟	؟	✓	✓	✓
Hammami et al (44)	✓	✓	؟	؟	؟	✓	؟	؟	✓	؟
Hammami et al (45)	✓	✓	✓	؟	؟	؟	؟	؟	✓	✓
Oi et al (46)	✓	✓	؟	؟	✓	؟	؟	؟	✓	✓
Lee et al (47)	✓	✓	x	؟	؟	؟	؟	✓	✓	✓
Abdullah et al (48)	✓	✓	✓	؟	؟	✓	؟	؟	✓	✓
Asadpour et al (49)	✓	✓	x	؟	؟	؟	؟	✓	✓	✓

Hammami and Abdelmalik (38) concluded that garlic contains phytoestrogens, which have a direct effect on estrogen. It is a precursor to testosterone production, so it is possible that garlic stimulates the sexual cells and sex hormones (38,43). The results in the study by Oi et al indicated that garlic supplementation boosts LH from the pituitary gland, and this stimulates testosterone secretion from the testicles (46). Nonetheless, in the study by Bahrami et al (7), it was recommended that the cooked garlic has better therapeutic effects and, while affecting the reproduction of the sexual cells in testes and epididymis, improves spermatogenesis (7).

Due to presence of dialyldisulfide in its biochemical structure, garlic affects the hypothalamic-pituitary axis. Diallyldisulfide stimulates the basophilic cells and secretion of LH sex hormones by affecting the anterior pituitary. LH stimulates Leydig cells in the testes, which in turn is a precursor to secretion and regulation of testosterone (50). Also, diallyldisulfide reduces oxygen free radicals, enhances and strengthens the blood-testis barrier and increases the circulation in the testicles, thus protects the sexual organs (39). By increasing blood flow to the testicles (due to the consumption of garlic), phenol and phenolic glycosides are released which increase the glutathione peroxidase enzyme. The role of this enzyme is to protect sperms in testicular and epididymal tissue (51). The enzyme protects the sperm from the damage of free radicals by placement in the plasma membrane and the nucleus of sperm, epididymal fluid and epididymis, and leads to ultimate maturation and development of the sperm (52). Also, garlic can repair and protect the DNA of the sperm, in addition to sperm maturation through vitamins C, B, E, which are its potent antioxidants (53). Approximately 45%-50% of infertility has a male cause, but nevertheless, 30-45% is due to idiopathic causes (54). Typically, infertility in men is indicated by oligozoospermia, asthenozoospermia, or teratozoospermia and varicocele (55). Recent studies have shown that, in physiological conditions, reactive oxygen species play a very important role in intracellular messaging processes. On the other hand, during the last decade, reactive oxygen species have been implicated in the development of male infertility, due to excessive production of reactive oxygen species or reduced ability of the antioxidant system of the genital system and sperm. In pathological conditions, reactive oxygen species result in male infertility through disruption of the spermatogenesis process, sperm function and structure, mobility, survival, acrosome reaction, sperm-to-oocyte coupling and even reduced fertilization and implantation (56).

Conclusion

Probably, due to the antioxidant power and the absence of side effects of garlic, it can be useful in enhancing fertility. Due to the limited number of clinical studies, there is no definite overall and reassuring result. In order to ensure the effects of this plant and its compounds, clinical studies with a larger statistical population, as well as an increase

Table 2. Effect of garlic on reproductive system and fertility

Effect of garlic	Type of extract	Duration of treatment	Dose	Administration	Sample study	Part used	Result	Ref.
Effects on sexual hormones	Hydro alcoholic extract	30 days	200 and 400 mg/kg	Orally	Rats	Leaves	↓Testosterone levels, ↓Estrogen, ↑Progesterone	(34)
	Aged garlic extract	7-14 days	250 mg/kg	Orally	Rats	Seeds	↑Testosterone leves, ↓MDA concentration, ↑GSH level, ↑GSH-Px, ↑CAT, and SOD activity	(35)
	Aged garlic extract	65 days	2 mL/kg	Orally	Rats	Leaves	↑Androgen levels	(36)
	Garlic oil	NM	4 mg/kg	Orally	Rats	NM	↓Testosterone levels, ↓Caspase-3, ↓Cytochrome P450 2E1	(37)
	NM	120 days	30 g	Orally	Rats	NM	↓Testosterone levels	(38)
Effects on spermatogenesis and testicular structure and other results	NM	14 days	50 g	Orally	Rabbits	Seeds	↑Sperm motility and viability, ↑Sperm speed, ↑White blood counts	(39)
	Garlic juice	30 days	60 and 120 mg/kg	Gavage	Rats	Seeds	↓Semen MDA activity, ↓TAS activity	(40)
	NM	30 days	5% and 15% of raw garlic and cooked garlic	Orally	Rats	Seeds	In cooked garlic, ↓Weight Loss, ↑Number of spermatocyte cells, ↑Number of spermatozoa, ↑Number of sperm cells, ↑Number of Sertoli cells, ↑Testicle weight, ↑External diameter of the epididymide, ↑The inner diameter of epididymide, ↑Sperm volume	(7)
	Alcoholic extract	30 days	0.05%, 0.1% and 0.2%	Orally	Rooster	Leaves	Garlic alcoholic extract 0.2%: ↑Semen volume, ↑Testicle weight, ↑Sperm counts, ↑Percentage of mobility and sperm biocompatibility, ↑Laydic cell count	(41)
	NM	Between 7-21 days	0.5 mL/100 g. BW	Gavage	Rats	Leaves	↑LOP, ↑Glutathione *S*-transferase, ↑GSH, ↑SOD, ↑CAT, ↑Epididymal sperm concentration, ↑Sperm progress motility, ↓Lipid peroxidation	(42)
	Aqueous Extract	28 days	500 and 100 mg/kg	Feeding tube	Rats	Leaves	↓Spermatozoa count, ↓SOD activity in the blood	(25)
	NM	NM	5%, 10% and 15%	Orally	Rats	Leaves	↑Number of tubules deprived of spermatozoa, ↓Apoptosis of testicular germ cells, ↓Testosterone levels	(43)
	NM	30 days	5%, 10% and 15% of 30 g	Orally	Rats	Seeds	↑CASP3 levels, ↑Caspase inhibitors BIRC3 and BIRC2, ↑IAP inhibitor DIABLO, ↓AMH, RHOX5 and CDKN1B, ↑GATA4	(44)
	NM	30 days	5%, 10%, 15% and 30% of 9 g	Orally	Rats	Seeds	↓Prostate weight, ↓Seminal vesicle weight, ↓Testosterone levels, ↑LH levels, ↑Phosphatase acid activity	(45)
	NM	28 days	8 g	Intraperitoneal injection	Rats	-	↑LH levels, ↑Testicular testosterone, ↓Plasma corticosterone	(46)
	Ethanolic extract	37 days	5, 10, 20 and 40 mg/kg/bw	Perorally	Rats	Leaves	↓Weight loss, ↓Testicular weight, ↑Spermatogenesis	(47)
	NM	90 days	100 mg/kg/d	Intraperitoneal injection	Mice	Leaves	↑Weight of seminal vesicles and epididymides, ↑Sperm count, ↑Weight loss, ↑WBC, ↓RBC	(48)
	NM	35 days	400 mg/kg	Gavage	Rats	Leaves	↑Sperm motility and viability, ↑MDA level, ↑ SOD activities	(49)

NM: not mentioned, MDA: malondialdehyde, GSH: glutathione, GSH-px: glutathione peroxidase, SOD: superoxide dismutase, CAT: catalase, TAS: total antioxidant status, BIRC3: baculoviral IAP repeat-containing protein 3, BIRC2: baculoviral IAP repeat-containing protein2, AMH: anti-Mullerian hormone, CDKN1B: cyclin-dependent kinase inhibitor 1B, LH: luteinizing hormone

in the duration of its administration, comparison with safe drugs and the determination of the exact molecular mechanism are recommended.

Authors' contributions

All authors contributed equally in planning and carrying out this work. All authors read the manuscript and confirmed the publication for final version.

Conflict of interests

None.

Ethical considerations

Not applicable.

Funding/Support

There is no financial support for this work.

References

1. Mohammadi F, Nikzad H, Taherian A, Amini Mahabadi J, Salehi M. Effects of herbal medicine on male infertility. Anat Sci J. 2013;10(4):3-16.
2. Kim SJ, Kim MR, Hwang SY, Bae WJ, Kim S, Hong SH, et al. Preliminary report on the safety of a new herbal formula and its effect on sperm quality. World J Mens Health. 2013;31(3):254-61. doi: 10.5534/wjmh.2013.31.3.254.
3. Roozbeh N, Rostami S, Abdi F. A review on herbal medicine with fertility and infertility characteristics in males. Iranian Journal of Obstetrics, Gynecology and Infertility. 2016;19(13):18-32.
4. Mascarenhas MN, Flaxman SR, Boerma T, Vanderpoel S, Stevens GA. National, regional, and global trends in infertility prevalence since 1990: a systematic analysis of 277 health surveys. PLoS Med. 2012;9(12):e1001356. doi: 10.1371/journal.pmed.1001356.
5. Direkvand Moghadam A, Delpisheh A, Sayehmiri K. The Prevalence of infertility in Iran, a systematic review. Iranian Journal of Obstetrics, Gynecology and Infertility. 2014;16(81):1-7.
6. Imai H, Suzuki K, Ishizaka K, Ichinose S, Oshima H, Okayasu I, et al. Failure of the expression of phospholipid hydroperoxide glutathione peroxidase in the spermatozoa of human infertile males. Biol Reprod. 2001;64(2):674-83.
7. Bahrami KH, Mahjor AA, Johary H, Bahrami R, Bahrami A. Comparative study on histopatological and histomorphometric effect of raw and cooked garlic on spermatogenesis in testis and epidydims of rats. J Fasa Univ Med Sci. 2014;3(4):371-9.
8. Fisher J, Hammarberg K. Psychological Aspects of Infertility Among Men. In: Simoni M, Huhtaniemi IT, eds. Endocrinology of the Testis and Male Reproduction. Cham: Springer International Publishing; 2017:1287-317.
9. Baniaghil AS, Zarei Abolkheir A, Keshavarz A, Ahmadi SM, Vakili MA. The effect of integrated third-party reproduction counseling on egg donation recipientsa attitude towards assisted reproductive techniques. Iranian Journal of Obstetrics, Gynecology and Infertility. 2016;19(36):1-10.
10. Kooti W, Moradi M, Peyro K, Sharghi M, Alamiri F, Azami M, et al. The effect of celery (*Apium graveolens* L.) on fertility: A systematic review. J Complement Integr Med. 2017;15(2). doi: 10.1515/jcim-2016-0141.
11. Anbari K, Ghanadi K. Use of complementary and alternative mediecine methods and its related factors in person referred to health centers in Khorramabad. Complementary Medicine Journal of Faculty of Nursing & Midwifery. 2015;4(4):987-99.
12. Aliakbari F, Gilani MA, Amidi F, Baazm M, Korouji M, Izadyar F, et al. Improving the efficacy of cryopreservation of spermatogonia stem cells by antioxidant supplements. Cell Reprogram. 2016;18(2):87-95. doi: 10.1089/cell.2015.0067.
13. Amidi F, Pazhohan A, Shabani Nashtaei M, Khodarahmian M, Nekoonam S. The role of antioxidants in sperm freezing: a review. Cell Tissue Bank. 2016;17(4):745-56. doi: 10.1007/s10561-016-9566-5.
14. Rezaeian Z, Yazdekhasti H, Nasri S, Rajabi Z, Fallahi P, Amidi F. Effect of selenium on human sperm parameters after freezing and thawing procedures. Asian Pac J Reprod. 2016;5(6):462-6. doi: 10.1016/j.apjr.2016.11.001.
15. Amidi F, Ebrahimi S, Abbasi M, Yazdani M, Ghasemi S. Effects of saffron extract on sperm parameters in rats with experimentally induced varicocele. J Qazvin Univ Med Sci. 2014;18(5):4-11.
16. Mansouri E, Ghasemiboroon M, Asadi-Samani M, Alamiri F, Ashtary-Larky D, Kafash-Farkhad N, et al. The effect of hydro-alcoholic extract of *Apium graveolens* L. leaf on delivery rate in female rats, weight and gender ratio of infants. Jundishapur J Nat Pharm Prod. 2017;12(1):e28802. doi: 10.5812/jjnpp.28802.
17. Kooti W, Moradi MT, Ali-Akbari S, Sharafi-Ahvazi N, Asadi-Samani M, Ashtary-Larky D. Therapeutic and pharmacological potential of *Foeniculum vulgare* Mill: a review. J Herbmed Pharmacol. 2014;4(1):1-9.
18. Kooti W, Hasanzadeh-Noohi Z, Sharafi-Ahvazi N, Asadi-Samani M, Ashtary-Larky D. Phytochemistry, pharmacology, and therapeutic uses of black seed (*Nigella sativa*). Chin J Nat Med. 2016;14(10):732-45. doi: 10.1016/s1875-5364(16)30088-7.
19. Golkhani S, Vahdati A, Modaresi M, Edalatmanesh MA. The effects of *Matricaria chamomilla* extract during neonatal period of rats on pituitary-gonadal hormone axis and changes in testicular tissue of male progenies. Middle East Journal of Family Medicine. 2017;15(6):126-32.
20. Modaresi M, Messripour M, Asadi Marghmaleki M, Hamadanian M. Effect of Saffron (*Crocus sativus*) extract on level of FSH, LH and testosterone in mice. J Zanjan Univ Med Sci. 2008;16(63):11-8.
21. Naseri M, Heydari Nasrabadi M, Khodarahmi P, Ahmadi F, Mojibi P, Abotalebei H. Study of the effect of *Fumaria parviflora* alcoholic extract on spermatogenesis in male rats. New Cellular and Molecular Biotechnology Journal. 2011;1(2):61-5.
22. Kazemi P, Jowhary H, Sharifi E, Zeraat PA. Androgenic effect of *Origanum vulgarel* l. spp viride extract on hormone level of pituitary-gonadal axis in mature male Wistar rats. J Arak Univ Med Sci. 2012;14(6):89-96. [Persian].
23. Nouri M, Khaki A, Fathi Azar F, Rashidi MR. The protective effects of carrot seed extract on spermatogenesis and cauda epididymal sperm reserves in gentamicin treated rats. Yakhteh. 2009;11(3):327-32.
24. Bastampoor F, Sadeghi H, Hosseini S. The *Petroselinum crispum* L. hydroalcoholic extract effects on pituitary- gonad axis in adult rats. Armaghane Danesh. 2014;19(4):305-13. [Persian].

25. Omotoso G, Oyewopo A, Kadir R, Olawuyi S, Jimoh A. Effects of aqueous extract of *Allium sativum* (garlic) on semen parameters in Wistar rats. Internet J Urol. 2010;7(2):1-5.
26. Block E. The organosulfur chemistry of the genus *Allium* – implications for the organic chemistry of sulfur. Angew Chem Int Ed Engl. 1992;31(9):1135-78. doi:10.1002/anie.199211351.
27. Freeman F, Kodera Y. Garlic Chemistry: Stability of S-(2-Propenyl)-2-Propene-1-sulfinothioate (Allicin) in Blood, Solvents, and Simulated Physiological Fluids. J Agric Food Chem. 1995;43(9):2332-8. doi: 10.1021/jf00057a004.
28. Rivlin RS. Historical perspective on the use of garlic. J Nutr. 2001;131(3s):951s-4s. doi: 10.1093/jn/131.3.951S.
29. Plata-Rueda A, Martinez LC, Santos MHD, Fernandes FL, Wilcken CF, Soares MA, et al. Insecticidal activity of garlic essential oil and their constituents against the mealworm beetle, *Tenebrio molitor* Linnaeus (Coleoptera: Tenebrionidae). Sci Rep. 2017;7:46406. doi: 10.1038/srep46406.
30. Rahman MS. Allicin and other functional active components in garlic: health benefits and bioavailability. Int J Food Prop. 2007;10(2):245-68. doi: 10.1080/10942910601113327.
31. Ledezma E, Apitz-Castro R. Ajoene the main active compound of garlic (*Allium sativum*): a new antifungal agent. Rev Iberoam Micol. 2006;23(2):75-80.
32. Moher D, Liberati A, Tetzlaff J, Altman DG. Preferred reporting items for systematic reviews and meta-analyses: the PRISMA statement. PLoS Med. 2009;6(7):e1000097. doi: 10.1371/journal.pmed.1000097.
33. Hooijmans CR, Rovers MM, de Vries RB, Leenaars M, Ritskes-Hoitinga M, Langendam MW. SYRCLE's risk of bias tool for animal studies. BMC Med Res Methodol. 2014;14:43. doi: 10.1186/1471-2288-14-43.
34. Hajiuon B. Effects of garlic (*Allium sativum* L) hydroalcoholic extract on estrogen, progesterone and testosterone levels in rats exposed to cell phone radiation. Zahedan Journal of Research in Medical Sciences. 2014;16(12):19-24.
35. Nasr AY. The impact of aged garlic extract on adriamycin-induced testicular changes in adult male Wistar rats. Acta Histochem. 2017;119(6):648-62. doi: 10.1016/j.acthis.2017.07.006.
36. Abu Zeid EH, Alam RTM, Abd El-Hameed NE. Impact of titanium dioxide on androgen receptors, seminal vesicles and thyroid hormones of male rats: possible protective trial with aged garlic extract. Andrologia. 2017;49(5). doi: 10.1111/and.12651.
37. El-Akabawy G, El-Sherif NM. Protective role of garlic oil against oxidative damage induced by furan exposure from weaning through adulthood in adult rat testis. Acta Histochem. 2016;118(5):456-63. doi: 10.1016/j.acthis.2016.04.008.
38. Abdelmalik SW. Histological and ultrastructural changes in the adult male albino rat testes following chronic crude garlic consumption. Ann Anat. 2011;193(2):134-41. doi: 10.1016/j.aanat.2010.12.003.
39. Ouarda M, Abdennour C. Evaluation of the therapeutic efficiency of raw garlic on reproduction of domestic rabbits under lead induced toxicity. Ann Biol Res. 2011;2(3):38993.
40. Ghiasi Ghalehkandi J. Garlic (*Allium sativum*) juice protects from semen oxidative stress in male rats exposed to chromium chloride. Anim Reprod. 2014;11(4):526-32.
41. Safaei Ayda, Gharejan lu Mitra, Rezvani Morvarid, Fahime A. The effect of garlic alcoholic extract in water on fertility and spermatogenesis, Golpayegan Native Cockroaches. Civilica; 2012. https://www.civilica.com/Paper-Agribiotech03-Agribiotech03_589.html.
42. Ola-Mudathir KF, Suru SM, Fafunso MA, Obioha UE, Faremi TY. Protective roles of onion and garlic extracts on cadmium-induced changes in sperm characteristics and testicular oxidative damage in rats. Food Chem Toxicol. 2008;46(12):3604-11. doi: 10.1016/j.fct.2008.09.004.
43. Hammami I, Nahdi A, Atig F, Kouidhi W, Amri M, Mokni M, et al. Effects of garlic fractions consumption on male reproductive functions. J Med Food. 2013;16(1):82-7. doi: 10.1089/jmf.2011.0335.
44. Hammami I, Amara S, Benahmed M, El May MV, Mauduit C. Chronic crude garlic-feeding modified adult male rat testicular markers: mechanisms of action. Reprod Biol Endocrinol. 2009;7:65. doi: 10.1186/1477-7827-7-65.
45. Hammami I, Nahdi A, Mauduit C, Benahmed M, Amri M, Ben Amar A, et al. The inhibitory effects on adult male reproductive functions of crude garlic (*Allium sativum*) feeding. Asian J Androl. 2008;10(4):593-601. doi: 10.1111/j.1745-7262.2008.00358.x.
46. Oi Y, Imafuku M, Shishido C, Kominato Y, Nishimura S, Iwai K. Garlic supplementation increases testicular testosterone and decreases plasma corticosterone in rats fed a high protein diet. J Nutr. 2001;131(8):2150-6. doi: 10.1093/jn/131.8.2150.
47. Lee SC, Hwang SY, Kim SW, Kim SK. Ethanol extract of *Allium sativum* attenuates testicular and liver toxicity induced by 2,3,7,8-tetrachlorodibenzo-p-dioxin in rats. J Med Food. 2009;12(1):93-9. doi: 10.1089/jmf.2007.0620.
48. Al-Bekairi AM, Shah AH, Qureshi S. Effect of *Allium sativum* on epididymal spermatozoa, estradiol-treated mice and general toxicity. J Ethnopharmacol. 1990;29(2):117-25.
49. Asadpour R, Azari M, Hejazi M, Tayefi H, Zaboli N. Protective effects of garlic aquous extract (*Allium sativum*), vitamin E, and N-acetylcysteine on reproductive quality of male rats exposed to lead. Vet Res Forum. 2013;4(4):251-7.
50. Ultee-van Gessel AM, Timmerman MA, de Jong FH. Effects of treatment of neonatal rats with highly purified FSH alone and in combination with LH on testicular function and endogenous hormone levels at various ages. J Endocrinol. 1988;116(3):413-20.
51. Pal R, Vaiphei K, Sikander A, Singh K, Rana SV. Effect of garlic on isoniazid and rifampicin-induced hepatic injury in rats. World J Gastroenterol. 2006;12(4):636-9.
52. Amin A, Hamza AA. Effects of Roselle and Ginger on cisplatin-induced reproductive toxicity in rats. Asian J Androl. 2006;8(5):607-12. doi: 10.1111/j.1745-7262.2006.00179.x.
53. Brooks DE. Activity and androgenic control of glycolytic enzymes in the epididymis and epididymal spermatozoa of the rat. Biochem J. 1976;156(3):527-37.
54. Jo J, Lee SH, Lee JM, Jerng UM. Semen quality improvement in a man with idiopathic infertility treated with traditional Korean medicine: A Case Report. Explore (NY). 2015;11(4):320-3. doi: 10.1016/j.explore.2015.04.007.
55. Kim KI, Jo J. The effectiveness of Korean medicine treatment in male patients with infertility: a study protocol for a prospective observational pilot study. Medicine (Baltimore). 2018;97(4):e9696. doi: 10.1097/md.0000000000009696.
56. Fanaei H, Azizi Y, Khayat S. A Review: Role of oxidative stress in male infertility. J Fasa Univ Med Sci. 2013;3(2):93-103.

The effects of *Urtica dioica* hydroalcoholic extract on the propylthiouracil induced hypothyroidism in rat

Fatemeh Abdolhosseinipoor[1], **Masoud Sadeghi-Dinani**[2], **Ali Hosseini-Sharifabad**[1*]

[1]Department of Pharmacology and Toxicology, School of Pharmacy and Pharmaceutical Sciences, Isfahan University of Medical Sciences, Isfahan, Iran
[2]Department of Pharmacognosy, School of Pharmacy and Pharmaceutical Sciences, Isfahan University of Medical Sciences, Isfahan, Iran

ARTICLE INFO

Keywords:
Hypothyroidism
Medicinal plants
Herbal medicine
Propylthiouracil
Urtica dioica

ABSTRACT

Introduction: Hypothyroidism is an important endocrine disorder determined by some depressed symptoms. *Urtica dioica* (Urticaceae) is a medicinal plant which has been traditionally used for treatment of a wide range of decreased functions of different organs. In the current study, we aimed to evaluate the effect of hydroalcoholic extract of aerial parts of *U. dioica* on thyroid hormones in propylthiouracil (PTU)-induced hypothyroidism in rats.
Methods: Forty-two male Wistar rats were randomly divided into 7 groups including control, PTU, different doses of *Urtica dioica* hydroalcoholic extract (UDHAE) treated and levothyroxine treated groups. The animals in various groups received water (control group) or water containing 0.1% W/V PTU and then injected saline (control group) or 25, 50, 100, 150 mg/kg UDHAE, respectively for 4 weeks. Positive control group was fed levothyroxine 0.5 mg/kg during the PTU treatment. Then, the blood samples were collected and the levels of thyroxine (T_4), triiodothyronine (T_3), free triiodothyronine (FT_3) and thyroid-stimulating hormone (TSH) measured via the Elisa method.
Results: The data showed that PTU decreased the blood level of thyroid hormones but increased TSH, significantly. The 50 or 100 mg/kg doses of UDHAE remarkably increased the blood level of T_3 and FT_3. The 50 mg/kg doses of UDHAE increased the blood level of T_4. None of the UDHAE doses showed significant change in the TSH levels. 25 and 150 mg/kg doses of UDHAE did not change the PTU- diminished level of thyroid related hormones.
Conclusion: The findings suggest that 50 mg/kg dose of UDHAE has stimulatory effect on thyroid gland function and raises plasma T_3 & T_4 & FT_3 levels. UDHAE at the dose of 50 or 100 mg/kg could enhance blood level of T_3 and FT_3 perhaps by increase in T_4 to T_3 transformation. Higher doses of UDHAE could not increase the level of these hormones probably due to the presence of inhibitory materials.

Implication for health policy/practice/research/medical education:
The extract of *Urtica dioica*, in some especial doses reversed the PTU-induced T_3 diminution. The results show that it might be effective in hypothyroidism disease.

Introduction

Thyroid hormones play an important role in the normal activity of all body tissues. Decrease in the thyroid hormone levels is known as hypothyroidism (1). It can occur because of the deficiency in iodine intake, thyroid gland lesions, autoimmune disorders and impaired activity of pituitary gland (2,3). The untreated hypothyroidism leads to a wide range of abnormalities including loss of energy, fatigue sensation, weight gain, dry skin, depression, behavioral fluctuations, hair loss, hands and face swelling and increased cholesterol (4). For the treatment of hypothyroidism the levels of thyroid hormones should be elevated to normal levels. The common way is the replacement of them with administration of "levothyroxine"(5). Beside levothyroxine, some medications like supplementations or plants are used to help the treatment of hypothyroidism. These components could decrease the peripheral hypothyroidism symptoms or increase the production of related hormones (6-8). Although the well-known hypothyroidism medication, levothyroxine, shows an

***Corresponding author**: Ali Hosseini-Sharifabad,
Email: hosseini_a@pharm.mui.ac.ir

excellent efficacy, it causes different side effects like tachycardia, heat intolerance and tremor (9). So, the use of medicinal plants instead of levothyroxine, or along with it, in treatment of hypothyroidism for better outcome or decrease of its side effects, is attractive for the researchers (10). It has been shown that some plants like Guggulu (*Commiphora mukul*), Marshmallow (*Althaea officinalis* L.), *Rhodiola rosea, Commiphora Muku, Bacopa monnieri* (Water Hyssop) improve the hypothyroidism by involving different mechanisms (1,11-13).

Nettle or *Urtica dioica* is a famous medicinal plant that grows in the tropical and warm regions from May to September. Nettle consists of a wild range of chemical compounds including sterols, terpenes, coumarins, lignans, ceramids and fatty acids. The flowers, leaves, stem and root of Nettle are used for medicinal purposes (14). For a long time it has been employed for treatment of urological problems like kidney stones and prostatic hyperplasia (14,15). In addition, Nettle has antimicrobial, anti-arthritis and glucose lowering effects (16-19). In traditional medicine, Nettle is known as a plant with hot and dry nature (20). This type of plants is able to increase the metabolism and activity in the body. In other words it possibly can improve the symptoms of hypothyroidism (21,22). In addition it is believed that the sterols and coumarins compounds can change the thyroid hormone (23,24) .The present study is going to evaluate the effect of hydroalcoholic extract of aerial parts of *U. dioica* on the level of thyroid hormones in PTU-induced hypothyroid in rats.

Materials and Methods

Animals

Male Wistar rats weighting 180 to 220 g were obtained from the animal house in Isfahan School of Pharmacy and Pharmaceutical Sciences, Isfahan, Iran. The animals were housed in polypropylene cages under standard laboratory conditions in a 12 h light/12 h dark cycles. The rats had free access to tap water and standard pellet diet.

Chemicals

Propylthiouracil (PTU) was purchased from Iran hormone Pharmaceutical Co, Tehran, Iran. The ELISA assay kits for measurement of serum T_4, T_3, FT_3 and TSH hormones were purchased from Pishgaman Sanjesh Research Co, Tehran, Iran.

Plant and preparation of extract

The aerial parts of *U. dioica* were gifted from Booalidaroo Co. (Qom, Iran). The firstly were evaluated and approved by an expert technician and then a voucher specimen of the plant was deposited in the herbarium collection of Isfahan School of Pharmacy.

The maceration method was used for preparation of hydroalcoholic extract. For this purpose, 1176 g of freshly dried aerial parts of *U. dioica* were crushed and incubated with a mixture of ethanol: water (70:30) solvent at room temperature for four day. The product was filtered and then concentrated under reduced pressure at 50°C in a rotary evaporator machine. The obtained extract was freeze-dried and 102.7 g powder was yielded.

Experimental protocol

Forty-two male Wistar rats were randomly divided into 7 equal groups. All of them except control group were treated with 0.1% W/V PTU via the drinking water for 4 weeks. In addition, they were treated according to the following schedule during the PTU exposure period:

Control: daily received i.p injection of saline for 4 weeks.

PTU: daily received i.p injection of saline for 4 weeks.

UDHAE treated: daily received i.p injection of 25, 50, 100 or 150 mg/kg doses of UDHAE for 4 weeks.

Levothyroxine: daily received 0.5 mg/kg levothyroxine by oral gavage for 4 weeks.

At the end of treatments, animals were slightly anesthetized and the blood samples were obtained from the angle eye vein. The plasma was separated and used for the further biochemical evaluations.

Measurement of plasma level of thyroid related hormones

The plasma level of T_4, T_3, FT_3 and TSH were measured via ELISA method using special kits (25). For determination of T4, 25 µL and for T3, FT3 and thyroid-stimulating hormone (TSH), 50 µL of sample was used. Fifty microliters of assay buffer and 50 µL of conjugate solution were added and incubated for 60 minutes in room temperature. Then, the product was rinsed with rinsing solution, 5 times. After that 100 µL of chromogenic substrate was added and kept in a dark place for 15 minutes. 100 µL of stop solution was added and the plate was shaken by hand for 15-20 seconds. At the end, the absorption of samples was read at 450 nm.

Statistical analysis

The data were presented as the mean ± SEM. Statistical analysis was performed by one-way analysis of variance (ANOVA) followed by Tukey post-hoc test using GraghPad Prism software version 4. The values of $P < 0.05$ were regarded to be statistically significant.

Results

Effect of PTU on the thyroid related hormones in rat

Administration of 0.1% PTU via drinking water for 4 weeks, significantly decreased the blood levels of T_4, T_3 and FT_3 but increased the level of TSH compare to the control group ($P < 0.001$) (Figure 1).

Effect of *Urtica dioica* hydroalcoholic extract on the blood level of T_4 in rat

While 25, 100 and 150 mg/kg doses of *U. dioica*

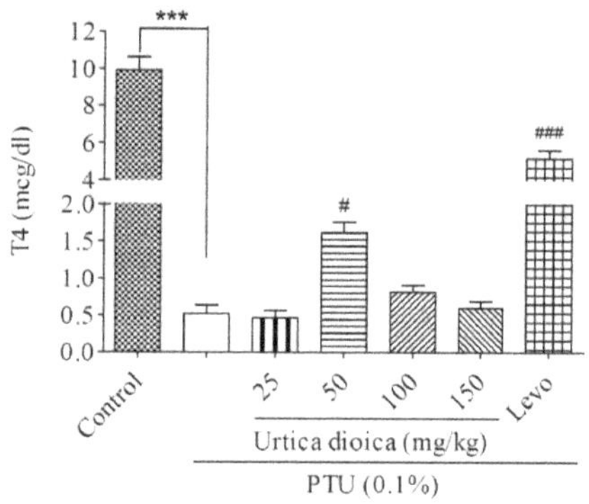

Figure 1. Effect of *Urtica dioica* extract on blood level of T_4 in PTU induced hypothyroidism. Values are presented as means ± SEM (n=6). ***P< 0.001 versus saline control group, ###P < 0.001 and #P < 0.05 versus PTU treated group.

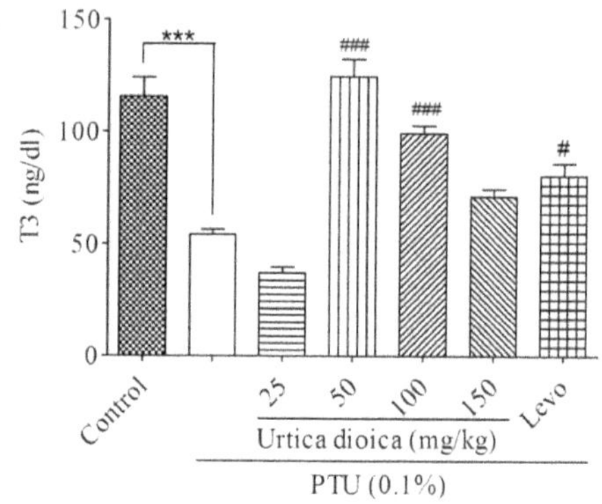

Figure 2. Effect of *Urtica dioica* extract on blood level of T_3 in Propylthiouracil (PTU) induced hypothyroidism. Values are presented as means ± SEM (n=6). ***P < 0.001 versus saline control group, ###P < 0.001 and #P < 0.05 versus PTU treated group.

hydroalcoholic extract (UDHAE) did not change the level of PTU-induced diminution in T_4, its administration at the dose of 50 mg/kg statistically increased the blood level of T_4 compared to the PTU-treated group (P<0.05; Figure 1).

Effect of UDHAE on the blood level of T_3 in rat

Animal treatment with 50 or 100 mg/kg doses of UDHAE for 4 weeks caused remarkably increase in the blood T_3 level compared to the PTU- treated rats (P<0.001). The low (25 mg/kg) or high (150 mg/kg) administered doses failed to prevent the PTU-induced decrease in the level of T_3 (Figure 2).

Effect of UDHAE on blood level of FT_3 in rat

A similar pattern of T_3 was occurred for the level of FT_3. While the 25 or 150 mg/kg doses of UDHAE didn't show an elevating effect in the level of FT_3 compared to the PTU-treated group, 50 or 100 mg/kg of UDHAE significantly increased the FT_3 level which had been decreased by PTU (P<0.001, P<0.01, respectively) (Figure 3).

Effect of UDHAE on the blood level of TSH in rat

Although the PTU increased the blood level of TSH, none of the studied doses of UDHAE changed the level of TSH compared to the PTU group (Figure 4).

Discussion

The current study evaluated the effect of hydroalcoholic extract of *Urtica dioica* aerial part on the serum level of thyroid related hormones in hypothyroidism rats. In the PTU treated animals which received PTU from drinking water for 4 weeks, the serum T_4, T_3 and FT_3 levels remarkably decreased and TSH level increased compared to that of control group. PTU is commonly used for the induction of hypothyroidism in the laboratory animals to evaluate the beneficial effects of agents in hypothyroidism treatment (26,27). PTU causes

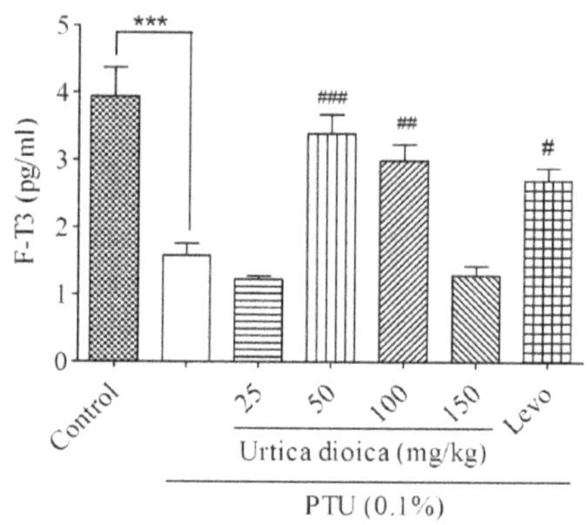

Figure 3. Effect of *Urtica dioica* extract on blood level of FT_3 in Propylthiouracil (PTU) induced hypothyroidism. Values are presented as means ± SEM (n=6). ***P< 0.001 versus saline control group, ###P < 0.001 and ##P < 0.01 and #P < 0.05 versus PTU treated group.

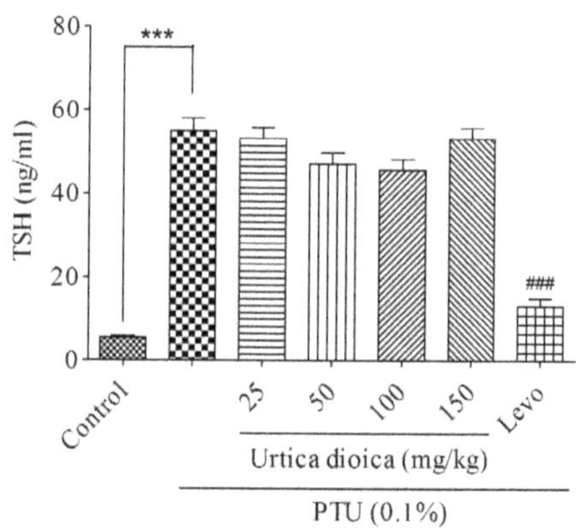

Figure 4. The level of TSH in propylthiouracil (PTU)-treated groups, alone or in combination with different doses of UDHAE and levothyroxine. Values are presented as means ± SEM (n = 6). ***P < 0.001 versus saline control group, ###P < 0.001 versus PTU treated group.

hypothyroidism by inhibition of thyroperoxidase (TPO) which is a key enzyme in production of thyroid hormones (28). In the levothyroxine treated animals, levothyroxine could prevent the decreasing effect of PTU in T_4, T_3 and FT_3 levels, also it prevented the increase in TSH level, indicating the animals and the method of measurement were reliable for this study. For the evaluation of UDHAE effect in different doses as well as its dose dependency on hypothyroidism, four increasing doses were chosen. This selection was according to the doses previously used to evaluate other effects of *U. dioica* like its antidiabetic effect (29,30).

UDHAE at the doses of 50 mg/kg and 100 mg/kg showed ameliorating effect in the PTU induced disruption of thyroid related hormones. This effect on T_3 and FT_3 was more significant than that of T_4 and TSH levels. On the other word, the levels of T_3 and FT_3 following administration of 50 and 100 mg/kg doses of UDHAE came back close to the normal level while T_4 level just showed a little increase compared to that of PTU treated animals. The level of TSH in different extract treated groups showed no significant effect compared to the PTU. The preventing effect against the hypothyroidism was most significant after 50 mg/kg dose of UDHAE. While the low dose of UDHAE did not show any ameliorating effect in the thyroid hormones levels, interestingly this effects were decreased following administration of the studied highest dose. The 150 mg/kg dose of UDHAE failed to prevent the hypothyroidism induced by PTU. From the findings, it can be deduced that UDHAE in especial doses can encounter to hypothyroidism by increase in transformation of T_4 to T_3. Because the level of T_3 was near to the normal but the T_4 level did not significantly change, it can be supposed that if these doses of UDHAE increased the production of T_4, all of them transformed to the T_3 form. The low dose of UDHAE was not enough to make any change in the thyroid related hormones. Also the studied high doses showed the opposite effect on the thyroid hormones compared to the moderate doses. This event illustrates that the anti-hypothyroidism effect of UDHAE do not follow a dose-dependent manner. The decreasing effect of the higher dose of UDHAE could be due to the presence of inhibitory components. These components overcome other benefit materials in this dose.

There are several phytochemical agents in the UDHAE. They include coumarins, stroles, triterpenes, ceramides and flavonoids (14). It has been previously reported that coumarin derivatives cause increase in the level of thyroid hormones which is in agreement to the current results (23). The specific mechanism of coumarins which increase the thyroid hormones is not well clarified.

In addition, the extract of *U. dioica* possesses a significant antioxidant property (14,31). This effect is resulted from the stimulating effect of extract on the antioxidant enzymes like super oxide dismutase and catalase (32-34). Some of the improving effect of UDHAE against PTU induced hypothyroidism could be related to its antioxidant properties.

Evidence demonstrates that estrol compounds increase the activity of thyroid gland. The stroles could increase the activity of 5'-deiodinase which in turn enhances the conversion of T_4 to T_3 (11,24). This effect agrees the obtained current results on thyroid hormones in this study.

Interestingly the flavonoid compounds decreased the thyroid hormones by inhibiting the TPO which is the key enzyme in biosynthesis of thyroid hormones (35,36). It is supposed that the effect of flavonoids is dominant in the high doses of UDHAE which leads to the opposing effects on the thyroid hormone levels.

Based on the researches, steroid compounds cause reduction of proteins which transfer Thyroid Hormones in serums (37). Consequently, because of steroids available in *U. dioica* extract, reduction of T_4, T_3 and FT_3 hormones in higher doses by reduction of proteins which transfer Thyroid Hormones is also justifiable.

Conclusion

The findings suggest that 50 mg/kg dose of UDHAE has stimulatory effect on thyroid gland function and raises plasma T_3, T_4 and FT_3 levels. UDHAE at the dose of 50 or 100 mg/kg could enhance blood level of T_3 and FT_3 perhaps by increase in T_4 to T_3 transformation. Higher doses of UDHAE could not increase the level of these hormones probably due to the presence of inhibitory materials. In sum, UDHAE can affect the thyroid action and the effect of this herb on thyroid function depends on the doses which can be effective in treatment of thyroid disorders.

Acknowledgments

The content of this paper was extracted from the Pharm. D dissertation of Fatemeh Abdolhosseinipoor.

Authors' contributions

AH: Statistical analysis, data interpretation, manuscript preparation. FA: Data collection, design of the study, literature search, funding collection. MS: design of the study, contributed to conducting the study. All read and confirmed the article ready for publication.

Conflict of interests

Authors declare no conflict of interests.

Ethical considerations

Ethical issues (including plagiarism, misconduct, data fabrication, falsification, double publication or submission, redundancy) have been completely observed by the authors.

Funding/Support

This research was financially supported by Isfahan University of Medical Sciences, Isfahan, Iran. (Grant No. 3941049).

References

1. Kar A, Panda S, Bharti S. Relative efficacy of three medicinal plant extracts in the alteration of thyroid hormone concentrations in male mice. J Ethnopharmacol. 2002;81(2):281-5.
2. Ott J, Promberger R, Kober F, Neuhold N, Tea M, Huber JC, et al. Hashimoto's thyroiditis affects symptom load and quality of life unrelated to hypothyroidism: a prospective case-control study in women undergoing thyroidectomy for benign goiter. Thyroid. 2011;21(2):161-7. doi: 10.1089/thy.2010.0191.
3. Ozturk BT, Kerimoglu H, Dikbas O, Pekel H, Gonen MS. Ocular changes in primary hypothyroidism. BMC Res Notes. 2009;2:266. doi: 10.1186/1756-0500-2-266.
4. Koumourou R. Running on Empty: hypothyroidism, introduction to an underactive thyroid gland. Australia: Cocoon Books; 2004.
5. Mistry D, Atkin S, Atkinson H, Gunasekaran S, Sylvester D, Rigby AS, et al. Predicting thyroxine requirements following total thyroidectomy. Clin Endocrinol (Oxf). 2011;74(3):384-7. doi: 10.1111/j.1365-2265.2010.03940.x.
6. Gartner R, Gasnier BC, Dietrich JW, Krebs B, Angstwurm MW. Selenium supplementation in patients with autoimmune thyroiditis decreases thyroid peroxidase antibodies concentrations. J Clin Endocrinol Metab. 2002;87(4):1687-91. doi: 10.1210/jcem.87.4.8421.
7. Costantini A, Pala MI. Thiamine and Hashimoto's thyroiditis: a report of three cases. J Altern Complement Med. 2014;20(3):208-11. doi: 10.1089/acm.2012.0612.
8. Vahabi Anaraki P, Aminorroaya A, Amini M, Momeni F, Feizi A, Iraj B, et al. Effect of vitamin D deficiency treatment on thyroid function and autoimmunity markers in Hashimoto's thyroiditis: A double-blind randomized placebo-controlled clinical trial. J Res Med Sci. 2017;22:103. doi: 10.4103/jrms.JRMS_1048_16.
9. Levothyroxine Side Effects. drugs.com website. 2017 [cited 2018 April 10]. Available from: https://www.drugs.com/sfx/levothyroxine-side-effects.html.
10. Ernst E. The efficacy of herbal medicine--an overview. Fundam Clin Pharmacol. 2005;19(4):405-9. doi: 10.1111/j.1472-8206.2005.00335.x.
11. Panda S, Kar A. Guggulu (*Commiphora mukul*) potentially ameliorates hypothyroidism in female mice. Phytother Res. 2005;19(1):78-80. doi: 10.1002/ptr.1602.
12. Roshangar F, Modaresi M, Toghyani M. Effect of marshmallow's root extract on thyroid hormones in Broilers Res J Appl Sci Eng Technol. 2014;7(1):161-4. doi: 10.19026/rjaset.7.234.
13. Lima STC, Merrigan TL, Rodrigues ED. Thyroid and parathyroid diseases-new insights into some old and some new issues. Croatia: InTech; 2012:221-8.
14. WHO. Radix Urticae. WHO Monographs on Selected Medicinal Plants. Geneva: World Health Organization; 2003:327-41.
15. Moradi HR, Erfani Majd N, Esmaeilzadeh S, Fatemi Tabatabaei SR. The histological and histometrical effects of *Urtica dioica* extract on rat's prostate hyperplasia. Vet Res Forum. 2015;6(1):23-9.
16. Motamedi H, Seyyednejad SM, Bakhtiari A, Vafaei M. Introducing *Urtica dioica*, a native plant of Khuzestan, as an antibacterial medicinal plant. Jundishapur J Nat Pharm Prod. 2014;9(4):e15904.
17. Roman Ramos R, Alarcon-Aguilar F, Lara-Lemus A, Flores-Saenz JL. Hypoglycemic effect of plants used in Mexico as antidiabetics. Arch Med Res. 1992;23(1):59-64.
18. Bnouham M, Merhfour FZ, Ziyyat A, Mekhfi H, Aziz M, Legssyer A. Antihyperglycemic activity of the aqueous extract of *Urtica dioica*. Fitoterapia. 2003;74(7-8):677-81.
19. Obertreis B, Giller K, Teucher T, Behnke B, Schmitz H. [Anti-inflammatory effect of *Urtica dioica* folia extract in comparison to caffeic malic acid]. Arzneimittelforschung. 1996;46(1):52-6.
20. Hughes RE, Ellery P, Harry T, Jenkins V, Jones E. The dietary potential of the common nettle. J Sci Food Agric. 1980;31(12):1279-86.
21. Parvinroo S, Zahediasl S, Sabetkasaei M, Kamalinejad M, Naghibi F. The effects of selected hot and cold temperament herbs based on Iranian traditional medicine on some metabolic parameters in normal rats. Iran J Pharm Res. 2014;13(Suppl):177-84.
22. Parvinroo S, Naghibi F, Zahediasl S, Kamalinejad M, Sabetkasaei M. The effects of seeds with hot and cold temperaments on serum thyroid hormones, corticosterone and urine vanillylmandelic acid concentrations of healthy rats. J Ethnopharmacol. 2014;156:216-21. doi: 10.1016/j.jep.2014.08.026.
23. Qin LP, Zhang HM, Zhang WD. [Effect of osthol and total coumarins of *Fructus cnidii* on thyroid hormone and thyrotropic hormone in kidney-yang deficiency rats]. Zhongguo Zhong Xi Yi Jie He Za Zhi. 1996;16(9):552-3.
24. Awaisheh SS, Khalifeh MS, Al-Ruwaili MA, Khalil OM, Al-Ameri OH, Al-Groom R. Effect of supplementation of probiotics and phytosterols alone or in combination on serum and hepatic lipid profiles and thyroid hormones of hypercholesterolemic rats. J Dairy Sci. 2013;96(1):9-15. doi: 10.3168/jds.2012-5442.
25. Shamsian AA, Ghazvini K, Sokhtanloo M, Moghaddam MS, Vakili R. Which quantitative method in determination of the thyroid hormone levels is more consistent with the clinical symptoms of the thyroid disorders? Comp Clin Path. 2016;25(1):101-6. doi: 10.1007/s00580-015-2148-2.
26. Mirazi N, Abdolmaleki N, Mahmoodi M. Study of salvia officinalis hydroethanolic extract on serum thyroid hormone levels in hypothyroid male rat. Avicenna J Clin Med. 2013;19(4):27-35.
27. Tousson E, Ali EM, Ibrahim W, Mansour MA. Proliferating cell nuclear antigen as a molecular biomarker for spermatogenesis in PTU-induced hypothyroidism of rats. Reprod Sci. 2011;18(7):679-86. doi: 10.1177/1933719110395401.
28. Bertram GK. Thyroid and antithyroid drugs. In: Shafiei A, ed. Basic and Clinical Pharmacology. Thehran: Andishe Rafih; 2012:883.
29. Kavalali G, Tuncel H, Goksel S, Hatemi HH. Hypoglycemic

activity of *Urtica pilulifera* in streptozotocin-diabetic rats. J Ethnopharmacol. 2003;84(2-3):241-5.

30. Ahangarpour A, Mohammadian M, Dianat M. Antidiabetic effect of hydroalcholic urticadioica leaf extract in male rats with fructose-induced insulin resistance. Iran J Med Sci. 2012;37(3):181-6.
31. Zengin H, Baysal AH. Antibacterial and antioxidant activity of essential oil terpenes against pathogenic and spoilage-forming bacteria and cell structure-activity relationships evaluated by SEM microscopy. Molecules. 2014;19(11):17773-98. doi: 10.3390/molecules191117773.
32. Houshmand F, Faghihi M, Zahediasl S. The role of oxytocin on cardiac ischemia-reperfusion-induced oxidative stress in rats. Iran J Endocrinol Metab. 2011;12(6):633-40.
33. Tahiliani P, Kar A. Role of Moringa oleifera leaf extract in the regulation of thyroid hormone status in adult male and female rats. Pharmacol Res. 2000;41(3):319-23. doi: 10.1006/phrs.1999.0587.
34. Tahiliani P, Kar A. Achyranthes aspera elevates thyroid hormone levels and decreases hepatic lipid peroxidation in male rats. J Ethnopharmacol. 2000;71(3):527-32.
35. Ferreira AC, Neto JC, da Silva AC, Kuster RM, Carvalho DP. Inhibition of thyroid peroxidase by *Myrcia uniflora* flavonoids. Chem Res Toxicol. 2006;19(3):351-5. doi: 10.1021/tx0501684.
36. Ferreira AC, Lisboa PC, Oliveira KJ, Lima LP, Barros IA, Carvalho DP. Inhibition of thyroid type 1 deiodinase activity by flavonoids. Food Chem Toxicol. 2002;40(7):913-7.
37. Cooper DS, Klibanski A, Ridgway EC. Dopaminergic modulation of TSH and its subunits: in vivo and in vitro studies. Clin Endocrinol (Oxf). 1983;18(3):265-75.

Effect of *Kelussia odoratissima* Mozaff essential oil on promastigot form of *Leishmania major* (*in vitro*)

Khodadad Pirali Kheirabadi[1*], Siavash Saei Dehkordi[2], Parviz Kheibari[3]

[1]Department of pathobiology, Faculty of Veterinary Medicine, Shahrekord University, Shahrekord, Iran
[2]Department of Food Hygiene and Quality Control, Faculty of Veterinary Medicine, Shahrekord University, Shahrekord, Iran
[3]Faculty of Veterinary Medicine, Shahrekord University, Shahrekord, Iran

ARTICLE INFO

Keywords:
Essential oil
In vitro
Kelussia odoratissima
Leishmaniasis
Promastigot form

ABSTRACT

Introduction: Leishmaniasis is a zoonotic disease caused by a protozoan of the genus *Leishmania*. In this study, the effects of *Kelussia odoratissima* Mozaff essential oil on the promastigot form of *Leishmania* major were studied.

Methods: In this study, the effects of *Kelussia odoratissima* Mozaff essential oil on the promastigot form of *Leishmania major* were assessed by calculating the average number of surviving promastigots after exposure to different concentrations of essential oil, relative to the control Glucantime, at different time intervals. To achieve this, various essential oil concentrations (7.5 µl, 15 µl, 25 µl, 35.25 µl, 50 µl) were added to parasites. Different groups in this study were kept in a 26°C incubator under identical conditions. 24, 48 and 72 hours after incubation, living promastigots were counted.

Results: The effect of the essential oil of *Kelussia odoratissima* Mozaff differed from the negative and positive controls and depended on the concentration: higher concentrations (35.25 µl, 50 µl) had a stronger effect on promastigots, causing total mortality.

Conclusion: This study showed that *Kelussia odoratissima* Mozaff essential oil had effects on promastigot form of *Leishmania major.* So it might be possible to use the essential oil of *Kelussia odoratissima* instead of chemical drugs.

Implication for health policy/practice/research/medical education:
It is possible to use the essential oil of *Kelussia odoratissima* instead of chemical drugs. The use of any concentration of essential oil of *Kelussia odoratissima* controlled *L. major* more effectively by increasing in essential oil concentration. Future research would assess the effect of this essential oil on the amastigote form of *L. major.*

Introduction

Medicinal herbs contain physiologically active principles that have been exploited in traditional medicine for the treatment of various ailments due to their anti-microbial properties (1,2). The antifungal and antibacterial activity exhibited by extracts and essential oils of medicinal plants is well proved (3).

Kelussia odoratissima Mozaff. (wild celery; Apiaceae) is a sweet-smelling, glabrous, perennial aromatic herb, which is traditionally consumed in Iran and grows to a height of 120 to 200 cm. The flowers are 1-2 mm in diameter and all are hermaphroditic. *K. odoratissima* is an Iranian endemic plant native to Zagros (central region of Iran) (4).

***Corresponding author**: Khodadad Pirali Kheirabadi, Department of Pathobiology, Faculty of Veterinary Medicine, University of Shahrekord, Shahrekord, Iran. Email: khpirali@yahoo.com

Kelussia grows in April and its aerial parts are harvested (5,6). Flavonoids have anti-inflammatory (7), anti-allergy (8), anti-diabetes, antihyperlipidemic and anti-hypercholesterolemic effects (9,10) and improves spatial memory (11). Phthalides constitute 70% of the *Kelussia* essence with several effects: liver protection, prostaglandin F2α inhibition, prevention of cancer tumors, treatment of epilepsy and liver disorders and reduction in blood viscosity (5,12,13). Despite this, there are no study related to the antileishmanial effect of the essential oil of *K. odoratissima*, this being the focus of our study.

Leishmaniasis affects more than 12 million people in 88 countries (14). Cutaneous leishmaniasis (CL), with 1 to 1.5 million annual cases, is the most common form of this disease (15). There is no vaccine available against any form of leishmaniasis and chemotherapy is the only currently available treatment (16,17). The standard treatment for

CL is antimoniate, which requires long-term injections, and resistance is emerging, which cause high dose usage, resulting side effects (17,18).
The search for new, safe and inexpensive drugs to treat and control CL, especially anthroponotic CL, is needed. Conventional healers are usually cheap and sometimes more effective than chemical drugs (19).
In this study, the effect of the essential oil of *K. odoratissima* on promastigot form of *Leishmania major* was studied. The results obtained from this study help us to find the alternative natural drug instead of chemical ones.

Materials and Methods

Plant material
A wild-growing plant from Kogiluye and Buyer Ahmad province located in the southwest of Iran, was collected in April and May, 2012. The samples, which were identified and confirmed as *K. odoratissima* Mozaff, were deposited in the Herbarium of the Research Institute of Jahade Keshavarzi of Shahrekord, Iran.

Isolation of the volatile oil
20 kg from aerial parts of the plant was dried in an oven equipped with warm air circulation. One hundred grams of the air-dried material was ground and powdered. The powder was subjected to hydro-distillation for 3 hours using a Clevenger-type system. Finally, 30 ml essential oil extracted. The oil was kept at 2°C to 4°C in a sealed brown vial.

Chemical analysis of the oil
Analysis of the essential oil was performed on a Hewlett-Packard Model 6890 GC-MS using a HP-5MS capillary column (30 m×0.25 mm i.d., 0.25 m film thickness). The injector temperature and detector temperature was 250°C. Helium was used as the carrier gas at a flow rate of 1.00 ml/min. The column temperature was programmed from 40°C to 280°C at a rate of 4°C/min. The EI mode was at 70 eV, while the mass spectra were recorded from 30 to 450 m/z. Confirmation of identity was carried out by comparing their retention indices with the Wiley 275 library data of the GC–MS system and with the mass spectra literature data (20).

Preparing the promastigot form of Leishmania major
The promastigot form of *Leishmania major* strain MRHO/IR/ER/75 was prepared from department of Parasitology Research, University of Medical Sciences of Isfahan, Iran. The promastigots were transferred to RPMI 1640 medium and incubated at 26°C for 72 hours.

Preparing the different concentrations and control groups
After the promastigots increased in the medium, they were counted using a Neobar chamber (0.100 mm, Tiefe, Depth, Profondeur, Neubauer Improved, Precicolor, HBG, Germany) in which 10 µl of this medium was mixed with 10 µl of formalin, which was used to kill the promastigots. 150 µl of medium contained 10^6 promastigots. Next, different concentrations of *K. odoratissima* essential oil (15, 30, 50, 75 and 100 mg/ml) were prepared, to achieve this, various essential oil concentrations (7.5 µl, 15 µl, 25 µl, 35.25 µl, 50 µl) were added to parasites. There was a negative control (no essential oil) and a positive control (Glucantime®, Specia, Paris, France) by mixing with sterile RPMI 1640 medium in different tubes. 10^6 promastigots (i.e., 150 µl of medium containing promastigots) were added to each tubes, as presented in Table 1. The total volume of all tubes was 500 µl after mixing.

Counting the number of living promastigots after the mixing
After mixing the promastigots with different concentrations of *K. odoratissima* essential oil, those tubes, as well as the negative and positive controls, were incubated in dark incubator and in 26°C for 72 hours. The number of living promastigots was counted at 24, 48 and 72 hours after incubation.

Statistical analysis
The data were analyzed by one-way analysis of variance (ANOVA) and significant differences ($P<0.05$) between means were assessed by Tukey's test using SPSS software version 19.0.

Results

Composition of essential oil
In the essential oil of *K. odoratissima*, the sesquiterpene hydrocarbons were the most abundant compounds (57.77%). In addition, the least quantitative percentage (2.7%) was belonged to monoterpene hydrocarbons. The major components were *Z*-ligustilide (34.5%), *E*-ligustilide (11.79%), 3-*Z*-butylidenephthalide (8.81%) and Dec-9-en-1-ol (5.86%).

24 and 48 hours after incubation
Effects of essential oil of *Kelussia odoratissima* Mozaff on promastigot form of *Lishmania major* differenced from

Table 1. Volume of materials in each tube prepared for different concentrations of essential oil

Tubes Materials	15 mg/ml	30 mg/ml	50 mg/ml	75 mg/ml	100 mg/ml	Negative control	Positive control (Glucantime)
Promastigots	150 µl	150 µl	150 µl	150 µl	150 µl	150 µl	150 µl
RPMI 1640	342.5 µl	335 µl	325 µl	314.75 µl	300 µl	350 µl	181 µl
Glucantime	-	-	-	-	-	-	169 µl
Essential oil	7.5 µl	15 µl	25 µl	35.25 µl	50 µl	-	-
Total volume	500 µl	500 µl	500 µl	500 µl	500 µl	500 µl	500 µl

Table 2. Mean number of living promastigots ± SEM 24, 48 and 72 hours after incubation

Tube	Mean number of living promastigots ± SEM						
	15 mg/ml	30 mg/ml	50 mg/ml	75 mg/ml	100 mg/ml	Negative Control	Positive Control
24 h	127.25±3.12 a	119.11±4.54 a	116.63±3.96 a	111.76±4.32 a	103.51±3.81 a	125.3±1.96 b	79.47±0.44 c
48 h	124.12±2.68 a	117.63±2.96 a	110.17±4.23 a	104.00±3.69 a	98.99±1.99 a	148.25±2.25 b	74.23±0.97 c
72 h	119.08±1.75 a	102.45±1.85 a	93.27±2.17 a	87.00±4.44 a	73.93±3.12 d	211.63±2.19 b	67.56±0.82 c
Mean of 3 Times	123.48±2.51 a	113.06±3.11 b	106.69±3.45 c	100.92±4.15 d	92.14±2.97 e	161.72±2.13 f	73.75±0.74 g

Different letters within each row (i.e., within each time interval) indicate significant differences (P<0.05) between mean of living promastigots number in each tube according to Tukey's test.

negative control and positive controls. However, there were no significant differences between groups with different concentrations of essential oil (Table 2).

72 hours after incubation

In this time decreasing in living promastigots in different tubes were more than past times. Same as past times, effect of essential oil of *Kelussia odoratissima* Mozaff on promastigot form of *Lishmania major* was differenced from negative control and positive control (Table 2).

Totally the *K. odoratissima* essential oil had a different effect on the promastigot form of *L. major* relative to the negative and positive control, but this depended on the essential oil concentration; higher concentrations (35.25 µl, 50 µl) had a stronger effect on promastigots, causing total mortality (Table 2). In all three-time intervals, the use of any concentration of essential oil of *Kelussia odoratissima* controlled *L. major* more effectively by increasing in essential oil concentration (Table 2).

Discussion

The application of natural plant products for control of bacterial, fungal and parasitic bee and brood diseases has several advantages over conventional means. In the specialized literature resistance of bacteria to essential oils has not yet been documented. In addition, natural substances in bee products decompose rapidly, their quantity in honey is low and they do not have an adverse effect on the health of consumers (21). Although in small amounts, essential oils and organic acids are normally contained in various types of honey. According to some authors their use as alternative means for prevention and control of bee diseases guarantees ecologically clean bee products (22).

This study showed antileishmanial effects of *Kelussia odoratissima* Mozaff essential oil on promastigot form of *Leishmania major.* The current treatment regimens for leishmaniasis, which are based on chemotherapy, are limited and are not ideal because they are often associated with severe side effects (23). In a case report from France, successful treatment of a 10-year-old boy with cutaneous leishmaniasis (*L. major*) was reported with oral azithromycin (24).

Pentavalent antimonials remain the drug of choice for the treatment of cutaneous and mucocutaneous leishmaniasis. Despite its availability in health facilities, its high toxicity and its parenteral use are limiting factors for the proper treatment of cases of CL. It should be noted that most of these cases occur in areas of difficult access, in rural areas, which complicates the parenteral application of the drug and monitoring of its side effects. Treatment of CL with the drugs currently available represents an obstacle to proper clinical handling of the cases of leishmaniasis, and efforts should be made in order to add the promising drugs to clinical trials and investigate the use of new alternative drugs (25)

Traditional alternatives to antimonials used in unresponsive cases are amphotericin B, which cause serious, toxic side-effects (26,27), and the emergence of drug-resistant parasites is a major problem (17). These limitations and factors emphasize the urgent need for new, inexpensive, safe and easy-to-administer substances for the treatment of this infectious disease, possibly through the form of traditional medicines which represent the accumulation of practices based on theories, beliefs and experiences of different cultures over a wide period of time (28).

Amphotericin B is the second drug of choice when antimonials fail or cannot be used. However, they are toxic and expensive drugs, which often require hospitalization for their administration (29). An alternative to the treatment with conventional amphotericin B is the use of liposomal amphotericin B, which has higher peak plasma levels and lower toxicity (30).

Traditional medicines are used for the maintenance of health and in the prevention, diagnosis, improvement and treatment of illnesses (31). Based on traditional medicine, new drugs of herbal origins discovered through ethnopharmacological studies have shown promising results.

Conclusion

By considering an increase in drug resistance against leishmania, it is possible to use the essential oil of *Kelussia odoratissima* instead of chemical drugs. The use of any concentration of essential oil of *Kelussia odoratissima* controlled *L. major* more effectively by increasing in essential oil concentration. Future research would assess the effect of this essential oil on the amastigote form of *L. major*.

Acknowledgments

Work in the laboratory was supported by University of Shahrekord. I would like to thank all of persons who help us to do this research.

Authors' contributions
All the authors wrote the manuscript equally.

Conflict of interests
The authors declared no competing interests.

Ethical considerations
Ethical issues (including plagiarism, misconduct, data fabrication, falsification, double publication or submission, redundancy) have been completely observed by the authors.

Funding/Support
This research was financially supported by Shahrekord University, Shahrekord, Iran.

References

1. Kelmanson JE, Jager AK, Van Staden J. Zulu medicinal plants with antibacterial activity. J Ethnopharmacol 2000; 69: 2416.
2. Srinivasan D, Sangeetha N, Suresh T, Perumalsamy PL. Antimicrobial activity of certain Indian medicinal plants used in folkloric medicine. J Ethnopharmacol 2001; 74: 217-20.
3. Fazeli MR, Amin GH, Ahmadian AM, Ashtiani H, Jamalifar H, Samadi N. Antimicrobial activities of Iranian sumac and avishan-e-shirazi (Zataria multiflora) against some food-borne bacteria. Food Control 2007; 18: 646-9.
4. Ahmadi F, Kadivar M, Shahedi M. Antioxidant activity of Kelussia odoratissima Mozaff. in model and food systems. Food Chem 2007; 105: 57-64.
5. Tehrani Z. Phytochemical chemical study on Kelussia odoratissima Mozaffarian: Pharmacy thesis. School of Pharmacy, Isfahan University of Medical Sciences. 1999; 42-48.
6. Gandomkar M. Phytochemistry of the essential oil of wild celery plant: Pharmacy thesis. School of Pharmacy, Isfahan University of Medical Sciences. 1999; 37-41.
7. Asgari S, Naderi GA, Garipour M, Dashti G, Sadjadian RA. Effect of Amirkabiria odoratissima on the development and progression of atherosclerosis in hypercholesterolemic rabbits. Iranian Journal of Diabetes and Lipid Disorders 2003; 3(1): 88-3.
8. Hashemi V, Ghannadi A, Soltani RL. Analgesic and anti-inflammatory effects of Amirkabiria odoratissima. Journal of Research in Medical Sciences 2003; 7(4): 121-5.
9. Asgari S, Naderi GA, Jafariyan A, Askari N, Behagh AR. Fibrinolytic activity of Amirkabiria odoratissima Mozaffarian. Journal of Medicinal Plants 2005; 4(13): 19-25.
10. Roghani M, Baluchnejadmojarad T, Ramazani M. The effect of chronic oral feeding of Apium graveolens on learning and memory in diabetic rats. Journal of Medicinal Plants 2008; 7(27): 98-105.
11. Cao YX, Zhang W, He JY, He LC, Xu CB. Ligustilide induces vasodilatation via inhibiting voltage dependent calcium channel and receptor- mediated Ca2+ influx and release. Vascul Pharmacol 2006; 45: 171-6.
12. Craker LE. Herbs species and medicinal plants. Encanto. Oxyx Press 1984; 2: 15-6.
13. Beck J. Investigation of the bioactive constituents of several herbal medicines [Doctoral dissertation]. Colorado State University; 1996.
14. WHO. Leishmaniasis. The global trend. [Accessed 30 January 2009]. http:// www.who.into /neglected_ disease/ integrated-media_ Leishmaniasis/ en/ index. html
15. Desjeux P. Leishmaniasis: Current situation and new perspectives. Comp. Immunol Microbiol Infect Dis 2004; 27: 305-18.
16. Noazin S, Khamesipour A, Moulton LH, Tanner M, Nasseri K, Modabber F. Efficacy of killed whole-parasite vaccines in the prevention of leishmaniasis-A meta-analysis. Vaccine 2009; 27: 474-5.
17. Croft SL, Sundar S, Fairlamb AH. Drug resistance in leishmaniasis. Clin Microbiol Rev 2006; 19: 111-26.
18. Hadighi R, Boucher P, Khamesipour A, Meamar AR, Roy G, Ouellette M, *et al.* Glucantime- resistant Leishmania tropica isolated from Iranian patients with cutaneous leishmaniasis are sensitive to alternative antileishmania drugs. Parasitol Res 2007; 101: 1319-22.
19. Sandhu DS, Heinrich M. The use of health foods, spices and other botanicals in the Sikh community in London. Phytother Res 2005; 19: 633-42.
20. Adams RP. Identification of Essential Oil Components by Gas Chromatography/Quadruple Mass Spectroscopy. 3rd ed. Carol Stream, IL: Allured Publishing Corporation; 2001. p. 456,.
21. Nozal MJ, Bernal JL, Jiménez JJ, González MJ, Higes M. Extraction of thymol, eucalyptol, menthol, and camphor residues from honey and beeswax. Determination by gas chromatography with flame ionization detection. Journal of Chromatography A 2002; 19: 207-15.
22. Zhelyazkova I, Gurgulova K, Malinova K, Ali AS. Investigation on the sti-mulating effect of plant preparations "Green TM" and "Ecophyl-P" upon bee families development. In: Proceedings of the International Scientific Conference. 2009; Union of Scientists Stara Zagora.
23. Tasdemir D, Kaiser M, Brun R, Yardley V, Schmidt TJ, Tosun F, Rüedi P. Antitrypanosomal and antileishmanial activities of flavonoids and their analogues: in vitro, in vivo, structure-activity relationship, and quantitative structure-activity relationship studies. Antimicrob. Agents Chemother 2006; 50(4): 1352-64.

24. Minodier P, Zambelli L, Mary C, Faraut F, Garnier JM, Berbis P. Cutaneous leishmaniasis treated with azithromycin in a child. Pediatr Infect Dis J 2008; 27 (1): 80-1.
25. Basano AS, Camargo LM. [American cutaneous leishmaniasis: history, epidemiology and prospects for control]. Rev Bras Epidemiol 2004; 7: 328-37.
26. Sereno D, Holzmuller P, Lemesre JL. Efficacy of second line drugs on antimonyl-resistant amastigotes of Leishmania infantum. Acta Trop 2000; 74: 25-31.
27. Croft SL, Seifert K, Yardley V. Current scenario of drug development for leishmaniasis. Ind J Med Res 2006; 123: 399-410.
28. Fennel CW, Makunga NP, Van Staden J. Medicinal plants and biotechnology: An integrated approach to healthcare. In: Teixeira da Silva JA, (Ed.). Floriculture, Ornamental and Plant Biotechnology: Advances and Topical Issues. 1st ed. Isleworth, UK: Global Science Books, Ltd.; 2006. p. 41-53.
29. Machado-Pinto J, Pinto J, da Costa CA, Genaro O, Marques MJ, Mobabber F. Immunochemotherapy for cutaneous leishmaniasis: a controlled trial using killed Leishmania (Leishmania) amazonensis vaccine plus antimonial. Int J Dermatol 2002; 41: 73-8.
30. Berman JD. Human leishmaniasis: clinical, diagnostic, and chemotherapeutic developments in the last 10 years. Clin Infect Dis 1997; 24: 684-703.
31. Firenzuoli F, Gori L. Herbal Medicine Today. Clinical and Research 2007; 4(S1): 37-40.

Cytotoxic effect of *Cousinia verbascifolia* Bunge against OVCAR-3 and HT-29 cancer cells

Seyed Ebrahim Sajjadi[1], Mustafa Ghanadian[2,1*], Mehrangiz Haghighi[1], Leili Mouhebat[3]

[1]Department of Pharmacognosy, School of Pharmacy and Pharmaceutical Sciences, Isfahan University of Medical Sciences, Isfahan, Iran
[2]Isfahan Pharmaceutical Sciences Research Center, Isfahan University of Medical Sciences, Isfahan, Iran
[3]Department of Microbiology, School of Medicine, Isfahan University of Medical Sciences, Isfahan, Iran

ARTICLE INFO

Keywords:
Asteraceae
Cousinia verbascifolia
Cytotoxicity
OVCAR-3
HT-29

ABSTRACT

Introduction: Little information is available about phytochemical and biological properties of *Cousinia* genus. In a primary study, seven *Cousinia* species including *C. verbascifolia* showed cytotoxic activity ranged between 18.4 ± 0.59 to 87.9 ± 0.58 µg/mL. To the best of our knowledge, no other biological studies have been conducted on this plant. Therefore, in this study the cytotoxic effect of *Cousinia verbascifolia* Bunge against OVCAR-3 and HT-29 cancer cells was evaluated.
Methods: Filtration and *in vacuo* concentration of methanol extract resulted in a green gum which was subjected on reverse column chromatography. Semi polar fraction (41.3 g) eluted with water: methanol (20:80), was then subjected on a silica gel column chromatography using hexane/acetone and resulted in 11 fractions. Finally, cytotoxic activities against ovarian and colon cancer cells were determined at a wavelength of 570 nm by Matrix metalloproteinase protein (MTT) standard method.
Results: None of the fractions showed highly cytotoxic activity. Based on NCI, fractions Fr. 1, Fr. 2, Fr. 4, Fr. 5, Fr. 6, Fr. 8 and Fr. 10 showed moderately cytotoxicity with IC_{50} values ranged between 119 to 190 µg/mL against OVCAR-3 cells. Fractions Fr. 1, Fr. 2, Fr. 6, Fr. 7 and Fr. 8 showed moderately cytotoxic activity ranged between 118 to 194 µg/mL against HT-29 cells. Fr. 10 and Fr. 11 showed no cytotoxic activity.
Conclusion: Due to the inhibitory properties of extract and its fractions on cancer cells, identification of responsible compounds possessing cytotoxic effects for generating possible new approach in medicinal chemistry are recommended.

Implication for health policy/practice/research/medical education:
In the present study, we evaluated the cytotoxicity properties of *Cousinia verbascifolia* fractions on cancer cells of ovarian and colon cancer cells. Moderated toxicity of fractions indicated that this plant has the value of more phytochemical consideration to found anti-cancer lead compounds and generating new achievements in medicinal chemistry.

Introduction

Cancer, a term applied to a group of different diseases can be generally described as an uncontrolled multiplication of cells at any part of the body. These abnormal cells can create expansive masses, spread to vital organs and eventually cause patient death (1). Cytotoxic compounds are the majority of drugs currently used for cancer chemotherapy. The first step of developing new antitumor compounds is testing a wide range of compounds both natural and synthetic with the aim of discovering molecules of useful properties. Plant kingdom provides a rich and wonderful source of biologically active compounds. There are about 250 000-500 000 plant species on earth, out of which only about 20% have been submitted to biological and phytochemical screening. Besides, plant species investigated for anticancer potentials are also a very small fraction (2,3). So, a huge number of plant species still remain to be studied and described in terms of biological and phytochemical profiles.

Cousinia, one of the largest genera of Asteraceae, with 600-

***Corresponding author**: Mustafa Ghanadian, Department of Pharmacognosy, School of Pharmacy, Isfahan University of Medical Sciences, Isfahan, Iran. Email: ghannadian@gmail.com

700 species, is one of the most diverse genera in central and south west Asia. About 250 species of the genus are distributed throughout Iran, comprising About 200 endemic species (4-7). *Cousinia verbascifolia* Bunge, is a monocarpic biennial plant, up to 45 cm high, stems simple or branched from the base, leaves lyrate with spiny-dentate margin, flowers 50-150; corolla pink, rose or purple, 20-35 mm long. The flowering period of the plant is May to July. This plant is endemic to Kopetdagh (NE Iran and S Turkmenistan), open areas, scrublands and stony slopes (6). Little information is available about its phytochemical and biological properties. Phytochemical studies on some *Cousinia* species provide some information about their chemical constituents including: acetylenes, triterpenes, steroids, sesquiterpene lactones, and flavonoids (8-17). In a previous study, the cytotoxic activity against Fibrosarcoma WEHI 164 cancer cells, as well as antibacterial and Matrix metalloproteinase protein (MMP) inhibitory effects of a total ethanol extract of seven *Cousinia* species including *C. verbascifolia* were tested (18). In this study total extract of these plants showed cytotoxic activity with IC_{50} values ranged between 18.4 ± 0.59 to 87.9 ± 0.58 µg/mL.
To the best of our knowledge, no other biological studies have been conducted on this plant. Therefore, in this study the cytotoxic effect of *Cousinia verbascifolia* Bunge against OVCAR-3 and HT-29 cancer cells was evaluated.

Materials and methods

Plant material

Flowering aerial parts of *C. verbascifolia* from Asteracea family were collected from Salehabad, Torbate-Jam, Khorassan-Razavi province, Iran in May 2013 and authenticated by Dr. Iraj Mehregan. A voucher specimen (No. 2838) was deposited at the Herbarium unit of the Pharmacognosy Department, School of Pharmacy, Isfahan University of Medical Sciences, Isfahan, I.R. Iran.

Extraction and fractionation

Aerial parts of plant material (3.5 kg) were air-dried in the shade and reduced to fine particles using an electric mill. The powdered plant was extracted exhaustively via percolation using methanol as solvent at a flow rate of 4 ml/min for 10 days. The extract was concentrated under reduced pressure by a rotary evaporator at a temperature not exceeding 50°C. The concentrated extract (450 g) was mixed with appropriate amount of Celite, left to dry, sieved to obtain fine homo sized particles. It was subjected to Medium Pressure Liquid Chromatography (MPLC) on C-18 column and water: methanol (0→100) as mobile phase. Aqueous fraction eluted with water: methanol (70:30) containing polar contents and fraction eluted by methanol (100%) containing fats and chlorophyll were excluded from the study. Semi-polar fraction (41.3 g) eluted with water: methanol (20:80), was subjected on a silica gel column chromatography (400 g silica gel, 7×30 cm) using hexane/acetone (97:3) as mobile phase with increasing acetone to 100%.

MTT viability assay

Human ovarian carcinoma cancer cell line OVCAR-3, and colon carcinoma cancer cell line HT-29 were obtained from Pasteur Institute of Iran. The cell lines were grown in RPMI-1640 media supplemented with 10% fetal calf serum, 100 U/ml + 100 µg/ml penicillin and streptomycin at 37°C in 5% CO_2 condition. Cell viability was determined by colorimetric assay, using 3-(4,5-dimethylthiazol-2-yl)-2,5-diphenyl tetrazolium bromide (MTT) and compared with untreated controls. Cells were seeded at 5×10^3 cells/well in 96-well plates. After incubation, compounds at concentrations of 5, 50, and 500 µg/ml were added and incubated again for 48 h. Then, MTT (5 mg/ml in PBS) was added to each well and the cells were incubated for 4 hours. The supernatants were aspirated and 200 µl of dimethyl sulfoxide was added to each well. The plates were shaken for 10 minutes and using colorimetric method, the absorbance was read by the microplate reader (Bio-Rad, Hercules, CA, USA) at 570 nm (19).

$$\text{Cell viability} = \frac{\text{Average absorbances of triplicate treated cells}}{\text{Average absorbances of control cells}} \times 100$$

The criteria used to categorize the cytotoxicity of *C. verbascifolia* fractions against OVCAR-3 and HT-29, based on U.S. National Cancer Institute (NCI) and Geran protocol was as follows: $IC_{50} \leq 20$ µg/ml = highly cytotoxic, IC_{50} ranged between 21 and 200 µg/ml = moderately cytotoxic, IC_{50} ranged between 201 and 500 µg/ml = weakly cytotoxic and $IC_{50} > 501$ µg/ml = no cytotoxicity (20-23).

Statistical analysis

All samples were presented as mean ± SD for three measurements. Unpaired Student's t test was used to calculate $P<0.05$ for each compound against the control (+ve). The dose-response curves were plotted to enable the calculation of IC_{50} for each sample.

Results

Semi-polar fraction obtained from MPLC was subjected to silica-gel column chromatography (CC) and eluted with n-hexane: acetone with increasing polarity. Isolated fractions were organized by TLC profile into 11 combined fractions (Fr. 1-Fr. 11). The fractions were concentrated by a rotary evaporator at 40°C and stored in refrigerator at -20°C before running biological assays (Table 1).
To investigate the cytotoxic effects of different factions of the *C. verbascifolia*, on the cell viability, OVCAR-3 and HT-29 cell lines were incubated with the concentrations of 5, 50, and 500 µg/mL of fractions 1-11. None of the fractions showed significant cytotoxic effect ($P<0.05$) at concentrations of 5, and 50 µg/ml against OVCAR-3 cell line. Fr. 1-Fr. 10 showed significant cytotoxic effect at concentration of 500 µg/ml against OVCAR-3 cell lines ($P<0.05$). Fractions 1-11 inhibited growth of HT-29 cells in a concentration-dependent manner. Fr. 1, Fr. 2 and Fr. 4-Fr. 11 showed significant cytotoxic effect at concentration of 50 and 500 µg/ml against HT-29 cell

Table 1. Solvent system employed for column chromatography

Combined Fraction	n-hexane: acetone
Fr. 1	93:7
Fr. 2	88:12
Fr. 3	80:20
Fr. 4	80:20
Fr. 5	70:30
Fr. 6	50:50
Fr. 7	50:50
Fr. 8	50:50
Fr. 9	0:100
Fr. 10	0:100
Fr. 11	Methanol (100%)

lines (P<0.05). Cytotoxicity activities of Fr. 1-11 against cancer cell lines: OVCAR-3 and HT-29 cells are displayed in Figure 1.

A fitted dose-response curve was plotted to enable the calculation of the concentrations that could kill 50% of the cells (IC_{50}). The IC_{50} was calculated for all of the fractions with cytotoxic activities (Table 2). The cytotoxicity data based on IC_{50} values are displayed in Table 2.

A fitted dose-response curve were plotted to enable the calculation of the concentrations that kill 50% of the cells (IC_{50}). The criteria used were as follows: IC_{50}<20 µg/ml (high cytotoxic activity), IC_{50}: 20-100 µg/ml (moderate cytotoxic activity), IC_{50}: 201-500 µg/ml (weak cytotoxic activity), IC_{50}>500 µg/ml (no cytotoxic activity).

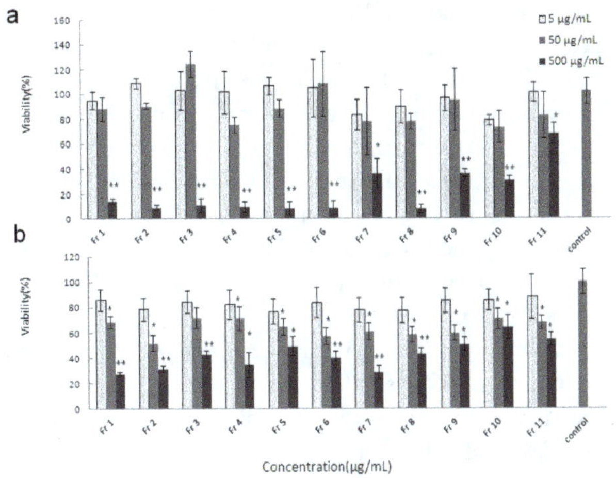

Figure 1. Cytotoxic effect of different fractions: F1-F11 of *C. verbascifolia* against ovarian OVCAR-3 (a) and colon HT-29 (b) cancer cell lines. Cells were treated with different concentrations of fractions 1-11 for 48 hours, and Cytotoxicity was assessed by MTT assay. Results (mean ± SD) were calculated as percent of corresponding control values. *P<0.05, **P<0.001 are significant. Statistical analysis was performed by unpaired Student's t test.

Discussion

Fr. 1-Fr. 10 inhibited growth of OVCAR-3 and HT-29 cells in a concentration-dependent manner. None of the fractions showed high cytotoxic activity. Fractions Fr. 1, Fr. 2, Fr. 4, Fr. 5, Fr. 6, Fr. 8 and Fr. 10 showed moderate cytotoxic activity against OVCAR-3 cells according to a criteria based on NCI and Geran protocols (22,23). Fractions Fr. 1, Fr. 2, Fr. 6, Fr. 7 and Fr. 8 showed moderate cytotoxic activity against HT-29 cells. The highest cytotoxic activities were observed for Fr. 4, and Fr. 8, with IC_{50} values of 120-121 µg/mL against OVCAR-3 and for Fr. 2 with IC_{50} values of 73.4 µg/mL against HT-29 colon cancer cells. The lowest cytotoxic effects were observed for Fr.10 against HT-29 and Fr. 11 against both cell lines with IC_{50} values more than 500 µg/mL.

Despite the large body of work on taxonomy, systematics, and phylogeny studies of *Cousinia* species, their biological and phytochemical studies are very limited. Based on previous studies, some species of *Cousinia* including *C. verbascifolia* as reported by Shahverdi *et al.*, have shown cytotoxic, MMP inhibitory and antbacterial activities (18). In this study ethanol extract of *C. verbascifolia* exhibited high cytotoxic effect against fibrosarcoma cell line (WEHI

Table 2. IC_{50} Values of *C. verbascifolia* fractions against ovarian (OVCAR-3) and colon (HT-29) cancer cell lines

	OVCAR-3		HT-29	
Fraction	IC_{50} ± SD (µg/mL)	Cytotoxic activity	IC_{50} ± SD (µg/mL)	Cytotoxic activity
Fr. 1	162.73±11.9	Moderate	125.4±8.3	Moderate
Fr. 2	138.68±0.84	Moderate	73.4±8.4	Moderate
Fr. 3	221.3±0.35	Weak	370.2±24.8	Weak
Fr. 4	119.92±12.15	Moderate	214.8.5±20.8	Weak
Fr. 5	149.26±10.61	Moderate	481.6±45.3	Weak
Fr. 6	190.09±63.64	Moderate	162.5±18.2	Moderate
Fr. 7	232.08±15.87	Weak	118±11.2	Moderate
Fr. 8	121.46±18.38	Moderate	194.6±15.2	Moderate
Fr. 9	289.52±28.78	Weak	392.3±38.9	Weak
Fr. 10	171±16.06	Moderate	>500	No
Fr. 11	>500	No	>500	No

A fitted dose-response curve were plotted to enable the calculation of the concentrations that kill 50% of the cells (IC_{50}). The criteria used were as follows: IC_{50}<20 µg/ml (high cytotoxic activity), IC_{50}: 20-100 µg/ml (moderate cytotoxic activity), IC_{50}: 201-500 µg/ml (weak cytotoxic activity), IC_{50}>500 µg/ml (no cytotoxic activity).

164) with IC_{50} value of 18.4 ± 0.59. In contrast, the ethanol extract of *C. shulabadensis*, exhibited weak cytotoxicity with IC50 value of 304.5 ± 0.61 μg/mL.

Comparatively, among the plants from the group "*Arctium-Cousinia* complex"; *Arctium*, the closely related genus to *Cousinia* (6), has showed considarable cytotoxic activity against cancer cell lines. Recently, arctigenin, a lignane-9,9'-olide structure isolated from *Arctium lappa*, showed tumor specific cytotoxicity against lung, liver and stomach cancer cells (23).

Phytochemical assessments in *Cousinia species* revealed the presence of sesquiterpene lactones (SLs) mainly guaianolides and oxygenated bisabolene derivatives, and flavonoids (11-13,18). SLs possess a wide range of biological activities including cycotoxic, and antitumor effects (9,10). So, the cytotoxic properties observed in *C. verbascifolia* less polar fractions like Fr. 2 and Fr. 4 could be contributed to the presence of SLs. Cytotoxic activities of semi polar fractions like Fr. 8 might be due to the presence of flavonoids, lignanes or other phenolic compounds. Fr. 10 and Fr. 11 as polar fractions showed no cytotoxicities.

Conclusion

Due to the inhibitory properties of extract and its fractions on cancer cells, identification of responsible compounds possessing cytotoxic effects for generating possible new approach in medicinal chemistry are recommended.

Acknowledgments

This paper is part of the thesis of Mehrangiz Haghighi submitted for the fulfillment of the degree of Pharm D in Faculty of Pharmacy and Pharmaceutical Sciences, Isfahan University of Medical Sciences, Isfahan, Iran.

Authors' contributions

SES participated in most of the study. MG carried out the design and contributed to data analysis and writing and finalizing the manuscript. MH participated in most of the experiments and in manuscript writing. LM carried out the MTT assay.

Conflict of interests

The authors declared no competing interests.

Ethical considerations

Ethical issues (including plagiarism, misconduct, data fabrication, falsification, double publication or submission, redundancy) have been completely observed by the authors.

Funding/Support

None.

References

1. Dutt R, Garg V, Madan AK. Can plants growing in diverse hostile environments provide a vital source of anticancer drugs? Cancer Therapy 2014; 10: 13-37.
2. Niño J, Narváez DM, Mosquera OM, Correa YM. Antibacterial, antifungal and cytotoxic activities of eight Asteraceae and two Rubiaceae plants from Colombian biodiversity. Brazilian Journal of Microbiology 2006; 37: 566-70.
3. Pan L, Chai H, kinghorne AD. Discovery of new anticancer agents from higher plants. Front Biosci 2013; 4: 142-56.
4. Attar F, Djavadi SB. A taxonomic revision of *Cousinia*, sect. Cynaroides (Asteraceae, Cardueae) in the flora of Iran. Iranian Journal of Botany 2012; 16(1): 130-84.
5. Mehregan,I. Systematics, phylogeny and biogeography of *Cousinia* (Asteraceae). *PhD thesis*, Fachbreich Biologie der Johannes Gutenberg-Universitat Mainz. 2008.
6. Mehregan I, Kadereit JW. Taxonomic revision of Cousinia sect. Cynaroideae (Asteraceae, Cardueae). Wildenowia 2008; 38: 293-362.
7. Zare M, Khosravi AR, Joharchi MR. Distribution patterns of the genus *Cousinia* (Asteraceae) in Iran. Iranian Journal of Botany 2013; 19: 127-41.
8. Bohlmann F, Burkhardt T, Zdero C. Naturally occurring Acetylenes. London: Academic press; 1973. p. 445.
9. Alberto Marco J, Sanz Juan F, Albiach R, Rustayian A, Habibi Z. Bisabolene derivatives and sesquiterpene lactones from *Cousinia* species. Phytochemistry 1993; 32: 395-400.
10. Rustaiyan A, Niknejad A, Sigari H, Ahmadi A. Guaianolides from *Cousinia onopordioides*. Fitoterapia 1981; 52: 31-2.
11. Rustaiyan A, Sharif Z, Sadjadi A. Two farnesol derivatives from *Cousinia adenostica*. Phytochemistry 1987; 26: 2635-6.
12. Turdumambetov K, Rakhimov DA, Malikova MK. Oligo-and polysaccharides from *Cousinia umbrosa*. Chemistry of Natural Compounds 2007; 43: 308-9.
13. Turdumambetov K, Plekhanova NV, Rakhimov DA, Yagudaev MR. Glucofructans of *Cousinia polycephala*. Chemistry of Natural Compounds 1989; 25: 371-2.
14. Plekhanova NV, Turdumambetov K, Sudnitsyna IG. Carbohydrates of *Cousinia*. Chemistry of Natural Compounds 1983; 19: 603-4.
15. Ulubelen A, Tuzlaci E, Mericli A. Triterpenic and steroidal compounds from *Cousinia canescens*. Fitoterapia 1986; 57: 269-70.
16. Ulubelen A, Tuzlaci E. Flavonoids and terpenoids from *Cousinia eriocephala*. Fitoterapia 1988; 59: 350.
17. Azimova S, Glushenkova A. Lipids, lipophilic components and essential oils from plant sources. London: Springer; 2012. p: 110-3.
18. Shahverdi AR, Khorramizadeh MR, Attar F, Saadat F, Vahid S, Ghahraman A. Concomitant chemopreventive and antibacterial effects of some

Iranian plants from the genus *Cousinia* (Asteraceae). Brazilian Journal of Pharmacognosy 2007; 17: 325-30.

19. Zarei SM, Ayatollahi AM, Ghanadian M, Aghaei M, Choudhary MI, Fallahian F. Unusual ingenoids from *Euphorbia erythradenia* Bioss. with pro-apoptotic effects. Fitoterapia 2013; 91: 87-94.
20. Srisawat T, Chumkaew P, Heed-Chim W, Sukpondma Y, Kanokwiroon K. Phytochemical screening and cytotoxicity of crude extracts of Vatica diospyroides Symington Type LS. Tropical Journal of Pharmaceutical Research 2013; 12: 71-6.
21. Goldin A, Venditti JM, Macdonald JS, Muggia FM, Henney JE, Devita VT Jr. Current results of the screening program at the Division of Cancer Treatment, National Cancer Institute. Eur J Cancer 1965; 17: 129-42.
22. Geran RI, Greenberg NH, MacDonald MM, Schumaker AM, Abbott BJ. Protocols for screening chemical agents and natural products against animal tumors and other biological systems. Cancer Chemother Rep 3 1972; 3: 59-61.
23. Susanti S, Iwasaki H, Itokazu Y, Nago M, Taira N, Saitoh S, Oku H. Tumor specific cytotoxicity of arctigenin isolated from herbal plant Arctium lappa L. J Nat Med 2012; 66: 614-21.

Total phenolic compounds and in vitro antioxidant potential of crude methanol extract and the correspond fractions of *Quercus brantii* L. acorn.

Ali Karimi[1], Mohammad-Taghi Moradi[2*]

[1]Faculty of Paramedicine, Shahrekord University of Medical Science, Shahrekord, Iran
[2]PhD student, Medical Plants Research Center, Shahrekord University of Medical Science, Shahrekord, Iran

ARTICLE INFO

Keywords:
Antioxidant
Phenolic compounds
Fraction
Medicinal plants
Quercus brantii Lindl.

ABSTRACT

Introduction: Due to their roles in the maintenance of human health, phytochemicals and antioxidants in plants are raising interest. Phenolic and flavonoids are components with potential to protect against human diseases such as cardiovascular disease and cancers. *Q. brantii* is one of the traditional folk medicinal plants widely used in Iran. In this study, crude methanol extract and four correspond fractions of this plant were used to evaluate the total phenolic, total flavonoids, total flavonol, and antioxidant activities.
Methods: The identification of phenolic, flavonoid, and flavonol components and assay of antioxidant activity were carried out using standard in vitro procedures.
Results: The n-butanol fraction (376.2±7.1) had the highest amount of total phenolic compounds and the n-butanol fraction exhibited the lowest IC50 value (6.5±0.6 μg ml). There was significant relationship between the total phenolic contents and the free radical scavenging property in the four fractions in this study ($R= -0.768$, $P< 0.01$).
Conclusion: The results indicate that at least, n-butanol fraction of this plant with high phytoconstituents and less toxicity could be a promising source of medicinally important natural compound.

Implication for health policy/practice/research/medical education:
This study indicates that, at least some fractions of methanolic extract of *Q. brantii* acorn can be used as an accessible source of natural antioxidants. However, further works might be needed to the other extracts of this plant to reveal and evaluate its antioxidant potential.

Introduction

As an available source of innovative active biological compounds, medicinal plants are increasingly analyzed to determine the components on the structural level (1). These new compounds are pivotal for the discovery of new herbal medicines. Some kinds of side effects such as carcinogenesis have been attributed to synthetic antioxidants and thus, there is increasing interest to replace them with naturally occurring antioxidants (2,3). Antioxidant activity is one of the most important biological properties of these natural compounds. As natural antioxidants are capable of promoting food quality and stability and could act as nutraceuticals to end free radical chain reaction in biological systems, an increasing attention has been recently paid to directly evaluating the antioxidant properties of plant extracts as the source of natural antioxidants (4,5).

Many of naturally occurring antioxidants have been found to be free radical or active oxygen scavengers (6) and thus plants have been investigated for their biological activities and antioxidant properties (7-10). Flavonoides which are of the largest group of herbal polyphenols (11) contain tannins (12). Recent reports about antioxidant activity and polyphenol contents of herbals, used for fighting cancer, show that polyphenols, i.e. flavonoids, tannins, and phenolic acids, have antioxidant properties.

Belongs to the family of Fagaceae, Genus Quercus contains 500 species, some of which such as *Quercus brantii L.* are

***Corresponding author**: Mohammad-Taghi Moradi, Medical Plants Research Center, Shahrekord University of Medical Science, Rahmatieh, Shahrekord, Iran. Email: mtmoradi65@gmail.com

predominant in central and northern regions of Iran (13). The fruit of Oak tree is called acorn and is placed within a cup called Gland. Vitamins, nutrients, and Carbohydrates have been reported to comprise a large portion (48%-85%) of acorn components. Acron also contains considerable amounts of phenolic, tannin, catechin, epicatechin, and gallocatechin components (13-16).

There are some reports indicating different biological activities of some species of Genus Oak include Iranian Oak with use of the acorn and bark in treatment of some diseases such as chronic dermatological diseases, eczema, and varis (2,7,14,17-19). Additionally, some of the biologically active substances of acorn are utilized in preparing functional foods (20-22). To the best of our knowledge, to date, there has been no reports on the phytochemical analysis and antioxidant potential of different fractions of *Q. brantii* acorn. The main aim of this work was to evaluate phytochemical screening and antioxidant activity of both crude methanol extract and four correspond fractions of *Q. brantii* acorn.

Materials and Methods

Plant collection

The fruits of Oak were gathered from southwest region of Iran. Then, in Herbarium of Medical Plants Research Center of Shahrekord University of Medical Sciences (Iran), genus and species of the plant were identified and confirmed.

Extraction and fractionation of plant material

The fruits were harvested and powdered three times per maceration method. The plant material was dissolved in 70% ethyl alcohol and kept at room temperature for 96 hours. After that, the mixture was filtered and concentrated under nearly vacuum pressure and at 40°C using rotary evaporator. Having crude methanol extract of the plant, four fractions of the crude extract, with different polarity through in-solution isolation and using the difference in various secondary metabolites' polarity, were prepared. To isolate hexane fraction, the extract concentrated, suspended in 70% ethyl alcohol, and mixed with equal volume of normal hexane with sufficient shaking. The remaining plant material, from which the methanol was removed, mixed with distilled water and with chloroform in equal volume, shaked, dried over anhydrous sodium sulfate and used as the chloroform fraction. To prepare butanol fraction, equal volume of butanol was added to the remaining aqueous phase of the material, shaked and concentrated at 40°C and in vacuum condition. The remaining aqueous phase was concentrated, with the similar condition, mentioned above and used as aqueous fraction. The extracts were kept in sterile bottles, under refrigerated conditions, until further use.

Determination of the free-radical scavenging activity

The free-radical scavenging activity was measured by the 2,2 diphenyl-1-picrylhydrazyl (DPPH) method described by Moon and Terao, with some modification (23). Different amounts of each extract and methanol were added to a solution of 0.3 mg/mL methanolic solution of DPPH to make up a total volume of 3.0 mL. After standing for 15 min at room temperature, the absorbance was measured at 517 nm using UV–Vis spectrophotometer (UNICO 2100: USA). High absorbance of the reaction mixture indicated low free radical scavenging activity. Butylated hydroxytoluene (BHT) was used as positive control. Inhibition of free radical by DPPH was calculated as follows: Antiradical activity (%) = $(A_{control} - A_{sample})/A_{control} \times 100$. The IC_{50} value, defined as the amount of antioxidant necessary to decrease the initial DPPH concentration by 50% and was calculated based on linear regression of plots of the percentage antiradical activity against the concentration of the tested compounds (24). The experiment was carried out in triplicate and the results are average values.

Determination of total phenolic content

The total phenolic content of the crude extract and four correspond fractions of *Q. brantii* fruits was determined using Folin-Ciocalteu method (25). Briefly, 0.1 ml of each of the diluted samples was added to 0.5 ml of 10% (v/v) Folin-Ciocalteu reagent. After 3-8 min, 0.4 ml of 7.5% (w/v) sodium carbonate solution was added to the mixture. After being kept in total darkness for 30 min, the absorbance of the reaction mixture was measured at 765 nm using a UV–Vis spectrophotometer (UNICO 2100: USA). Amounts of total phenolic were calculated using a gallic acid calibration curve. The results were expressed as gallic acid equivalents (GAE) g/g of dry plant matter.

Determination of total flavonol content

The total flavonol content was measured following a previously reported method (26). Briefly, 0.5 ml of each diluted plant material was independently mixed with 1.5 ml of methanol, 0.1 ml of 10% (w/v) aluminum chloride, 0.1 ml of 1M potassium acetate, and 2.8 ml of distilled water. After incubation at room temperature for two and a half h absorbance of the reaction mixture was read at 440 nm using a UV-Vis spectrophotometer (UNICO 2100: USA). The results were expressed in mg of rutin equivalents of dry plant matter by comparison with the standard curve, which was made in the same condition. All measurements were done in triplicate and statistical analysis was done by statistical software using one-way analysis of variance (ANOVA) and the post-hoc Tukey's test. All the data are expressed as ± SEM.

Results

DPPH radical scavenging activity

Our results showed that the scavenging effect of the fractions increases as the concentration increases. The four fractions of *Q. brantii* fruit significantly reduced the DPPH. The concentration of each fraction which showed inhibition of higher than 50% were found to be significant ($P<0.05$; Table 1). The n-butanol fraction exhibited the lowest IC_{50} value (6.5±0.6 µg ml) as compared to the other fractions under study. The crude extract, chloroform fraction, and aqueous fraction had IC_{50} values of 15±3, 12.7±1, and 22.4±1.7 μg/ml, respectively, and the n-hexane fraction showed highest value (144.54±5). The results are expressed relative to butylated hydroxytoluene (BHT), a reference standard having IC_{50} of 25.41±1.89 μg/ml. The IC_{50} values of the chloroform fraction, the n-butanol fraction, the crude extract, and the n-hexane fraction were found to be significant (P<0.05) while that of the aqueous soluble fraction non-significant (P>0.05) as compared with BHT (Table 2).

Total phenolic content

The total phenolic content of the *Q. brantii* extract and the four fractions were expressed as gallic acid equivalent and are presented in Table 2. The results showed total phenolic content of the fractions ranged from 24.4 to 376.2 mg gallic acid equivalent (mgGAE/g). Among the four fractions, the n-butanol (376.2±7.1) and the n-hexane (24.4±3.5) had the highest and the lowest amount of total phenolic compounds, respectively. The total phenolic contents of the crude extract, the chloroform fraction, the n-butanol fraction, and the aqueous fraction were significantly different from that of the n-hexane fraction (P<0.05; Table 2). There was good relation between the total phenolic contents and the free radical scavenging property in the four fractions in this study (R= -0.768, P<0.01).

Total flavonoid and flavonol content

The total flavonoid and flavonol contents of the crude extract and the four fractions of *Q. brantii* fruit were expressed as gallic acid equivalent, as rutin equivalent (mg/g) and are presented in Table 2. The most amount of flavonoid and flavonol (91.6 and 105 mg/mL, respectively) was extracted in chloroform fraction and the lease amount (5.8 and 1.1 mg/mL, respectively) was extracted in aqueous fraction (P<0.05).

Discussion

In this study, crude methanol extract and the four correspond fractions of fruit of *Q. brantii* with different polarities were prepared through in-solution isolation and using the difference in different secondary metabolites' polarity. Also, the ability of these plant materials to inhibit

Table 1. DPPH radical-scavenging activity of the crude extract and various fractions of *Quercus brantii* L. acorn.

Sample	Concentration (μg/ml)	Scavenging of DPPH radical activity inhibition (%) (main ± SEM)
Crude extract	25	80.9±0.5
	20	66.4±1.1
	15	49.7±0.9
	10	34.5±0.3
	5	19±1
n-hexane fraction	150	55.3±1.5
	125	47.5±2
	100	40±2/1
	75	37.7±.08
	50	17.4±.3
Chloroform fraction	25	91.5±1.5
	20	80.1±1.4
	15	62.5±0.8
	10	40.2±1.3
	5	22.9±2.4
n-Butanol fraction	10	75±1.5
	7.5	58.2±1.2
	5	47.3±0.3
	2.5	25.8±1.3
	1	8.6±1.2
Remaining aqueous fraction	40	86.8±2.5
	30	66.5±1.9
	20	44.3±0.7
	10	19±0.9
	5	11.8±1.4
BHT	50	90.8±1.5
	40	78.3±1.2
	30	55.5±0.7
	20	40.09±1.7
	10	22±1.06

All results are presented as mean ± standard mean error of three assays. DPPH: 1,1-Diphenyl-2-picrylhydrazyl, BHT; Butylated hydroxytoluene

Table 2. DPPH-radical scavenging activity IC_{50}, total phenolics, flavonoid, and flavonol values of the different fractions of *Quercus brantii* L. acorn.

Sample	DPPH-radical scavenging activity IC_{50}/(μg/ml)	Total phenolics (mg GAE/g)	Flavonoid content (mg/g)	Flavonol content (mg/g)
Crude extract	$15±3^{\#a}$	201.6±4	$14.7±2.2^{a}$	33.6±2
n-hexane fraction	$144.5±5^{\#}$	24.4±3.5	$16.8±2^{a}$	$2.4±0.5^{a}$
Chloroform fraction	$12.7±1^{\#ab}$	222.5±2.5	91.6±1.5	105±4.5
n-Butanol fraction	$6.5±0.5^{\#b}$	376.2±7.1	22±2	70.9±55
Remaining aqueous fraction	22.4±1.7	120±3.5	5.8±0.5	$1.1±0.4^{a}$
P-value*	<0.01	<0.01	<0.01	<0.01

All results are presented as mean ± standard mean error of three assays.
*In terms of analysis of variance; [a,b] values with the same letter in each column are not significantly different according to Tukey test (P< 0.05); # Significant when compared with the reference standard (BHT, IC_{50} of 25.41±1.89 μg/ml).
Abbreviations: DPPH, 1,1-Diphenyl-2-picrylhydrazyl; IC_{50}, the concentration of a sample at which 50% inhibition of free radical activity is observed; GAE, gallic acid equivalent.

free radicals was assessed using DPPH method.

Among the 4 fractions, the n-butanol (376.2±7.1) and the n-hexane (24.4±3.5) had the highest and the lowest amount of total phenolic compounds, respectively. Based on the scavenging capacity of the free radicals, the n-butanol exhibited the highest antioxidant activity with the highest percent inhibition of the DPPH radical, followed by the chloroform fraction with higher percent inhibition of the DPPH radical compared to that of BHT. Also, the n-hexane fraction contained lower percent inhibition of the DPPH radical compared to BHT and the other fractions, indicating proper relation between the total phenolic contents and the free radical scavenging property, given that as IC_{50} value decreases, the ability to inhibit free radicals increases.

Similar to our study, some authors (27,28) have demonstrated a linear relation between the content of total phenolic compounds and their antioxidant capacity of some plant extracts. Therefore, the antioxidant potential of our plant extracts most probably is due to presence of phenolic components (376.2±7.1). Additionally, as tannins have been reported to be considerable components of phenolics in *Q. brantii* fruit (12), notable antioxidant potential of our fractions could be also due to the tannins. Our results, based on the DPPH method, showed that with increasing the polarity of the extracts, their radical scavenging activity will increase. Similar findings were reported on the rate of antioxidant property of the bark of *Quercus robur* (14). In this study, the crude methanol extract of *Q. brantii* fruit and some of the fractions showed promising antioxidant activity, by inhibiting DPPH, which is related to its total phenolic content. The presence of phenols and flavonoids in the plant, as its major constituents, plays a major role in controlling antioxidants. Phenolic compounds are very important plant constituents because their phenolic groups are responsible for high antioxidant activity and their hydroxyl groups confer scavenging ability.

Conclusion

The results of this study showed that at least some fractions of methanolic extract of *Q. brantii* acorn could be used as easily accessible source of natural antioxidants. However, as some of the fractions show lower activity in DPPH and total phenol content as compared with standard, further works may be taken up to the other extracts of this plant to reveal and evaluate its antioxidant potential.

Acknowledgments

Authors are thankful to the Director of Medical Plants Research Center and to the Deputy of Research of Shahrekord University of Medical Sciences, Shahrekord, Iran for financial support.

Authors' contributions

All authors contributed equally.

Conflict of interests

The authors declare that there are no conflicts of interests.

Ethical considerations

Ethical issues (including plagiarism, misconduct, data fabrication, falsification, double publication or submission, redundancy) have been completely observed by the authors.

Funding/Support

Deputy of Research and Technology of Shahrekord University of Medical Sciences, Shahrekord, Iran.

References

1. Clark AM. Natural products as a resource for new drugs. Pharm Res 1996; 13(8): 1133-44.
2. Karimi A, Moradi MT, Saeedi M, Asgari S, Rafieian-Kopaei M. Antiviral activity of Quercus persica L.: High efficacy and low toxicity. Adv Biomed Res 2013; 2: 36.
3. Znati M, Hichem BJ, Cazaux S, Bouajila J. Chemical composition, biological and cytotoxic activities of plant extracts and compounds isolated from Ferula lutea. Molecules 2014; 19(3): 2733-47.
4. Ito N, Fukushima S, Hagiwara A, Shibata M, Ogiso T. Carcinogenicity of butylated hydroxyanisole in F344 rats. J Natl Cancer Inst 1983; 70(2): 343-52.
5. McClements DJ, Decker EA. Lipid Oxidation in Oil-in-Water Emulsions: Impact of Molecular Environment on Chemical Reactions in Heterogeneous Food Systems. J Food Sci 2000; 65(8): 1270-82.
6. Zheng W, Wang SY. Antioxidant activity and phenolic compounds in selected herbs. J Agric Food Chem 2001; 49(11): 5165-70.
7. Basri D, Fan S. The potential of aqueous and acetone extracts of galls of Quercus infectoria as antibacterial agents. Indian J Pharmacol 2005; 37(1): 26-9.
8. Rafieian-Kopaei M, Baradaran A, Rafieian M. Oxidative stress and the paradoxical effects of antioxidants. J Res Med Sci 2013; 18(7): 629.
9. Rafieian-Kopaei M, Baradaran A, Rafieian M. Plants antioxidants: From laboratory to clinic. J Nephropathol 2013; 2(2): 152-3.
10. Riaz T, Abbasi A, Aziz-Ur-Rehman A, Shahzadi T, Ajaib M, Khan M. Phytochemical screening, free radical scavenging, antioxidant activity and phenolic content of Dodonaea viscosa. J Serb Chem Soc 2012; 77(4): 423-35.
11. Kovacevic N. Basic Pharmakognosy. Belgrade: University of Belgrade–Faculty of Pharmacy; 2000.
12. Rakic S, Petrovic S, Kukic J, Jadranin M, Tešević V, Povrenović D, *et al.* Influence of thermal treatment on phenolic compounds and antioxidant properties of oak acorns from Serbia. Food Chem 2007; 104(2): 830-4.
13. Saffarzadeh A, Vincze L, Csapo J. Determination of the chemical composition of acorn (Quercus branti), Pistacia atlantica and Pistacia Khinjk seeds as non-conventional feedstuffs. Acta Agr Kapos. 1999; 3(3): 59-69.
14. Andrensek S, Simonovska B, Vovk I, Fyhrquist P,

Vuorela H, Vuorela P. Antimicrobial and antioxidative enrichment of oak (Quercus robur) bark by rotation planar extraction using ExtraChrom. Int J Food Microbiol 2004; 92(2): 181-7.
15. Cadahia E, Munoz L, Fernandez de Simon B, Garcia-Vallejo MC. Changes in low molecular weight phenolic compounds in Spanish, French, and American oak woods during natural seasoning and toasting. J Agric Food Chem 2001; 49(4): 1790-8.
16. Popovic BM, Stajner D, Zdero R, Orlovic S, Galic Z. Antioxidant characterization of oak extracts combining spectrophotometric assays and chemometrics. Scientific World Journal. 2013; 2013: 134656.
17. Aslani A, Emami S, Ghannadi A, Ajdari M. Formulation and physicochemical evaluation of an herbal antihemorrohid ointment from Quercus, Black cumin and Fenugreek for the treatment of internal anal hemorrhoids. J Pharm Sci Tabriz Univ Med Sci 2009; 14: 247-57.
18. Kaur G, Hamid H, Ali A, Alam MS, Athar M. Antiinflammatory evaluation of alcoholic extract of galls of Quercus infectoria. J Ethnopharmacol 2004; 90(2-3): 285-92.
19. Khosravi A, Behzadi A. Evaluation of the antibacterial activity of the seed hull of Quercus brantii on some gram negative bacteria. Pak J Med Sci 2006; 22(4): 429-32.
20. Cantos E, Espin JC, Lopez-Bote C, de la Hoz L, Ordonez JA, Tomas-Barberan FA. Phenolic compounds and fatty acids from acorns (Quercus spp.), the main dietary constituent of free-ranged Iberian pigs. J Agric Food Chem 2003; 51(21): 6248-55.
21. Rakić S. Effect of oak acorn extracts on lipide oxidation kinetics. J Agric Sci 2000; 45(2): 139-43.
22. Rakić S, Maletić RO, Perunović MN, Svrzić G. Influence of thermal treatment on tannin content and antioxidation effect of oak acorn Quercus cerris extract. J Agric Sci 2004; 49(1): 97-107.
23. Moon JH, Terao J. Antioxidant Activity of Caffeic Acid and Dihydrocaffeic Acid in Lard and Human Low-Density Lipoprotein. J Agric Food Chem 1998; 46(12): 5062-5.
24. Nahak G, Sahu RK. In vitro antioxidative acitivity of Azadirachta indica and Melia azedarach Leaves by DPPH scavenging assay. Nat Sci 2010; 8(4): 22-8.
25. Folin O, Ciocalteu V. On tyrosine and tryptophane determinations in proteins. J Biol Chem 1927; 73(2): 627-50.
26. Rabiei Z, Rafieian-kopaei M, Heidarian E, Saghaei E, Mokhtari S. Effects of zizyphus jujube extract on memory and learning impairment induced by bilateral electric lesions of the nucleus basalis of meynert in rat. Neurochemical research 2014; 39(2): 353-60.
27. Rahnama S, Rabiei Z, Alibabaei Z, Mokhtari S, Rafieian-kopaei M, Deris F. Anti-amnesic activity of Citrus aurantium flowers extract against scopolamine-induced memory impairments in rats. Neurological Sciences Neurol Sci 2014 Nov 4.
28. Shirzad H, Taji F, Rafieian-Kopaei M. Correlation between antioxidant activity of garlic extracts and WEHI-164 fibrosarcoma tumor growth in BALB/c mice. J Med Food 2011; 14(9): 969-74.

PERMISSIONS

All chapters in this book were first published in JHP, by Shahrekord University of Medical Sciences; hereby published with permission under the Creative Commons Attribution License or equivalent. Every chapter published in this book has been scrutinized by our experts. Their significance has been extensively debated. The topics covered herein carry significant findings which will fuel the growth of the discipline. They may even be implemented as practical applications or may be referred to as a beginning point for another development.

The contributors of this book come from diverse backgrounds, making this book a truly international effort. This book will bring forth new frontiers with its revolutionizing research information and detailed analysis of the nascent developments around the world.

We would like to thank all the contributing authors for lending their expertise to make the book truly unique. They have played a crucial role in the development of this book. Without their invaluable contributions this book wouldn't have been possible. They have made vital efforts to compile up to date information on the varied aspects of this subject to make this book a valuable addition to the collection of many professionals and students.

This book was conceptualized with the vision of imparting up-to-date information and advanced data in this field. To ensure the same, a matchless editorial board was set up. Every individual on the board went through rigorous rounds of assessment to prove their worth. After which they invested a large part of their time researching and compiling the most relevant data for our readers.

The editorial board has been involved in producing this book since its inception. They have spent rigorous hours researching and exploring the diverse topics which have resulted in the successful publishing of this book. They have passed on their knowledge of decades through this book. To expedite this challenging task, the publisher supported the team at every step. A small team of assistant editors was also appointed to further simplify the editing procedure and attain best results for the readers.

Apart from the editorial board, the designing team has also invested a significant amount of their time in understanding the subject and creating the most relevant covers. They scrutinized every image to scout for the most suitable representation of the subject and create an appropriate cover for the book.

The publishing team has been an ardent support to the editorial, designing and production team. Their endless efforts to recruit the best for this project, has resulted in the accomplishment of this book. They are a veteran in the field of academics and their pool of knowledge is as vast as their experience in printing. Their expertise and guidance has proved useful at every step. Their uncompromising quality standards have made this book an exceptional effort. Their encouragement from time to time has been an inspiration for everyone.

The publisher and the editorial board hope that this book will prove to be a valuable piece of knowledge for researchers, students, practitioners and scholars across the globe.

LIST OF CONTRIBUTORS

Marzieh Mousavi
Young Researchers and Elite Club, Mashhad Branch, Islamic Azad University, Mashhad, Iran

Javad Baharara
Research Center for Animal Development Applied Biology, Mashhad Branch, Islamic Azad University, Mashhad, Iran

Majid Asadi-Samani
Medical Plants Research Center, Shahrekord University of Medical Sciences, Shahrekord, Iran

Mohammad Kiani and Shirin Moradkhani
Medicinal Plants and Natural Products Research Center, Hamadan University of Medical Sciences, Hamadan, Iran
Department of Pharmacognosy and Pharmaceutical Biotechnology, School of Pharmacy, Hamadan University of Medical Sciences, Hamadan, Iran

Farzin Firoozian
Department of Pharmaceutics, School of Pharmacy, Hamadan University of Medical Sciences, Hamadan, Iran

Javad Baharara and Marzieh Mousavi
Research Center for Animal Development Applied Biology, Mashhad Branch, Islamic Azad University, Mashhad, Iran

Tayebeh Ramezani
Faculty of Biological Sciences, Kharazmi University, Tehran, Iran

Majid Asadi-Samani
Medical Plants Research Center, Shahrekord University of Medical Sciences, Shahrekord, Iran

Mohammad-Ali Kohanpour
PhD Candidate, Department of Exercise Physiology, Islamic Azad University, Central Tehran Branch, Iran

Maghsoud Peeri and Mohammad-Ali Azarbayjani
Professor, Department of Exercise Physiology, Islamic Azad University, Central Tehran Branch, Iran

Daniel M. Gaichu, Amos M. Mawia, Godfrey M. Gitonga, Mathew P. Ngugi and David N. Mburu
Department of Biochemistry and Biotechnology, School of Pure and Applied Sciences, Kenyatta University, Nairobi, Kenya

Abdolshakoor Raissi
Faculty of agriculture, Department of Horticulture, Velayat University, Iranshahr, Iran

Mina Arbabi
PhD Student of Medicinal Plant, Islamic Azad University, Science and Research Branch, Tehran, Iran

Javad Roustakhiz
Higher Educational Complex of Saravan, Saravan University, Saravan, Iran

Masih Hosseini
Medical Plants Research Center, Shahrekord University of Medical Sciences, Shahrekord, Iran

L.D.A. Menuka Arawwawala and D.L.S. Madushani Jayaratne
Industrial Technology Institute, Bauddhaloka Mawatha, Colombo7, Sri Lanka

Mustapha A Tijjani, Thiza B Adamu and Fanna I Abdurahaman
Department of Chemistry, Faculty of Science, University of Maiduguri, P.M.B 1069, Maiduguri, Borno State, Nigeria

Garba T Mohammed
Department of Pharmaceutical Chemistry, Faculty of Pharmacy, University of Maiduguri, P.M.B 1069, Maiduguri, Borno State, Nigeria

Yagana T Alkali
Department of Biological Sciences, Faculty of Sciences, University of Maiduguri, P.M.B 1069, Maiduguri, Borno State, Nigeria

Amit Gupta
School of Sciences, P.P. Savani University, Kosamba, Surat, Gujarat, India
Department of Microbiology, Vidya Pratishthan's, Arts, Science and Commerce College, Baramati, Maharashtra, India

Samrat S Patil and Nilima Pendharkar
Department of Microbiology, Vidya Pratishthan's, Arts, Science and Commerce College, Baramati, Maharashtra, India

Ette Okon Ettebong and John Akpan Udobang
Department of Clinical Pharmacology and Therapeutics, Faculty of Clinical Sciences, University of Uyo, Uyo, Nigeria

Paul Alozie Nwafor
Department of Pharmacology and Toxicology, Faculty of Pharmacy, University of Uyo, Uyo, Nigeria

Peace Edwin Ubulom
Pharmaceutical Microbiology and Parasitology Unit, Department of Pharmaceutics and Pharmaceutical Technology, Faculty of Pharmacy, University of Uyo, Uyo, Nigeria

Amit Gupta and Sushama R Chaphalkar
Vidya Pratishthan's School of Biotechnology (VSBT, Research centre affiliated to Savitribai Phule Pune University), Baramati-413133, Maharashtra, India

Anosike Nnamdi
Department of Pharmacology and Toxicology, Faculty of Pharmacy, University of Uyo, Uyo, Nigeria

Ette Ettebong
Department of Clinical Pharmacology and Therapeutics, Faculty of Clinical Sciences, University of Uyo, Uyo, Nigeria

Koofreh Davis
Department of Physiology, Faculty of Basic Medical Sciences, University of Uyo, Uyo, Nigeria

Dara Shirzadi and Ali Zanbouri
Physiology Department, Maragheh Branch, Islamic Azad University, Maragheh, Iran

Saeid Abbasi-Maleki
Pharmacology & Toxicology Department, Urmia Branch, Islamic Azad University, Urmia, Iran

Hojjatollah Shokri
Department of Pathobiology, Faculty of Veterinary Medicine, Amol University of Special Modern Technologies, Amol, Iran

Aghil Sharifzadeh
Mycology Research Center, Faculty of Veterinary Medicine, University of Tehran, Tehran, Iran

Shubham S Gaikwad
Department of Biotechnology, Vidya Pratishthan's, Arts, Science and Commerce College, Baramati, Maharashtra, India

Amit Gupta and Bharat Shinde
Department of Biotechnology, Vidya Pratishthan's, Arts, Science and Commerce College, Baramati, Maharashtra, India
Department of Zoology, Vidya Pratishthan's, Arts, Science and Commerce College, Baramati, Maharashtra, India

Yurii Aleksandrovich Boiko and Alexey Antonovich Shandra
Department of Physiology, Odessa National Medical University, Odessa, Ukraine

Irina Anatolievna Kravchenko
Department of Pharmaceutical Chemistry, Odessa National University I.I. Mechnikova, Odessa, Ukraine

Irina Anatolievna Boiko
Department of Pharmacognosy, Odessa National Medical University, Odessa, Ukraine

Mohammad-Ali Kohanpour
PhD Candidate, Department of Exercise Physiology, Islamic Azad University, Central Tehran branch, Iran

Maghsoud Peeri and Mohammad-Ali Azarbayjani
Professor, Department of Exercise Physiology, Islamic Azad University, Central Tehran Branch, Iran

Kossivi Issa Saloufou, Pakoupati Boyode, Oudjaniyobi Simalou, Outéndé Toundou and Kafui Kpegba
Laboratoire de chimie organique et des substances naturelles (Lab COSNat), Départements de Chimie, Faculté Des Sciences, Université de Lomé, 01 BP 1515 Lomé 01, Lomé, TOGO

Kodjo Eloh
Department of Life and Environmental Sciences, Unversity of Cagliari, Via Ospedale 72, 09124, Cagliari, Italy

Kokou Idoh and Amegnona Agbonon
Laboratoire de Physiologie, Pharmacologie et Toxicologie, Faculté des Sciences, Université de Lomé, 01 BP 1515 Lomé 01, Lomé, TOGO

Mamatchi Melila
Département de Biochimie, Université de Lomé, 01 BP 1515 Lomé 01, Lomé, TOGO

Shahrbanoo Alami-Rostami
Department of Biology, Islamic Azad University, Gomishan Center, Gorgan Branch, Gorgan, Iran

Maryam Rafieirad
Department of Biology, Faculty of Sciences, Izeh Branch, Islamic Azad University, Izeh, Iran

Hassan Sadraei
Department of Pharmacology and Toxicology, School of Pharmacy and Pharmaceutical Sciences, Isfahan University of Medical Sciences, Isfahan, Iran

Mostafa Ghanadian and Gholamreza Asghari
Isfahan Pharmaceutical Sciences Research Center, School of Pharmacy and Pharmaceutical Sciences, Isfahan University of Medical Sciences, Isfahan, Iran

Nastaran Sekhavati
Department of Pharmacology and Toxicology, School of Pharmacy and Pharmaceutical Sciences, Isfahan University of Medical Sciences, Isfahan, Iran
Isfahan Pharmaceutical Sciences Research Center, School of Pharmacy and Pharmaceutical Sciences, Isfahan University of Medical Sciences, Isfahan, Iran

Dipa Islam, Amdadul Huque, Liton Chandra Mohanta, Sadhan Kumar Das and Evena Parvin Lipy
Biomedical and Toxicological Research Institute (BTRI), Institute of Food Science and Technology, Bangladesh Council of Scientific and Industrial Research (BCSIR), Dhaka, Bangladesh

Sheuly
Science, Secondary Education Quality and Access Enhancement Project (SEQAEP), Ministry of Education, Dhaka, Bangladesh

Abida Sultana
Department of Food Technology, Kishoreganj Polytechnic Institute, Kishoreganj, Bangladesh

U. K. Prodhan
Department of Food Technology and Nutritional Science, Mawlana Bhashani Science and Technology University, Bangladesh

Fatemeh Jamshidi-Kia, Zahra Lorigooini and Hossein Amini-Khoei
Medical Plants Research Center, Basic Health Sciences Institute, Shahrekord University of Medical Sciences, Shahrekord, Iran

Siamak Beheshti and Bahareh Shahmoradi
Department of Biology, Faculty of Sciences, University of Isfahan, Isfahan, Iran

Oludele John Olanlokun and Olufunso Olabode Olorunsogo
Laboratories for Biomembrane Research and Biotechnology, Department of Biochemistry, Faculty of Basic Medical Sciences, College of Medicine, University of Ibadan

Vandana Mohan and Ashwani Koul
Department of Biophysics, Basic Medical Science Block II, South campus, Panjab University, Chandigarh, India

Hamidu Usman, Muhammad Awwal Tijjani, Abdulkarim Hassan and Zainab Babagana Aji
Department of Chemistry, University of Maiduguri, P.M.B. 1069 Maiduguri, Nigeria

Hanieh Torabi-Pour
MSc in Medical Entomology, Department of Medical Entomology and Vector Control, School of Public Health, Tehran University of Medical Sciences, Tehran, Iran

Mansoureh Shayeghi, Hassan Vatandoost and Mohammad-Reza Abai
Department of Medical Entomology and Vector Control, School of Public Health, Tehran University of Medical Sciences, Tehran, Iran

Moosa Javdani
Department of Clinical Sciences, Faculty of Veterinary Medicine, Shahrekord University, Shahrekord, Iran

Mojtaba Ahmadi Dastjerdi
Faculty of Veterinary Medicine, Shahrekord University, Shahrekord, Iran

Sadegh Shirian
Department of Pathobiology, Faculty of Veterinary Medicine, Shahrekord University, Shahrekord, Iran

Emmanuel Ayodeji Ayeni, Ahmed Abubakar, Garba Ibrahim and Zainab Muhammad
Department of Pharmacognosy and Drug Development, Ahmadu Bello University Zaria, Nigeria

Vallada Atinga
Department of Pharmacognosy and Drug Development, Gombe State University, Gombe, Nigeria

Leila Safaeian
Department of Research and Development, Vice Chancellery for Food and Drug, Department of Pharmacology and Toxicology, School of Pharmacy and Pharmaceutical Sciences, Isfahan University of Medical Sciences, Isfahan, Iran

Bahar Baniahmad
Department of Pharmacology and Toxicology, Isfahan Pharmaceutical Sciences Research Center, School of Pharmacy and Pharmaceutical Sciences, Isfahan University of Medical Sciences, Isfahan, Iran

Zahra Esfandiari
Department of Research and Development, Vice-Chancellery for Food and Drug, Isfahan University of Medical Sciences, Isfahan, Iran

Sayed Ali Alavi
Hakiman Shargh Investigative Corporation, Isfahan Science and Technology Town, Isfahan, Iran

Kafui Kpegba, Etonam Tété Kondo, Oudjaniyobi Simalou, Pakoupati Boyode, Outéndé Toundou and Nagba Yendoubé Gbandjaba
Laboratoire de Chimie Organique et des Substances Naturelles (Lab COSNat), Faculté des Science, Université de Lomé, 01 BP 1515 Lomé 01, Lomé-Togo

Komlatsè Togbenou, Amegnona Agbonon and Messanvi Gbeassor
Laboratoire de Physiologie et de Pharmacologie, Faculté des Science, Université de Lomé; 01 BP 1515 Lomé 01, Lomé-Togo

Atefeh Araghi and Mohaddeseh Abouhosseini Tabari
Faculty of Veterinary Medicine, Amol University of Special Modern Technologies, Amol, Iran

Hannaneh Golshahi
Department of Pathology, Faculty of Veterinary Medicine, University of Tehran, Tehran, Iran

Farshad Baghban
Department of Veterinary Medicine, Yasooj Branch, Islamic Azad University, Yasooj, Iran

Saeid Valipour Chahardahcharic and Mahbubeh Setorki
Department of Biology, Izeh Branch, Islamic Azad University, Izeh, Iran

Hadis Musavi
Department of Biochemistry, Faculty of Basic Science, Razi University Kermanshah, Kermanshah, Iran

Malihe Tabnak
Department of Basic Sciences, East Tehran Branch, Islamic Azad University, Tehran, Iran

Farzaneh Alaei Sheini
Department of Biology, Shahrekord Branch, Islamic Azad University, Shahrekord, Iran

Maryam Hasanzadeh Bezvan
Department of Microbiology, Shahr-e-Qods Branch, Islamic Azad University, Tehran, Iran

Fardin Amidi
Department of Anatomy, School of Medicine, Tehran University of Medical Sciences, Tehran, Iran

Mojtaba Abbasi
Veterinary Medicine, Faculty of Veterinary Medicine, Shahrekord Branch, Islamic Azad University, Shahrekord, Iran

Fatemeh Abdolhosseinipoor and Ali Hosseini-Sharifabad
Department of Pharmacology and Toxicology, School of Pharmacy and Pharmaceutical Sciences, Isfahan University of Medical Sciences, Isfahan, Iran

Masoud Sadeghi-Dinani
Department of Pharmacognosy, School of Pharmacy and Pharmaceutical Sciences, Isfahan University of Medical Sciences, Isfahan, Iran

Khodadad Pirali Kheirabadi
Department of pathobiology, Faculty of Veterinary Medicine, Shahrekord University, Shahrekord, Iran

Siavash Saei Dehkordi
Department of Food Hygiene and Quality Control, Faculty of Veterinary Medicine, Shahrekord University, Shahrekord, Iran

Parviz Kheibari
Faculty of Veterinary Medicine, Shahrekord University, Shahrekord, Iran

Seyed Ebrahim Sajjadi and Mehrangiz Haghighi
Department of Pharmacognosy, School of Pharmacy and Pharmaceutical Sciences, Isfahan University of Medical Sciences, Isfahan, Iran

Mustafa Ghanadian
Department of Pharmacognosy, School of Pharmacy and Pharmaceutical Sciences, Isfahan University of Medical Sciences, Isfahan, Iran
Isfahan Pharmaceutical Sciences Research Center, Isfahan University of Medical Sciences, Isfahan, Iran

Leili Mouhebat
Department of Microbiology, School of Medicine, Isfahan University of Medical Sciences, Isfahan, Iran

Ali Karimi
Faculty of Paramedicine, Shahrekord University of Medical Science, Shahrekord, Iran

Mohammad-Taghi Moradi
Medical Plants Research Center, Shahrekord University of Medical Science, Shahrekord, Iran

Javad Baharara
Research Center for Animal Development Applied Biology & Department of Biology, Mashhad Branch, Islamic Azad University, Mashhad, Iran

Elaheh Amini
Department of Animal Biology, Faculty of Biological Sciences, Kharazmi University, Tehran, Iran

Hassan Moghim, Simin Taghipoor, Najmeh Shahinfard and Hamideh Khabbazi
Medical Plants Research Center, Shahrekord University of Medical Sciences, Shahrekord, Iran

Soleiman kheiri
Social Health Determinants Research Center, Shahrekord University of Medical Sciences, Shahrekord, Iran

Ghazal Sami
Student Research Committee, Hamadan University of Medical Sciences, Hamadan, Iran

Ebrahim Khoshraftar
Department of Anesthesiology, Medical faculty, Hamadan University of Medical Sciences, Hamadan, Iran

Tavakol Heidary Shayesteh and Akram Ranjbar
Department of Toxicology and Pharmacology, School of Pharmacy, Hamadan University of Medical Sciences, Hamadan, Iran

Mohammad Ali Shahtalebi, Majid Tabbakhian and Sina Koosha
Department of Pharmaceutics, School of Pharmacy and Pharmaceutical Sciences, Isfahan University of Medical Science, Isfahan, Iran

Index

www.ingramcontent.com/pod-product-compliance
Lightning Source LLC
LaVergne TN
LVHW081038210926
848485LV00004B/1051